SYSTEMIC PATHOLOGY / THIRD EDITION

Volume 3 Alimentary Tract

SYSTEMIC PATHOLOGY / THIRD EDITION

General Editor

W. St C. Symmers

MD(Belf), PhD(Birm), DSc(Lond), FRCP(Lond, Irel, Ed), FRCS(Eng), FACP(Hon), FRCPA(Hon), FRCPath, FFPathRCPI

Emeritus Professor of Histopathology, University of London; Honorary Consulting Pathologist, Charing Cross Hospital, London, UK

System Editors

M. C. Anderson   **Gynaecological and Obstetrical Pathology**

T. J. Anderson and D. L. Page   **Breasts**

B. Corrin   **Lungs**

M. J. Davies, R. H. Anderson, W. B. Robertson and N. Woolf   **Cardiovascular System**

I. Friedmann   **Nose, Throat and Ears**

K. Henry   **Thymus, Lymph Nodes and Spleen**

B. C. Morson   **Alimentary Tract**

K. A. Porter   **Urinary System**

R. C. B. Pugh   **Male Reproductive System**

H. A. Sissons   **Bone, Joints and Soft Tissues**

D. Weedon   **Skin**

K. Weinbren   **Liver, Biliary Tract and Pancreas**

R. O. Weller   **Nervous System, Muscle and Eyes**

S. N. Wickramasinghe   **Blood and Bone Marrow**

E. D. Williams   **Endocrine System**

SYSTEMIC PATHOLOGY / THIRD EDITION

Volume 3

Alimentary Tract

EDITED BY

Basil C. Morson

VRD, MA(Oxon), DM(Oxon), FRCP(Lond), FRCS(Eng), FRCPath

Consulting Pathologist, St Mark's Hospital, London; Emeritus Civilian Consultant in Pathology, Royal Navy, UK

CHURCHILL LIVINGSTONE

EDINBURGH LONDON MELBOURNE AND NEW YORK 1987

CHURCHILL LIVINGSTONE
Medical Division of Longman Group UK Limited

Distributed in the United States of America by Churchill
Livingstone Inc., 1560 Broadway, New York, N.Y. 10036, and
by associated companies, branches and representatives
throughout the world.

First published 1987

ISBN 0-443-03095-2

British Library Cataloguing in Publication Data

Systemic pathology—3rd ed.
  Vol 3: Alimentary tract
  1. Pathology
  I. Morson, Basil C.
  616.07   RB111

Library of Congress Cataloging in Publication Data

Alimentary tract.

  (Systemic pathology; v. 3)
  Includes index.
  1. Digestive organs—Diseases. I. Morson, Basil C.
(Basil Clifford) II. Series. [DNLM: 1. Digestive
System Diseases. 2. Mouth Diseases. QZ 4 S995 1986 v.3]
RB111.S97 vol. 3 [RC802.9] 616.07 s   87–767
                  [616.3]

Typeset, printed and bound in Great Britain by
William Clowes Limited, Beccles and London

Preface

When I was invited by Professor Symmers and the late Professor Payling Wright over 25 years ago to write the chapters on the Alimentary Tract for the first edition of this book it was not unreasonable to expect one pathologist to write all these chapters other than the one on the teeth and gums which was provided by Professor R. B. Lucas. In the expanded second edition, published in 1978, the chapters on the Mouth and Salivary Glands were written by Professor R. B. Lucas and Professor A. C. Thackray; the Teeth and Periodontal Tissues by Professor Lucas and the remainder by myself with the exception of the one on the Small Intestine which was contributed jointly with Professor I. M. P. Dawson.

During the past 30 years there has been an enormous increase in our knowledge of alimentary tract pathology, mostly because of greater availability of surgical and biopsy material. This has provoked much new research and increasing specialization in different levels of the alimentary tract. It is not surprising then that this third edition has had to be further expanded and written by six authors. To them I must express my appreciation for their wholehearted collaboration in the production of this book. The result is a comprehensive and up-to-date account of the pathology of the alimentary tract which I trust will prove to be valuable as a source of reference for senior pathologists and a useful text for trainees in histopathology. Also, there is much in this volume, aside from histopathological detail, which could be useful to gastrointestinal surgeons and physicians including those studying for postgraduate qualifications.

The authors of this volume wish to express their appreciation to the general editor, Professor W. St C. Symmers, for his valuable criticisms. This volume is also the product of the skills of the secretaries to whom we owe a debt of gratitude for their devoted work. They include Miss Collette Youd (Dr D. W. Day), Mrs Maysuri Patani (Dr J. R. Jass) and Miss Cynthia Bury (Professor Cawson). We also thank Mr Alan Williams, Mr Alex Woodman and Miss Jill Maybee for photographic assistance.

London, January 1987   B.C.M.

Contributors

R. A. Cawson
MD(London), FDSRCS(Eng),
FDSRCPS(Glasg), FRCPath

Emeritus Professor of Oral Medicine and Pathology in the University of London, London, UK

I. M. P. Dawson
MA(Cambridge), MD(Cambridge),
FRCP(Lond), FRCPath

Emeritus Professor of Pathology, Nottingham University Medical School; Honorary Consultant Pathologist, Trent Regional Health Authority, UK

D. W. Day
MA(Cambridge), MB BChir(Cambridge),
MRCPath

Senior Lecturer in Pathology, University of Liverpool; Honorary Consultant Pathologist, Liverpool Health Authority, Liverpool, UK

Jeremy R. Jass
BSc(London), MD(London), MRCPath

Consultant Histopathologist, St Mark's Hospital; Senior Lecturer in Histopathology, St Bartholomew's Hospital Medical College, London, UK

R. B. Lucas
MD(Edinburgh), FRCP(Lond), FRCPath,
FDSRCS(Eng)

Emeritus Professor of Oral Pathology, University of London, London, UK

A. C. Thackray
MA(Cambridge), MD(Cambridge),
FRCS(Eng), FRCPath

Emeritus Professor of Morbid Histology, University of London; formerly Consultant Pathologist, The Middlesex Hospital, London, UK

Geraint T. Williams
BSc(Wales), MD(Wales), MRCP(UK),
MRCPath

Senior Lecturer in Pathology, University of Wales College of Medicine; Honorary Consultant Pathologist, University Hospital of Wales, Cardiff, UK

Contents

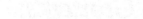

The mouth

Examination of the mouth is essential to a complete physical investigation, for many systemic disorders have oral manifestations and, on occasion, these may be the first sign of disease. It is not feasible to refer here to all these manifestations: it must suffice to point out that there is a great variety and that the investigator must be prepared to encounter them. This chapter deals principally with diseases that primarily affect the soft tissues of the mouth, including systemic conditions in which the local manifestations are of particular importance or prominence.

THE ORAL MUCOSA

NORMAL STRUCTURE[1]

The mucous membrane of the mouth consists of squamous epithelium covering a well-vascularized layer of connective tissue. This vascularity, due to an abundant plexus of blood vessels, permits the ready detection of cyanosis by inspection of the buccal mucosa. The epithelium is keratinized over the hard palate, the lips and the gingivae; elsewhere it is non-keratinized. It is thicker over the tongue than elsewhere in the mouth: this and the presence of the lingual papillae account for the roughness of the surface. The epithelium of the lower part of the pharynx is of stratified squamous type; towards the roof of the pharynx the epithelium becomes columnar.

Mucous glands—the minor salivary glands—are distributed throughout the oral mucosa. Sebaceous glands are often present, particularly in the area lateral to the angles of the mouth and also in the lips. They can be seen by the naked eye as small yellow spots (Fordyce's spots). Lymphoid tissue is present in large aggregations as the palatine tonsils and in smaller aggregations as the adenoid in the nasopharynx and the lingual tonsil in the posterior third of the tongue.

DEVELOPMENTAL AND MISCELLANEOUS ANOMALIES[2]

Thyroid tissue may be present in the tongue and, if actively functioning, may present as a tumour-like mass. It may give rise to symptoms of thyrotoxicosis. Rarely, myxoedema has followed excision of a lingual goitre; it is likely that in such cases the cervical thyroid was hypoplastic or absent. Adenoma and carcinoma have, rarely, arisen in lingual thyroid tissue.

Teratoma

Teratomas of the mouth and pharynx are rare. They are often referred to by the term epignathus, which literally means 'on the jaw' and should not be used of lesions elsewhere: most teratomas in fact arise from the region of the sphenoid bone or Rathke's pouch and bulge into the mouth or pharynx between the two halves of the palate. Less often, teratomas originate from cheek, tongue or jaw. They are usually found in the fetus or stillborn infant, since, as a result of their situation, they are seldom compatible with life. Very occasionally they are seen in older children.

Teratomas vary in structure and consist of a mixture of different tissues. So far as is known, and apart from any possible mechanical effects, they are benign.

Dermoid cysts are referred to on page 70.

Facial and palatal clefts

Various congenital deformities of the face and jaws may result from failure of the embryonic facial processes to complete their normal development. The commonest are clefts of the upper lip and palate, either alone or, more usually, both together. Many infants with these defects also have other anomalies, such as umbilical hernia and abnormalities of the limbs.

Enlargement of the tongue (macroglossia)

Congenital enlargement of the tongue is usually due to lymphangioma or haemangioma. Congenital neurofibromatosis is another cause. The tongue may also be enlarged in Down's syndrome. Enlargement due to muscular hypertrophy is a rarity; hemihypertrophy may be associated with hemihypertrophy of the facial muscles.

When the enlargement is due to lymphangioma the appearance is quite characteristic, the surface of the tongue being irregular and covered with many lymph-filled vesicles or bullae. Microscopically, the lesion consists of large intercommunicating lymphatic spaces lined by endothelium; there is no capsule and the lymphatic channels extend irregularly into the muscle. The lesion is hamartomatous and not a neoplasm. It tends to enlarge until puberty and then ceases to grow, although intermittent attacks of ulceration and infection, resulting in temporary enlargement, are common. Similar lesions are frequently present also in the floor of the mouth and in the neck. In the latter site the condition is commonly known as cystic hygroma.

In adults, additional causes of macroglossia include myxoedema, acromegaly and amyloidosis.

Reduction in the size of the tongue

Microglossia and aglossia are rare congenital abnormalities.

Atrophy of the tongue may be unilateral or bilateral. It results from damage to one or both hypoglossal nerves by inflammation or trauma.

Fissured tongue

Pronounced fissuring of the tongue ('scrotal tongue') appears to be a genetically-determined condition. It may be an isolated anomaly but is often seen in Down's syndrome and is a feature of Melkersson–Rosenthal syndrome. It is often also associated with benign migratory glossitis ('geographical tongue'), in which irregular, pink, smooth areas, with yellowish margins, appear from time to time on the dorsum of the tongue. In these patches the epithelium is thinner than normal and there are no papillae.

Median rhomboid glossitis

See page 28.

Torus palatinus and torus mandibularis

Torus palatinus is a bony overgrowth of the palate, forming a nodule or ridge in the midline. Torus mandibularis is a ledge-like or lobulate bony protrusion on the lingual aspect of the mandible. These lesions are exostoses and consist of normally structured bone; they grow very slowly. The palatal growth is usually noted in adolescents and young adults, the mandibular one oftener in the middle-aged. They are probably genetically determined and are frequently unremarked by the patient, being first noted by the doctor or dentist.

VIRAL INFECTIONS

Herpetic stomatitis

Herpetic stomatitis is usually caused by herpes simplex virus (HSV) type I. Rarely, type II may be responsible. Though traditionally regarded as a disease of infancy there has been a steady decline in incidence in recent years. This has been shown, for example, by Dudgeon[3] over a period of 20 years in London children. Since then, studies mainly among students have shown the proportion of seropositives in this age group to be as low as 30% while an extensive study[4] in a dental school in Michigan showed a similar low rate for staff and students with an appreciably higher average age.

It has been suggested that the increasing prevalence of genital herpes may be partly due to the decline in type I infections since the two types are believed to share some cross-immunity. Certainly, there has also been a great increase in HSV type I infections of the genitals.

Herpetic stomatitis is now as likely to be seen among adults as in children and produces an acute febrile illness with soreness of the mouth as the dominant feature. The earliest recognizable lesions are 2–3 mm, sharply defined, dome-shaped vesicles which affect any part of the oral mucosa and are often seen intact in the vault of the palate.

Histopathology

Microscopically, the vesicles are intra-epithelial with a roof several cells thick and with viral-damaged cells in the floor (Fig. 1.1). With rupture of the vesicles, viral damage spreads through the whole thickness of the epithelium within a sharply

circumscribed area and with remarkably well-demarcated margins. This pre-ulcerative phase is followed by shedding of the viral-damaged cells to leave an equally sharply defined ulcer (Fig. 1.2). Inflammatory changes in the corium are slight when the ulcers first form but increase later.

Rupture of vesicles produces flat coin-like lesions (the pre-ulcerative phase described above) and then circular ulcers which may coalesce to form rosette-shaped or more irregular lesions. The gums are often inflamed, swollen and sometimes haemorrhagic. The regional lymph nodes are enlarged and tender, and there is a febrile systemic upset which can be severe.

Smears from the lesions show epithelial cells whose nuclei are distended by the proliferating virus which pushes the chromatin to the nuclear margin (ballooning degeneration). Division of these nuclei but not of the cytoplasm produces multinucleated giant cells. Typical eosinophilic

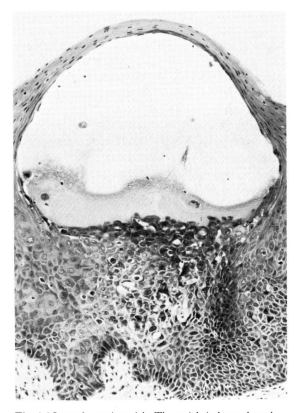

Fig. 1.1 Intact herpetic vesicle. The vesicle is dome-shaped with a thick roof but the floor is crowded with virus-infected epithelial cells.

Haematoxylin-eosin × 150

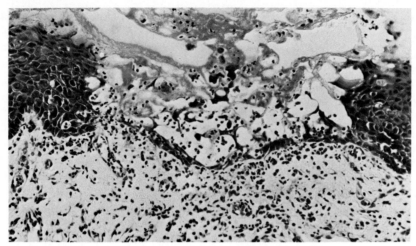

Fig. 1.2 Herpetic ulcer at a later stage than Figure 1. The epithelium has broken down completely leaving a sharply defined ulcer with vertical walls.

Haematoxylin-eosin   × 180.

inclusion bodies are (for unknown reasons) rarely, if ever, seen in these smears but can be seen in tissue sections.

Since there can be symptomless carriage of herpes simplex virus in the mouth the only reliable way of confirming the diagnosis is by showing a rising titre of neutralizing antibodies in acute phase and convalescent sera. In practice, the diagnosis is usually made on clinical grounds since in most cases the infection has resolved by the time that the second serum sample should have been taken.

After resolution of the primary infection about 30% of patients are susceptible to recurrent infections in the form of herpes labialis.

Herpes labialis

After the primary infection the herpes virus can persist in latent form[5] in the trigeminal ganglia and in susceptible subjects may be reactivated by a variety of stimuli, particularly febrile illnesses ('cold sores', or 'fever blisters') or exposure to strong sunlight or sea air.

Clinically, the mucocutaneous borders of the skin of the upper lip as far as the nostrils are affected. There is localized prodromal soreness or paraesthesia, quickly followed by the appearance of a cluster of vesicles. The latter soon rupture, weep infective exudate and then, after a few days, scab over. Further lesions may appear, however, before the previous ones have resolved but the

attack is self-limiting and there is wide individual variation in the frequency and severity of attacks.

Histopathology

Microscopically, the picture is the same as that of the primary infection and smears also show the same appearance. Diagnosis is by the distinctive clinical picture and history. There is no serological test of value since there is already a high titre of antibodies. Though a defect of cell-mediated immunity is often postulated as being responsible for recurrences, most patients remain healthy enough to suffer them for many years.

VARICELLA ZOSTER INFECTIONS: CHICKENPOX AND SHINGLES

The varicella zoster virus (VZV) causes chickenpox in the non-immune and zoster (shingles) as a reactivation infection comparable in many respects to herpes labialis.

Varicella typically affects children causing a vesiculating rash and stomatitis. The latter is not usually a conspicuous feature but infective saliva is an important vehicle for spread of the infection.

Trigeminal zoster

Zoster results from reactivation of the varicella zoster virus, typically late in life. Less commonly, zoster can develop earlier and, rarely, even in infants.

At the time of writing, the latency of the varicella zoster virus in the trigeminal ganglion had not (unlike herpes simplex) been confirmed by tissue culture explant methods. However, detection of VZV DNA sequences in tissue cells has been reported in both acute infections and in normal trigeminal ganglia.[6,7]

Though herpes zoster and herpes labialis are reactivation infections and share the same histopathological features, zoster tends to produce only a single attack and repeated recurrences are rare. Herpes zoster is commonly also said to be more frequently associated with significant underlying immunodeficiency states, and particularly with lymphomas. However, a study[8] involving no fewer than 9389 person-years showed no greater frequency of development of tumours in patients who had had shingles than in an unaffected population, apart from a slight increase in tumours of the colon and bladder in women. The trigeminal sensory area is second only to involvement of the intercostal area in frequency and accounts for 12–25% of cases. All three, or only the second and third divisions, may be affected. In the latter case there is a prodromal sensory disturbance which, in older patients especially, can produce pain indistinguishable from toothache since the same area of cortex receives the pain impulses. Misdiagnosis of the 'toothache' has prompted inappropriate dental extractions before the rash has become obvious and has led to the myth that extractions can precipitate trigeminal zoster.

The lesions are clinically and histologically the same as those caused by herpes simplex virus, namely clusters of vesicles (Fig. 1.3), but are widely distributed in the sensory area affected. In the mouth the lesions tend to be more severe than on the skin and can be confluent, but stop sharply at the midline. Bilateral zoster in this region is exceedingly rare.

When the first division is affected, the significant risk of damage to sight needs specialist attention.

Diagnosis

Biopsy is rarely performed and even if it were the changes are the same as those of herpes simplex. Diagnosis mainly depends, therefore, on the clinical picture. The combination of the vesiculating lesions in the mouth and on the skin sharply limited to trigeminal sensory areas, in association with aching pain are characteristic. Serological investigation is of no value because of the high titre of antibodies already present. However, it may be advisable to look for some cause of defective cell-mediated immunity and it is said that in 10% of

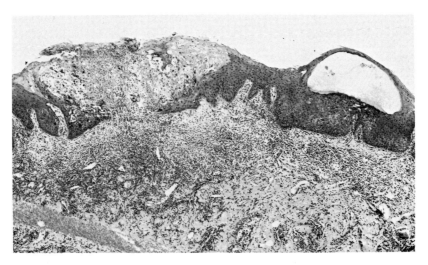

Fig. 1.3 Herpes zoster. There is both an intact vesicle and, nearby, an ulcer. The similarities to herpes simplex infection will be apparent.

Haematoxylin-eosin   × 40

cases of zoster there is an underlying lymphoma—most commonly Hodgkin's disease—but evidence to the contrary has also been produced.[9]

Herpetic infections in immunodeficient patients

Both herpes simplex and, to a lesser extent, zoster are common complications of heavy immunosuppressive treatment, particularly for organ transplantation, and can be severe. However, even before the advent of systemically-acting antiviral drugs, these infections usually resolved eventually of their own accord and withdrawal of immunosuppressive treatment is not thought to be necessary. Dissemination of and death from these infections in immunosuppressed patients is far less common than might be expected.[10]

Infectious mononucleosis

Infectious mononucleosis can produce minor oral lesions and pharyngitis is a common feature. The most common oral manifestation is the formation of small petechiae on the palate.

Involvement of oral lymphoid tissue of the foliate papillae is exceedingly rare but can happen and produce a lymphoma-like picture. More common is persistent enlargement of the cervical lymph nodes which has also been misdiagnosed histologically as lymphoma.

Hand, foot and mouth disease

Hand, foot and mouth disease is a common and usually minor infection caused by Coxsackie A viruses, particularly type A 16. The disease is highly infectious: an epidemic estimated to affect more than 800 children in South Wales[11] and a minor outbreak among members of staff of a dental hospital[12] have been reported.

Hand, foot and mouth disease is characterized by mild oral ulceration, clinically resembling that of herpetic stomatitis, associated with a vesicular rash on the extremities. Systemic symptoms are usually minimal and affected children seem more likely to notice the rash than the oral lesions. The latter can, however, appear in isolation and are likely then to be mistaken for mild herpetic stomatitis.

The histopathology of the lesions of hand, foot and mouth disease does not appear to have been described in detail.

BACTERIAL INFECTIONS

Tuberculosis

In spite of the decline in incidence of pulmonary tuberculosis and the availability of effective treatment, the proportion of patients with open infection who develop oral lesions appears from analysis of tens of thousands of cases to have remained unchanged at 0.2% since the pre-antibiotic era.[13, 14]

Oral ulcers secondary to pulmonary tuberculosis are seen virtually exclusively in middle-aged males and mainly affect the dorsum of the tongue or, less often, the lip. Classically, the ulcer is stellate or angular with overhanging edges and a pale floor. Pain is often absent. A chronic cough is associated but has usually been misinterpreted either as due to smoking or of no significance.

Histopathology

Microscopically, the typical overhanging edges of the ulcer may be obvious while in the floor and undermining the edges there are multiple granulomas with Langhans giant cells (Fig. 1.4) and some caseation. Acid-fast bacilli are unlikely to be found, however, irrespective of the staining method. Though oral ulceration with extensive granuloma formation is, in Britain at least, most likely to be tuberculous in nature, the diagnosis must be confirmed by sputum culture and chest radiographs.

Ulceration of this type associated with granuloma formation is unlikely to be a feature of sarcoidosis but one of the deep mycoses should be considered if there is any history suggestive of exposure.

Syphilis

Primary and secondary lesions in the mouth are unlikely to be biopsied and, if they are, the appearances are frequently insufficiently specific to make a diagnosis.

Tertiary lesions, particularly syphilitic leukoplakia, are virtually only of historical interest, but even in these the appearances may be unhelpful.

FUNGAL INFECTIONS

Candidosis

Candida albicans is the only important cause of fungal infections in the mouth in Britain and produces a variety of manifestations, as follows:

1. Acute candidosis
   a. Thrush
   b. Angular stomatitis
2. Chronic candidosis
   a. Denture stomatitis
   b. Limited hyperplastic candidosis (candidal leukoplakia)
   c. Chronic mucocutaneous candidosis syndromes
   d. Angular stomatitis.

It will be noted that angular stomatitis can be associated with either acute or chronic infections and can indeed be associated with any type of oral candidosis. This is the result of infected saliva leaking from the mouth and tracking along the small skinfold at the angle of the mouth. In the elderly, where the skinfold is larger due to the age-related sagging of the facial tissues, candidal infection produces a more conspicuous intertriginous infection.

Angular stomatitis is also a classical sign of iron deficiency, which in turn is a predisposing factor for candidosis. To what extent angular stomatitis in iron deficiency is mediated by candidal infection is not known.

Thrush

Thrush in infancy has been recognized since antiquity. The soft creamy-yellow plaques have the unusual feature that they can readily be wiped off, leaving an erythematous but intact epithelium. Angular stomatitis is commonly associated. The main aetiological factors are as follows:

1. Immunodeficiency
   a. Immaturity
   b. Primary (genetic or developmental)
   c. Secondary to tumours or other diseases
   d. As a result of immunosuppressive treatment
2. Antibacterial treatment, particularly with tetracycline
3. Haematological abnormalities—particularly iron deficiency

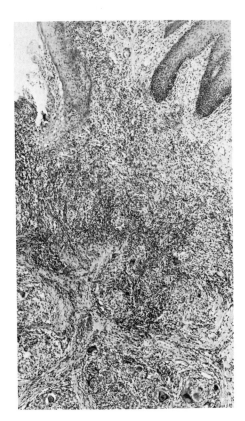

Fig. 1.4 Tuberculosis of the tongue. Only one edge of the ulcer with its overhanging margin is seen. Tuberculous granulomas extend deeply in the underlying tissue. The association of giant cell granulomas with ulceration in the mouth is seen virtually only in tuberculosis but occasionally also in the deep mycoses.

Haematoxylin-eosin   × 50

Since they are so numerous in different types of oral lesions, an abundance of plasma cells is not necessarily suggestive of a syphilitic lesion, as it might be in other tissues, and endarteritis may not be present.

It is necessary to make a direct smear since the diagnosis cannot be made serologically early in the primary stage. In the mouth, diagnosis is made difficult, however, by the presence of morphologically similar spiral commensal bacteria, though these are not normally numerous in superficial smears. It is important, therefore, first to wipe the lesion firmly, then to scrape the surface gently and to examine the wet material by dark field or phase contrast microscopy. In primary and secondary lesions the smear should show many spiral bacteria with the regular morphology of *Treponema pallidum* and its characteristic rotational movements.

4. Hormonal causes, e.g. pregnancy.

Often there may be a combination of factors, and in immunodeficiency states in particular the use of antibacterial drugs increases the likelihood of candidal infection. In young adult males, especially, persistent oral candidosis should prompt the suspicion that acquired immune deficiency syndrome (see p. 16) may be the underlying cause though this is (as yet) uncommon in Europe.

Histopathology

Microscopically, the plaque of thrush is produced by active epithelial proliferation and nuclear detail is well preserved even in the most superficial cells of the plaque (Fig. 1.5). The latter is infiltrated throughout by inflammatory exudate and leukocytes which separate the epithelial cells. This

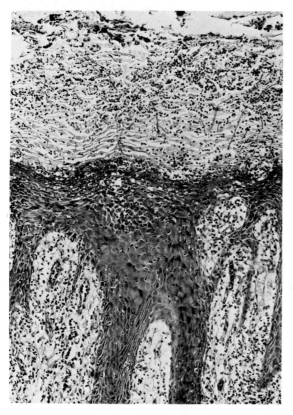

Fig. 1.5 Thrush. There is a parakeratotic plaque infiltrated by hyphae and inflammatory exudate. Micro-abscesses have formed at the junction between the plaque and the spinous layer.

Periodic acid-Schiff   × 150

exudate is particularly concentrated at the junction of the plaque with the glycogen-rich zone of the spinous layer, where micro-abscesses tend to form.

Periodic acid-Schiff staining shows that the plaque is invaded by many candidal hyphae which grow almost vertically downwards but do not invade the spinous layer below (Fig. 1.6). Deeply, the epithelium is mildly acanthotic with slender downgrowths around which there is a predominantly mononuclear inflammatory infiltrate.

It will be seen that the plaque of thrush is not a slough—hence the term 'pseudomembranous' candidosis is totally inappropriate—but the plaque is made friable by the widespread inflammatory infiltrate, the concentration of which, along its base, forms a plane of cleavage. As a consequence the plaque is readily wiped off.

Diagnosis

This is readily confirmed by making a Gram-stained smear which shows masses of long tangled hyphae (often with some yeast forms) and epithelial and inflammatory cells (Fig. 1.7).

Denture stomatitis

Denture stomatitis is probably the most common form of oral candidosis in adults, and is a minor iatrogenic infection produced by occlusion of the mucosa by a well-fitting upper denture. *C. albicans* colonizes the denture base and proliferates in the interface between the denture and mucosa. Inflammation and varying degrees of proliferation of the epithelium are produced and are probably mediated by enzymes such as proteases and phospholipases, secreted by the fungus.[15] There is no evidence for the reaction being immunologically mediated.

Clinically, there is bright or dusky erythema of the whole upper denture-bearing area and not extending beyond its margins. Usually the condition is asymptomatic but the patient is likely to complain mainly of associated angular cheilitis.

Histopathology

Typical findings are acanthosis, sometimes with long epithelial downgrowths, and intra-epithelial

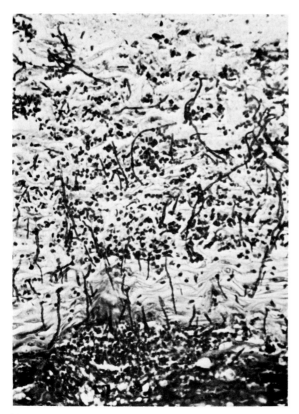

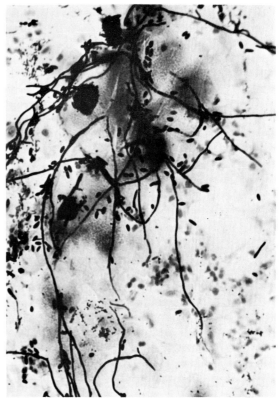

Fig. 1.6 Thrush. The large numbers of fungal hyphae are characteristic.

Periodic acid-Schiff   × 300

Fig. 1.7 Thrush. Smears show large numbers of long, tangled hyphae usually with a few yeast forms throughout.

Gram   × 400

oedema. Unlike other candidal lesions there is no plaque formation and hyphal invasion of the epithelium is typically absent or shows only superficial penetration. In the corium there is a predominantly mononuclear inflammatory infiltrate of variable density.

The histopathological features of denture stomatitis are not therefore specific and the diagnosis can only be made by the clinical features and direct smears showing candidal hyphae. However, biopsies are rarely submitted for diagnostic purposes.

Chronic hyperplastic candidosis

In contrast to chronic infection promoted by the artificial conditions under the denture, chronic candidosis of the exposed mucosa of the tongue or other sites can produce a tough adherent plaque,[16] clinically quite different from that of thrush and

indistinguishable except by biopsy from other leukoplakia-like conditions discussed later.

Adults, typically males of middle age or over, are affected. The most frequently affected sites are the dorsum of the tongue and the post-commissural buccal mucosa. The plaque is variable in thickness (probably dependent on the length of time it has been present) and often rough or irregular in texture, or nodular with an erythematous background, producing a speckled appearance. This plaque cannot be wiped off but fragments can be detached by firm scraping and, if Gram-stained, show clumps of epithelial cells from which hyphae protrude (Fig. 1.8).

Biopsy shows many features in common with thrush but altered mainly by the long duration of the infection. Like thrush, the plaque is parakeratotic but more coherent, containing only beads of inflammatory exudate which give it a psoriasiform appearance. Since oral psoriasis is so rare, this

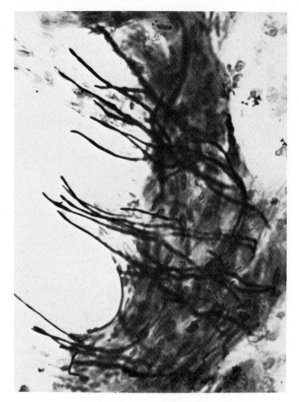

Fig. 1.8 Chronic hyperplastic candidosis. In contrast to thrush, scrapings of the lesion detach fragments of epithelium in which the hyphae are firmly embedded.

Gram   × 500

appearance should alert one to the possibility of candidosis even though hyphae are not obvious. Examination even of haematoxylin and eosin stained sections under high power is likely, however, to show hyphae, which appear as clear or faintly basophilic tracks through the epithelium (Fig. 1.9). Periodic acid-Schiff stain shows the hyphae clearly which, as in thrush, extend through the full thickness of the plaque to the glycogen-rich zone (Fig. 1.10), where the inflammatory exudate tends to be concentrated and can form micro-abscesses.

More deeply, the epithelium shows acanthosis, which can be massive with rounded downgrowths, and varying degrees of dysplasia (Fig. 1.11). If dysplasia is pronounced, there is a possibility ultimately of malignant change. Though there is typically a dense inflammatory infiltrate in the corium this frequently does not break up the deeper epithelium; the basement membrane then remains

intact and may appear to be thickened. This unusual feature in an oral keratotic lesion seems to be peculiar to chronic candidosis.

The diagnosis having been confirmed by biopsy, treatment should be by means of a systemically acting antifungal agent such as ketoconazole. Treatment may need to be prolonged for several months but in some cases some residual uninfected plaque may persist, and it seems that once the process has been initiated it becomes (as in syphilitic leukoplakia) to some degree autonomous. That the epithelial proliferation is induced by invasion by the fungus is shown by the fact that it has been reproduced experimentally.[17] Moreover, ultrastructural studies show that *C. albicans* is an intracellular parasite that grows within the cytoplasm of epithelial cells.[18] Understandably, therefore, the hyphae grow in relatively straight lines and do not pursue a tortuous path along the intercellular spaces.

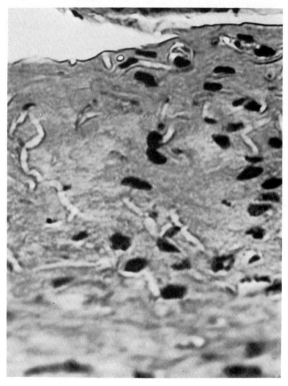

Fig. 1.9 Chronic candidosis. Haematoxylin and eosin do not stain fungal hyphae but these, however, can often be seen as clear tracks through the superficial epithelial plaque.

Haematoxylin-eosin   × 600

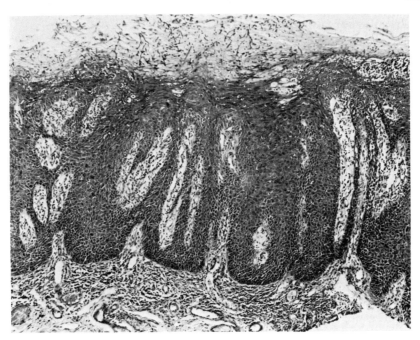

Fig. 1.10 Chronic candidosis. There is a parakeratotic plaque invaded by hyphae and micro-abscesses at the junction with the spinous layer. There is a close resemblance to psoriasis apart from the presence of the fungi.

Periodic acid-Schiff   × 70

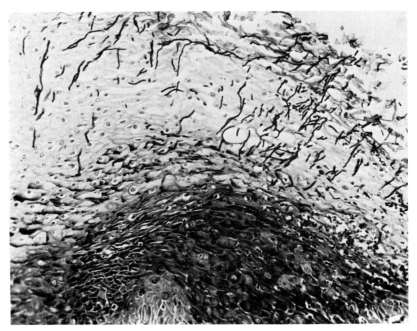

Fig. 1.11 Chronic candidosis. At higher power, stained with PAS, the fungi in the plaque are readily seen.

Periodic acid-Schiff   × 180

Chronic mucocutaneous candidosis syndromes

These syndromes are all rare but present a variety of features which make them of considerable interest in several specialities and particularly to immunologists. The following classification is mainly based on that of Higgs & Wells:[19]

1. Familial (limited) type
2. Diffuse type (candida 'granuloma')
3. Endocrine candidosis syndrome
4. Late onset type (thymoma syndrome).

Clinically these syndromes differ from each other mainly in their extra-oral features. Only the diffuse type shows significantly more severe candidal infection and may therefore be distinguishable from the others microscopically. Otherwise the microscopic features are the same as those described in the preceding section. The essential features of these variants are as follows.

Familial mucocutaneous candidosis

This condition is inherited as an autosomal recessive trait, though a family showing a dominant pattern of inheritance has been reported. The oral lesions are indistinguishable from those of the sporadic cases described above, but sideropenia is characteristic and there may be mild cutaneous involvement. The onset, however, is in infancy with thrush-like lesions which progress to form leukoplakia-like lesions in childhood.

Diffuse type mucocutaneous candidosis

Most cases are sporadic but affected families have been reported. This is the most severe type and was earlier termed 'Candida granuloma' by Hauser & Rothman[20] because of the often disfiguring and massive overgrowths on the skin. These, however, are produced by epithelial proliferation and are no more than an extreme expression of the same process that produces oral epithelial plaques in response to candidal invasion.

In addition to the severe mucocutaneous candidal lesions these patients usually also have abnormal susceptibility to bacterial diseases, particularly pulmonary and superficial suppurative infections.

Endocrine candidosis syndrome

In this bizarre variant, chronic mucocutaneous candidosis is associated with multiple glandular deficiencies and organ-specific autoantibody production. There is no direct aetiological relationship between the two features of this disorder and the candidal infection can precede the onset of endocrine deficiency by as much as 15 years. Occasionally, however, this sequence is reversed.

The most common associated endocrine deficiency is hypoparathyroidism and since (for quite different reasons) hypoparathyroidism and chronic candidosis may be associated in Di George's syndrome a myth has arisen that hypoparathyroidism produces susceptibility to candidosis.

Recently[21,22] it has been shown that there are two variants of the polyendocrinopathy syndrome, chronic mucocutaneous candidosis being associated with type I. In type I, Addison's disease and hypoparathyroidism are present in the great majority of patients, and many other glandular deficiencies can develop, but thyroiditis and insulin-dependent diabetes are rare. In type II neither candidosis nor hypoparathyroidism is found but Addison's disease is associated with thyroiditis or insulin-dependent diabetes in the majority of cases.

Although Thorpe & Handley[23] described chronic candidosis in association with early onset hypoparathyroidism as early as 1929, the presence of candidosis has not been mentioned in many reports of polyglandular deficiency. This is probably because type II appears to be considerably more common, but even when candidosis is present (in type I) it is often mild and either passes unnoticed or is thought merely to be a complication of the endocrine disorder.

Late onset mucocutaneous candidosis

This syndrome has a clearer immunological basis than those described above, in that there is a persistent defect of cell-mediated immunity produced by a thymoma. The syndrome comprises thymoma, myasthenia gravis, pure red cell aplasia and chronic mucocutaneous candidosis.

Immunological aspects

The immunological basis for susceptibility to

chronic candidosis has been the subject of extensive study but remains far from clear. It seems unjustifiable to categorize chronic mucocutaneous candidosis as an immunodeficiency disorder *per se*, in view of the number of cases where there is no detectable immunological defect and in view of the absence of any significantly greater susceptibility to other infections in most cases, even when there is an associated defect. In addition, when a defect of immunity is present, the fungal infection, though persistent, remains superficial and does not disseminate. Microscopically, infection does not extend more deeply than in the sporadic cases of oral chronic hyperplastic candidosis described earlier. Any immune defect is, thus, typically limited in nature.

The main immunological findings can be summarized as follows:

1. Immunological deficits, when detectable, are mainly of cell-mediated immunity, rarely of humoral immunity, and there is no consistent pattern.
2. The immunological defect is typically selective (except in the diffuse type syndrome) and there is a poor delayed response to *C. albicans* only.
3. Approximately 25% of patients have no significant defect of humoral or cellular immunity.
4. The immunological defect may be secondary and cases have been reported of reversal of the defect after adequate antifungal treatment.
5. Generally speaking, the more severe the candidal infection the more frequently immunological defects are found, but they are by no means invariably detectable even in diffuse type mucocutaneous infection.[24]

The deep mycoses

The deep mycoses produce a variety of pathological features and clinical pictures but a common pattern is acquisition of infection from spores, often from the soil, particularly the moist soil of warm river valleys. These diseases are therefore more frequent in such parts of the world as South America and, to a lesser degree, in some of the more southerly of the United States. The deep mycoses are rare in Britain and a history of visiting or residence in an endemic area is an important diagnostic clue.

Histoplasmosis, aspergillosis or mucormycosis can be seen as opportunistic complications of immunodeficiency states and various mycoses can complicate the acquired immune deficiency syndrome (see p. 16). Candidosis, unlike other mycoses, can cause either superficial (mucocutaneous) or disseminated infections but the two are hardly ever associated and oral lesions are rarely a feature of systemic candidosis.

Most of the deep mycoses can produce oral lesions. In blastomycosis it has been reported that 25% of patients have oral or nasal mucosal lesions while in paracoccidiodomycosis oral lesions are even more common. In histoplasmosis they can be an initial feature in as many as 30% of fatal cases. Oral lesions are infrequent, however, in cryptococcosis and sporotrichosis. Rhinocerebral phycomycosis typically starts in the antrum but can cause necrotizing ulceration of the palate and this may be an important feature which may make early diagnosis possible. Aspergillus species are common commensals in the mouth but painful lesions of the tongue and palate have been reported in disseminated aspergillosis. Other lesions, such as invasive aspergillosis of the cheek following dental extractions or lacerations of the face, are rare.

Aspergilloma (usually *A. fumigatus*) of the maxillary antrum is a rare finding in healthy persons and can sometimes follow displacement of a root of a tooth, which introduces the infection into the antrum.

The deep mycoses tend otherwise to produce nondescript proliferative or ulcerative lesions when they involve the oral tissues and the clinical features contribute little to the diagnosis. The latter therefore depends on the histopathological findings and often, as in histoplasmosis and cryptococcosis for example, there is formation of tuberculosis-like granulomas. Sometimes the characteristic tissue phases of the fungus can be seen, but often these are few and difficult or impossible to find. Wherever possible fresh material should therefore be taken for culture if the clinical or histopathological findings suggest a mycosis.[25]

ACQUIRED IMMUNE DEFICIENCY SYNDROME (AIDS)

Acquired immune deficiency syndrome (AIDS) can be defined as severe immunodeficiency, apparently infective and characterized by opportunistic infections, particularly by *Pneumocystis carinii*, and by otherwise uncommon tumours, particularly Kaposi's sarcoma, in previous healthy persons. The immunodeficiency has so far proved irreversible and is characterized by reduced numbers of T-helper (OKT4) lymphocytes, with a consequent reversal of the normal T-helper to suppressor cell ratio, and lymphopenia. The prevalence of AIDS and the opportunistic infections and neoplasms associated with this immunodeficiency are shown in Tables 1.1 and 1.2, and in 'Clinical features' below. In some respects, therefore, the pattern of disease is similar to but more severe than that which results from immunosuppressive treatment in transplant patients.

The disease is potentially lethal and can produce oral infections and tumours as early signs.[26-37]

Epidemiology

AIDS was first reported in 1981 among promiscuous male homosexuals in the United States and, in particular, in San Francisco and New York. These remain the most frequently affected group outside Africa but others at risk are indicated in Table 1.1. As shown there it is apparent that recipients of blood products are also vulnerable to this disease and this, among other features, suggested the now generally accepted concept that AIDS is transmissible. However, there has inevitably been uncertainty about its mode of acquisition by some patients sometimes as a result of reticence about their sexual habits or drug abuse. More recently it has become apparent that AIDS can also be transmitted by heterosexual intercourse, though rarely as yet, and to the fetus of mothers with the disease or carrying the virus.

In terms of scale, in addition to the numbers of known cases, at the time of writing, in Britain and the United States shown in Table 1.1, several hundred cases have been reported from most countries in Europe[38] and the disease has spread as far as Australia and Japan. Inevitably the infor-

mation recorded here will be out of date by the time it is read, but the incidence of AIDS has increased exponentially since it was first recognized and it is predicted[39] that 270 000 persons will have AIDS or will have died from the disease by 1991 in the United States alone.

An indication of the probable rate of increase in the disease in Britain is shown by the more than five-fold increase, from 3.7–21% between 1982 and 1984, in the prevalence of seropositivity to the putative AIDS virus (HTLV III) among homosexuals in a London sexually-transmitted disease clinic.[40] Since this group represents only a proportion of those at risk it is probable that several thousands have been exposed to the virus in the country as a whole.

AIDS has also been recognized in Central Africa where it appears to differ from the disease in the rest of the world only in that promiscuous heterosexual activity appears to be the chief mode of transmission. In addition, there has been suspicion that the causative virus originated in Africa and these beliefs have been supported by such reports as that of a Danish woman surgeon who had been working in Africa and who died of a disease fulfilling the criteria of AIDS as long ago as 1976.[41] About 5% of apparently healthy Zairians are reported to be antibody positive to the presumed causative agent.[42]

Table 1.1 Prevalence of AIDS (as at 28 February 1985) showing chief groups at risk*

Patient group	Total cases in USA Number	%	Total cases in UK Number	%
Homosexual/bisexual	6293	72	117	89
Intravenous drug abusers	1478	17	0	0
Haemophiliacs and blood transfusion recipients	166	2	3	2
Female sexual partners of men at risk	68	1	1	1
Children of affected mothers	104	1	0	0
Caribbean or Central African connection	280	3	7	6
Insufficient data or unknown	308	4	4	3
Totals	8697		132	

* Modified from: Anonymous. Acquired immune deficiency syndrome. London: Department of Health & Social Security, 1985.

Aetiology

A putative causative virus was first isolated in France in 1983, where it was named the Lymphadenopathy Associated Virus (LAV)[43] and later in the same year in the United States where the organism was named the Human T cell Lymphotropic Virus Type III (HTLV III).[44,45] Another term for the same or similar virus is the AIDS-Related Virus (ARV).[46] These viruses are closely related in structure[47] and since then other related viruses have been identified, with the result that the term 'Human Immunodeficiency Viruses (HIV)' is being increasingly used. Tests for antibodies in AIDS or its prodromes are, currently, for HTLV III/LAV, and those who develop AIDS but are seronegative for HTLV III/LAV may have the disease as a result of infection by another HIV or have failed to produce antibodies.

Evidence that these viruses are causative includes the findings that, of those with the syndrome, approximately 95% are seropositive for HTLV III, that apparently healthy, high-risk groups have a slightly lower (but still high frequency of seropositivity) and that prospective studies have shown that seroconversion to HTV III positivity is frequently followed by the appearance of serum markers of immunodeficiency and later (in a lesser number within the period of follow-up) of full-blown AIDS.[45,48-50]

HTLV III has also been isolated from blood, semen and saliva of patients with AIDS though the first two are regarded as the chief vehicles of transmission.

Nevertheless, acquisition of HTLV III alone seems relatively infrequently to be followed by AIDS since, for example, haemophiliacs who have long been exposed to the virus in blood or blood products have a low incidence of AIDS compared with other high-risk groups and there is some evidence to suggest that pre-existing immunodeficiency is an important predisposing factor. Male homosexual activity itself appears to have an immunodepressant effect, partly at least because of the stress imposed on the immune system by the multitude of infections acquired as a result of such habits. Even among male homosexuals, however, the chief risk for AIDS appears to be receptive anal intercourse.

In addition, HLA haplotypes may affect the level of risk of acquiring this disease and HLA DR5 is significantly more frequent among those who develop Kaposi's sarcoma.[51]

Generally speaking, therefore, it seems likely that exposure to HTLV III usually leads to production of antibodies against these viruses and a variable degree of risk of developing AIDS. It is not clear, however, whether it is possible to eliminate the virus as it has been shown that some, who are seropositive to HTLV III, also carry the virus.[52] Since also the incubation period of the disease can sometimes be exceptionally long (cases have been recorded as long as $5\frac{1}{2}$ years after a blood transfusion as the sole risk factor)[53] it will take a long time before the level of risk, after exposure to the virus, can be accurately assessed.

Following exposure to the virus a spectrum of disease may develop. Whatever the cause and associated factors necessary to produce the disease, the process appears to comprise an incubation period leading to a prodromal phase of gradually increasing immune dysfunction and, eventually, outward signs of immunodeficiency. As in transplant patients, neoplasms may not develop until some years after immune responses have become impaired, as shown by in vitro testing.

Clinical features

The features of the effects of exposure to HIV and AIDS are now widely known[54] but they are summarized here (Table 1.2) for convenience. Malignant tumours in AIDS are as follows:

1. Kaposi's sarcoma
2. Non-Hodgkin's lymphomas
3. Oral squamous cell carcinoma
4. Carcinoma of rectum.

There is wide individual variation. Many remain asymptomatic but the main manifestations are acute transient glandular fever-like syndrome,[55] persistent generalized lymphadenopathy syndrome and AIDS itself.

Persistent generalized lymphadenopathy syndrome
Persistent generalised lymphadenopathy syndrome (PGLS)[56] is characterized by lymphadenopathy

Table 1.2 Opportunistic infections in AIDS

Site	Infections*
1. Pneumonia, meningitis or encephalitis	*Pneumocystis carinii* Aspergillus *Candida albicans* *Cryptococcus neoformans* *Histoplasma capsulatum* Nocardia *Petrellidium boydii* Zygomycosis (mucormycosis) Strongyloides *Toxoplasma gondii* *Mycobacterium avium-intracellulare* Cytomegalovirus Progressive multifocal leukoencephalopathy Legionella sp.
2. Chronic enterocolitis	Cryptosporidium *Isospora belli* *Giardia lamblia*
3. Mucocutaneous	*Candida albicans* Herpes simplex Varicella zoster virus
4. Disseminated	Cytomegalovirus Herpes simplex *Candida albicans* *Cryptococcus neoformans* *Histoplasma capsulatum* *Mycobacterium avium-intracellulare*

* Often recurrent and/or mixed infections; may be recurrent and/or mixed infections.

due to follicular hyperplasia and is associated with lymphopenia and abnormal T-lymphocyte ratios. There is also loss of weight, splenomegaly, low fever, night sweats and fatigue. Though PGLS is a prodromal AIDS syndrome in some cases, as shown by its progression to typical AIDS, unlike the latter it may, in some cases, apparently resolve spontaneously.[57]

Acquired immune deficiency syndrome

Typical early symptoms are non-specific, namely lethargy, loss of weight, fever and night sweats. Widespread symmetrical lymphadenopathy is an important finding. Joint pains, rashes and diarrhoea are also common but the most common and more specific manifestations are either opportunistic infections, and in particular *P. carinii* pneumonia (60%), or Kaposi's sarcoma (25%) or both.

With regard to opportunistic infections the clinical picture will depend on the systems chiefly involved, namely, respiratory, central nervous or gastrointestinal, or generalized (see Table 1.2) and causing pyrexia of unknown origin.

Manifestations of the disease are common in the head and neck region and particularly in the mouth.[32-35, 58] Oral manifestations of AIDS include:

1. Infections
   a. Persistent candidosis
   b. Herpetic infection
2. Tumours
   a. Kaposi's sarcoma
   b. Squamous cell carcinoma.

One report[36] suggests that head and neck manifestations are present in up to 95% of patients. The development of unexplained oral candidosis (thrush), was reported in one of the earliest papers[26] and is now known to be an important prodromal feature of AIDS[32,37,57,59] while the finding of Kaposi's sarcoma in the mouth of a previously healthy young male is virtually pathognomonic of the disease.

Another oral lesion which appears strongly predictive of AIDS is a peculiar form of white lesion named 'hairy leukoplakia'[60] or, alternatively, oral condyloma plana. Herpetic infection can cause minor or severe intra- or perioral ulceration and several of these lesions may be concurrent.

Prognosis

The prognosis of AIDS is exceedingly poor and about 90% die within three years of diagnosis. The majority of deaths result from uncontrollable opportunistic infections. The response of AIDS-associated tumours to treatment is also poor.[61,62]

Immunological findings[62]

In addition to the depressed numbers of T-helper lymphocytes, there appears to be depressed interleukin 2 and interferon production. By contrast, the number of B-lymphocytes in lymph nodes appears to be increased and despite depressed B-cell function there is (paradoxically) polyclonal activation of these cells leading to raised levels of immunoglobulins, particularly IgG and IgA. In addition, natural killer cell activity is diminished and autoimmune phenomena such as thrombo-cytopenia may be associated.[63]

Antibody to HTLV III can now be detected using enzyme-linked immune assay (ELISA) and, if false positives can be excluded, indicates possible infectivity of blood or blood products. However, a few AIDS patients are not seropositive and it seems that infection with HTLV III virus may not always lead to antibody production[62] or the latter may only appear at a late stage. Alternatively, the infection may have been caused by another HIV.

Histopathology

Various abnormalities of lymph node structure have been reported. Such changes depend on the stage of development of the disease but may include florid follicular hyperplasia with atrophy of the mantle zone and disruption of adjacent follicles, reactive follicular and sinusoidal proliferation, follicular involution with expansion of the para-cortical zone, a mixed pattern of follicular hyper-plasia and involution, and, in two cases, angioimmunoblastic lymphadenopathy (diffuse loss of nodal architecture but preservation of the subcapsular sinus) with dysproteinaemia.[64]

Further, studies with monoclonal antibodies have shown destruction of the dendritic reticulum in patients with persistent glandular lymphadeno-pathy syndrome. It is suggested that this may lead to release of non-specifically activated B lympho-cytes into the blood and is of poor prognostic significance.[65]

It may be noted that somewhat similar lymph node changes had been described in association with Kaposi's sarcoma before the recognition of AIDS as an entity.[66]

The microscopic findings in the various infec-tions and tumours found in AIDS patients do not seem to differ significantly from those in other patients, especially those with other types of immunodeficiency.[67,68] However, the age inci-dence, distribution and behaviour of Kaposi's sarcoma, in particular, differ from those given in earlier descriptions.

In brief, the tumour as described by Kaposi (1872)[69] among elderly persons in Central Europe is predominantly cutaneous, mainly affects the lower extremities, and visceral lesions are rarely clinically apparent. The African form of Kaposi's sarcoma is most common in Zaire where it forms about 12% of all malignant tumours and is about half as common in neighbouring Uganda, Kenya, Rwanda and Tanzania.[70] Though children can be affected, the mean age of patients is 43, but this is regarded as elderly for this population. The African form of Kaposi's sarcoma is predominantly also cutaneous, affecting the lower extremities and having both an indolent course and a good response to chemotherapy. Head and neck involvement is exceedingly rare.

Though a variety of infections are often associ-ated, the possibility of underlying immunodefi-ciency had not been investigated until recently.

One feature shared by African Kaposi's sarcoma and AIDS is that about 60% in both groups are HLA DR5[51] and it is believed therefore that there is some underlying genetic susceptibility.

In AIDS, by contrast, Kaposi's sarcoma fre-quently involves the head and neck region. This may be oropharyngeal, cutaneous or in the cervical lymph nodes. Within the mouth the palate is the most commonly affected site and the tumour typically produces a flat or nodular purplish lesion. The response to chemotherapy is poor.

In AIDS patients, incidentally, Kaposi's sar-coma is most common among male homosexuals but relatively rare in haemophiliacs.[71]

A more aggressive form of Kaposi's sarcoma has been described in Zambia[72] and has many features in common with that seen in typical AIDS patients, including the distribution of the lesions and poor response to chemotherapy. Further, it has been found that there are cases of AIDS-like disease in Rwanda and Zaire differing from typical AIDS only in that males and females are virtually equally affected. In both Rwanda and Zaire heterosexual promiscuity seemed to be the most probable mode of spread.[73-75]

Kaposi's sarcoma originates from endothelial cells (as shown by the presence of the factor VIII marker)[76] and produces florid angiomatoid prolif-eration with some resemblance to granulation tissue. Recognition of the tumour may therefore be difficult, particularly in the early stages.

Three stages of development of the microscopic changes have been described. In the earliest ('presarcomatous') stage there is angiomatous proliferation with formation of irregular vascular spaces in the upper dermis and perivascular cuffing by lymphocytes and plasma cells. In the intermediate stage the angiomatoid changes are more widespread with slit-like, irregular vascular spaces (Fig. 1.12). In addition there is perivascular proliferation of spindle-shaped or angular cells. In the later stages the picture is increasingly dominated by the proliferation of the interstitial spindle-shaped (Fig. 1.13) and angular cells and mitotic activity may be prominent (Fig. 1.14). There is typically also extravasation of erythrocytes and deposition of haemosiderin. Central necrosis may develop.

In contrast to the figures frequently quoted for the incidence of Kaposi's sarcoma detected in AIDS during life, an autopsy study[77] has suggested a far higher frequency, namely 94% of 52 cases.

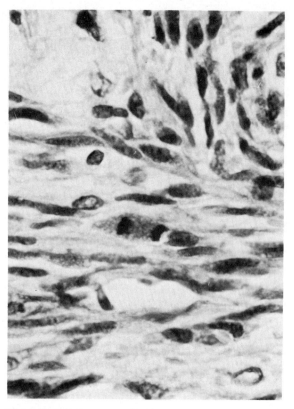

Fig. 1.13 Kaposi's sarcoma. At higher power the characteristic spindle-shaped cells with a few minute vascular spaces and a mitotic figure are shown.

Haematoxylin-eosin   × 650

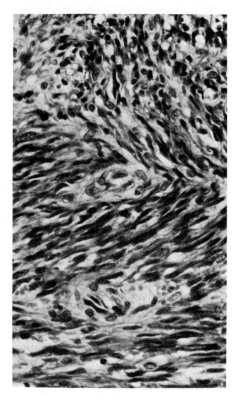

Fig. 1.12 Kaposi's sarcoma. Angiomatous proliferation is seen as spindle-shaped cells separated by slit-like spaces in longitudinal section (below) or as minute circular lumens (above) when cut transversely.

Haematoxylin-eosin   × 450

These had the inflammatory variant of the tumour in association with typical Kaposi's sarcoma while 36.5% had the latter alone. Many organs could be affected but the tumour was most frequently found in the lymph nodes and spleen. It appeared from these findings that the inflammatory variant was no less aggressive than classical Kaposi's sarcoma.

At the ultrastructural level[78] the vascular spaces lack or have a fragmented basal lamina and pericytes, or their processes are sparse or absent. The endothelium tends also to be discontinuous and intercellular junctions are small and sparse.[48] In rapidly progressive tumours, neoplastic endothelial cells may undergo necrosis or give rise to processes which infiltrate the surrounding collagen fibres and entrap them. These features are so distinctive as to enable Kaposi's sarcoma to be differentiated from other vascular proliferative lesions.

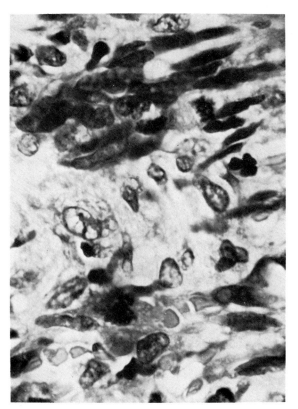

Fig. 1.14 Kaposi's sarcoma. The cellular picture is more pleomorphic here. There are several mitoses and a few extravasated erythrocytes among the tumour cells.

Haematoxylin-eosin   × 900.

NON-INFECTIVE DISORDERS

Recurrent aphthae

Recurrent aphthae are by far the most common disease of the oral mucosa and affect 10–20% of the population. Usually these ulcers are no more than a troublesome nuisance, but in a few cases major aphthae can produce disablingly painful ulcers several centimetres across, persisting for months and leaving fibrotic scars when they eventually heal.[79,80]

Notwithstanding the plethora of reports of immunological abnormalities in patients with recurrent aphthae (as discussed below in relation to Behçet's syndrome), there is no firm evidence that the disease is immunologically mediated. Recurrent aphthae typically affect young otherwise healthy persons, have no association with any of the recognized autoimmune diseases, do not re-

spond reliably to immunosuppressive treatment and, in the vast majority, are a self-limiting disorder. There are also no immunological tests which are useful in diagnosis.

In a minority of patients latent iron, folate or vitamin B_{12} deficiency appears to be a contributory factor[81] and in such patients appropriate replacement treatment is followed by remission or reduction of ulceration in the majority of cases.

Clinically, aphthae often start in childhood or adolescence, usually with only a few ulcers a year. Most patients who have sufficiently severe symptoms to seek specialist treatment have ulcers regularly every few weeks or so. Frequently the new ulcers appear before the previous crop has healed. An ulcer typically heals after about 10 days and the most common type is round or elliptical and shallow with a yellowish floor and a rim of erythema. The distribution is characteristic in that the masticatory ('keratinized') mucosa is spared and ulcers never appear, for example, in the vault of the palate.

Histopathology

Microscopically, aphthae show non-specific ulceration. There is no preceding vesiculation but the epithelium is infiltrated with mononuclear cells and destroyed (Fig. 1.15). Once this has happened, neutrophils tend to dominate the infiltrate, which extends deeply.

Biopsy is of little value in diagnosis except to exclude more serious conditions—this may be necessary in the case of major aphthae whose clinical appearance can closely resemble malignant ulcers. Though a history of repeated recurrences is the main diagnostic feature of aphthae, cancer can supervene in a patient as in anyone else.

Behçet's syndrome

Behçet's syndrome comprises oral and genital aphthae associated with uveitis or other ocular disease. Young men are predominantly affected and there is wide geographical variation in incidence. The disease is common in Turkey and, particularly, in Japan.[82]

Oral and genital ulceration are the most constant features. Skin lesions comprise ulceration of the

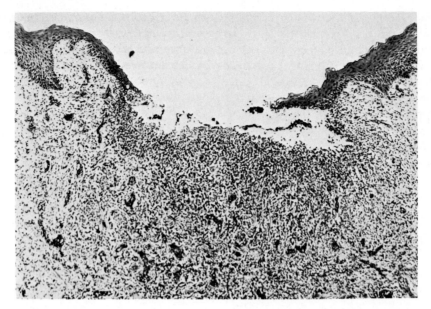

Fig. 1.15 Recurrent aphthae. The features are non-specific with localized destruction of the epithelium and a mixed inflammatory infiltrate extending deeply.

Haematoxylin-eosin   × 60

genital area, as well as erythema nodosum and pustular lesions in other areas. Other features can be neurological disease, arthralgia or arthritis, vascular, gastrointestinal and renal lesions. The incidence of these manifestations apparently varies from country to country. The variety of associated systemic disorders is such that there are no absolute criteria of diagnosis[83] and ulcerative colitis (for example) can also be associated with arthralgia, oral ulcers and erythema nodosum. Specialized investigation of the systems involved is therefore necessary, both as an aid to diagnosis and to ensure optimal management.

The oral ulcers can be minor or major and are not in themselves distinguishable from 'simple' aphthae. The histopathological features are equally non-specific.

Many immunological abnormalities have been reported.[80,84,85] They are generally similar to those in simple recurrent aphthae and include raised levels of IgA and acute phase proteins including C9, but falls in C2, C4 and C9, particularly before an attack of uveitis. Circulating immune complexes have also been reported but their association with increased disease activity is unconfirmed. It has been suggested that HLA B5 is significantly associated with ocular involvement and HLA DR7 may be associated with both ocular and neurological disease. HLA B12 and HLA DR7 may be associated with the milder, mucocutaneous and arthritic forms. More recently, and in contrast to earlier reports (as with many other of the immunological findings) abnormalities of T-lymphocyte subsets have been reported.[86] These changes comprise significantly decreased numbers of T-helper cells and a concomitant increase in T-suppressor cells. Such a finding, as the authors[86] point out seems, to say the least, incompatible with auto-antibody production but might be consistent with cytotoxic tissue damage. As in simple aphthae there is no reliable response to immunosuppressive treatment and there are no immunological diagnostic tests of value.

Lichen planus

Lichen planus is a common, chronic mucocutaneous disease which affects women rather more frequently than men, typically in middle age or later.

The aetiology of lichen planus is unknown but the histological appearances suggest a cell-mediated attack on the epithelium which can become progressively thinned until completely destroyed. Also suggestive of an immunopathogenesis are clinically identical lesions induced by drugs and as a feature of chronic graft-versus-host disease.[87] Lichen planus responds reliably to treatment with immunosuppressive drugs.

The oral lesions consist of striae, atrophic areas or erosions. Bullae are more frequently mentioned than seen and it seems that, though the microscopic picture shows otherwise, many believe that the erosions are produced by rupture of bullae. An additional source of confusion is that the fibrin-covered granulation tissue forming the floor of an erosion can bulge upwards above its surroundings to simulate a bulla.

The oral striae, unlike those on the skin, are grossly obvious, sharply defined, bluish-white and can extend over several square centimetres forming a net-like pattern. The buccal mucosa, usually of both sides, is most frequently affected. The dorsum of the tongue is another common site but the lesions are more varied in appearance.

The chief cause of symptoms are atrophic areas, which appear red and shiny, or erosions, which are irregular, sharply defined and covered with yellow exudate. These are usually but not necessarily associated with striae and all three types of lesion are distinguishable microscopically. It is important to take into account both the clinical and microscopic features in making a diagnosis.

Histopathology

Striate lesions can show the 'classical' histological features of lichen planus at least as clearly as cutaneous lesions, namely a saw-tooth profile to the deep margin of the epithelium, liquefaction degeneration of the basal cell layer and a dense band-like mononuclear infiltrate which hugs the dermo-epidermal junction (Fig. 1.16). The white appearance is caused by hyperortho- or parakeratosis. Frequently, however, absolutely distinctive features are lacking and the picture is often no more than consistent with lichen planus. Andreasen[88] has reviewed the variation in the microscopic picture and found the most constant feature to be liquefaction degeneration of the basal cell layers. Atrophic lesions have a much thinned, flat epithelium with an even more dense band of inflammatory cells (Fig. 1.17) while the erosions show complete destruction of the epithelium and, as a consequence, non-specific ulceration. More

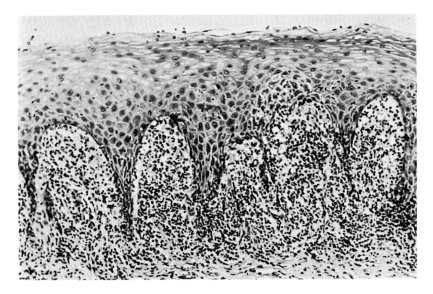

Fig. 1.16 Oral lichen planus. The saw-tooth rete ridges with liquefaction degeneration of the basal cell layer and a band-like infiltrate of mononuclear cells are 'classical' features but infrequently seen.

Haematoxylin-eosin   × 110

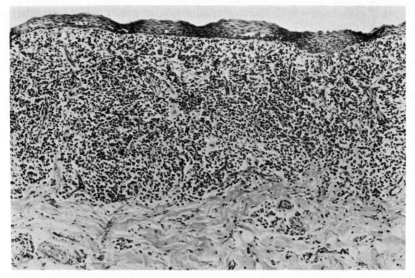

Fig. 1.17 Atrophic lichen planus. The epithelium has become thin and flattened but the band-like infiltrate of mononuclear cells is retained.

Haematoxylin-eosin   × 110

typical changes of lichen planus may be apparent at the margins, however.

Civatte ('colloid') bodies are rounded eosinophilic featureless bodies usually seen in the basal cell layer. They appear to be degenerate epithelial cells which sometimes undergo phagocytosis. They are not specific to lichen planus. By use of monoclonal antibodies it has been shown that T lymphocytes predominate in the subepithelial infiltrate.

Immunofluorescence studies with antifibrinogen show brilliant staining along the basement membrane. This reaction is shared with lupus erythematosus but is negative in erythema multiforme and mucous membrane pemphigoid. Unlike lupus erythematosus, deposition of immunoglobulins in the basement membrane zone is not seen in lichen planus but C3 may be detectable in a granular pattern.

Malignant change in lichen planus

The prevalence of oral lichen planus is impossible to assess since it is often asymptomatic. As a result the incidence of malignant change is equally impossible to assess accurately and estimates have varied widely.[89–91] However, carcinoma is occasionally seen in an area that has been for long affected by lichen planus and rarely malignant change can be seen in association with microscopic features of lichen planus.

Pemphigus vulgaris

Pemphigus has a better defined immunopathogenesis than any other oral disease and appears to be mediated by circulating autoantibodies directed against the intercellular substance of squamous epithelium.[92]

Women, usually between the ages of 40 and 50, are predominantly affected and the formation of vesicles in the mouth is often the first sign. The vesicles are, however, fragile and not often seen intact. The appearances, according to the severity of the disease, therefore range from somewhat nondescript-looking, shallow ulcers to widespread sloughing of the oral epithelium. Stroking of the oral mucosa may lead to formation or extension of existing vesicles (Nikolsky's sign). Spread to the skin follows after a variable period and, if untreated, leads to widespread formation of flaccid bullae.

Histopathology

Diagnosis must be confirmed by biopsy, which must include perilesional tissue. This shows char-

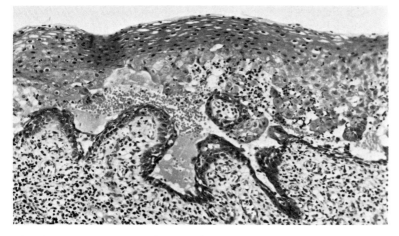
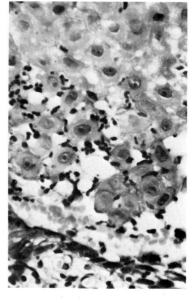

Fig. 1.18a, b Pemphigus vulgaris. (**a**) At this early stage of vesicle formation the basal cells are intact but many of the spinous cells are starting to separate from one another. (**b**) The acantholytic cells have become rounded and there is partial separation of the more superficial cells.

Haematoxylin-eosin   (**a**) × 160; (**b**) × 300

acteristic acantholysis with separation of the epithelial cells from one another to produce a suprabasal cleft (Fig. 1.18a). The latter extends to form a vesicle with an increasingly attenuated roof which soon ruptures. The detached epithelial cells round-up and can be seen floating in isolation or in small clusters in the vesicle fluid (Fig. 1.18b).

Circulating autoantibodies are detectable in most patients and can, if necessary, be demonstrated by immunofluorescence on a sample of epithelium. From the viewpoint of diagnosis, however, it is simpler and more satisfactory to use a frozen section to demonstrate the binding of immunoglobulin (usually IgG) along the intercellular junctions (Fig. 1.19) and coating separated acantholytic cells.[93] Complement components, particularly C3, can usually also be detected and there is evidence that complement activation by autoantibody complexes leads in turn to activation of epidermal proteases which degrade the intercellular cement substance. Basal cells are less vulnerable to this process by virtue of attachment to their neighbours by hemidesmosomes and their fibrillar attachment to the basement membrane.

Confirmation of the diagnosis at the earliest possible stage by these means is essential to initiate immunosuppresive treatment in this potentially lethal disease.

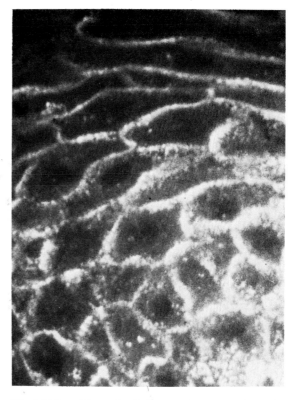

Fig. 1.19 Pemphigus vulgaris. Immunofluorescence shows the typical pattern of antibody bound at the intercellular junctions.

Fluorescein isothiocyanate   × 550

Pemphigus has an infrequent but significant association with other autoimmune diseases (particularly myasthenia gravis and lupus erythematosus) and with HLA D/DR4.

Pemphigus variants. Pemphigus vulgaris is the most common type. Other rare types are pemphigus vegetans, pemphigus foliaceous, pemphigus erythematosus (Senear-Usher syndrome), drug-induced pemphigus and Brazilian pemphigus (fogo selvagem). All are characterized by autoantibodies similar to those found in pemphigus vulgaris.

Mucous membrane (cicatricial, ocular) pemphigoid

Mucous membrane pemphigoid is not satisfactorily distinguishable either microscopically or immunologically from bullous pemphigoid, but the target tissues differ. In short, mucous membrane pemphigoid affects the mouth, eyes and sometimes the oesophagus or larynx but skin lesions are typically absent or minor. By contrast, oral lesions in bullous pemphigoid are rare.

Women, usually past middle age, are mainly affected. The oral lesions consist of bullae often one or two centimetres across which, unlike those of pemphigus vulgaris, may often be seen intact or recently ruptured with residual tags of epithelium (from the vesicle roof) at their margin. Scarring after healing is not significant in oral lesions.

Histopathology

There is separation of the full thickness of the epithelium from the underlying connective tissue to form subepithelial bullae (Fig. 1.20). There is a variable inflammatory infiltrate in the corium but this becomes more intense and acute in character after the bullae rupture. Non-specific ulceration is then produced but the diagnosis may be suggested by subepithelial oedema and early separation of the epithelium along the line of the basement membrane in the perilesional tissue. However, it is important to distinguish the latter appearance from artefactual epithelial detachment.

Since the histological appearances may be inadequate for firm diagnosis, immunological studies are particularly important. However, only a minority of patients have circulating autoantibodies and immunofluorescence studies are less frequently positive than in pemphigus vulgaris. Nevertheless, in most cases, there is linear deposition of C3 along the line of the basement membrane (Fig. 1.21), while in about 40% of patients immunoglobulin,

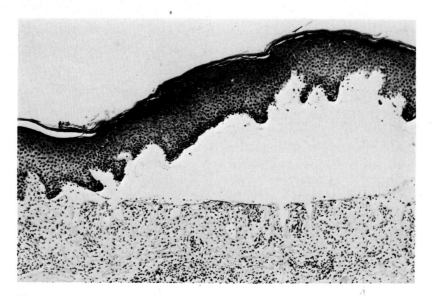

Fig. 1.20 Mucous membrane pemphigoid. Separation of the full thickness of the epithelium from the underlying connective tissue with the formation of a thick-roofed vesicle is characteristic.

Haematoxylin-eosin   × 40

Darier's disease and warty dyskeratoma (isolated dyskeratosis follicularis)

Darier's disease is characterized microscopically by acantholytic lesions producing suprabasal clefts in the epithelium. It is usually hereditary. Warty dyskeratoma appears to be unrelated to Darier's disease but produces lesions which are histologically closely similar. Lesions of Darier's disease and warty dyskeratoma can occasionally affect the mouth.[95-97]

Clinically, oral lesions of Darier's disease and warty dyskeratoma consist of white plaques, sometimes with a corrugated surface. They are typically asymptomatic.

The epithelium is hyperkeratotic with a crater-like depressed central area filled with keratin. There is intra-epithelial vesiculation in the form

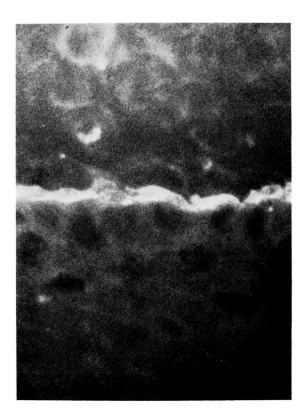

Fig. 1.21 Mucous membrane pemphigoid. Direct immunofluorescence frequently shows deposition of C3; immunoglobulins are found infrequently.

Fluorescein isothiocyanate ×550

particularly IgG, is detectable there.[94] There is no association with other autoimmune diseases.

'Desquamative gingivitis'

Desquamative gingivitis is a clinical term used in dentistry for lesions produced by mucous membrane pemphigoid or atrophic lichen planus, both of which frequently affect the gingivae, or by pemphigus vulgaris, which rarely involves this site. The term has no histopathological significance. In the past, desquamative gingivitis was thought to be the result of hormonal disturbances associated with the menopause. There is no evidence that this is the case, but women at or near menopausal age happen to be the group most frequently affected by oral lichen planus or mucous membrane pemphigoid.

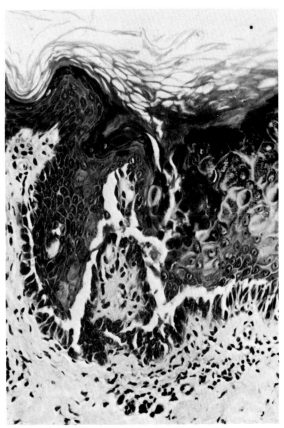

Fig. 1.22 Warty dyskeratoma. There is hyperkeratosis with intra-epithelial, suprabasal clefting and dyskeratotic cells superficially.

Haematoxylin-eosin ×250

of suprabasal clefting with villous proliferation from the floor (Fig. 1.22). Within the prickle-cell layer may be seen large rounded dyskeratotic cells (corps ronds) with a pyknotic nucleus and peripheral halo. Hyaline bodies (grains) may be seen in the keratin layer. Corps ronds, and particularly hyaline bodies, seem to be seen less often in oral than in cutaneous lesions. Distinction from early oral manifestations of pemphigus vulgaris may therefore be difficult. It is essential, therefore, to carry out immunofluorescence studies to exclude the intercellular deposition of immunoglobulin and complement which is characteristic of the affected epithelium of pemphigus vulgaris.

Bullous erythema multiforme

Only the bullous form of erythema multiforme is likely to affect the oral mucosa, which is the most commonly and often the only affected site. In such cases there may be doubts about the diagnosis but the clinical picture is often distinctive and the microscopic findings can be helpful. The diagnosis may also be confirmed by the development of typical generalized Stevens–Johnson syndrome in a later attack.

The aetiology of erythema multiforme is unknown but the fact that it may follow infections (particularly herpetic or mycoplasmal) or use of drugs (particularly sulphonamides) has led many to believe that it is immunologically mediated. In addition, leakage of immune components has been shown microscopically by immunofluorescence.[98] Nevertheless, in the great majority of cases no precipitating factor is evident and despite the immunofluorescence findings, vasculitis is not evident microscopically.

Young males are mainly affected and the most consistent feature is severe swelling, bleeding and crusting of the lips associated with widespread, ill-defined oral erosions. In addition, there may be conjunctivitis or vesiculation, genital ulceration, bullous or other rashes and rarely renal involvement.

Histopathology

Microscopically, the oral epithelium often shows severe eosinophilic colloid changes or vacuolation in its superficial layers (Fig. 1.23a), though this is not specific. Rarely, intra- or subepithelial vesiculation (Fig. 1.23b) may be seen and there is necrosis of keratinocytes. There is a scattered, predominantly mononuclear cellular infiltrate in the corium which in some cases shows a striking perivascular distribution. All accounts of the histopathology,[99–101] however, agree on the absence of true vasculitis.

Dermatitis herpetiformis

Oral lesions are present in dermatitis herpetiformis in an unknown proportion of patients. Reported estimates have ranged from zero to 70%[102,103]— possibly because oral lesions can be asymptomatic. These oral lesions can be highly variable in appearance ranging from erythematous or purpuric areas to vesicular lesions and erosions.

Histopathology

The characteristic feature is the accumulation of granulocytes at the tips of the papillary corium. Neutrophils are predominant at first, but with the formation of micro-abscesses eosinophils become prominent. Rupture of micro-abscesses leaves erosions which are likely to lack any distinctive features, but papillary micro-abscesses may be present in adjacent intact mucosa.

Pyostomatitis vegetans

Pyostomatitis vegetans is a rare mucocutaneous disorder originally described by Hallopeau in 1898 as *pyodermite végétante*, among the features of which were oral lesions. Pyostomatitis vegetans is typically associated with ulcerative colitis.[104]

Macroscopic features

Pyostomatitis vegetans produces, most characteristically, soft hyperplastic mucosal folds with minute superficial miliary abscesses and erosions. In addition to the fissuring between the mucosal folds some patients may have multiple yellow pustules.

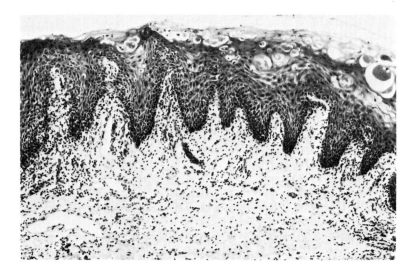 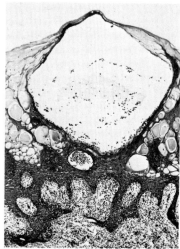

Fig. 1.23a, b Bullous erythema multiforme. (**a**) Biopsy frequently shows this pattern of eosinophilic colloid change in the superficial epithelium. Inflammatory cells both infiltrate the epithelium and are also scattered widely and deeply in the underlying connective tissue, often with perivascular concentrations. (**b**) Very occasionally an intact intra-epithelial vesicle can be seen in association with the more frequently found eosinophilic colloid change in the surrounding superficial epithelium.

Haematoxylin-eosin   (**a**) ×120; (**b**) ×50

Histopathology

The main feature is the presence of multiple miliary intra-epithelial and/or subepithelial abscesses containing many eosinophils (Fig. 1.24). A dense inflammatory infiltrate of similar character also fills the corium. The epithelium is acanthotic with blunt-tipped downgrowths. In addition to micro-abscesses at the tips of the papillary corium or within the epithelium, the latter may be diffusely infiltrated with leukocytes among which eosinophils predominate.[104]

In differentiating these lesions from those of pemphigus vegetans it should be noted that acantholysis is absent in pyostomatitis vegetans, which also lacks the characteristic immunofluorescence pattern of pemphigus.

Reiter's syndrome

Oral lesions may be present in 30%[105] of cases but are typically transient and asymptomatic.

The characteristic clinical appearance is that of red areas with slightly raised, white circinate borders resembling those of migratory glossitis. Exactly similar lesions may be seen on the penis.

Microscopically, the lesions have been reported to be closely similar to those of psoriasis.[106]

Migratory glossitis (erythema migrans linguae, geographical tongue)

Migratory glossitis is probably a minor developmental anomaly. It is found in a high proportion of infants and its appearance in several generations in a family has been described. In most cases, however, no complaint is made until middle age.

One form of migratory glossitis is that of irregular, partially depapillated, red areas with white intervening areas produced by thickening of the filiform papillae. The other consists of red areas with slightly raised, white circinate or scalloped borders. The most characteristic feature is the way in which the pattern changes from day to day.

Microscopically, there is thickening of the keratin layer of the filiform papillae at the periphery of the patches while, centrally, there is relative atrophy of the papillae with migration of neutrophils and inflammatory exudate into the epithelium to produce a psoriasiform appearance. There is also a mixed inflammatory infiltrate in the corium.

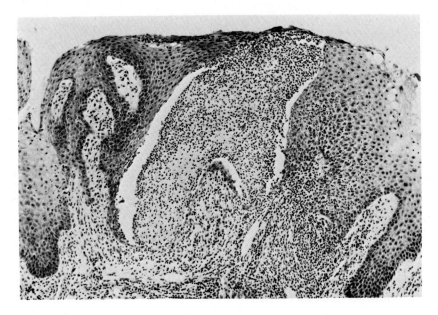

Fig. 1.24 Pyostomatitis vegetans. Intra-epithelial abscess formation, typically with many eosinophils, but absence of acantholysis is characteristic.

Haematoxylin-eosin   × 110

Median rhomboid glossitis

Median rhomboid glossitis has been traditionally regarded as a developmental anomaly produced by failure of submergence of the tuberculum impar. Some credence to this developmental theory is given by the site and symmetry of the lesion. It is typically lozenge-shaped and situated in the midline of the tongue at the junction of the anterior two-thirds with the posterior third. The appearances are otherwise variable and the lesion may simply consist of a red area of depapillation, a white patch, or it may be of normal colour but nodular.

Microscopically, the appearances are also variable but many show chronic candidal infection with the typical microscopic appearances that this produces (see p. 10). Otherwise there is usually loss of filiform papillae and a highly irregular pattern of acanthosis. The corium is typically very vascular and contains an inflammatory infiltrate.

Perhaps most important is the fact that some of the appearances of median rhomboid glossitis have in the past been mistaken histologically for squamous cell carcinoma. In some of these cases there was a granular cell myoblastoma with typical pseudo-epitheliomatous hyperplasia. The midline of the dorsum of the tongue is, however, virtually never the site of cancer and this diagnosis should not be made without the utmost care being taken to be certain of the facts.

Lupus erythematosus

Oral ulceration can be a feature of both discoid and systemic disease. In the latter it is present in 20% of patients and is now one of the American Rheumatism Council's criteria of diagnosis.[107]

Macroscopic appearances

The lesions slightly resemble lichen planus in that there is typically ulceration with a tendency to formation of white striae. In lupus erythematosus, however, the striae are far less well defined and tend to form a relatively faint pattern radiating from the periphery of ulcers. The latter also tend to appear indented. In other patients there is hyperkeratotic plaque formation without ulceration.

In systemic lupus the oral lesions usually consist of shallow erosions, sometimes linear ulceration along the gingival margin and superficial keratosis. Such lesions are occasionally among the earliest signs.

Histopathology

Microscopically, discoid and systemic lupus erythematosus cannot be distinguished except by immunofluorescence or (the rarely seen) vasculitis in the deeper zones.

Characteristic features, however, are as follows:[108-111]

1. Acanthosis and atrophy of the epithelium. Acanthosis is typically grossly irregular and may have an unusual flame-like profile or it may extend in long slender strands deeply into the corium. Occasionally pseudo-epitheliomatous hyperplasia is produced (Fig. 1.25). Elsewhere the epithelium is thin or ulcerated
2. Keratotic plugging (Fig. 1.26). This is unusual but may be conspicuous. In addition, there may be deep cell keratinization which may simulate cell nest formation but for the lack of epithelial atypia
3. Liquefaction degeneration of the basal cell layer

4. Variable thickening of the basement membrane with deposition of immunoglobulins
5. Hyalinization of the superficial zones of the connective tissue of the corium
6. A widely scattered inflammatory infiltrate of mononuclear cells which can extend remarkably deeply but is often attenuated.

Direct immunofluorescence should show deposition, in a band-like pattern and with a granular texture, of immunoglobulins and complement components along the basement membrane. Such changes are detectable only in the lesions of discoid lupus erythematosus but in systemic disease are also detectable in clinically normal epithelia. The role of immune complexes in the production of mucocutaneous lesions is therefore difficult to reconcile with these findings.

In some cases, however, there can be close resemblance to lichen planus and some believe that intermediate forms exist. There is no evidence otherwise that this is the case and such 'intermediate' forms are probably no more than an expression of the limited repertoire of microscopically visible changes possible in this tissue.

In systemic lupus erythematosus particularly, a firm diagnosis may not be possible on the basis of

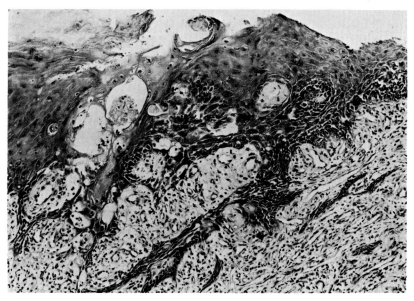

Fig. 1.25 Discoid lupus erythematosus. The irregularity of the epithelial proliferation is in extreme form here. The widely scattered inflammatory infiltrate is, however, typical.

Haematoxylin-eosin   × 180

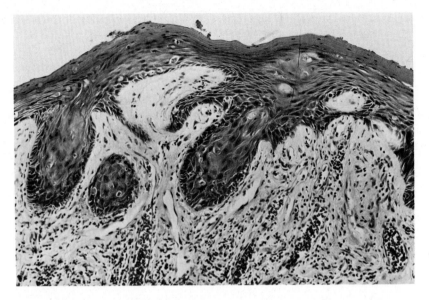

Fig. 1.26 Lupus erythematosus. There is keratotic plugging and the characteristic hyalinization of the subepithelial corium.

Haematoxylin-eosin   × 180

an oral biopsy alone. Account must therefore be taken of lesions in other systems and the immunological findings.

Systemic sclerosis

Systemic sclerosis can affect the oral tissues but usually less severely than the skin, and oral involvement is unlikely to be an early or major feature of the disease. In addition to limitation of opening of the mouth caused by fibrosis of the lips and facial skin, the tongue and, less conspicuously, the buccal mucosa can become fibrotic and stiff.

Microscopically, there is thickening of the connective tissues and hyalinization of the collagen of the corium. The epithelium may be thinned and there is atrophy of the underlying muscle, particularly evident in the tongue where muscle fibres normally extend into the corium.

In fewer than 10% of patients there is widening of the periodontal ligament space in radiographs.

Oral submucous fibrosis

This disease is histologically similar to systemic sclerosis but differs in the following respects:

1. Virtually only those from the Indian subcontinent are affected
2. The oral changes are more severe than those in systemic sclerosis but the skin is not involved
3. There is sometimes dysplasia associated with the epithelial atrophy and there is probably a significant risk of carcinomatous change[112]
4. There are no associated immunological abnormalities.

Clinically, the buccal mucosa, inner aspects of the lips and soft palate are most commonly affected. The fibrotic areas become strikingly blanched and so hard as not to be indentable with the finger. Fibrous contracture of the cheeks can become so severe that the mouth cannot be opened and tube-feeding becomes necessary. The overlying epithelium may appear normal or there may be blistering and ulceration.

Microscopically, there is epithelial atrophy, sometimes with dysplasia. The characteristic feature is, however, thickening and hyalinization of the collagen of the corium with atrophy of underlying muscle (Fig. 1.27). There is typically a patchy mononuclear cell infiltrate irregularly scattered in the hyperplastic connective tissue.[113–115]

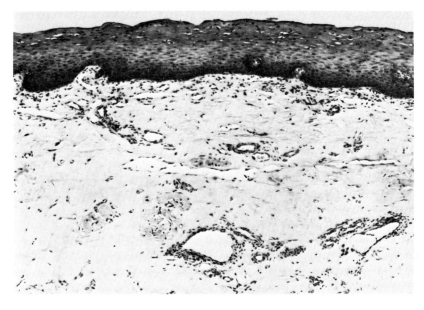

Fig. 1.27 Oral submucous fibrosis. The epithelium of the buccal mucosa has become thin and flattened. Underlying it there is dense hyaline fibrous tissue containing the remnants of degenerating muscle fibres.

Haematoxylin-eosin   × 140

Solar (actinic) elastosis

Solar elastosis can be seen in the lips, particularly in the elderly but also in young, fair-complexioned persons exposed to tropical sunlight.

The condition is important as lip cancer may be a later sequel.

Microscopically, there is patchy basophilic change in the collagen of the corium. The collagen also tends to lose its fibrous character and becomes more homogeneous in appearance. Positive staining for elastin is increased and the postively staining material is sometimes referred to as cholastin.

CHRONIC ORAL KERATOSES AND LEUKOPLAKIA

Keratinization of any great degree is abnormal in the mouth and since the keratin becomes sodden in this site, it appears white. Leukoplakia means, of course, no more than a white plaque but since, in the past, it was widely believed that most such lesions were premalignant, the term 'leukoplakia' should be used with circumspection. Since this term also often leads to quite unjustifiable assump-

tions as to the underlying histopathology, a World Health Organization committee has defined leukoplakia as 'a white patch or plaque which cannot be characterized clinically or pathologically as any other condition'.

As to the risk of malignant change, keratosis *per se* is of no significance except in so far as a minority of oral keratotic lesions also show epithelial dysplasia. Thus a minority of white lesions can undergo malignant change but this is not to say that all leukoplakias are premalignant or that all premalignant lesions are white; indeed, erythroplastic lesions more frequently show dysplasia than white lesions, as discussed later. There is also no evidence that the majority of cancers are preceded by detectable premalignant change and probably only a few develop in patches of leukoplakia.

Once dysplasia appears in an oral lesion, prognostication is as difficult as in any other site, but it appears that in the mouth milder degrees of dysplasia than are seen in the uterine cervix are of more serious significance and the gross top-to-bottom changes seen in the latter are rare in oral lesions. Malignant change, therefore, not infrequently develops in oral lesions showing (in so far as it can be quantified) no more than moderately severe dysplasia. Moreover, once cancer develops in such a lesion the 5-year survival rate (approximately 40%) is significantly lower than in the case of cervical cancer (approximately 55%).

Idiopathic leukoplakia and premalignant change

For the majority of persistent white plaques, no aetiological factor can be identified. The histopathology is also highly variable, ranging from simple hyperkeratosis and hyperplasia to severe dysplasia.

The most extensive studies on leukoplakia so far carried out, however, suggest[116] that this idiopathic group has a higher risk of developing cancer than the other types described. In most lesions of definable cause the risk of malignant change is very low, especially now that late stage syphilis forms a negligibly small group.

Though there is no doubt about the potentialities of leukoplakias to undergo malignant change[113-115], the level of risk cannot be accurately assessed from the histopathology. One of the largest single studies was carried out in Sweden and based on no fewer than 782 cases of histologically unspecified oral white lesions followed for an average of 12 years;[116] of these only 2.4% underwent malignant change in 10 years and less than 5% after 20 years. Even this low rate, however, represents a risk of malignant change 50–100 times that in the normal mouth. It may be noted incidentally that, in this very large study, the rate of malignant change in oral leuokoplakias was 10 times higher in non-smokers than in smokers. Illustrative of the difficulties in quantifying the risk of malignant change and hence of assessing the prognosis in oral white lesions, however, is a recent report of 257 patients who had been followed for an average of 8 years, where Silverman and his colleagues[117] found a transformation rate of no less than 17.5%. Again, malignant change was more frequent among non-smokers. Silverman had, however, reported earlier rates of 0.12% in India and of 6% in the USA. Other, smaller, series have suggested transformation rates of 30% or more, though in many cases no time scale has been indicated.

It should perhaps be emphasized that these large-scale studies have been on histologically unspecified oral keratoses. Because of the relative rarity of dysplastic oral lesions there are very few studies, and none on a large scale, that have followed their progress for adequate periods. In one such study,[118] 45 patients with oral lesions showing dysplasia were followed for up to eight years. Only 11% underwent malignant change in this period. Much less is therefore known about the behaviour of dysplastic oral lesions than those of similar histological appearance of the uterine cervix, simply because the latter are far more common. The incidence of cervical carcinoma is 10 times greater than that of mouth cancer and only a minority of cases of the latter appear to go through a recognizable premalignant phase.

These difficulties are further increased by the fact that some 30% of dysplastic lesions in both the mouth and cervix can regress or even ultimately disappear spontaneously. It must be emphasized, therefore, that the assessment of dysplasia is essentially subjective and it is not possible to prognosticate solely on the basis of the histopathological changes. An additional problem is that there is no satisfactory way of sampling such lesions. If part is taken for biopsy purposes there is no certainty that it is representative of the whole.[119]

Macroscopic features

Idiopathic leukoplakias and dysplastic lesions do not have any specific clinical appearance. Small and innocent-looking white patches are as likely to show epithelial dysplasia as large and irregular ones.

Histological features

The epithelium may or may not be hyperplastic and is often thinner than normal. The surface usually shows keratosis (though this may be slight), usually in the form of parakeratosis.

A plaque may show both hyperortho- and parakeratosis in different parts and the two may alternate along the length of the specimen. A chronic inflammatory cellular infiltrate of highly variable intensity is usually present in the corium. In addition, the epithelium itself may show any of the cytological changes of dysplasia (Fig. 1.28).

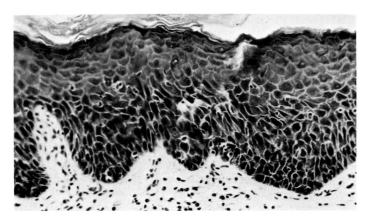

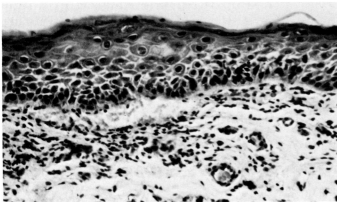

Fig. 1.28a, b Oral leukoplakia. (**a**) There is only mild hyperkeratosis but obvious dysplasia. (**b**) The epithelium is atrophic, with a tendency of the epithelial cells to separate, and well-marked dysplasia. The patient subsequently developed several carcinomas.

Haematoxylin-eosin   × 180

'Carcinoma-in-situ'

Carcinoma-in-situ is a controversial term used for dysplasia where the abnormalities extend throughout the thickness of the epithelium; a state sometimes graphically called 'top-to-bottom change'. All the cellular abnormalities characteristic of malignancy may be present; only invasion of the underlying connective tissue is absent.

Top-to-bottom dysplasia is rarely seen in the mouth and, like other dysplastic lesions, has no absolutely characteristic clinical appearance. Erythroplasia, however, as discussed below, often proves to be 'carcinoma-in-situ' or early invasive carcinoma.

Erythroplasia (erythroplakia)

In contrast to the foregoing lesions, erythroplasias are red. The surface is usually also velvety in texture and the margin may be sharply defined. Lesions of this type typically do not form plaques and the surface is often depressed below the level of the surrounding mucosa. Erythroplasia is uncommon in the mouth.

Histopathology

Erythroplastic lesions frequently show dysplastic epithelial changes which are often severe. In other cases there may be micro-invasive or frankly invasive carcinoma.

Speckled leukoplakia is the term that has been given to lesions consisting of white flecks or nodules on an atrophic erythematous base. It can be regarded as a combination of leukoplakia and erythroplasia and it has been shown that speckled leukoplakia more frequently shows dysplasia than the more homogeneous-looking lesions. The histological characteristics are usually therefore intermediate between leukoplakia and erythroplasia.

Many cases of chronic candidosis have this appearance.

Other types or causes of persistent white plaques

These are as follows:

1. White sponge naevus
2. Frictional keratosis
3. Smoker's keratosis
4. Syphilis (tertiary)
5. Chronic candidosis
6. Lichen planus
7. Sublingual keratosis
8. Dyskeratosis congenita
9. Psoriasis
10. Pachyonychia congenita
11. Oral keratosis of renal failure
12. Early carcinoma.

White sponge naevus

White sponge naevus is a developmental anomaly inherited as an autosomal dominant.[120] The appearance is characteristic in that virtually the whole of the oral mucosa can be affected by white, soft and irregular thickening.[121] Part of the irregularity of the surface is caused by patients chewing off protruding tags and where this happens a thinner white layer of parakeratin is exposed.

Unlike other white lesions, the edges merge imperceptibly with the normal mucosa without well-defined borders. The anus and vagina can also be affected.

Histopathology

The epithelium is hyperplastic, showing uniform acanthosis with the ridges having a regular outline. The macroscopic white appearance of the lesion is produced by gross hyperparakeratosis and intracellular oedema, which also makes the cell membranes abnormally prominent and produces a so-called basket-weave appearance (Fig. 1.29). There is no dysplasia and inflammatory infiltration in the corium is typically also absent.

Frictional keratosis

This is caused by continued abrasion of the mucous membrane by such irritants as a sharp tooth, cheek biting or, in elderly patients, prolonged denture wearing.

In their early stages these lesions are pale and translucent rather than white, but later become dense and white, sometimes with a rough surface. Cheek biting, a nervous habit, causes a lesion with

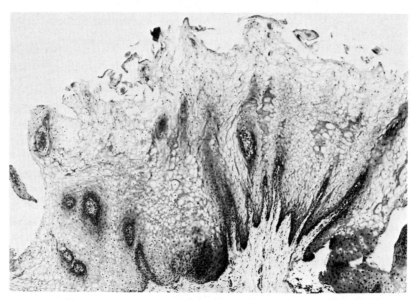

Fig. 1.29 White sponge naevus. The epithelium is irregularly hyperplastic with gross and widespread intra-epithelial oedema of the spinous cells.

Haematoxylin-eosin   × 50

a more uneven surface, patchily red and white in colour.

Histopathology

Biopsy usually shows a moderately hyperplastic epithelium with a prominent granular cell layer and thick keratin on the surface. There is often a scattered infiltrate of chronic inflammatory cells in the corium.

Removal of the source of friction causes the patch quickly to disappear and this confirms the diagnosis. True frictional keratosis is completely benign and there is no evidence that continued minor trauma of this sort alone has any carcinogenic effect.

Smoker's keratosis ('stomatitis nicotina')

Smoker's keratosis is only seen in Britain among heavy, long-term pipe smokers and is therefore only seen in men. The appearances are characteristic in that the palate is affected but any part covered by a denture is spared. In a full denture wearer, therefore, only the soft palate is affected. The lesion has two components, namely hyperkeratosis and inflammatory swelling of minor mucous glands; either component may predominate but a characteristic appearance is white thickening of the palatal mucosa in which there are small umbilicated swellings with a red centre.

Histopathology

The microscopic features of the white areas are not specific but show hyperorthokeratosis and acanthosis with a variable inflammatory infiltrate in the corium. The diagnostic feature is the inflamed mucous glands with hyperkeratosis extending up to the duct orifice and producing, as a result of the inflammatory swelling, a volcano-in-miniature appearance (Fig. 1.30).

However, the clinical appearances in association with the history are so distinctive that biopsy should not be necessary and malignant change does not develop in the keratotic area.

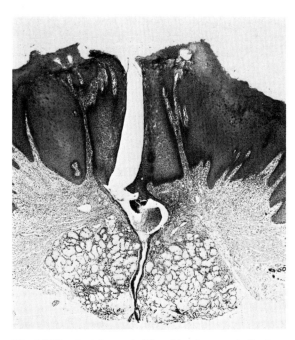

Fig. 1.30 Smoker's keratosis. The white plaque typically shows unremarkable hyperkeratosis but inflammation of the subepithelial minor salivary glands and hyperplasia of the periductal epithelium produces the typical umbilicated palatal swellings.

Haematoxylin-eosin × 30

Syphilis (tertiary)

Keratosis of the dorsum of the tongue is one of the characteristic changes that may be seen in tertiary syphilis. It is of little more than historical interest now.

Histopathology

In addition to the hyperkeratosis and acanthosis often present in dysplasia, the characteristic changes of the late syphilitic granuloma may be seen in the connective tissue with a chronic inflammatory cellular infiltrate mainly, of plasma cells. Giant cells and, rarely, more or less well-formed, tubercle-like granulomas may be seen. Endarteritis of the small arteries is particularly characteristic. One or more foci of malignant change may be found in the epithelium. However, distinctive features of the syphilitic inflammatory reaction may be lacking.

Antibiotic treatment of syphilis does not cure

the keratosis, which persists and may undergo malignant change despite normal serology. Syphilitic keratosis is usually regarded as having a high risk of malignant change. Carcinoma developing at or near the centre of the dorsum of the tongue is virtually always related to syphilitic keratosis and, as a consequence of the great decline in late-stage syphilis in recent years, is exceedingly rare now.

Chronic candidosis (candidal) leukoplakia

Candidal infection of mucocutaneous surfaces typically provokes epithelial proliferation and plaque formation. Plaques caused by chronic candidosis are distinguishable from other keratoses by their microscopic features, as discussed earlier.

Lichen planus

Lichen planus occasionally causes plaque-like lesions, particularly on the dorsum of the tongue. These plaques may be thick, are characteristically snowy-white and may have ill-defined margins with a fluffy or cotton wool-like appearance. The microscopic features have been discussed earlier.

Sublingual keratosis

An irregular, but frequently symmetrical, white soft plaque with a wrinkled surface and an irregular but well-defined margin may appear in the sublingual region. The plaque typically extends from the anterior floor of the mouth to the undersurface of the tongue and may have a roughly butterfly shape. There are usually no associated inflammatory changes.

Sublingual keratosis was at one time thought to be a naevus but the clinical appearance alone readily enables sublingual keratosis to be distinguished from true white sponge naevus.

Histologically, sublingual keratosis is not distinctive but the frequency of dysplasia or malignant change has been reported to be exceptionally high and may be as great as 15%.[122,123]

Dyskeratosis congenita

Dyskeratosis congenita is a rare syndrome which may be inherited as a recessive or dominant trait characterized by dysplastic lesions of the oral mucosa, dermal pigmentation, dystrophies of the nails and, occasionally, aplastic anaemia.[124]

Oral lesions typically consist of white patches or of inconspicuous erythematous areas. The cutaneous pigmentation is greyish-brown and predominantly affects the trunk. The nails may become dystrophic early and be completely destroyed before adolescence. There may also be alopecia. Aplastic anaemia is rare but can be a cause of early death.

Histopathology

However innocent the oral lesions may appear macroscopically and however slight the symptoms, typically there is severe dysplasia and the risk of carcinomatous change is high. Multiple oral carcinoma formation can therefore result and the expectation of life is poor. Close observation and further biopsies should be prompted by the slightest symptoms to enable each tumour to be treated as early as possible.

Fanconi's anaemia is also associated with oral cancer but, unlike dyskeratosis congenita, there is a characteristic chromosomal anomaly.[124]

Psoriasis

Though psoriasis is a common skin disease, estimated to affect 2% of the population, and can affect the mouth, it is nevertheless, for unknown reasons, a rarity in this site.

Oral psoriatic lesions are most often associated with severe pustular psoriasis[125] and only occasionally with psoriasis vulgaris.

The macroscopic appearance of the oral lesions is variable. Whitish translucent plaques or circinate lesions resembling migratory glossitis may form but macules, diffuse erythema and pustules have also been reported. Oral lesions are frequently asymptomatic and it may be, therefore, that they are more common than is generally believed.[126]

Histopathology

Oral lesions can sometimes closely resemble the dermal lesions with parakeratosis, superficial spongiosis and an inflammatory infiltrate which can form Monro abscesses. There may also be the characteristic, but unusual, pattern of acanthosis with long, slender, square-tipped epithelial downgrowths (Fig. 1.31). The inflammatory infiltrate in the corium is sparse.[127]

Several oral mucosal lesions can have a psoriasiform appearance in some respects. The main examples are chronic candidosis, migratory glossitis and Reiter's syndrome. The diagnosis of oral psoriasis should not therefore be made unless most of the characteristic microscopic features can be seen (as described above) and the patient has undoubted cutaneous psoriasis.

Pachyonychia congenita

Pachyonychia congenita is an uncommon congenital disorder characterized by hypertrophy of the

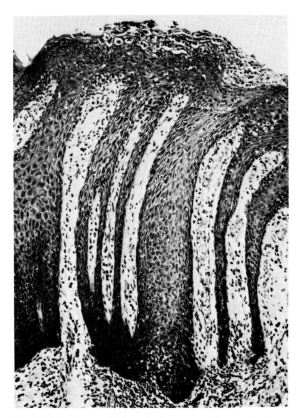

Fig. 1.31 Oral psoriasis. In typical cases, usually associated with pustular psoriasis, epithelial plaques show superficial spongiosis and abscess formation together with this somewhat unusual pattern of acanthosis with long, slender, square-tipped epithelial downgrowths.

Haematoxylin-eosin   × 100

nail bed, skin lesions (particularly hyperkeratosis of the palms and soles) and oral white lesions. Premature eruption producing natal teeth has also been reported.

The oral lesions typically comprise limited areas of soft white thickening of the epithelium of the tongue, gingivae or buccal mucosa. Microscopically, these plaques show acanthosis and parakeratosis with widespread intracellular vacuolization (Fig. 1.32)—an appearance similar to that of white sponge naevus.[128,129] The latter, however, produces considerably more gross and widespread white thickening of the oral mucosa and lacks ungual or cutaneous abnormalities.

Oral keratosis of renal failure

The development of oral white plaques is an occasional and unexplained complication of long-standing renal failure.[130,131]

The plaques are soft, have a crenated surface and are typically symmetrically distributed. With restoration of normal renal function by means of effective dialysis or renal transplantation the lesion clears spontaneously.

Histopathology

The features do not appear to be sufficiently distinctive to enable a diagnosis to be made without knowledge of the underlying disease; there is irregular acanthosis with mild atypia of the epithelial cells and moderate parakeratosis (Fig. 1.33). However, biopsy may be useful to distinguish these lesions from other adherent white plaques which may also develop in patients with renal failure but which are bacterial in nature.

Early squamous cell carcinoma

Occasionally carcinomas produce sufficient surface keratin in their early stages to appear as white plaques. These are always small lesions (5–7 mm across), since further progress produces a mass or ulcer more typical of these tumours.

MUCOSAL PIGMENTATION

Pigmentation of the oral mucosa has various causes.

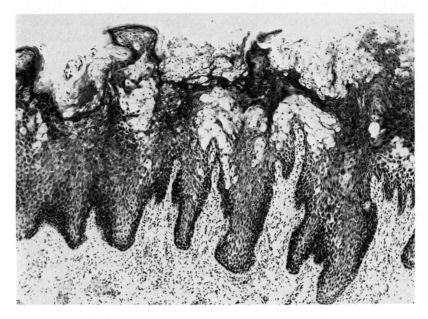

Fig. 1.32 Pachyonychia congenita. There is acanthosis and parakeratosis with intracellular vacuolization but of a lesser degree than that seen in white sponge naevus.

Haematoxylin-eosin ×60

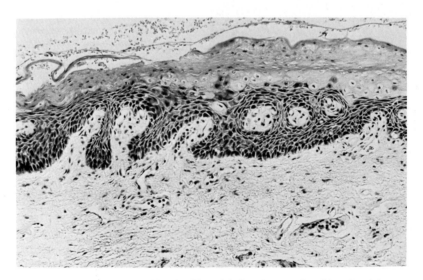

Fig. 1.33 Oral keratosis of renal failure. The epithelium is somewhat thinned and shows a minor degree of atypia. There is superficial plaque with a minor degree of spongiosis and no inflammatory infiltrate in the corium. Other areas were considerably more hyperplastic but the lesion disappeared after renal function was re-established by dialysis.

Haematoxylin-eosin ×140

Provided by Professor Bertram Cohen.

Endogenous pigmentation

Melanin is often normally present in the mucosa of the mouth in dark-skinned people. It is also present, although less frequently, in light-skinned people.

Pathological endogenous pigmentation may be seen in neurofibromatosis, fibrous dysplasia, Addison's disease, haemochromatosis and other conditions. In the Peutz-Jeghers syndrome freckle-like pigmentation affects the circumoral skin as well as the oral mucosa and is associated with the characteristic intestinal polyposis.

Exogenous pigmentation

Exogenous pigmentation is caused by various inorganic and organic chemical substances. The best known are lead and bismuth. The 'lead line', due to the deposition of lead sulphide, appears as a bluish-black discoloration along the gingival margin. The gums are not inflamed. Bismuth may be deposited in the gingivae as a dark-blue line, similar to that produced by lead, but accompanied by pronounced gingivitis.

Swelling, redness and bleeding of the gingivae, loosening of the teeth and ultimately necrosis and sloughing are seen in mercurial poisoning, in which mercury is present in the saliva, secretion of which is much increased (ptyalism).

Amalgam tattoos

Fragments of mercury amalgam sometimes become embedded in the oral mucosa during the filling of teeth and produce a bluish patch which can be mistaken for a melanoma.

Histologically, amalgam tattoos show the amalgam as black material within the connective tissue, generally unassociated with inflammatory or other reactive changes. A foreign-body reaction is only rarely seen.

'Black hairy tongue'

In this condition the filiform papillae are elongated and become yellow, brown or black. There appears to be a variety of causes, including smoking, the use of oxidizing agents, and changes in the oral microbial flora as a result of antibiotic therapy.

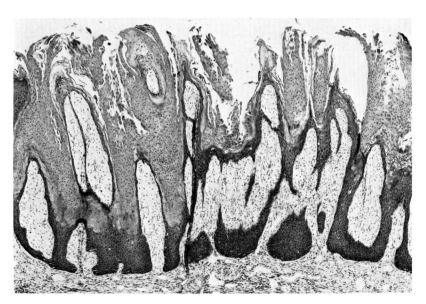

Fig. 1.34 Verruciform xanthoma. The surface of the epithelium shows the characteristic verrucous outline and there is sharp demarcation of the parakeratin layer from the immediately underlying spinous cells. Between the folds of the epithelium there are foamy cells.

Haematoxylin-eosin   × 50

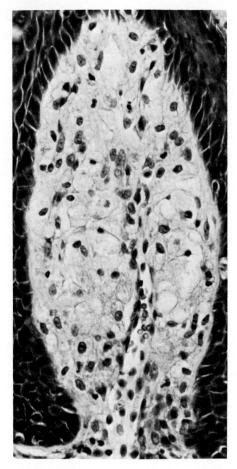

Fig. 1.35 Verruciform xanthoma. The characteristic foam cells fill the papillary corium.

Haematoxylin-eosin   × 350

Often no cause can be found. The condition is harmless.

Verruciform xanthoma

Verruciform xanthoma is a rare oral lesion with a distinctive histopathological appearance.

Adults over 50 are predominantly affected and the most common site is the gingiva. The clinical appearances are very variable and descriptions range from 'white and warty' to 'red and ulcerated'. In some cases these lesions have been mistaken for papillomas.

Histopathology

The surface of the epithelium is verrucous and parakeratinized. This parakeratin is sharply demarcated from the underlying spinous cells but tends to extend deeply into the acanthotic epithelial processes (Fig. 1.34) and to have an unusual orange colour in haematoxylin and eosin preparations.

The papillary corium is filled with large foamy cells (Fig. 1.35), the granules of which stain positively with periodic acid-Schiff and are diastase-resistant. Lipid can also be detected. The foam cells extend only as far as the tips of the elongated rete ridges. The same histopathological findings have rarely also been reported in vulval lesions.

There is no apparent association with the hyperlipidaemias or any other systemic disease.[132–134]

XEROSTOMIA AND SJÖGREN'S SYNDROME

Failure of salivary secretion causes distressing symptoms and also fundamentally impairs oral defences against infection.

The main causes of xerostomia are as follows:

1. Drugs. Drugs with sympathomimetic or anticholinergic activity are responsible and among the most potent in this respect are the tricyclic antidepressants
2. The Sjögren syndromes
3. Radiation damage
4. Dehydration.

Now that care is taken to prevent postoperative dehydration, drugs and the Sjögren syndromes have become more important as causes of severe xerostomia. The effects are accelerated dental caries and periodontal disease, diffuse erythematous candidosis, causing soreness of the mucosa, and the risk of acute ascending parotitis. Among ambulant patients, the Sjögren syndromes are probably now the main predisposing cause of acute parotitis.

Sjögren and sicca syndromes

Sjögren's syndrome comprises dry mouth, dry eyes and rheumatoid arthritis or other connective-tissue disease[135,136] (Table 1.3).

Table 1.3 Estimated frequency of association of diseases with secondary Sjögren's syndrome

Disease	%
Rheumatoid arthritis	30
Raynaud's phenomenon	21
Chronic pulmonary fibrosis	15
Primary biliary cirrhosis	6
Systemic lupus erythematosus	5
Systemic sclerosis	5
Chronic thyroiditis	4
Myopathy	3
Graft-versus-host disease	?

Sicca syndrome differs in the absence of associated connective-tissue disease, in the immunological findings[137] and in the prognosis. Lymphoma can be a complication of either syndrome but particularly of sicca syndrome.

Sicca syndrome is frequently now also termed primary Sjögren's syndrome and Sjögren's syndrome proper is termed secondary Sjögren's syndrome. Quite apart from the obvious rationale for these terms it also happened that Sjögren[138] himself first noted the association between dry mouth and dry eyes and only later found that these were often associated with rheumatoid arthritis.

These syndromes therefore have common features but important differences. They are frequent in that Sjögren's syndrome affects approximately 15% of patients with rheumatoid arthritis, up to 30% of patients with systemic lupus erythematosus, at least 70% of patients with primary biliary cirrhosis[139] and variable numbers of patients with chronic active (lupoid) hepatitis and progressive systemic sclerosis. The prevalence of sicca syndrome is unknown but it appears to be as common as Sjögren's syndrome in otherwise healthy persons and is also a recognized feature of chronic graft-versus-host disease.[140,141]

Immunological aspects

The main findings are summarized in Table 1.4. One curious feature is that though antithyroid autoantibodies are a relatively common finding in these syndromes and, histologically, Sjögren's syndrome is not dissimilar to Hashimoto's thyroiditis, the two are only rarely associated clinically.

Histopathology

The features of fully developed Sjögren's syndrome are those of benign lymphoepithelial lesion (Ch. 3). Earlier changes can be seen in biopsies and for this purpose the lip[142,143] is a convenient site since the changes there correlate well with the parotid lesion. Lip biopsy also lacks the operative hazards of parotid biopsy and there is no risk of persistent fistula formation. Lip biopsy is now an important aid in confirming the diagnosis of graft-versus-host disease.

The earliest changes are mononuclear, predominantly lymphocytic, infiltration and replacement of the acinar tissue starting from the periductal area. The ducts, however, survive but formation of epimyoepithelial islands is uncommon in labial glands. Since these glands are removed entire, it can also be seen that the mononuclear infiltrate is confined by the capsule and perilobular septa.

Labial gland biopsy using a standardized technique and a semi-quantitative estimation of the inflammatory infiltrate has been shown to be one of the more reliable and simple techniques for the diagnosis of Sjögren's syndrome.

In the assessment of these biopsies a grading system may be used but care should be taken to exclude non-specific inflammatory changes, par-

Table 1.4 Typical patterns of circulating autoantibodies in sicca and Sjögren syndromes

Autoantibody	% of patients with autoantibody	
	Sicca syndrome	Sjögren's syndrome
Rheumatoid factor (anti-immunoglobulin G)	50	90
Antinuclear factors	40	55
Antisalivary duct antibodies	10	65
Antibodies to smooth muscle, thyroid antigens, gastric parietal cells, etc.	+ but variable	+ but variable
SS-A*	50	50
SS-B*	50	50

* Widely varying figures reported in different series.

ticularly neutrophil infiltration, mild scattered infiltrates, acinar atrophy and ductal dilatation.

The method of grading[142] is usually by counting the number of foci of 50 or more mononuclear cells per 4 mm^2 of the section as follows:

Grade 0. No infiltrate
Grade 1. Slight infiltrate
Grade 2. Moderate infiltrate—less than one focus per 4 mm^2
Grade 3. One focus per 4 mm^2
Grade 4. More than one focus per 4 mm^2.

Several gland lobules should be assessed since the cellular infiltrate varies from one to another. By using such methods it has been shown that an infiltrate justifying a grade of 2 or 3 by the above criteria correlates with the presence of sicca syndrome, other connective-tissue disease, or both, in about 50% of cases. The correlation is increasingly close as the number of foci increases so that if there are more than five foci per 4 mm^2 the accuracy of diagnosis is over 95%.[144]

Immunopathogenesis

The microscopic appearances are far from informative. Since autoantibodies against acinar components are not a feature of these syndromes it seems unlikely that antibody-mediated cytotoxicity is involved. There are no features indicative of the immune complex (type 3) reactions which appear to play a major role in associated connective tissue diseases. There is also little to suggest a type 4 reaction and indeed cell-mediated immunity tends to be depressed. Antisalivary duct antibodies do not appear to play any role in the immunopathogenesis since their titre does not correlate with the severity of the disease and ductal tissue tends to persist or may even proliferate.

Relation between benign lymphoepithelial lesion and the Sjögren syndromes

The traditional distinction between the Sjögren syndromes and benign lymphoepithelial lesion is that the latter lacks the immunological abnormalities and functional effects of the Sjögren syndromes. However, benign lymphoepithelial lesion is usually noticed as a tumour-like swelling and

treated as such and there appear to have been no adequate immunological studies of patients presenting in this way. Moreover, it is impossible to conceive that the total acinar destruction produced by benign lymphoepithelial lesion does not cause failure of salivary function. It does not appear, therefore, that any fundamental difference between the Sjögren syndromes and benign lymphoepithelial lesion has been convincingly established. However, it is important to establish the diagnosis because of the risk of involvement of the lacrimal glands in the Sjögren syndromes with ensuing damage to sight. Early keratoconjunctivitis sicca is asymptomatic but early treatment with artificial tears can prevent damage to the cornea.

Lymphoma in the Sjögren syndromes

Lymphoma is a recognized complication of long-standing Sjögren's syndrome and is somewhat more common in sicca syndrome. The bulk of evidence, however, suggests that such lymphomas are predominantly extrasalivary.[145] The incidence of such change is estimated to be approximately 5%.

Radiation damage

The most important long-term complications of irradiation of the oral tissues are damage to salivary glands, obliterative endarteritis leading to ischaemia of the bone and the risk of intractable osteomyelitis. In addition there is a risk of radiation-induced tumour formation, particularly sarcoma of the tongue or other sites.

Such hazards have been considerably reduced by appropriate preparation of the patient and by modern radiotherapy techniques. However, salivary tissue is particularly vulnerable and damage is not always avoidable.

Histopathology

The main features are disappearance of salivary acini but relative persistence of ductal tissue, for a time at least, and progressive fibrous replacement. There is usually an associated, light, scattered lymphocytic infiltrate. Typical radiation-induced obliterative endarteritis may be seen in any vessels that remain.

Functional effects. Xerostomia secondary to radiation damage to salivary glands has the effects described earlier. However, the damage to the teeth and their supporting tissues is of special importance since it may make dental extractions necessary and there is then a high risk of precipitating osteomyelitis in the ischaemic jaw.

Intra-oral salivary gland tumours

The same tumours that affect the major glands can affect the minor intra-oral glands. However, the trabecular or canalicular adenoma of the lip (see p. 111) is peculiar to the mouth and in the past has been mistaken for adenoid cystic carcinoma or other malignant tumours. In addition, the proportion of malignant salivary gland tumours within the mouth is significantly higher than in the parotid glands.

OTHER SYSTEMIC DISORDERS WHICH MAY BE RECOGNIZABLE FROM ORAL BIOPSIES

Oral manifestations are uncommon in, or form only a minor feature of the following diseases. However, it is important to know that such manifestations may be the first sign of disease.

1. Acute myelomonocytic leukaemia
2. Amyloidosis
3. Crohn's disease
4. Histiocytosis X
5. Polyarteritis nodosa
6. Sarcoidosis
7. Melkersson Rosenthal syndrome
8. Wegener's and other midline granulomas.

Acute myelomonocytic leukaemia

In adults, acute leukaemia can produce striking gingival changes, namely gross swelling which may progress to necrotizing ulceration as a result of massive infiltration of the gums by leukaemic cells. This is an abnormal reaction to the gingival flora. Usually other features of acute leukaemia such as anaemia or purpura will prompt haematological examination to confirm the diagnosis. In

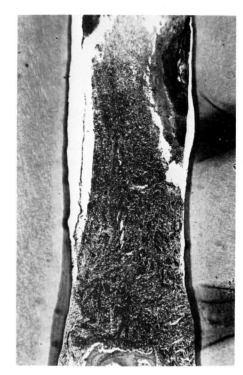

Fig. 1.36 Acute myelomonocytic leukaemia. This is an interdental papilla between two adjacent teeth. The normal structure has been completely destroyed (see Fig. 2.10 for comparison) and is replaced by leukaemic cells which extend down to the alveolar bone.

Haematoxylin-eosin   × 40

the event that a gingival biopsy is taken, however, there is a characteristic microscopic picture with a massive uniform infiltration of the periodontal tissues by leukaemic cells and necrosis of the gingival epithelium (Fig. 1.36). Sharply localized inflammatory infiltrate in simple gingivitis is shown for contrast in later illustrations (Figs 1.54 and 1.55). Similar leukaemic infiltrates can also produce tumour-like oral swellings.

Amyloidosis

Although the gingivae have, in the past, been said to be a good site for biopsy when amyloidosis is suspected, this is only true when there are visible oral lesions. The most striking of these is macroglossia and the tongue is then typically flabby, or firm and pale and may have a nodular border. Gingival lesions consist of small swellings or tags of pale tissue. Histologically, the amyloid is recognizable by standard techniques.

Macroglossia is most often a feature of primary amyloidosis and is also seen in amyloid secondary to myelomatosis.[146,147] Though it is usually a late feature, it can be the earliest physical sign. In such cases the tongue is typically grossly enlarged, pale and firm and indented by the teeth so that the border has a crenated appearance. Oral purpura may be associated.

Crohn's disease

In Crohn's disease oral lesions may closely resemble the intestinal changes, with cobblestone-like proliferation of the oral mucosa (Fig. 1.37), miliary ulceration and typical granuloma formation microscopically[148,149] (Fig. 1.38). These changes may or may not be associated with intestinal involvement. In the case of isolated oral Crohn's type lesions it is controversial whether it is justifiable to use the term 'localized oral Crohn's disease' but intestinal involvement can develop in such patients after a delay, sometimes of several years.

Histiocytosis X, eosinophilic granuloma

Solitary and multifocal eosinophilic granuloma can affect the jaws and oral manifestations can produce early symptoms.[150,151] Though oral soft tissue lesions have been reported, some cases are somewhat suspect in view of possible confusion with the so-called traumatic eosinophilic granuloma described below. Oral lesions include periodontal tissue destruction exposing the roots of the teeth and tumour-like areas of bone destruction. Males are predominantly affected.

Histopathology

The characteristic features are osteolytic lesions containing abundant histiocyte-like cells which often have a reddish tinge with routine staining,

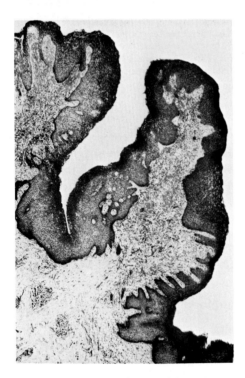

Fig. 1.37 Crohn's disease. Proliferation of the oral mucosa, as here, can produce characteristic ridging or a cobblestone appearance.

Haematoxylin-eosin   × 30

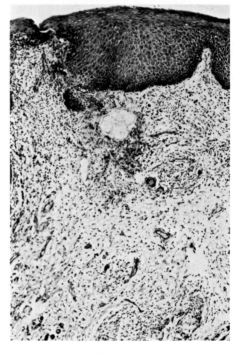

Fig. 1.38 Crohn's disease. Granulomas such as these are typically found irregularly scattered in the submucosal connective tissue or more deeply but are not usually numerous.

Haematoxylin-eosin   × 100

variable but occasionally large numbers of eosino-phils and a poorly fibrillar matrix with a typically granular appearance.

It has been reported that the cellular picture depends on the stage of development. Thus there may be many eosinophils in early lesions, increasing numbers of histiocyte-like cells in more mature lesions (Fig. 1.39) and finally fibrous tissue prolif-eration and diminishing numbers of eosinophils in the later stages. Electron microscopy suggests that the histiocyte-like cells are Langerhans cells since they contain Birbeck granules and also carry the T6 antigen.[152]

Though jaw changes may be the prominent feature, the possibility of involvement of other bones should be excluded by radiography or bone scans. Monostotic lesions have a very good prog-nosis with chemotherapy.

Jaw involvement has been reported as an early feature of multifocal eosinophilic granuloma (Hand-Schüller-Christian disease) but when Let-terer-Siwe disease involves the mouth it seems more likely to affect the soft tissues, particularly the gingivae and, like Hand-Schüller-Christian disease, can cause loosening or exfoliation of the teeth as an early feature. Dental involvement has been reported to be as high as 28% in a large series.

Traumatic eosinophilic granuloma of the tongue

In the mouth, the differential diagnosis of histio-cytosis X is complicated by the existence of what has been termed traumatic eosinophilic granuloma of the tongue. However, these rare lesions have also been reported in the gingiva[153] and the traumatic origin has also been questioned. Never-theless, it is clear that they are not a manifestation of histiocytosis X, not least because they heal spontaneously, usually in less than 10 weeks. The tongue is the most commonly affected site and the typical appearance is a solitary painless swelling which may ulcerate and produce a tumour-like, fungating mass.

Histopathology

The picture is one of a dense aggregation of eosinophils and histiocytes (Fig. 1.40). The latter show no atypia and lack the characteristic electron microscopic features of Langerhans cells. These cells extend into the papillary corium and even infiltrate the epithelium. In the tongue the myo-fibrils are also infiltrated, widely separated and tend to degenerate. This lesion also lacks the amorphous granular matrix so commonly seen in true histiocytosis.[154,155] If ulcerated, there is slough and a mixed inflammatory cellular picture super-ficially.

In order to avoid the unnecessary hazards of excessive treatment it is important to bear in mind the possibility of this condition, especially when the lesion is isolated and affects the tongue.

Polyarteritis nodosa

This disease rarely produces oral lesions,[156,157] but just as subcutaneous nodules form at the sites of vasculitis so, very occasionally, submucosal nod-ules can form in the mouth at an early stage.

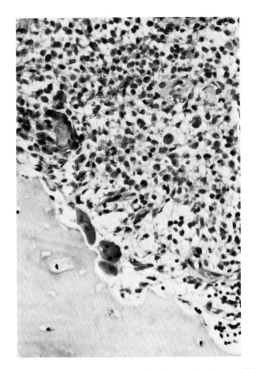

Fig. 1.39 Eosinophilic granuloma. This lesion in the mandible shows many eosinophils and histiocyte-like cells in a finely fibrillar matrix together with bone destruction at the periphery.

Haematoxylin-eosin × 300

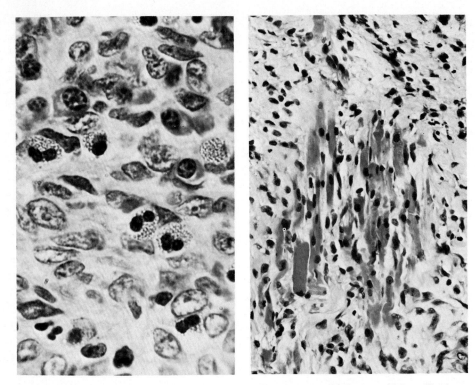

Fig. 1.40a, b 'Traumatic' eosinophilic granuloma. (**a**) There are many histiocytes which, unlike those in eosinophilic granuloma, are normal in appearance but associated with eosinophils. (**b**) Degeneration of muscle fibres both within and peripheral to the main concentration of histiocytes and eosinophils is a frequent finding.

Haematoxylin-eosin   (**a**) ×1300; (**b**) ×300

Damage to the blood vessels can also lead to severe ulceration. The features of biopsy are characteristic (Fig. 1.41). Leakage of immunoglobulins and complement components through the damaged vessel wall can be seen by immunofluorescence microscopy. Such changes are regarded as typical manifestations of immune complex reactions, but the antigen can rarely be identified. An exception is hepatitis B, where vasculitis is a recognized complication and the surface antigen can be identified in the exudate in approximately 30–40% of cases of polyarteritis nodosa.

Sarcoidosis

Sarcoid granulomas may be found in the mouth and can produce gingival[158] or salivary gland swellings[159] in association with pulmonary and other manifestations of sarcoidosis. Oral lesions can also precede systemic manifestations or be found in isolation. The possibility that more widespread sarcoidosis can ultimately develop cannot be excluded but, if this does not happen, it is controversial (having excluded all other possible causes of granuloma formation) whether these lesions are a localized form of sarcoidosis or merely a 'sarcoid-like' reaction. Since the aetiology and pathogenesis of sarcoidosis remain obscure it seems academic to make such a distinction, but from the practical viewpoint all that is necessary is to keep the patient on recall to detect systemic disease if it develops.

Sarcoidosis has a tendency to involve salivary glands and biopsy of minor salivary glands of the lip has been suggested[160] as a simple method of confirming the diagnosis which might reduce the necessity for invasive procedures such as trans-bronchial lung biopsy. Positive results have been reported in a high proportion of patients with systemic disease and this very minor procedure

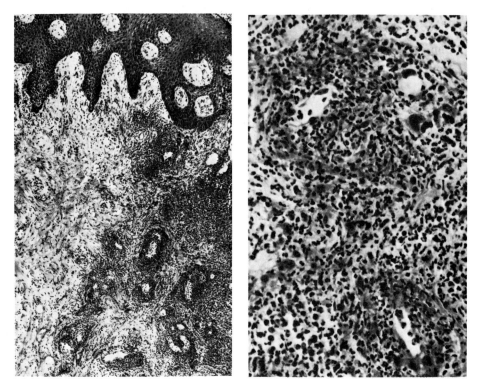

Fig. 1.41a, b Polyarteritis nodosa. (**a**) The necrotizing vasculitis involves many arterioles in the wall of this oral ulcer. (**b**) There is necrotizing arteritis in this submucosal lesion. The normal structure of the arterioles has been destroyed. Their walls are infiltrated with inflammatory cells but a few swollen endothelial cells remain attached.

Haematoxylin-eosin   (**a**) ×50; (**b**) ×350

may therefore have a useful confirmatory role, but only if associated with positive clinical and radiographic findings.[161]

Melkersson-Rosenthal syndrome

Melkersson Rosenthal syndrome is mentioned here because of its histological similarities to sarcoidosis or Crohn's disease. The syndrome, which is rare, comprises recurrent facial paralyses and swelling, particularly of the lip, and fissured tongue. The aetiology is unknown but a genetic trait appears to be involved. There is no relationship to sarcoidosis. The onset is most often in the second or third decades but sometimes earlier and the facial palsy can become permanent.

Histologically, Melkersson-Rosenthal syndrome is characterized by oedema of the corium of the affected mucosa together with non-caseating epithelioid granulomas.[162] These are typically small and loosely arranged, and occasionally contain multinucleate giant cells. In long-standing cases there is increasing fibrosis which can extend into and replace the underlying muscle. Proliferative gingival lesions with the characteristic granuloma formation are a rare feature of the disease.[163]

Cheilitis granulomatosa (*cheilitis glandularis*) is the name given to facial swelling, particularly of the lips, with the same histological appearances as Melkersson-Rosenthal syndrome but lacking the other clinical features.[164]

Wegener's granulomatosis and other forms of midline granuloma

Several forms of non-healing midline granuloma have been described[165], each with more or less distinctive histopathological appearances and with more or less severe destructive changes appearing in the nasopharynx or mouth at an early stage.

Two main types of midfacial granuloma syndrome, namely Wegener's granulomatosis and the Stewart type of non-healing necrotizing granuloma, have been described in Chapter 3 of Volume 1.

Wegener's granulomatosis is perhaps the best defined of these diseases in that the histopathological picture and, usually, the course are characteristic and a peculiar form of proliferative gingivitis, pathognomonic of the disease, can be an early feature. The nature of several other types of midline granuloma tends to be rather more controversial in that the microscopic appearances may be more difficult to interpret and the subsequent courses of these disorders are more variable. These differences may be considered either to be due to inherent characteristics or the results of variations in severity or the effects of treatment.

The following brief account of these diseases is not definitive. There is still controversy as to the precise nature of many of these cases and intermediate forms may also exist.

Though several of the conditions, particularly Wegener's granulomatosis, are thought to be immunologically mediated, there are no useful immunological tests and diagnosis depends in the early stages on the histological findings.

Wegener's granulomatosis

This disease can occasionally produce a form of gingivitis which is pathognomonic in both its clinical and pathological features and is frequently then the initial sign of the disease.

The gingivae are livid or bright red and undergo proliferative changes producing a granular or, in extreme cases, a raspberry-like texture.[166–169] Another possible finding is ulcerative stomatitis, as mentioned by Wegener in his original description of the disease,[168] but it is not so specific in character as the gingivitis.

Microscopically, in addition to the irregular hyperplasia of both the gingival epithelium and connective tissue (Fig. 1.42), there is a dense mononuclear infiltrate in which the characteristic giant cells are found (Fig. 1.43). Epithelial granuloma formation is not a feature and necrotizing arteritis is not seen in this site because the gingival vessels are too small to show inflammation in and damage to their walls. If, however, changes involve the maxillary antrum, typical arteritis may be seen.

Early diagnosis can be made from the findings in an oral biopsy from such cases and this is particularly important in view of the sharp deteri-

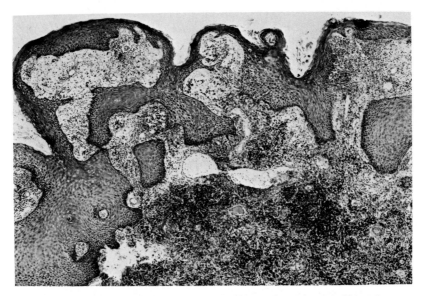

Fig. 1.42 Wegener's granulomatosis. This gingival biopsy shows the typical irregular hyperplasia which produces a characteristic strawberry-like texture clinically. More deeply there is an intense mixed inflammatory infiltrate.

Haematoxylin-eosin   × 50

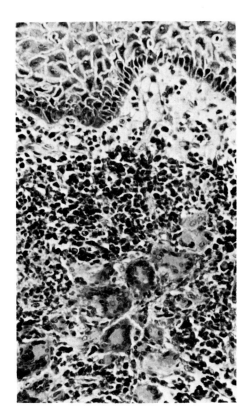

Fig. 1.43 Wegener's granulomatosis. The characteristic, irregularly-shaped giant cells are an important diagnostic feature.

Haematoxylin-eosin   × 350

oration in the prognosis associated with spread of the disease and in particular as a result of renal involvement.

Extensive mutilating necrosis of the face is not characteristic of Wegener's disease, but necrosis and perforation of the nasal septum and a saddle nose deformity may develop.

Lymphomatoid granulomatosis

It has been pointed out that the pleomorphic cellular picture seen in the Stewart-type midfacial granuloma may be indistinguishable from that of lymphomatoid granulomatosis[165]. The latter is a lymphoreticular disease which is angiocentric and angiodestructive, and though it predominantly affects the lungs, midfacial granuloma syndrome can be one of its less common manifestations.[170]

There is increasing evidence that lymphomatoid granulomatosis is a T-cell lymphoma. Some cases are, however, of low grade and lymphomatoid granulomatosis can therefore have a highly variable course; some cases are indolent or even apparently undergo temporary or permanent remission. Vasculitic manifestations may in rare cases persist for as long as 15 years before lymphoma has been recognized and it has therefore been suggested that, in such cases, a non-neoplastic inflammatory process gave rise to a peripheral T cell lymphoma.[171]

There is also evidence that polymorphic reticulosis which can also cause the midline granuloma syndrome is the same entity as lymphomatoid granulomatosis.[172]

Nasopharyngeal lymphoma

An unusual form of lymphoma can produce, as an early manifestation, destructive midline lesions of the upper respiratory tract and ulceration and necrosis of the palate in particular.[173,174] The palate can then have a peculiar boggily oedematous appearance and anterior teeth may become slightly extruded.

Microscopically, the appearances in the early stages may be readily mistaken for inflammatory changes, which as a result of the ulceration may, in fact, be superimposed. Particularly careful assessment of the cellular picture and, if need be, use of lymphocyte markers is therefore necessary in the attempt to confirm the diagnosis before the disease becomes disseminated and more obviously lymphomatous in nature. The cellular changes may be such that it has been suggested that the lesion is an 'atypical lymphoma', outside the accepted classifications. However, this view has not been generally accepted. The prognosis is poor, especially as the diagnosis may not be suspected or confirmed until the disease has become widespread.

Summary

In brief, then, current evidence suggests that the midfacial granuloma syndrome can be a manifestation of a variety of diseases. If those of known cause, such as chronic infections, are excluded, the remainder appear to be divisible into Wegener's granulomatosis and lymphoreticular diseases. The main example of the latter may be lymphomatoid granulomatosis, which appears to be a T-cell lymphoma. Nasopharyngeal lymphoma is more readily recognisable as such, but may originate in either T or B cells. Both lymphomatoid granulomatosis and other nasopharyngeal lymphomas can disseminate, but lymphomatoid granulomatosis may do so only after remaining localized for a very long period. Moreover, lymphomatoid granulomatosis can have an indolent or remittant course and it seems possible that it may also be the cause of another type of midfacial granuloma termed 'idiopathic midline destructive disease' which is reported[175] to have a benign course and a good response to low-dose radiotherapy. Palatal necrosis has been described in approximately 50% of such cases. Moreover, despite having been reported as a distict entity, idiopathic midline destructive disease shares with lymphomatoid granulomatosis the perivascular distribution of the mononuclear cellular infiltrate.

It is conceivable, therefore, that the apparently overlapping nature of the pathological processes underlying some cases of the midfacial granuloma syndrome may be due to the fact that both Wegener's granulomatosis and lymphomatoid granulomatosis are angiodestructive. In addition, T-cell lymphomas, of which lymphomatoid granulomatosis is an example, can have a variable microscopic picture and course; it seems likely that some of these lymphomas have not, initially at least, been recognized as such but 'transition' to lymphoma has been described as a late complication.

Another possible cause of malignant granuloma syndrome is malignant histiocytosis.[176–177] However, the small numbers of cases of midline granuloma syndrome in the many different reports and the fact that more specific methods of identification of cells of lymphoreticular origin have only become available relatively recently leaves considerable areas of uncertainty about some of the diseases causing this syndrome.

REFERENCES

1. Squier CA, Johnson NW, Hopps RM. Human oral mucosa: development, structure and function. Oxford: Blackwell Scientific, 1976.
2. Sperber GH. Craniofacial embryology. 2nd ed. Bristol: Wright, 1976.
3. Dudgeon JA. In: Heath RB, Waterson AP, eds. Modern trends in medical virology. 2nd ed. London: Butterworth, 1970.
4. Brooks SL, Rowe NH, Drach JC et al. JADA 1981; 102: 31–34.
5. Jordan MC (Moderator). Ann Intern Med 1984; 100: 866–880.
6. Hyman RW, Ecker JR, Tenser RB. Lancet 1983; ii: 814–816.
7. Gilden DH, Vafai A, Shtram Y et al. Nature 1983; 306: 478–480.
8. Ragozzino MW, Melton LJ, Kurland LT et al. N Engl J Med 1982; 307: 393–397.
9. Winston DJ, Gale RP, Meyer DV et al. Medicine (Baltimore) 1979; 58: 1–31.
10. Peterson PK, Ferguson R, Fryd DS et al. Medicine (Baltimore) 1982; 61: 360–372.
11. Evans AD, Waddington EBJ. Dermatol 1967; 79: 309–317.
12. Cawson RA, McSwiggan DA. Oral Surg 1969; 27: 451–459.
13. Cawson RA. Br J Dis Chest 1960; 54: 40–53.
14. Weaver RA. JAMA 1976; 235: 2418.
15. Pugh D, Cawson RA. Sabouraudia 1977; 15: 29–35.
16. Cawson RA. Oral Surg 1966; 22: 582–591.
17. Cawson RA. Br J Dermatol 1973; 89: 497–503.
18. Cawson RA, Rajasingham KC. Br J Dermatol 1972; 87: 435–443.
19. Higgs JM, Wells RS. Br J Dermatol 1973; 89: 179–190.
20. Hauser FV, Rothman S. Arch Dermatol Syph 1950; 61: 297–310.
21. Neufeld M, Maclaren NK, Blizzard RM. Medicine (Baltimore) 1981; 60: 355–362.
22. Eisenbarth GS, Rassi N. In: Davies TF, ed. Autoimmune endocrine disease, ch. 10. New York: Wiley, 1983.
23. Thorpe ES, Handley HE. Am J Dis Child 1929; 38: 328–334.
24. Valdimarsson H, Higgs JM, Wells RS et al. Cell Immunol 1973; 6: 348–352.
25. McCracken AW, Cawson RA. Clinical and oral microbiology. Washington: Hemisphere Publishing, McGraw-Hill, 1983.
26. Gottlieb MS, Schroff R, Schanker HM et al. N Engl J Med 1981; 305: 1425–1431.
27. Jaffe HW, Choi K, Thomas PA et al. Ann Intern Med 1983; 99: 145–151.
28. Gottlieb MS (Moderator). Ann Intern Med 1983; 99: 208–220.
29. Jaffe HW, Bregman DJ, Selik RM. J Infect Dis 1983; 148: 339–345.
30. Selik RM, Haverkos HW, Curran JW. Am J Med 1984; 76: 493–500.
31. Fauci AS (Moderator). Ann Intern Med 1984; 100: 92–106.
32. Lozada F, Silverman S, Migliorati CA et al. Oral Surg 1983; 56: 491–494.
33. Napier BL, McTighe AH, Snow JF et al. Laryngoscope 1983; 93: 1466–1469.
34. Gnepp DR, Chandler W, Hyams V. Ann Intern Med 1984; 100: 107–114.

35. Abemayor E, Calcaterra TC. Arch Otolaryngol 1983; 109: 536–542.
36. Rosenberg RA, Schneider KL, Cohen NL. Laryngoscope 1984; 94: 642–646.
37. Klein RS, Harris CA, Small CB et al. N Engl J Med 1984; 311: 354–358.
38. Centers for Disease Control Atlanta; Morbidity & Mortality Weekly Report 1985; 34: 1161–1163.
39. Barnes DM. Science 1986; 232: 1589–1590.
40. Carne CA, Sutherland S, Ferns R B et al. Lancet 1985; ii: 1261–1262.
41. Bygbjerg K. Lancet 1983; 1: 676.
42. Greenwood BM. Immunol Today 1984; 5: 293–294.
43. Barré-Sinoussi F, Cherman JC, Rey F et al. Science 1983; 220: 868–871.
44. Broder S, Gallo RC. N Engl J Med 1984; 311: 1292–1297.
45. Gallo RC. Cancer 1985; 55: 2317–2323.
46. Levy J, Hoffman A, Kramer S et al. Science 1984; 225: 840–842.
47. Ratner L, Gallo RC, Wong-Staal. Nature 1985; 313: 636–637.
48. Gallo RC, Salahuddin SZ, Popovic M et al. Science 1984; 224: 500–503.
49. Montagnier L, Barre-Sinoussi F, Chermann JC. Elsevier Science, 1984: 367–372.
50. Laurence J, Brun-Vezinet F, Stevens E et al. N Engl J Med 1984; 311: 1269–1273.
51. Pollack MS, Gold J, Metroka et al. Hum Immunol 1984; 11: 99–103.
52. Salahuddin SZ, Markham PD, Redfield RR et al. Lancet 1984; 2: 1418–1420.
53. Maloney MJ, Cox F, Wray BB et al. N Engl J Med 1985; 312: 1256.
54. Anonymous. Acquired immune deficiency syndrome. London: Department of Health & Social Security, 1985.
55. Cooper DA, Maclean P, Finlayson R et al. Lancet 1985; i: 537–540.
56. Abrams DI, Lewis BJ, Beckstead JH et al. Ann Intern Med 1984; 100: 801–808.
57. Mathur-Wagh V, Enlow RW, Spigland I et al. Lancet 1984; 1: 1033.
58. Marcusen DC, Sooy CD. Laryngoscope 1985; 95: 401–405.
59. Romanowski B, Weber J. Ann Intern Med 1984; 101: 400–401.
60. Greenspan D, Conant M, Silverman S Jr et al. Lancet 1984; ii: 831–834.
61. Reichert CM, O'Leary TJ, Levens DL et al. Am J Pathol 1983; 112: 357–361.
62. Seligman M, Chess L, Fahey JL et al. N Engl J Med 1984; 311: 1286–1290.
63. Pinching AJ. Clin Exp Immunol 1984; 56: 1–13.
64. Blumenfeld W, Beckstead JH. Arch Pathol Lab Med 1983; 107: 567–569.
65. Janossy G, Pinching AJ, Bofill M et al. Clin. Exp Immunol 1985; 59: 257–266.
66. Symmers W St C. The lymphoreticular system. Systemic pathology. 2nd ed. Edinburgh: Churchill Livingstone, 1978: vol. 2.
67. Hui AN, Koss MN, Meyer PR. Hum Pathol 1984; 15: 670–676.
68. Millard PR. J Pathol 1984; 143: 223–239.
69. Kaposi M. Arch Dermatol Syphilol 1872; 4: 265.
70. Hutt MSR. Br Med Bull 1984; 40: 355–358.
71. Cohn DL, Judson FN. Ann Intern Med 1984; 101: 401.
72. Bayley AC. Lancet 1984; i: 1318–1320.
73. Clumeck N, Sonnet J, Taelman H et al. N. Engl. J Med 1984; 310: 492–497.
74. Van de Perre P, Lepage P, Kestelyn P et al. Lancet 1984; ii: 62–65.
75. Piot P, Quinn TC, Taelman H et al. Lancet 1984; ii: 65–69.
76. Guarda LG, Silva EG, Ordonez NG, Smith JL. Am J Clin Pathol 1981; 76: 197–199.
77. Moskowitz LB, Hensley GT, Gould EW et al. Hum Pathol 1985; 16: 447–456.
78. McNutt NS, Fletcher V, Conant MA. Am J Pathol 1983; 111: 62–77.
79. Sircus W, Church R, Kelleher J. Quart J Med 1957; XXVI (new series): 235–249.
80. National Institutes of Health. J Oral Pathol 1978; 7: 341–440.
81. Hutcheon AW, Dagg JH, Mason DK, Wray D, Ferguson MM, Lucie NP. Postgrad Med J 1978; 54: 779–783.
82. Oshima Y, Shimizu T, Yokohari R et al. Ann Rheum Dis 1963; 22: 36–45.
83. Haim S, Gilhar A. Br J Dermatol 1980; 102: 361–363.
84. Shimizu T, Katsuta Y, Oshima Y. Ann Rheum Dis 1965; 24: 494–500.
85. Dilsen N, Konice M, Ovul C, eds. Proceedings of an International Symposium on Behcet's Disease, Istambul, 29–30 Sept. 1977. Amsterdam: Excerpta Medica, 1979.
86. Lim SD, Haw CR, Kim NI, Fusaro RM. Arch Dermatol 1983; 119: 307–310.
87. Rodu B, Gockerman JP. JAMA 1983; 249: 504–507.
88. Andreasen JO. Oral Surg 1968; 25: 158–166.
89. Andreasen JO, Pindborg JJ. Nord Med 1 VIII 1963; 70: 866.
90. Koveski G, Banoczy J. Int J Oral Surg 1973; 2: 13–19.
91. Fulling H-J. Arch Dermatol 1973; 108: 667–669.
92. Ahmed AR (Moderator). Ann Intern Med 1980: 92: 396–405.
93. Meurer M, Millns JL, Rogers RS, Jordan RE. Arch Dermatol 1977; 113: 1520–1524.
94. Provost TT. Dermatologic diseases. In: Stites DP, Stobo JD, Fudenberg H, Wells JV, eds. Basic & clinical immunology, ch 32. 4th ed. Los Altos, California: Lange, 1982: 576–592.
95. Weathers DR, Sharpe LO. Arch Dermatol 1969; 100: 50–53.
96. Prindiville DE, Stern D. J Oral Surg 1976; 34: 1001–1006.
97. Basu MK, Moss N. Br J Oral Surg 1979–1980; 17: 57–61.
98. Kazmeirowski JA, Wuepper KD. J Invest Dermatol 1978; 71: 366–369.
99. Ackerman AB, Penneys NS, Clark WH. Br J Dermatol 1971; 84: 554–566.
100. Bedi TR, Pinkus H. Br J Dermatol 1976; 95: 243–250.
101. Buchner A, Lozada F, Silverman S. Oral Surg 1980; 49: 221–228.
102. Russotto SB, Ship II. Oral Surg 1971; 31: 42–48.
103. Fraser NG, Kerr NW, Donald D. Br J Dermatol 1973; 89: 439–450.
104. Sciubba JJ. Oral Surg 1983; 55: 363–373.
105. Willkens RF, Arnett FC, Bitter T et al. Arth Rheum 1981; 24: 844–849.
106. Perry HO, Mayne JG. Arch Dermatol 1965; 92: 129.
107. Tan EM, Cohen AS, Fries JF et al. Arth Rheum 1982; 25: 1271–1277.

108. Andreason JO, Poulsen HE. Acta Odontol Scand 1964; 22: 389–400.

109. Urman JD, Lowenstein MB, Abeles M, Weinstein A. Arth Rheum 1978; 21: 58–61.

110. Shklar G, McCarthy PL. Arch Dermatol 1978; 114: 1031–1035.

111. Schiodt M, Pindborg JJ. Oral Surg 1984; 57: 46–51.

112. McGurk M, Craig GT. Br J Oral Maxillofac Surg 1984; 22: 56–64.

113. Mani NJ, Singh B. Oral Surg 1976; 41: 203–214.

114. Millard PR. Br J Dermatol 1966; 78: 305–307.

115. Moos KF, Madan DK. Br Dent J 1968; 124: 313–317.

116. Einhorn J, Wersall J. Cancer 1967; 20: 2189–2193.

117. Silverman S, Gorsky M, Lozada F. Cancer 1984; 53: 563–568.

118. Mincer HH, Coleman SA, Hopkins KP. Oral Surg 1972; 33: 389–399.

119. Cawson RA. Br Med Bull 1975; 31: 164–169.

120. Browne WG, Izatt MM, Renwick JH. Ann Hum Genet 1969; 32: 271–281.

121. Jorgensen RJ, Levin LS. Arch Dermatol 1981; 117: 73–76.

122. Kramer IRH, El-Labban N, Lee KW. Br Dent J 1978; 144: 171–180.

123. Pogrel MA. J Oral Pathol 1979; 8: 176–178.

124. Sirinavin C, Trowbridge AA. J Med Genet 1975; 12: 339–354.

125. Wagner G, Luckasen JR, Goltz RW. Arch Dermatol 1976; 112: 1010–1014.

126. Hietanen J, Salo OP, Kanerva L, Juvakoski T. Scand J Dent Res 1984; 92: 50–4.

127. Fischmann SL, Barnett ML, Nisengard RJ. Oral Surg 1977; 44: 253–260.

128. Young LL, Lenox JA. Oral Surg 1973; 36: 663–666.

129. Maser ED. Oral Surg 1977; 43: 373–378.

130. Jaspers MT. Oral Surg 1975; 39: 934–944.

131. Kellett M. Br Dent J 1983; 154: 366–368.

132. Zegarelli DJ, Zegarelli-Schmidt EC, Zegarelli EV. Oral Surg 1974; 38: 725–734.

133. Buchner A, Hansen LS, Merrell PW. Arch Dermatol 1981; 117: 563–565.

134. Neville BW, Weathers DR. Oral Surg 1980; 49: 429–434.

135. Whaley K, Webb J, McAvoy BA et al. Quart J Med 1973; XLII (new series): 513–548.

136. Manthorpe R, Frost-Larsen, Isager H, Prause JU. Allergy 1981; 36: 139–153.

137. Elkon KB, Gharavi AE, Hughes GRV, Moutsoupoulos HM. Ann Rheum Dis 1984; 43: 243–245.

138. Sjögren H. Acta Ophth 1935; 13: 1.

139. Penner E, Reichlin M. Arth Rheum 1982; 25: 1250–1253.

140. Gratwhol AA, Moutsopoulos HM, Chused TM et al. Ann Intern Med 1977; 87: 703–706.

141. Schubert MM, Sullivan KM, Morton TH et al. Arch Intern Med 1984; 144: 1591–1595.

142. Chisholm DM, Waterhouse JP, Mason DK. J Clin Pathol 1970; 23: 690–694.

143. Greenspan JS, Daniels TE, Talal N, Sylvester RA. Oral Surg 1974; 37: 217–229.

144. Daniels TE. Arth Rheum 1984; 27: 147–156.

145. Batsakis JG. Head & Neck Surg 1982; 5: 150–163.

146. Kyle RA, Greipp PR. Mayo Clin Proc 1983; 58: 665–683.

147. Van der Waal I, Fehmers MCO, Kraal ER. Oral Surg 1973; 36: 469–481.

148. Cohen C, Krutchkoff D, Eisenberg E. J Oral Surg 1981; 39: 613–618.

149. Brook IM, King DJ, Miller ID. Oral Surg 1983; 56: 405–408.

150. Hartman KS. Oral Surg 1980; 49: 38–54.

151. Jones RO, Pillsbury HC. Laryngoscope 1984; 94: 1031–1035.

152. Favara BE, McCarthy RC, Mierau GW. Hum Pathol 1983; 14: 664–676.

153. Tornes K, Bang G. Oral Surg 1974; 38: 99–102.

154. Tang TT, Glicklich M, Hodach AE, Oechler HW, McCreadie SR. Am J Clin Pathol 1981; 75: 420–425.

155. Elzay RP, Oral Surg 1983; 55: 497–506.

156. Plumpton S. Br Dent J 1965; 118: 249–254.

157. Cowpe JG, Hislop WS. Oral Surg 1983; 56: 597–601.

158. Hogan JJ. Br Dent J 1983; 154: 109–110.

159. Howarth RI. Br Dent J 1981; 150: 130–132.

160. Hughes GRV, Gross NJ. Br Med J 1972; 3: 215.

161. Postma D, Fry TL, Malenbaum BT. Arch Otolaryngol 1984; 110: 28–30.

162. Worsaae N, Christensen KC, Schiodt M, Reibel J. Oral Surg 1982; 54: 404–413.

163. Worsaae N, Pindborg JJ. Oral Surg 1980; 49: 131–138.

164. Azaz B, Nitzan DW. Oral Surg 1984; 57: 250–253.

165. Friedmann I. Nose, throat and Ears. Systemic pathology (Ed. W. St. C. Symmers) Vol. 1. 3rd. ed. Edinburgh: Churchill Livingstone; 1986.

166. Cawson RA. Br Dent J 1965; 118: 30–32.

167. Cohen PS, Meltzer JA. JAMA 1981; 246: 2610–2611.

168. Israelson H, Binnie WH, Hurt WC. J Periodontol 1981; 52: 81–87.

169. McDonald TJ, DeRemee RA. Laryngoscope 1983; 93: 220–231.

170 Crissman JD, Weiss MA, Gluckman J. Am J Surg Pathol 1982; 6: 335–346.

171. Weis JW, Winter MW, Phyliky RL, Banks PM. Mayo Clin Proc 1986; 61: 411–426.

172. DeRemee RA, Weiland LH, McDonald TJ. Mayo Clin Proc 1978; 53: 634–640.

173. Michaels L, Gregory MM. J Clin Pathol 1977; 30: 317–327.

174. Ishii Y, Yamanaka N, Ogawa K et al. Cancer 1982; 50: 2336–2344.

175. Tsokos M, Fauci AS, Costa J. Am J Clin Pathol 1982; 77: 162–168.

176. Kassel SH, Eschevarria RA, Guzzo FP. Cancer 1969; 23: 920–935.

177. Aozasa K, Inoue A. J Pathology 1982; 138: 241–249.

178. Kassel SH, Echevarria RA, Guzzo FP. Cancer 1969; 23: 920–935.

2

R.A. Cawson and R.B. Lucas

The teeth and supporting tissues
Tumours of the mouth and jaws

NORMAL STRUCTURE

The teeth are composed of three calcified tissues—enamel, dentine and cementum—and the connective-tissue pulp (Fig. 2.1). Most of the tooth consists of dentine, of which 30% is organic material and water and 70% is inorganic material. The organic element of dentine consists of collagen fibrils bound together by a mucopolysaccharide cementing substance; the inorganic material (as in bone, enamel and cementum) consists mainly of calcium phosphates deposited in the form of apatite crystals. Thus, dentine resembles bone in its physical and chemical composition, although it differs in cellular organization: in bone the osteocytes are distributed throughout the tissue, but in dentine the cells are all arranged in a layer over the surface that adjoins the pulp. Each dentine cell, or odontoblast, has a process that runs through the entire thickness of the dentine; dentine thus contains a very large number of tubules, 2–3 μm in diameter, each containing an odontoblast process.

The dentine of the crown of the tooth is covered by enamel. Enamel is almost wholly inorganic in composition (96%), consisting of long rods or prisms, about 4 μm in diameter, that pass through its entire thickness. The rods are held together by a small amount of inter-rod substance that is also calcified. The small quantity of organic material in enamel contains keratin-like proteins, glycoproteins, fats and other substances. Since part of this fraction as well as all of the inorganic fraction is soluble in acid, enamel is usually entirely lost in decalcified sections. It can therefore be reliably demonstrated microscopically only in ground sections.

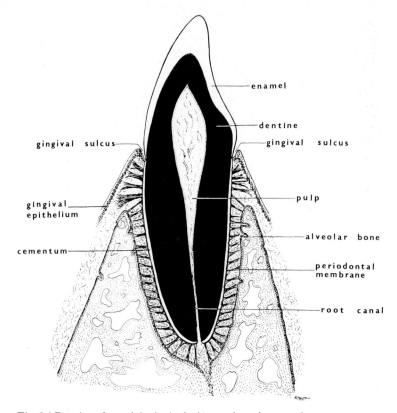

Fig. 2.1 Drawing of a tooth in situ in the jaw, to show the normal structure.

The dentine of the root is covered by a thin layer of cementum. This tissue, which is very similar to bone in composition and morphology, gives attachment to the periodontal ligament. The ligament consists of collagen fibres that attach the tooth to the bony wall of its socket.

The dental pulp consists of connective tissue and contains the vessels and nerves of the tooth. It occupies the pulp cavity and root canals.

The gingiva, or gum, is the portion of the oral mucosa that surrounds the teeth. The gingiva is firmly attached like a cuff to the surface of the tooth, but the arrangement is such that there is a shallow groove or sulcus between them.

NORMAL DEVELOPMENT

The teeth are compound structures, developing from ectoderm and mesoderm. The ectodermal element, the enamel, is formed by the enamel organ. The enamel organ develops as a solid bud of cells growing into the jaw from the basal layer of the oral epithelium: the cells soon differentiate to form a bell-shaped or cap-shaped structure comprising a core of stellate cells and a peripheral layer of cubical or columnar cells. Its deep aspect is concave: the cells that cover this aspect become the ameloblasts. At first, the enamel organ retains a connection with the oral epithelium by a strand of cells, the dental lamina; later, this breaks up and for the most part disappears, although isolated groups of the cells remain indefinitely as rests. The mesenchyme deep to the enamel organ condenses to form the dental papilla, which later becomes the dental pulp. The cells of the papilla in contact with the enamel organ differentiate into odontoblasts and begin to lay down dentine matrix. This is followed by the deposition of enamel matrix by the ameloblasts. Calcification of the pre-dentine and pre-enamel soon follows (Fig. 2.2).

Dentine and enamel continue to be laid down in this manner until the form of the tooth is

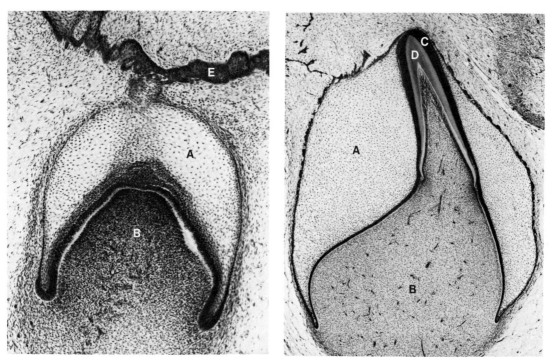

Fig. 2.2a,b Developing teeth. The tooth germ on the right (**b**) is at a later stage of development than that on the left (**a**), and is forming enamel and dentine. A = enamel organ; B = dental papilla; C = enamel; D = dentine; E = dental lamina.

Haematoxylin-eosin   × 35

completed. By this time the dental papilla has become enclosed by dentine to form the pulp, and the enamel organ, which has gradually diminished in size as the amount of enamel laid down has increased, is finally reduced to a thin layer of cells covering the enamel. In addition, some isolated cell remnants, both of the enamel organ itself and of the dental lamina, remain in the tissues round the tooth. These epithelial rests persist throughout life, and although usually of no importance they may become involved in certain pathological conditions.

The other dental tissue, cementum, is laid down on the surface of the root dentine by cementoblasts which have differentiated from the surrounding connective tissue.

DEFECTS IN DEVELOPMENT

A wide variety of developmental defects can be found in teeth; many of them are of local significance only and are primarily of interest to the dental surgeon. However, some defects are associated with systemic disease[2] and come within the purview of the medical practitioner.

Enamel hypoplasia. The two processes involved in the formation of enamel—the laying down of matrix by the ameloblasts, and the subsequent deposition of mineral salts in it—may be affected by systemic disturbances or nutritional deficiencies during the formative period. The results are seen when the teeth erupt. Defects in the matrix are indicated by irregularities in the enamel. When the damage has been mild there may be little more than a few tiny pits in the surface—in more severe cases the pits are deeper and are arranged in one or more horizontal rows stretching across the surface of the tooth. In other cases there may be deep furrows or grooves in the enamel. The enamel is typically qualitatively normal; sometimes, however, it may also be insufficiently calcified.

Enamel hypoplasia can affect both the deciduous and the permanent teeth, involving only those that were forming enamel at the time of the causal disturbance. It is thus possible to determine when this happened from the distribution of the lesions. The possible causes of hypoplasia are very varied and include genetic defects, severe birth injury, severe intercurrent disease (particularly the infectious fevers in the first year or two of life), hypocalcaemia resulting from vitamin D deficiency, congenital syphilis and ingestion of fluorides. Congenital syphilis and fluorides give rise to distinctive lesions (see below).

In congenital syphilis the permanent incisors and first molars are affected, due to the presence of *Treponema pallidum* in the developing dental tissues. When the teeth erupt, the incisors are peg-shaped and the incisal edge is often notched (Hutchinson's incisors). The crowns of the first molars may have a mulberry-like appearance, owing to irregularity of the enamel or be dome-shaped (Moon's molars).

Dental fluorosis develops in localities where the drinking water contains more than one part per million of fluorides; it affects those who have taken the water during the period of enamel formation. In mild cases there are no more than opaque paper-white areas in the enamel. With increasing severity there is mottled brown staining and in extreme cases pitting and roughening of the enamel surface. Despite these defects, resistance to dental caries is increased.

Amelogenesis imperfecta. Amelogenesis imperfecta is the term given to several different defects of enamel formation which are inherited in a variety of patterns. The two main variants are the hypoplastic type in which enamel matrix formation is defective but calcification is essentially normal, and the hypocalcified type in which the matrix is normal but calcification is defective.

The hypoplastic type of amelogenesis imperfecta is characterized by deficiency of enamel which may be almost absent or merely irregular and pitted. The enamel is, however, hard and translucent though it is often heavily stained by material which accumulates in the defects. In the hypoplastic type by contrast, the enamel is, initially at least, morphologically normal but soft, chalky, opaque and typically yellowish in colour. As a consequence it readily chips away leaving a characteristic shouldered form to the incisor teeth.

Defects of dentine. Systemic disturbances during the period of dental development may affect dentine formation as well as enamel formation. Rickets, scurvy, hypoparathyroidism and severe intercurrent disease may all result in defective dentine formation. In some cases there may be underdevelopment of the roots of the teeth and delayed eruption, as in rickets, but generally dentinal defects are only detected microscopically.

One particular type of dentine dysplasia is genetically determined. This is *dentinogenesis imperfecta*, in which the normal pattern of tubule formation in the dentine is upset and continued deposition of dentine leads to more or less complete obliteration of the pulp chamber. Clinically, the crowns of the teeth typically appear morphologically normal but have a purplish or brownish tinge (hence the earlier name, hereditary opalescent dentine). The enamel is, however, weakly attached to the dentine and tends to flake off. In severe cases loss of the enamel allows the softer dentine to become worn down to the gum margins by early adolescence. Obliteration of the pulp chamber by the abnormal dentine, however, prevents infection of the pulp though the teeth are of little functional value at this stage. The condition may be an isolated defect or associated with osteogenesis imperfecta.

Dental defects in systematized inherited diseases. In addition to the conditions already mentioned there are many defects of the teeth, in terms of form, structure or number, as a feature of inherited diseases. This subject requires reference to a specialized textbook.[2]

Pigmentation. Pigmentation of the teeth is relatively common. Extrinsic stains, which affect only the surface of the teeth, can be removed by local measures. Such stains include the common green—sometimes brown or black—discoloration of children's teeth by chromogenic bacteria, and staining by constituents of tobacco smoke or other chemical substances.

Intrinsic pigmentation cannot be removed by local treatment, since it affects the calcified tissues of the teeth. It may be of local origin or blood-borne. There are many causes, including endogenous systemic disorders such as alkaptonuria, congenital porphyria and erythroblastosis fetalis, and absorption of various exogenous substances, including tetracycline antibiotics.

Tetracycline pigmentation. Since tetracycline antibiotics are taken up by calcifying tissues, they are incorporated into the teeth if given during the period of dental development. The developing teeth of the fetus incorporate tetracyclines when these drugs are given to the mother during pregnancy; the permanent teeth incorporate tetracyclines when these are given during infancy and childhood. As the crowns of the permanent anterior teeth calcify between the fourth month of extra-uterine life and the sixth year, tetracyclines should be avoided, when possible, during this time. The antibiotic accumulates in dentine and, to some extent, in enamel, giving the teeth a more or less bright-yellow colour that gradually becomes brown or grey; the different tetracyclines differ in the tint and intensity of the discoloration that they cause. The discoloration is permanent. Microscopical examination in ultraviolet light shows conspicuous fluorescence along the incremental lines of the dentine. Some degree of hypoplasia of the teeth may be associated with the pigmentation in severe cases.

DISEASES OF THE TEETH AND THEIR SUPPORTING TISSUES

Dental caries

This destructive lesion of the calcified tissues of the teeth is the result of a prolonged attack by acid-forming bacteria. Although dental enamel, by virtue of its high mineral content, is the hardest body tissue and offers no pathways for bacterial invasion, it is vulnerable to acid, which can cause it to disintegrate. Dentine, however, like bone, contains an appreciable proportion of organic material which provides a substrate for bacteria and in addition contains tubules which provide pathways for invasion.[3,4,5]

Aetiology

Dental caries has been shown by means of germ-free and gnotobiotic studies in animals to be bacterial in nature and to depend on the presence of specific strains of *Streptococcus mutans*. These bacteria have at least two essential properties, namely the ability to form insoluble polysaccharides which are tenaciously adherent to the teeth

and to form acids rapidly from sugars. Sugar (sucrose) is the main bacterial substrate and must be available to cariogenic bacteria at frequent intervals for tooth destruction to progress at a significant rate.

It is probable that strains of *Strep. mutans* are also responsible for human dental caries (as suggested by Clarke as long ago as 1924)[6] although it has not yet been possible to establish this point unequivocally. The destructive effects of bacterial acid are made possible by the physicochemical properties of the plaque on the teeth. Bacterial plaque consists essentially of bacteria enmeshed in the glucan-like polysaccharides that they have produced. The bacterial population of plaque is mixed and complex. Light microscopy shows filamentous forms to be conspicuous, but their role is uncertain. The numbers of bacteria present can, however, be judged by the fact that their concentration is little less than that of a centrifuged bacterial pellet. This plaque, therefore, contains a massive concentration of bacterial enzymes which degrade sugar to acid within minutes of its having entered the mouth and it also prevents the acid from being leached out or buffered by the saliva to any significant degree. This is so effective that plaque pH does not return to resting levels for up to 45 minutes from the ingestion of a single dose of sugar.

Macroscopic features

The early changes of dental caries are submicroscopic and little is visible to the naked eye until the process is well advanced.

The two main areas of attack are interstitially, that is at the contact points where adjacent teeth are contiguous (smooth surface caries) and the occlusal pits, particularly of molar teeth. In such sites bacterial plaque forms in sufficient thickness to concentrate bacterial acid production and to protect it from salivary buffering. These sites are also inaccessible to disturbance by tooth-brushing.

The earliest visible enamel lesion, which can only be seen if the adjacent tooth is removed, consists of a white spot less than 2 mm in diameter in the otherwise translucent enamel at the point where the tooth was in contact with its neighbour. Pit and fissure caries develops so deeply in the enamel that nothing can be seen until it is so far advanced as to cause the surrounding enamel to appear chalky.

Interstitial caries can, however, be visualized at an early stage by intra-oral radiographs which show a triangular area of decalcification, first of the enamel and later of the dentine also. In the late stages, where there is formation of a grossly visible cavity as a result of enamel destruction, the pulp will already have become infected and inflamed even though symptoms may be absent.

Enamel caries

Pathogenesis and pathology

The pre-invasive phase. As mentioned earlier, acid production by plaque bacteria mediates the attack and bacteria invade the tissue only at a relatively late stage. Enamel, though very dense, has a minute organic content which is keratin-like and permits the passage of hydrogen ions. Since this organic matrix surrounds the apatite crystallites, the hydrogen ions gain access to the crystallites and gradually erode them. Although these changes take place at the ultrastructural level, a series of zones can be discerned by light microscopy, beneath a physically intact surface zone (Fig. 2.3). These zones can be shown by imbibition studies using polarized light to be produced by the formation of submicroscopic pores in the enamel.

A molecular sieve is thus formed and the different degrees of decalcification in each zone can be estimated by microradiography. The ability of the process to go on for a considerable time without destruction of the surface is due to remineralization of the latter, since calcium ions are being removed from the enamel and, by unknown mechanisms, are transported outwards into the bacterial plaque which, since it does not become calcified, must in some way complex the calcium ions and dispose of them. Some of these ions are, however, re-incorporated into the enamel and the degree of remineralization considerably affects the rate of progress of the attack.

The phase of bacterial invasion. Progressive dissolution of the enamel crystallites eventually produces apertures large enough for bacteria to penetrate. Once this has happened the relatively permeable amelodentinal junction can be reached and the bacteria are then able to spread laterally and attack both the dentine, on a wide front, and also the enamel from its under-surface. The enamel thus becomes undermined as well as decalcified from beneath (secondary enamel caries) so that it becomes chalky in appearance and texture, greatly weakened and eventually crumbles away.

Dentine caries

Since dentine has a relatively high organic content and is also permeated by tubules extending to the pulpal surface, there are thus ready-made pathways for bacterial invasion. Bacterial invasion is, however, preceded by softening of the dentine by acid diffusing from the overlying enamel lesion.

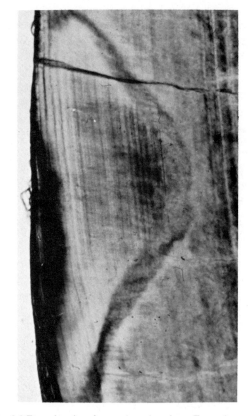

Fig. 2.3 Dental caries, the pre-invasive phase. Enamel structure remains apparently intact but a series of zones are seen as a result of submicroscopic demineralization and formation of minute pores in the tissue.

Ground, unstained section   × 100

The dentine is then invaded along a broad front by bacteria which have spread along the amelodentinal junction and a conical lesion with its apex towards the pulp is formed. In this, bacteria can be seen advancing via the tubules until they fill the latter. Since the matrix has been softened by decalcification, the proliferating bacteria produce spindle-shaped swellings with distortion of the neighbouring tubules (Fig. 2.4). Breakdown of intervening matrix leads to ragged liquefaction foci and progressive, macroscopic destruction.

Pulpal and dentinal reactions to dental caries

As mentioned earlier, the enamel is unable to react to attack but if the progress of the disease is not too acute the dentine is capable of limited reaction. In slowly advancing disease the dentinal tubules can become sclerotic and progressively obliterated by calcification. Under a more acute attack the underlying odontoblasts can be killed and the pulpal ends of the tubules become sealed by a layer of calcified tissue. More obvious, however, is the formation of reactionary (secondary) dentine which, if the disease is sufficiently chronic, resembles normal dentine in structure and is laid down underneath the original dentine (Fig. 2.5).

These reactions no more than delay the progress of the attack but secondary dentine formation, by allowing the pulp to escape infection, can permit the tooth to be repaired even though destruction is well advanced. In children, however, the process of carious attack can be so acute that the pulp has no time to mount any significant reaction.

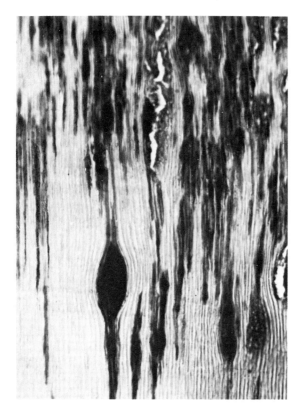

Fig. 2.4 Dentine caries. Most of the dentinal tubules are filled with bacteria and some are dilated as a result of the decalcification of the surrounding matrix by proliferation of the bacteria and their metabolites.

Haematoxylin-eosin   × 200

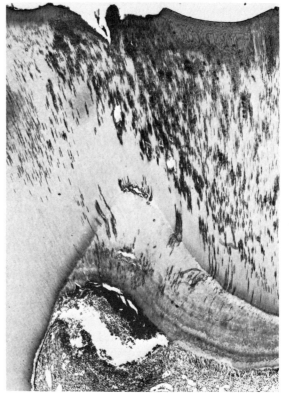

Fig. 2.5 Dentine caries and pulpal reactions. Bacteria have spread widely through the dentine and have also invaded the reactionary dentine beneath. A minute abscess has formed in the cornu of the pulp where bacteria have reached it.

Haematoxylin-eosin   × 30

Resistance to dental caries

The nature of the host factors that may develop in response to caries is far from certain. There is no convincing evidence that there is any natural immunity and children with Down's syndrome, for example, are singularly free from this disease, despite natural immunodeficiencies leading to increased susceptibility to infection in general, and despite gross oral plaque formation. With the exception of fluoride no aspect of tooth formation has been shown to affect susceptibility to caries. Neither severe morphological defects nor poor calcification (as was once believed) have been shown to make teeth more vulnerable. Similarly, no dietary deficiency (in the usual sense) has been shown to increase the vulnerability of the teeth and none of the so-called protective foods such as dairy products have been shown to have any benefit in this respect. Dental caries is, in general, a disease of relatively opulent communities and not a disease of the poverty-stricken or malnourished.

The sole agent of proven protective value is the fluoride ion,[7] which is most effective when ingested during dental development from a water supply with a fluoride content of one part per million. The main effect is then that hydroxy-apatite in the enamel is replaced by fluorapatite which appears to be more resistant to solution by acid. Though the mechanism of the protective effect of fluorides on the teeth has been discussed since 1867[8] its mode of action remains far from certain.

Pulpitis and other sequelae of dental caries[3]

The inevitable consequence of dental caries, if uncontrolled, is infection and inflammation of the dental pulp. Other causes of pulpitis such as irritant filling materials are relatively uncommon but, in children especially, the pulp can become exposed to the exterior when a tooth is fractured.

Otherwise, most cases of pulpitis are closed, that is, have no macroscopic opening into the pulp chamber. This rigid enclosure limits the response of the pulp since it cannot swell and the pressure of inflammatory exudate is likely to limit the blood flow.

Nevertheless, all stages of pulpal inflammation can be seen from mere hyperaemia, highly localized

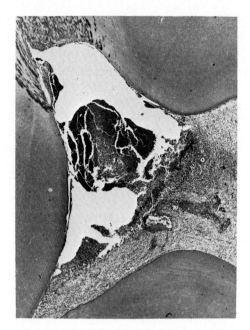

Fig. 2.6 Acute pulpitis. Bacteria have spread through the dentine so rapidly that no reactionary dentine has had time to form. Having reached the pulp the bacteria have caused the formation of a large abscess and spreading inflammatory changes.

Haematoxylin-eosin × 25

collections of inflammatory cells and abscess formation (Fig. 2.6) to generalized cellulitis of the pulp. Such changes have no clear relation to symptoms and though intense pain can result from acute pulpitis, abscess formation can be painless. Sooner or later, however, pulpitis leads to death of the pulp and extension of inflammation to the periapical tissues (apical periodontitis) and thence a variety of changes are possible.

Open pulpitis

Occasionally, in spite of gross infection of most of the overlying dentine, the dental pulp survives until it becomes exposed to the mouth as a result of the crown of the tooth having largely decayed away. By this time the pulp has been replaced by granulation tissue which can acquire an epithelial covering (Figs 2.7 and 2.8). Thus protected, inflammatory changes tend to subside and the pulp proliferates as a fibrous nodule surrounded by the remains of the crown of the tooth. This condition is painless and is visible in the mouth as a pink or

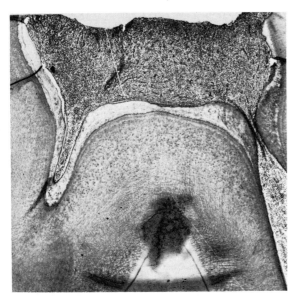

Fig. 2.7 Open pulpitis. The crown of the tooth has been destroyed and though the pulp has survived it has become replaced by granulation tissue and none of its specialized cells survive.

Haematoxylin-eosin   × 15

red swelling (a pulp polyp). Contrary to the traditional view, this is not particularly a phenomenon of immature teeth with open apices and an unrestricted blood supply, but can develop in fully formed mature teeth.

Apical periodontitis

Acute periodontitis is a typical acute inflammatory reaction in the minute space between the apex of the tooth and the surrounding alveolar bone. Hardly surprisingly, the process is intensely painful and the tooth becomes exquisitely tender to contact.

If undrained, this infection can perforate the nearest cortical plate of the jaw to produce acute oedema of the face and a sinus, or spreading inflammation such as acute perioral cellulitis or acute osteomyelitis of the jaw. Severe infections of this latter sort are now so rare as to be of little more than of historical interest in Britain, but fatal dental infections (usually caused by extension of the infection to produce cellulitis of the parapharyngeal spaces) are still occasionally reported from the United States.[9]

Chronic periodontitis is common. In many cases

pulpitis and subsequent periodontitis are entirely asymptomatic until complications develop. Dental caries is usually the initiating cause but often a blow to a tooth during childhood, severing the apical vessels, produces no significant effect until adult life. However, when the dental pulp is killed in this way leakage of blood products into the dentinal tubules causes the tooth to become obviously darkened.

Histopathology

Chronic apical periodontitis is an unremarkable chronic inflammatory reaction apart from the fact that it may lead to proliferation of epithelial rests in the periodontal ligament and cyst formation. This is the origin of the great majority of cysts of the jaws.

In addition to any element of epithelial proliferation, chronic periodontitis is also characterized by connective tissue proliferation and the gradual formation of a nodule of granulation tissue (an *apical granuloma*) with resorption of the surrounding bone to accommodate it (Fig. 2.9). Such granulomas appear as sharply defined, rounded areas of radiolucency typically less than a centimetre in diameter at the apex of the tooth.

Though granulation tissue is the predominant

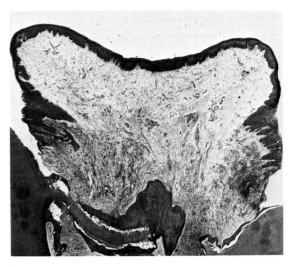

Fig. 2.8 Open pulpitis (pulp polyp). Open pulpitis may progress in this way, by proliferation of the connective tissue, to form a prominent nodule which becomes epithelialized

Haematoxylin-eosin   × 10

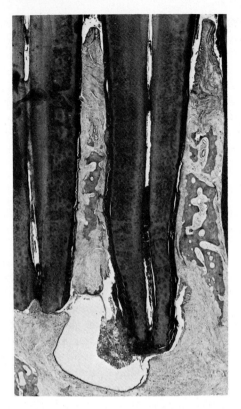

Fig. 2.9 Apical periodontitis. Death of the dental pulp has been followed by spread of inflammatory changes to the periapical tissues and resorption of bone round the tooth apex. The tip of the root canal of the affected tooth is filled with bacteria.

Gram haematoxylin-eosin   × 10

component of these lesions, they vary, (1) in the nature of the cellular infiltrate which ranges from an almost pure plasma cell picture to abscess formation and chronic suppuration, and (2) in the epithelial content. This may be absent (presumably destroyed by infection and inflammation), scanty or vigorously proliferating to form a microcyst with a hyperplastic lining.

There is, however, little clinical significance in these findings as all such lesions will resolve once the focus of infection in the dead tooth is eliminated by effective root canal treatment. If this happens, removal of the apical granuloma is rarely necessary, though it is frequently done.

Despite the readily visible area of bone destruction, there is no evidence that apical granulomas are a significant source of infection capable of dissemination. Several aspiration studies have shown these lesions to be sterile and their disappearance following treatment of the causative tooth suggests that bacteria from the latter are well localized.

Periodontal abscesses and skin sinuses

Suppuration from a chronic periapical abscess, if untreated, usually forms a sinus on the gum. In the case of the more anterior lower teeth, however, the sinus can point on the overlying skin in the region of the chin or more posteriorly. Sinuses in such sites should always be suspected as being of dental origin as they are recalcitrant to any treatment other than extraction or disinfection (root canal treatment) of the tooth of origin. The latter is quickly identified by radiography.

Gingivitis and periodontal disease

Periodontal disease is a term which includes any disease of the dental supporting tissues but in practice usually refers to gingivitis and periodontitis associated with the accumulation of bacterial plaque on the teeth. Gingivitis is a state of inflammation of the gingival margins only, while periodontitis refers to inflammation and destructive changes extending into the periodontal ligament and alveolar bone.[3]

Gingivitis is a virtually universal disease, preventable only by effective tooth-brushing (Fig. 2.10). Nevertheless, since strong local immunity develops, periodontal disease usually progresses so slowly that it may take half a century for the tissues to become so greatly damaged that the teeth are loosened.

Aetiology

Gingivitis develops in childhood if bacterial plaque is allowed to accumulate in the angle between the gingival margin and the crown of the teeth (the gingival sulcus). The microbial flora of this bacterial plaque is predominantly Gram-positive and aerobic initially, but with the passage of years there are increasing numbers of Gram-negative and anaerobic species. These, which include many recognized pathogens such as *Fusobacterium nucleatum* and *Bacteroides* species, are believed to play a

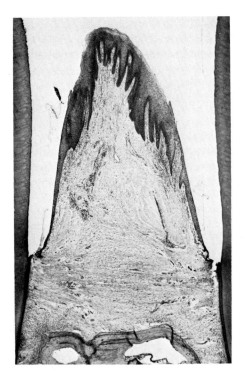

Fig. 2.10 Early chronic gingivitis. The interdental tissues are virtually normal and only a thin and patchy inflammatory infiltrate involves the superficial corium.

Haematoxylin-eosin   × 30

major role in the pathogenesis of destruction of the periodontal tissues.

Since there is inevitably an immunological response to the many antigens of the vast and varied flora in contact with the periodontal tissues, this has led to the widespread assumption that periodontal tissue damage is immunologically mediated. However, gnotobiotic studies[3] and more especially the histopathological features in humans do not provide strong support for such assumptions. Though it seems likely that antigen-antibody complexes as well as endotoxin are important in activation of complement and inflammation, there is no more evidence that periodontal tissue damage is immunologically mediated than is the case with most other infectious diseases.

Most cases of gingivitis, unless rigorously controlled, progress over the course of years to chronic periodontitis, where there is destruction of the dental supporting tissues. However, the course of the disease is highly variable and not entirely

predictable, as there are unidentified factors which affect the rate of progress. Epidemiological studies on a large scale have confirmed that there is no simple and uniform relationship between the level of oral neglect and the course of periodontal destruction. Some, therefore, believe that rapidly progressive periodontal destruction depends on the presence of certain pathogens such as Capnocytophaga, *Actinobacillus actinomycetemcomitans*, or *Bacteroides* species (particularly *B. gingivalis* (*asaccharolyticus*)) but, though there is some association, it is by no means absolute.

Histopathology[3]

Bacterial plaque is seen on the tooth surface, particularly where it is in apposition to the soft tissues of the gingiva. This plaque appears as a dense mat of microorganisms which, when Gram stained, appears to be knitted together by filamentous organisms enmeshing cocci and bacilli. However, the role of filamentous bacteria in periodontal disease is unclear.

Calcification of bacterial plaque forms calculus, which can be identified in decalcified sections by its layered structure and a typically yellowish tinge in haematoxylin and eosin stained preparations.

Calculus forms initially on the crowns of teeth, particularly on the lower teeth adjacent to the ducts of the submandibular glands whose secretions have a high calcium content. Once pockets have formed round the teeth, plaque continues to be deposited on the root surfaces and in this site inflammatory exudate and extravasated blood cells from the pocket wall contribute to its composition. This subgingival plaque can also become calcified and forms an additional factor preventing healing of periodontal tissue damage.

Gingivitis is characterized by inflammation restricted to the gingival margins. The inflammatory infiltrate is dense and is mainly mononuclear in character, often with a predominance of plasma cells. The inflammatory infiltrate is contiguous with and limited to the vicinity of the bacterial plaque, which can be seen on the tooth surfaces as a dense mat of organisms among which filamentous forms are conspicuous (Fig. 2.11).

The epithelial attachment where the gingival epithelium adjoins the tooth surface is strongly

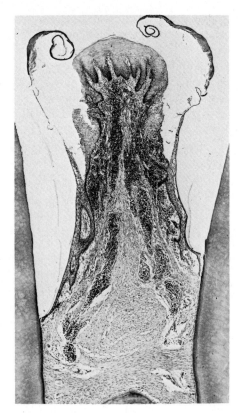

Fig. 2.11 Chronic gingivitis. The interdental papilla has become densely infiltrated with chronic inflammatory cells but the deeper tissues (the periodontal ligament and alveolar bone) are unaffected.

Haematoxylin-eosin   × 40

adherent to the latter and forms a mechanical seal protecting the underlying tissue. In the normal state the epithelial attachment is on the enamel or at the amelocemental junction and remains at this level until periodontitis develops.

Periodontitis is characterized by the following changes:

1. Gingivitis
2. Destruction of periodontal ligament fibres
3. Resorption of the alveolar bone from the crest towards the root
4. Rootward migration of the epithelial attachment
5. Formation of pockets between the tooth and the gingival soft tissue (Fig. 2.12).

The result, in most patients, is slowly progressive but inexorable destruction of the tissues supporting the teeth until they become so mobile as to make mastication increasingly difficult. Natural exfoliation is usually forestalled by extraction of the increasingly uncomfortable and useless teeth. The process is otherwise asymptomatic.

The inflammatory changes in chronic periodontitis remain sharply localized to the immediate vicinity of the bacterial plaque which, as pockets form, extends *pari passu* in a rootward direction. In the protected environment of the pockets, proliferation of bacteria proceeds unhampered save

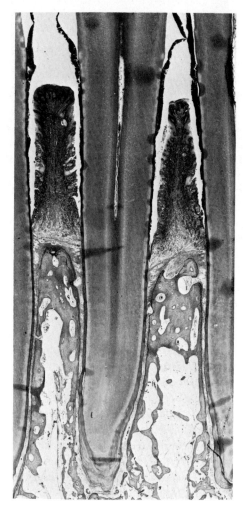

Fig. 2.12 Chronic periodontitis. Destruction of the periodontal ligament and alveolar bone has progressed. In addition, pockets filled with bacterial plaque have formed between the surviving gingiva and the tooth surface. Inflammatory changes are, however, restricted to the soft tissues of the interdental papilla.

Haematoxylin-eosin   × 15

by competition for nutrients and by the activity of phagocytic cells which migrate through the pocket wall.

Below the level of the pocket floor there is a zone free from inflammatory cells and none of the latter invest the more superficial of the remaining periodontal ligament fibres of the crest of the alveolar bone. This absence of leukocytes from the zone of tissue destruction tends to make the concept of immunologically-mediated tissue destruction difficult to credit (Fig. 2.12).

It may be worth noting, incidentally, that few people have access to any significant amounts of suitable autopsy material to study the microscopic features of this common condition, and many statements about its histopathology are based on assumption rather than observation.

The mechanism of destruction of the alveolar bone appears mainly to depend on humoral factors, as osteoblasts or even Howship's lacunae are rarely seen (Fig. 2.13). Though the fibres of the periodontal ligament are progressively destroyed, the connective tissue of the immediately adjacent gingiva survives and the gingival epithelium grows downwards to line the pocket thus formed. This epithelium retains its attachment to the tooth and thus also forms the floor of the pocket.

An enclosed, protected environment favourable to the proliferation of bacteria is thus created and, once pockets have formed, the disease is self-perpetuating. In view of the vast numbers of bacteria harboured in periodontal pockets, it is remarkable that in the average patient tissue destruction proceeds so slowly. Approximately one centimetre's depth of alveolar bone needs to be destroyed for the teeth to become loosened and, since gingivitis typically starts in childhood, the *average* rate of bone destruction in the majority of patients is no more than 0.2 mm a year. In view of the number of pathogens in direct contact with the tissues, the indolence of this disease process forms a remarkable tribute to the defensive powers of the immune response.

These periodontal bacteria are, incidentally, one source of infection in infective endocarditis and septicaemias in immunodepressed patients. Even in otherwise healthy persons these bacteria can also give rise to lung and brain abscesses if aspirated into the airways.

Juvenile periodontitis

Juvenile periodontitis ('periodontosis') is a rare form of early onset periodontal destruction which is typically rapidly progressive and can lead to loss of the teeth in early adolescence. Currently it is widely believed that in juvenile periodontitis and rapidly progressive periodontitis, an important contributory cause is *Actinobacillus actinomycetemcomitans* which is frequently found in these lesions and invades the periodontal connective tissue. It also secretes collagenase and other virulence factors which could contribute to tissue destruction. Elimination of this bacterium will sometimes greatly reduce tissue destruction. However, *Actinobacillus actinomycetemcomitans* is not invariably found in this condition and, in some cases, there may be a limited defect of cell-mediated immunity or of neutrophil function. Any such defect is of limited scope, however, since increased susceptibility to other infections is not generally associated.

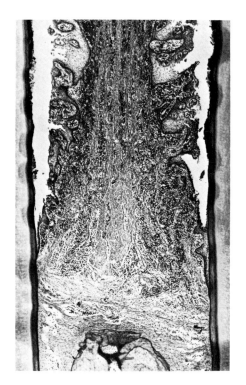

Fig. 2.13 Chronic periodontitis. Inflammatory cells are concentrated in the vicinity of the periodontal pocket and bacterial plaque. The alveolar bone, though greatly resorbed, is not involved in the inflammatory process.

Haematoxylin-eosin   × 50

Juvenile periodontitis can also be a prominent manifestation of systemic disorders, mainly as a result of immunodeficiency or defective collagen formation, as for example:

1. Uncontrolled diabetes mellitus (maturity onset type can also greatly accelerate periodontal destruction late in life)
2. Neutropenia (any cause)
3. Down's syndrome
4. Hyperkeratosis palmaris et plantaris (Papillon-Lefèvre syndrome)
5. Ehlers-Danlos syndrome (type VIII)
6. Histiocytosis X (see p. 44)
7. Hypophosphatasia. In this condition early loosening and exfoliation of the teeth may be the most prominent and sometimes the only sign. This is a result of failure of cementum formation and absence, therefore, of adequate anchorage of periodontal ligament fibres.

Acute ulcerative (Vincent's) gingivitis

Acute ulcerative gingivitis is an anaerobic infection of the gingivae. It was widespread particularly during the two World Wars but has declined sharply in incidence since then. Little is known of the aetiology; otherwise healthy young adults, particularly males, are predominantly affected, but the necrotic tissues are teeming with a fusospirochaetal complex which morphologically appears to be *Borrelia vincenti* and *Fusobacterium nucleatum*. Though this infection has been reported[10] in immunosuppressed children (who are otherwise exempt from this disease in the Western world) there is nothing to suggest that typical patients are in any way immunodeficient.

Clinically, the disease typically starts in dirty, neglected mouths and produces necrotizing ulceration at the tips of the interdental papillae, spreading along the gingival margins and, if untreated, extends deeply to destroy the interdental soft tissues and bone to leave triangular gaps between the teeth. Despite the rapidity of this destruction, patients typically remain otherwise well and there is rarely even lymphadenopathy.

Microscopically, there is a slough of necrotic material overlying tissue which is densely infiltrated by inflammatory cells and in which invading spirochaetes can be shown by electron microscopy. Direct Gram-stained smears show a characteristic picture dominated by Gram-negative spirochaetes and fusiform bacteria together with leukocytes. The infection responds rapidly to metronidazole.

Vincent's angina

This is a pharyngeal infection apparently caused by the same organisms responsible for ulcerative gingivitis (which may be associated) but causing necrotizing ulceration of the pharynx. This clinically resembles diphtheria but usually causes no significant systemic effects. Like ulcerative gingivitis, Vincent's angina was common among the armed forces in the War periods. An outbreak was reported among American troops in 1977[11] but it has apparently disappeared from Britain.

Cancrum oris

Cancrum oris has not been seen in Britain for many decades but has in more recent years been most often reported in children in West Africa. The infection appears to begin in a similar manner to Vincentiform gingivitis but the precise microbial cause and predisposing factors are unknown, apart from the likelihood that malnutrition is probably contributory.

Gingival fibromatosis

Fibrous hyperplasia of the gingivae is either familial or drug-induced.

By far the most important drugs causing gingival hyperplasia are phenytoin and, less frequently, cyclosporin and nifedipine. This type of hyperplasia predominantly affects the interdental papillae which become bulbous, overlap the labial and buccal surfaces of the teeth and can thus become contiguous.

The pathogenesis of phenytoin-induced hyperplasia, which affects 30–50% of patients on long-term treatment, possibly depends on the fact that (among its multifarious effects) phenytoin is a collagenase inhibitor. The mechanism of other drug-induced gingival hyperplasias is unknown.

The most common type of familial gingival hyperplasia is the syndrome of gingival hyperplasia, hypertrichosis, epilepsy and mental retardation. In this disorder, inherited as an autosomal dominant, the fibrous overgrowth of the gums starts typically before the eruption of the teeth, which as a consequence may appear to fail to erupt since only their extreme tips may be visible through the thickened gums. The gingival hyperplasia also differs from the drug-induced type in that it affects the entire gingival margin so that the whole of the alveolar ridge becomes uniformly thickened. The edentulous mouth can also be affected. In addition to the hypertrichosis there can be gross thickening of the facial features, indistinguishable at first glance from that of acromegaly. Epilepsy is uncommon (there appears to be no information on the effects on the gums if such patients are treated with phenytoin) and mental defect is rare.

Although hypertrichosis is a regular feature of this genetic syndrome it is also another side-effect of phenytoin and more strikingly of cyclosporin. No mechanism has been suggested for the association between fibrous gingival hyperplasia and hypertrichosis.

Histopathology

There appears to be no significant difference in the microscopic appearances of these different types of gingival hyperplasia. There is massive proliferation of fibrous connective tissue but because of the continuity between the periosteum and papillary corium in the attached gingiva, the rete ridges tend to be slender and elongated since they are compressed by connective tissue. Despite the deep pockets formed round the teeth by the hyperplastic connective tissue, inflammatory changes are frequently slight and may be virtually absent.

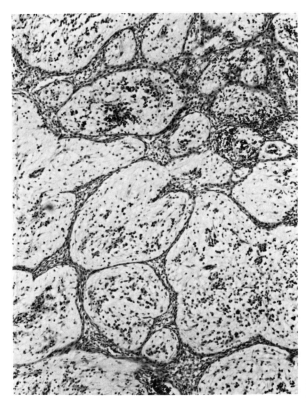

Fig. 2.14 Apical granuloma. A network of epithelium permeates the lesion.

Haematoxylin-eosin   × 40

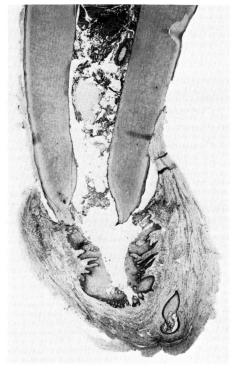

Fig. 2.15 Apical granuloma. A chronic inflammatory focus at the apex of a tooth, which has replaced the alveolar bone and contains a microcyst lined by hyperplastic squamous epithelium.

Haematoxylin-eosin   × 14

CYSTS OF THE ORAL TISSUES[12]

Cysts in the oral region arise from both dental and non-dental tissues. Odontogenic cysts comprise the radicular cyst which is of inflammatory origin, and several others of developmental origin. The non-odontogenic cysts are also of developmental or non-developmental origin.

ODONTOGENIC CYSTS

Radicular cyst (periapical cyst; dental cyst)

This is the most common of the odontogenic cysts and indeed of all the cysts that may appear in the mouth. It may appear at any age, although it is rare in children.

The radicular cyst originates in an apical granuloma (Fig. 2.14) and is thus the result of infection. It has already been noted that apical granulomas frequently become permeated by epithelium from epithelial rests. The central cells of a focus of this proliferating epithelium (Fig. 2.15) may undergo degeneration with the formation of a cavity, and in this way a cyst is formed.[13]

If small, radicular cysts may, like granulomas, adhere to the root of the tooth on extraction. Others form quite large lesions in the jaw and require separate operative intervention. Radicular cysts usually contain clear, amber fluid in which numerous cholesterol crystals may be found; sometimes the contents are a thicker, pultaceous material. The wall consists of fibrous tissue of variable thickness, with a lining of squamous epithelium. Chronic inflammation is practically always present and there is usually considerable epithelial proliferation, forming a relatively thick, irregular, squamous lining, with many epithelial processes penetrating the underlying connective tissue (Fig. 2.16). Clefts at the site of cholesterol crystals, dissolved during histological processing, are frequently to be seen, both in the wall of the cyst and in its inspissated contents; they are often surrounded by foreign body giant cells. Lipid-laden histiocytes (foam cells) are often numerous. Occasionally, cysts in the maxilla may be lined by epithelium of respiratory type.

Radicular cysts may persist in the jaws almost indefinitely, increasing very slowly in size until they produce an obvious swelling. Not infrequently, however, acute infection supervenes, with pain, increased swelling and suppuration.

Dentigerous cyst (follicular cyst)[14]

The dentigerous cyst arises in connection with the enamel organ and is thus developmental in origin. In most cases the cystic change takes place when the enamel has more or less completely formed and the enamel organ has been reduced to the thin layer of epithelial cells that remains over the crown of the tooth. Fluid forms in this layer, or between it and the enamel, and this produces a cyst into which the crown of the tooth protrudes. Dentigerous cysts are much less common than radicular cysts. They are the most common type of jaw cyst in children but overall are more common in adults, and show the highest incidence between the ages of 20 and 50. These cysts are particularly associated with the maxillary canine and mandibular third molar teeth. They may enlarge to a considerable size. Structurally, the dentigerous cyst is similar to the radicular cyst, with a wall of fibrous tissue lined by stratified squamous epithelium, though this is typically flat rather than irregular or arcaded. However, the chronic inflammatory changes seen so characteristically in the radicular cyst are generally absent, except when the dentigerous cyst has opened into the mouth (Fig. 2.17).

Odontogenic keratocyst (primordial cyst)

The odontogenic keratocyst, like the dentigerous cyst, arises in connection with the tooth-forming epithelium. It may possibly arise from the enamel organ itself, at an early stage before enamel has begun to form, as in the tooth germ at the left in Figure 2.2 (p. 55). Cystic change in the area of the stellate cells causes them to disintegrate and leave a cystic space bounded by the peripheral layer of enamel epithelium, which comes to be of stratified squamous type. As a tooth cannot now develop, the keratocyst takes its place; most commonly the missing tooth is a mandibular third molar. In other, and more frequent, instances, the keratocyst has no special relation to any tooth: in such cases

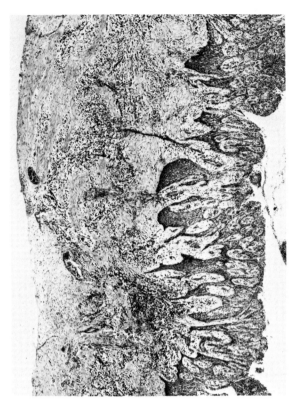

Fig. 2.16 Radicular cyst. The cyst wall consists of fibrous tissue lined by stratified squamous epithelium, and shows chronic inflammatory infiltration.

Haematoxylin-eosin   × 40

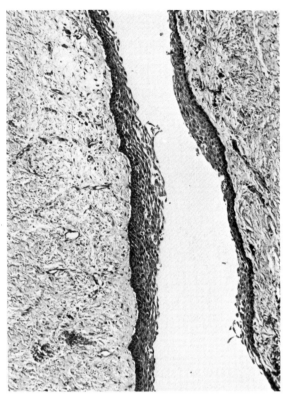

Fig. 2.17 Dentigerous cyst. The lining is a layer of stratified squamous epithelium, fairly uniform in thickness. There is no inflammatory infiltrate.

Haematoxylin-eosin   × 80

it has probably arisen from the germ of a supernumerary tooth or from the dental lamina (see p. 54).

The keratocyst is normally found in older adults, probably because its growth is slow, allowing it to remain undetected for many years. In time, it may become quite large, but it tends to infiltrate the cancellous bone rather than expand the jaw. Radiologically, there is a well-defined area of radiolucency in the jaw: if the cyst is large and of irregular shape, the defect may appear multiloculated, thus simulating an ameloblastoma.

The lining of a keratocyst is a relatively thin and regular layer of stratified squamous epithelium. The basal layer is typically very distinct since its nuclei stain quite intensely. There is nearly always some degree of keratinization although this is very often of minor degree. Gross keratinization, as for example in an epidermoid cyst, is present in only a minority. As in the dentigerous cyst, inflammatory

infiltration is generally absent (Fig. 2.18). If, however, infection supervenes, inflammatory changes can destroy the characteristic appearances of the epithelial lining of these cysts with the result that they can become indistinguishable from a periodontal cyst. A search of the remainder of the lining is therefore necessary in the hope of finding residual uninflamed areas where the characteristic features of keratocyst lining remain.

Unlike other oral cysts the epithelial lining of the keratocyst tends to separate rather easily from the underlying connective tissue: while this may partly be artefactual, it is also possible that the epithelium may separate readily during operation, and this may account for the frequency of recurrence, which is much greater than for other types of cysts of dental tissues. The rate of recurrence of keratocysts after surgical removal ranges from 6–60% in different published series.[15]

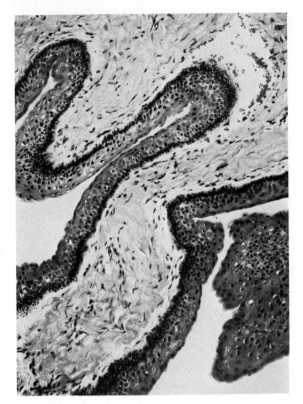

Fig. 2.18 Keratocyst. The cyst is lined by a thin, regular layer of keratin-forming squamous epithelium. There is no inflammation.

Haematoxylin-eosin   × 100

Multiple keratocysts and basal cell carcinomas (Gorlin-Goltz syndrome)[16]

Multiple keratocysts are associated with multiple basal cell carcinomas of the skin as a familial syndrome (the Gorlin-Goltz syndrome). Other abnormalities that may be present in this condition include bifurcation of ribs and other skeletal abnormalities, a characteristic facies with parietal and frontal bossing, calcification of the falx cerebri, ocular defects and occasionally mental retardation.

NON-ODONTOGENIC CYSTS

Developmental facial and jaw cysts[12]

Cysts may appear in those areas where, during the development of the face and jaws, the embryonic facial and other processes were in contiguity. It is presumed that such cysts have arisen in epithelial rests at these sites, but there is considerable doubt as to the real nature and aetiology of many of them. Lesions in this category include cysts at or near the midline of the palate (nasopalatine cyst, median palatal cyst), the midline of the mandible (median mandibular cyst), the nasolabial fold (nasolabial or nasoalveolar cyst) and the lateral incisor-canine region (globulomaxillary cyst).

These cysts are usually lined by squamous epithelium, though the nasopalatine may be lined at least in part by respiratory type epithelium. They do not generally attain any great size, and can be eradicated by simple enucleation.

Dermoid cyst

Dermoid cysts may form in the floor of the mouth. They are lined by stratified squamous epithelium and may contain sebaceous glands, sweat glands, hair follicles and occasionally other tissues in the cyst wall.[17]

Thyroglossal cyst

The remnants of the thyroglossal duct, which in embryonic life runs from the base of the tongue to the thyroid gland, may give rise to cysts. They may originate at any point, those above the level of the hyoid bone often being lined by squamous epithelium and those below this level by columnar epithelium. Both types of lining may be present in the same cyst.

Lympho-epithelial cyst

Cysts lined by squamous or in part by columnar epithelium with a subjacent layer of lymphoid tissue may be found, often incidentally since they are frequently asymptomatic, in the floor of the mouth, the tongue, or less often elsewhere in the oral tissues. They are similar to the branchial cysts of the neck.[18]

Bone cysts

Solitary bone cyst (traumatic cyst; haemorrhagic cyst) is seen most often in the humerus. Infrequently, it may form in the jaws, where it appears as a circumscribed cavity with a thin connective tissue lining and containing a small amount of fluid, sometimes blood-stained[19].

Aneurysmal bone cyst affects particularly the long bones and vertebrae. It is rare in the jaws. Like the lesions in other bones, jaw cysts contain blood and connective tissues in which there are numerous capillaries and larger blood-filled spaces. Multi-nucleated giant cells are usually numerous and areas of osteoid may be seen. In a significant proportion of these lesions in the jaws there are also other lesions of bone, including fibrous dysplasia, ossifying fibroma or giant cell granuloma[20].

Salivary cysts

These cysts are discussed in Chapter 3.

TUMOURS[21]

Tumours of the mouth and jaws are relatively common, although many of the lesions that are often included under this general designation are not neoplasms but are hyperplastic or other non-neoplastic tumour-like proliferations. These are generally readily recognized both clinically and pathologically, although debatable or borderline lesions are inevitably encountered from time to time. These non-neoplastic tumour-like lesions are considered here together with the neoplasms.

Another basic distinction is between those tumours that arise from the dental tissues—the odontogenic tumours—and those that arise from other tissues of the oral region. The odontogenic tumours all have some resemblance, in varying degree, to the developing dental tissues, and practically all of them are benign or, at most, locally aggressive.[22] Nevertheless, situated as they are in an area that creates many problems for the surgeon because of the close proximity of vital structures, together with the need to use procedures that are as conservative as possible so as to lead to the minimum of disfigurement, accurate diagnosis is essential.[14] The non-odontogenic tumours of the oral region resemble their counterparts elsewhere in the body, although there are often special features related to their site.

ODONTOGENIC TUMOURS

Ameloblastoma (adamantinoma)

This tumour arises as an intra-osseous growth, much more commonly in the mandible (80% of cases) than in the maxilla, appearing most often in the third and fourth decades. The molar region is the most frequent location. Its origin is from dental epithelium, the enamel organ itself or its epithelial residues, or in some cases possibly the basal layer of the oral epithelium, although this is not a widely held view. It is also thought that the tumour may sometimes arise in a dentigerous cyst, but this must be infrequent. However, some of the tumours present as cystic lesions that include a tooth, and they may thus resemble a dentigerous cyst clinically and radiologically. Rarely, the tumour may be entirely intraosseous and in the gingiva.

Grossly, the tumour appears as a greyish-white solid mass replacing the bone and expanding it. In some case cystic areas may be present, sometimes conspicuously so, giving rise to a multilocular appearance. Microscopically, the tumour consists of follicles or islets of epithelial cells separated by a moderate amount of fibrous tissue.[21,22] The follicles have a structure somewhat similar to that of the enamel organ, since they consist of a central area of stellate cells resembling the stellate reticulum, with a peripheral row of cubical or columnar cells resembling ameloblasts. The follicles vary in size and shape. Degenerative changes in the stellate cells are common, and may result in cyst formation (Fig. 2.19). Sometimes the epithelium is arranged in a plexiform manner, in continuous interlacing strands rather than in discrete follicles (Fig. 2.20). Not infrequently follicular and plexiform growth patterns may be seen in the same tumour. Squamous metaplasia may sometimes be seen, usually in the central area of the follicles, but infrequently it may be so extensive as to involve large areas of the tumour. Tumours consisting almost entirely of squamous epithelium have been reported under the designation of *squamous odontogenic tumour*,[23] but the relationship, if any, of these very uncommon lesions to ameloblastoma is still problematical. Granular cells, similar to those of granular cell myoblastoma, may be present in ameloblastoma, in the stellate reticulum-like areas. There may be

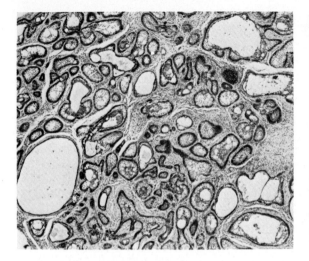

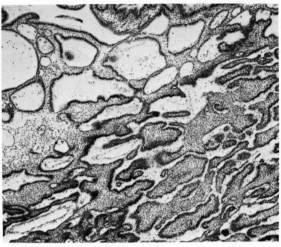

Fig. 2.19 Ameloblastoma. The follicular type of tumour, consisting of follicles or islets of epithelium in a fibrous stroma.

Haematoxylin-eosin   × 25

Fig. 2.20 Ameloblastoma. The plexiform pattern of growth, in which the tumour epithelium is disposed in continuous interlacing strands.

Haematoxylin-eosin   × 40

only small numbers of such cells, or they may be sufficiently numerous as to replace large areas of the tumour.

These histological variations do not appear to affect the course or prognosis of ameloblastoma. Rarely, however, tumours have grown more rapidly and behaved more aggressively than usual, and have shown cellular pleomorphism, mitotic activity and other histological features of malignancy. Such tumours, however, are exceedingly rare and almost certainly some that have been described as malignant ameloblastoma have been squamous or other carcinomas, which can sometimes have some superficial resemblance to ameloblastoma.[24]

Ameloblastoma is a slowly growing tumour that although mainly expansive is also locally invasive; this results in a pronounced tendency to local recurrence if treated by such measures as curettage. Excision of the tumour with a surrounding margin of normal tissue is therefore the appropriate treatment and effects a cure. In the mandible this can often be done while at the same time preserving the continuity of the lower border of the bone, since the tumour spreads much more readily through cancellous bone than through the compact bone of the cortex. The much less common maxillary tumours are more difficult to deal with,

the bony walls being thinner and the general anatomical arrangement being more complex than in the mandible. The monocystic tumours that appear clinically and radiologically as dentigerous cysts, and that are seen more often in children and adolescents, are possibly in a different category with respect to treatment. There is evidence that tumours of this type need rather less radical surgery than the usual type of tumour.[25]

The differential histological diagnosis of ameloblastoma includes other odontogenic tumours, salivary gland tumours and other non-odontogenic neoplasms. Since some odontogenic tumours or hamartomatous lesions such as adenomatoid odontogenic tumour or the odontomes are of limited growth potential, erroneous diagnosis could result in insufficiently radical treatment for an ameloblastoma. Confusion with a salivary tumour, most probably adenoid cystic carcinoma, might have the opposite effect. The possibility that a tumour of the jaws or of the soft tissues might be a metastasis from an as yet undiscovered primary growth should always be kept in mind. Lesions of this nature have on occasion been mistaken for ameloblastoma. Non-neoplastic epithelial proliferation such as takes place occasionally in the walls of odontogenic cysts may sometimes suggest ameloblastoma.

Ameloblastoma rarely metastasizes. In most of

the cases in which this has been reported there was a history of repeated local recurrences and consequent treatment, and the metastases have been pulmonary, due almost certainly to aspiration. More distant haematogenous metastases are very rare indeed.

Tumours with some histological resemblance to ameloblastoma are found occasionally in long bones, particularly the tibia (the so-called 'adamantinoma of the tibia'). Although these tumours have been described as ameloblastomas, it is now generally agreed that they are not related to the tumour of the jaws. The histological resemblance is coincidental and usually slight.

The craniopharyngioma, which arises in the region of the pituitary gland from remnants of the hypophyseal recess (Rathke's pouch), is also structurally similar to the ameloblastoma. As the hypophyseal recess develops from stomatodeal ectoderm, it has sometimes been thought that these two varieties of tumour may be related: this view is not generally supported.

Adenomatoid odontogenic tumour

This tumour is seen mainly in adolescents and young adults, more often in the maxilla than in the mandible and usually in the lateral incisor, canine or premolar region. It is often associated with an unerupted tooth and since it frequently produces a well-demarcated area of radiolucency in association with such a tooth, the clinical diagnosis is usually dentigerous cyst.[26]

Most of these tumours are quite small and they are generally removed completely. The growth has a fibrous capsule and there may be one or more associated cysts. Microscopically, the characteristic feature is the presence of tubule-like structures composed of columnar cells enclosing a central space that generally contains a small amount of homogeneous eosinophil material (Fig. 2.21). As well as forming tubule-like structures the columnar cells are also arranged in bands composed of double rows of the cells. These would appear to represent tubule-like structures that have not yet expanded to include a central space. Smaller ovoid or spindle cells, disposed in whorls between the pseudotubules and bands of columnar cells, form the remainder of the tumour, together with a scanty connective-

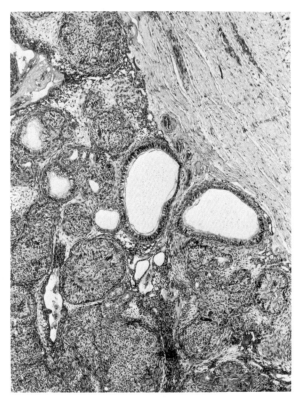

Fig. 2.21 Adenomatoid odontogenic tumour. Duct-like structures are a feature of this tumour.

Haematoxylin-eosin   × 40

tissue stroma and the frequent presence of small areas of calcification. The apparently tubular structures in the tumour led to the former designation adenoameloblastoma, the lesion being assumed to be a variant of ameloblastoma with glandular differentiation. It is now considered that the glandular appearance is fortuitous and that the tumour is not a variant of the ameloblastoma. Its behaviour is also quite different from that of ameloblastoma: the adenomatoid odontogenic tumour is not invasive and does not tend to recur. Simple enucleation is generally curative.

Calcifying epithelial odontogenic tumour

As its name implies, a characteristic feature of this tumour is the presence of more or less extensive areas of calcification, although variants with little or no calcification are relatively common. The tumour appears in the mandible more often than in the maxilla, usually in the premolar region, giving rise to a progressive swelling. There is often an associated unerupted tooth.[27]

Macroscopically, the calcifying epithelial odontogenic tumour may appear well circumscribed or it may be obviously invasive. Microscopically, it consists of sheets and strands of polyhedral cells with eosinophilic cytoplasm. Nuclear pleomorphism is a feature and giant nuclei are often present but mitotic figures are rare. Cases of this type have sometimes been diagnosed as squamous cell carcinoma. The stroma often has areas of homogeneous hyaline appearance, which give the reactions of amyloid. This amyloid or amyloid-like material appears to be the matrix in which the calcification that is so striking a feature of the tumour takes place. The calcium is laid down concentrically round and in the epithelial cells; large masses may form in this way (Fig. 2.22).

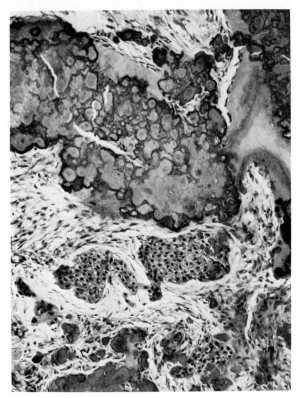

Fig. 2.22 Calcifying epithelial odontogenic tumour. The tumour consists of epithelial strands and sheets of variable size in a fibrous stroma. Concentrically calcified masses are characteristic of its structure.

Haematoxylin-eosin   × 100

In the non-calcifying variant of the tumour the epithelial element is similar to that in the calcifying tumour, but calcification is minimal or absent. In another variant the tumour cells have completely clear cytoplasm, and if a large area of the tumour has this appearance the diagnosis may be difficult. However, with thorough examination, more typical areas may be found.

Excision of the tumour with a margin of surrounding normal tissue should be curative; incomplete removal is likely to be followed by recurrence.

Calcifying odontogenic cyst

Like other odontogenic tumours this lesion generally produces a slowly progressive, usually painless, swelling of the jaw. The mandible is involved more often than the maxilla and the most common site is the molar-premolar area. In an appreciable number of cases the lesion is extra-osseous, being situated in the gingival tissues.[28] It is frequently cystic but may be solid. The name, calcifying odontogenic cyst, is not always appropriate, therefore, and has the further disadvantage that it may lead to confusion with the calcifying odontogenic epithelial tumour.

Microscopically, the cavity, which may be potential only, is lined by epithelium very similar to that of the ameloblastoma (Fig. 2.23). A characteristic feature is the presence of 'ghost' cells, similar to those seen in the calcifying epithelioma of Malherbe. These ghost cells are epithelial cells that have undergone an aberrant type of keratinization—the keratin stains poorly and the outlines of the cells are indistinct. The keratin gains access to the adjacent supporting fibrous tissue, where it excites a foreign body reaction, with numerous multinucleated giant cells. Calcification may be seen, both in the stroma and in the tumour cells, but not usually to any great degree.

The lesion is benign. Enucleation is generally sufficient treatment.

Ameloblastic fibroma

The ameloblastic fibroma is a rare benign tumour that consists of epithelial and connective tissue

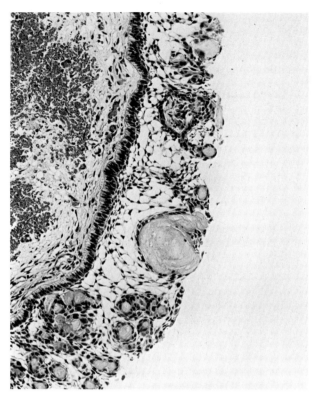

Fig. 2.23 Calcifying odontogenic cyst. The cyst is lined by epithelium resembling that of ameloblastoma. Some of the cells show aberrant keratinization ('ghost' cells) : this is a characteristic feature.

Haematoxylin-eosin   × 100

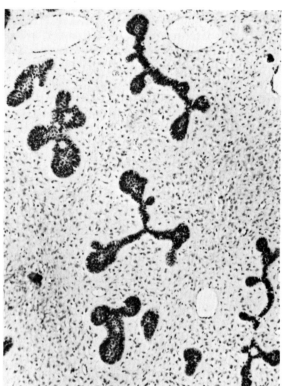

Fig. 2.24 Ameloblastic fibroma. The tumour consists of irregularly branching islets of epithelial cells in a cellular fibroblastic tissue.

Haematoxylin-eosin   × 80

derived from the corresponding elements of the dental primordium. It is generally seen in children or young adults, in the mandible more often than the maxilla and usually in the canine-molar region. It may be associated with an unerupted tooth. Growth is slow, with gradual, painless expansion of the jaw.[29]

Macroscopically, the tumour is circumscribed and well defined. Microscopically, it consists of epithelial follicles, somewhat similar to those of the ameloblastoma, set in very cellular fibroblastic tissue that resembles the papilla of the developing tooth (Fig. 2.24). Foci of dentine may be present. Tumours in which this is a prominent feature have been termed ameloblastic fibro-odontoma.

Although ameloblastic fibroma is a benign tumour, recurrence after local removal has been reported in an appreciable number of cases. However, it is probable in many of these cases that removal was not complete, and the well-circumscribed appearance of the tumour may have encouraged enucleation or other procedures that cannot be relied upon to remove all tumour tissue.

Ameloblastic fibrosarcoma

This rare tumour resembles ameloblastic fibroma in consisting of epithelial strands and follicles in a cellular fibroblastic tissue. However, while the epithelial component is not greatly different from that in ameloblastic fibroma, the fibroblastic element contains numerous pleomorphic cells with many mitoses. Tumour giant cells are also present. Although this tumour appears to be of relatively low-grade malignancy, with metastases being very rare, it can show pronounced local invasive activity.[30]

Odontoma

Odontomas are hamartomatous lesions that consist mainly of fully formed enamel and dentine. The *compound odontome* consists of small teeth ('denticles') in a fibrous capsule, while the *complex odontome* is a tumour-like mass of enamel, dentine, cementum and connective tissue arranged in a quite irregular manner, although the normal relationship of these tissues to each other is nevertheless preserved (Fig. 2.25).

During the period of active growth ameloblastic epithelium and odontoblasts are present, but when growth has ceased these cellular elements atrophy, leaving only the calcified dental tissues together with connective tissue. Both the compound and the complex odontome appear as hard masses in the jaw and are usually discovered during childhood. When found in adults, they have been present since childhood. The odontomes are devel-

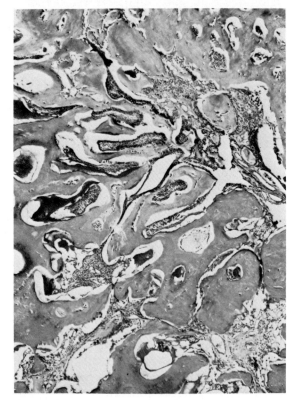

Fig. 2.25 Complex odontome. The lesion consists of irregularly arranged masses of dentine and cementum in a fibrous matrix. Enamel, lost in the process of decalcification, formerly occupied the clear spaces.

Haematoxylin-eosin   × 40

opmental anomalies of the teeth and are not neoplasms. They cease to enlarge when the development of the normal teeth has been completed, but they may erupt and can become infected.[31]

Odontogenic fibroma and myxoma

Although tumorous lesions of fibrous tissue are frequent in the soft tissues of the mouth, they are much less common in the jaws. Some of the fibromas that are found in the jaws are comparable to fibromas arising in other bones: there is also a specific type of fibroma that is almost certainly of dental origin. This tumour, the odontogenic fibroma, generally appears in childhood or early adult life and is frequently related to unerupted or missing teeth. It causes expansion of the jaw and consists of fibroblastic connective tissue, often very similar in appearance to the developing dental pulp. Sometimes appreciable amounts of collagen are formed: in other cases the tissue appears myxomatoid. Accordingly, these odontogenic tumours are often referred to as fibromas, fibromyxomas and myxomas, as best corresponds with their structure.[32] In addition to the connective-tissue element, groups and strands of epithelial cells may also be present (Fig. 2.26).

Cementomas

The term cementoma has been applied to a variety of tumours and tumour-like conditions characterized by the presence of cementum or cementum-like tissue.[21,22,33]

Periapical cemental dysplasia

Small masses consisting of cementum or cementum-like tissue are found quite commonly in the apical region of teeth, particularly anterior mandibular teeth. They are often multiple and are found most frequently in women who are past the menopause. They are usually symptomless, generally being detected in the course of radiological examination.

Cementoblastoma

This solitary lesion develops in connection with a premolar or molar tooth, usually in the mandible, and is seen most often in adolescent and young adult males. Unlike the multiple periapical lesions mentioned above, the cementoblastoma forms a

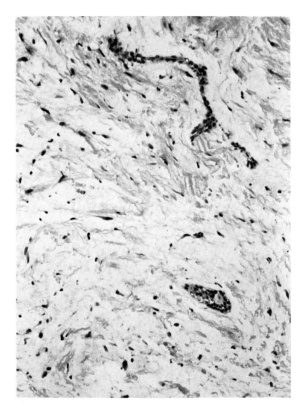

Fig. 2.26 Odontogenic fibromyxoma. Strands of odontogenic epithelial cells are present in a fibromyxomatous matrix.

Haematoxylin-eosin   × 100

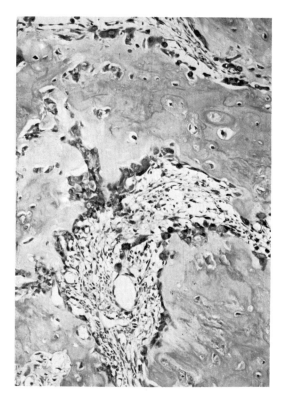

Fig. 2.27 Cementoblastoma, showing the mass of cementum-like tissue with numerous osteoblast-like cells that surrounded the root of a tooth.

Haematoxylin-eosin   × 100

mass of hard tissue around the root of the affected tooth and in time causes expansion of the jaw. The tumour is usually removed complete with the related tooth and is seen to consist of a mass of calcified cementum-like tissue with deeply-stained reversal lines. The cementum has been laid down in vascular connective tissue which generally still persists in places and contains osteoblast-like cells. These may be numerous, large and hyperchromatic in actively growing areas, but there is little pleomorphism, and mitoses are not seen (Fig. 2.27).

Cementoblastoma is a benign tumour. It can usually be enucleated without difficulty; recurrence is rare.[34]

Gigantiform cementoma

This cemental lesion is characteristically multiple, appearing most often in middle-aged women, especially negroes, and there may be a familial incidence. The lesions produce swellings of the jaw which, although the rate of growth is slow, can in time become large. They consist of dense irregular masses of cementum in which many empty lacunae may be seen.[35]

NON-ODONTOGENIC TUMOURS

Epidermoid tumours

Squamous papilloma

Papillomas may appear anywhere in the mouth, and show the usual macroscopic and microscopic features.[36] They are generally solitary, but multiple lesions are occasionally seen, sometimes concomitantly with verruca vulgaris of the skin. Multiple papillomatous lesions may also appear in *Down's syndrome* and in certain rarer syndromes. In *naevus unius lateris* there are multiple papillomas in the skin of the limbs and trunk on one side of the body. When oral papillomas are present they practically always affect the left side. Various dental abnormalities may be associated. In *Cowden's multiple hamartoma syndrome* papillomas may appear in the oral tissues. In *focal dermal hypoplasia* there is atrophy of the skin and other defects, including syndactyly, ocular abnormalities and microcephaly. Multiple papillomas may be present on the skin and mucosae, including the oral mucosa. Abnormalities of the teeth are also common.

In the infrequent condition of *papillary hyperplasia*, papillary growths of the palate are very numerous and may be almost confluent. The resulting warty growth may present an alarming appearance but there is no tendency to malignant change. The condition is often associated with a poorly-fitting denture but can appear in its absence.[37]

Squamous carcinoma

This is the most common malignant tumour of the mouth, accounting for nearly 90% of all malignant growths of the oral mucosa and adjacent tissues.[38] The majority of patients are middle-aged or elderly, and men are more commonly affected than women. In carcinoma of the lip the sex difference is pronounced, although there is wide international variation. In Britain the male–female ratio is nearly 10:1, but the ratio for other oral sites is much lower, and has been diminishing over the past few decades, due to a decline in the general incidence of oral cancer in men while the incidence in women has not changed to any great extent.

Smoking and spirit drinking are important aetiological factors in some parts of the world, the combination appearing to be particularly potent. Despite this belief it is noteworthy that in Britain, where reliable figures for both the incidence of and mortality from oral cancer are available on a national scale, the disease has steadily declined since about 1920. This decline in the incidence of oral cancer has been associated with a great increase in cigarette smoking and of alcohol consumption, and of other diseases known to be associated with these habits. The role of cigarette smoking and of alcohol in the aetiology of oral cancer is, in Britain at least, somewhat questionable.

Surveys have also shown that in other countries oral leukoplakias in non-smokers show a higher frequency of malignant change than such lesions in smokers (p. 32).

Syphilitic glossitis was formerly an important cause, as has already been mentioned (p. 35). Long-standing dental infection and poor oral hygiene may also be factors.

Oral cancer is a very frequent form of malignant disease in India, Sri Lanka and some other eastern countries. This is very probably due to habits such as betel-nut chewing and reversed smoking (smoking with the lighted end of the cigarette inside the mouth). In the case of betel chewing it is probably the tobacco, and possibly the slaked lime and other ingredients of the quid, that are carcinogenic rather than betel (the leaves of *Piper betle*) or the areca nut.

Long continued exposure to sunlight predisposes to carcinoma of the lip in fair-skinned people, and in countries where a large proportion of the white population are engaged in outdoor occupations such as fishing and farming this type of oral cancer accounts for a relatively high proportion of all cancers.

Other possible aetiological factors in oral cancer include some lesions of the oral mucosa, but although malignancy may indeed follow some of them, this happens very infrequently. These conditions include herpes simplex, lichen planus, discoid lupus erythematosus and candidosis. The *Kelly-Paterson syndrome* (*Plummer-Vinson syndrome*) has been more often associated with carcinoma. The syndrome almost solely affects women and is characterized by iron deficiency anaemia, achlorhydria and dysphagia. There is atrophy of the lingual mucosa, atrophic pharyngitis and atrophic gastritis. Squamous carcinoma has been reported in a significant proportion of such patients, the usual site being at the junction of the pharynx and oesophagus (post-cricoid region); in some cases the carcinoma develops in the mouth.

Carcinoma of the lip

Cancer of the lip begins as a small ulcer, fissure or warty protuberance on the external mucosal surface. The early lesion may have a deceptively insignificant appearance: it is therefore a wise rule that all such lesions that do not heal within three to four weeks should be examined histologically. The majority of the tumours are well differentiated (Fig. 2.28). Anaplastic growths are rare.

Carcinoma of the lip has a more favourable outlook than any other type of oral cancer. It is, or should be, diagnosed early, since it affects a visible and easily accessible surface. It metastasizes to the regional lymph nodes less frequently, and at a later stage, than tumours arising within the mouth. The submandibular and submental lymph nodes are usually the first to be involved, followed by the upper deep cervical nodes.

In neglected cases there is ultimately great destruction locally. Visceral metastases appear in some of these cases, but death from aspiration pneumonia or from haemorrhage caused by invasion of a large blood vessel in the ulcerated area often supervenes before metastases have spread widely.

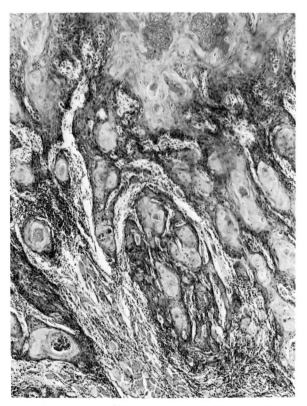

Fig. 2.28 Squamous cell carcinoma. A well-differentiated tumour, with prominent keratinization.

Haematoxylin-eosin   × 40

Intra-oral squamous carcinoma

Squamous carcinoma within the mouth can affect the tongue, floor of the mouth, cheek, palate or gingiva. Tumours of the tongue usually arise on the lateral border of its middle third. The posterior third is the next most common site. The tip, ventral surface or, rarely, the dorsum may also be affected. Leukoplakia may be present. In the floor of the mouth, tumours are most common close to the midline: at first they may spread superficially rather than in depth, but more often a tumour in this region is deeply situated and appears at the surface only as an ulcerated fissure.

Carcinoma is more common in the soft palate than in the hard palate; occasionally the uvula is its site of origin.

Carcinoma of the buccal mucosa usually appears opposite the lower third molar tooth; in many of the cases there has been long-standing leukoplakia in this area. Carcinoma of the gingiva also affects most frequently the molar region, in the lower jaw more often than the upper. Intra-oral squamous carcinomas are usually well differentiated, whatever their site. However, their duration before they spread to lymph nodes and the stage at which the growth is detected vary. Tumours of the tongue tend to metastasize to the regional nodes very early, and they have the least favourable prognosis of all intra-oral squamous carcinomas. The prognosis for carcinoma varies from site to site within the mouth; the tongue has the lowest 5-year survival rate of 37% for men and 46% for women. For the latter, therefore, the prognosis of cancer of the mouth is worse than that for the breast which has a 5-year survival rate of about 57%.

Verrucous carcinoma

This type of squamous carcinoma is considered separately because it has a characteristic clinical course and gross and microscopic appearances.[39] It mainly affects those over the age of 60. Its sites include the buccal mucosa, gingivae, palate, tongue, tonsils and nasopharynx. Similar tumours arise in the larynx, glans penis, vagina, scrotum and perineum.

The tumour appears as a warty growth that enlarges only slowly, but ultimately invades adjoining tissues, including bone. The regional lymph nodes are often enlarged and tender, but this is usually due to infection and not to metastasis. Microscopically, the tumour is composed of very well-differentiated squamous epithelium, with minimal cellular atypia (Fig. 2.29). There is nearly always heavy chronic inflammatory infiltration of the adjacent connective tissue.

Because of the slow growth of the tumour and the absence or very late appearance of metastases, the prognosis is very good, provided that the lesion can be completely eradicated surgically. Local recurrence is common in inadequately treated patients. Radiotherapy is contra-indicated as it is frequently followed by local recurrence and by a change in the character of the tumour, which may become anaplastic and metastasize.

Spindle cell carcinoma

This variant of squamous cell carcinoma is seen (though rarely) in the oral mucosa, parotid glands, oesophagus, bronchi, uterine cervix and skin. Macroscopically, lesions of this type tend to be fleshy and polypoid; microscopically, they may be mistaken for sarcoma because of the predominance of spindle-shaped cells. Immunocytochemistry may be needed for confirmation of their epithelial origin. The prognosis of these tumours when they arise in the mouth may be relatively good, since metastasis is less frequent than in the more usual type of squamous carcinoma. However, this is not always the case.[40]

Basal cell carcinoma

Basal cell carcinoma is seen occasionally in the lip, nearly always the upper. The tumour has almost certainly arisen in skin, although it may be very close to, or have extended to involve, the muco-cutaneous area of the lip. It is questionable whether basal cell carcinoma ever arises intra-orally, although histologically similar tumours have been reported from various sites in the mouth. Such tumours cannot readily be distinguished from the rare extra-osseous ameloblastomas (p. 71).

Intra-osseous carcinoma

Carcinoma may appear as a wholly intra-osseous tumour in the jaw.[41] However, many tumours that would seem to be intra-osseous are found on further investigation to have arisen in adjacent tissues and to have involved the bone by subsequent extension. Alternatively, intra-osseous tumours may be metastatic deposits from distant primary growths. If such sources can be excluded, an intra-osseous carcinoma may have arisen from epithelial rests or from aberrant salivary tissue within the jaws, or from an odontogenic cyst. All these tumours are rare and require detailed clinicopathological investigation to determine their exact origin.

Multicentric carcinoma

Multicentric squamous carcinomas are not uncommon in the mouth, particularly in heavy smokers in some countries. Multiple primary tumours are found in about 10% of patients with oral cancer.

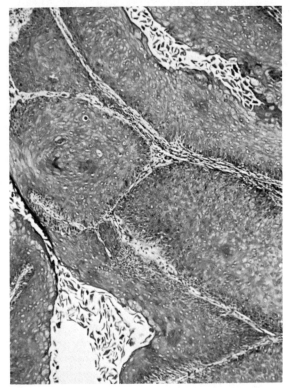

Fig. 2.29 Verrucous carcinoma. The tumour consists of well-differentiated epithelium

Haematoxylin-eosin   ×50

TUMOURS AND TUMOUR-LIKE LESIONS OF CONNECTIVE TISSUE

Fibrous growths

Fibrous growths of the soft tissues of the mouth are common. The majority are not true neoplasms, which are comparatively rare, but hyperplastic fibromatoids of inflammatory or irritative origin. For example, a nodule of fibrous tissue frequently forms in the cheek or tongue opposite the line of occlusion of the teeth, due to repeated biting of a fold of mucosa during mastication (Fig. 2.30) or to habitual sucking of mucosa into a gap in the dental arcade. In other cases small fibrous growths arise in relation to carious teeth or gingival calculus, or in the absence of any obvious cause.

When such lesions are on the gingivae they are often termed fibrous epulides (the name epulis signifies a growth 'on the gum').[42] Other synonyms for such growths on the gums and elsewhere include fibro-epithelial polyp and fibrous hyperplasia. The term 'fibroma' is also frequently, although usually inaccurately, employed.

All these lesions have similar microscopic appearances, consisting of bundles of collagen covered by stratified squamous epithelium. The epithelium is often acanthotic and keratinized. Gingival lesions are often more fibroblastic than those in other areas, and metaplastic formation of bone or cementoid tissue is not uncommon (Fig. 2.31).

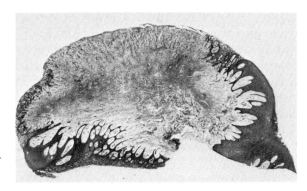

Fig. 2.31 Fibrous epulis. This gingival lesion consists of cellular fibrous tissue in which there are areas of metaplastic ossification. The covering epithelium is ulcerated over a wide area.

Haematoxylin-eosin   × 10

While most epulides are fibrous, a minority are giant cell or pyogenic granulomas and a few are metastatic tumours. These different entities may not be distinguishable clinically.

Lesions associated with irritation from dentures generally form in the buccal sulcus and are due to the flange of the denture pressing into the tissue and causing a groove, with overgrowth of the surrounding tissue to form a redundant mucosal flap.

Pyogenic granuloma

This lesion can appear anywhere in the oral mucosa but is most common in the gingivae and is similar to pyogenic granuloma of the skin.[43] It consists of very vascular fibrous and granulation tissue, often with superficial ulceration. It not infrequently appears during pregnancy. This 'pregnancy tumour' usually appears about the third month: it often grows rapidly, but seldom exceeds 1.5 cm in diameter. Once developed it may persist indefinitely until removed surgically, although occasionally it regresses spontaneously after childbirth. An identical lesion appears more rarely in women who are not pregnant and in men. Like the lesion of the skin, it is an inflammatory or reactive condition and not neoplastic.

Fibroma of the jaws

Odontogenic fibroma is described on page 76. Non-odontogenic fibroma, which arises from the

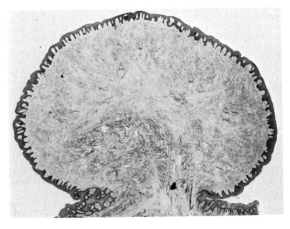

Fig. 2.30 A fibrous nodule of the buccal mucosa, the result of cheek biting.

Haematoxylin-eosin   × 5.5

mesenchyma of the jaw but is not necessarily related to the dental tissues, corresponds to the intra-osseous fibroma of other bones. It is not a bone-forming tumour and thus is distinct from the much more common fibrous lesions of the jaws in which there is also osteogenic activity and which fall into a different category. They are considered in the context of fibrous dysplasia (see below).

The non-odontogenic, or desmoplastic, fibroma appears especially in younger people up to the age of 30 and much more often in the mandible than the maxilla. The tumour is well defined and consists of fibroblasts and a prominent collagenous element. The fibroblasts are characteristically small, with narrow, elongated, well-stained nuclei. There is little or no mitotic activity. No bone is formed.[44]

Desmoplastic fibroma is a benign lesion and is adequately treated by complete excision.

Fibrosarcoma

This tumour is rare in the mouth. It may develop in the soft tissues or in the jaws.[45] Macroscopically and microscopically, it has the features of fibrosarcoma arising elsewhere in the body. Soft tissue tumours, which at first may clinically resemble the benign hyperplasias, tend to grow rapidly, ulcerate and infiltrate locally, but metastasis is uncommon. Intra-osseous tumours mainly involve the mandible, where they give rise to pain, swelling and loosening of the teeth. Again, local invasion is the principal feature, metastasis being unusual.

Fibrous histiocytoma

Tumours in this group are rare in the mouth. Although they have been noted in the soft tissues, in most of the reported cases the tumour has been intra-osseous. The macroscopic and microscopic features are as for comparable lesions elsewhere in the body.[46]

TUMOURS OF BONE

Osteoma

The osteomas are benign tumours that consist of cancellous or compact bone and increase in size by the continuous formation of bone. They are seen occasionally in the jaws, where they appear as hard, circumscribed lumps growing outward from the bone.[47]

Both types of osteoma, cancellous and compact, usually present as rounded or ovoid masses with a smooth or lobulated surface. The cut surface of the cancellous growths has the appearance of spongy bone while that of the compact osteomas is homogeneous and whitish-yellow like ivory. Microscopically, the cancellous osteomas are composed of trabeculae of lamellar bone with intervening fatty or fibrous marrow. The compact osteomas consist of dense lamellar bone with very little in the way of marrow spaces.

The *tori* are non-neoplastic bony overgrowths, histologically similar to compact osteoma. Torus mandibularis is a ridge or ridges of bone projecting symmetrically from the inner aspect of the mandible, and torus palatinus is a bony projection along the midline of the hard palate. These lesions may have a genetic basis. They are of very slow growth and do not usually cause any problems unless traumatized by a denture.

Osteoid osteoma and osteoblastoma

These tumours are rare in the jaws.[48] Cementoblastoma often closely resembles osteoblastoma histologically, but its association with a tooth is distinctive.

Osteosarcoma

Osteosarcoma is rare in the jaws. The prognosis is, however, rather better than in other bones, partly because it tends to metastasize later and because most tumours are mandibular, where radical excision can often be readily achieved.[49]

Fibrous dysplasia of bone and ossifying fibroma

Fibrous dysplasia may be characterized by involvement of various bones (polyostotic fibrous dysplasia) or there may be only a single lesion (monostotic fibrous dysplasia). In most cases of fibrous dysplasia of the jaws the lesion is solitary. Less often, there may be multiple jaw lesions: these may be accompanied by lesions in the skull. Least common is the association of lesions of the jaws with lesions of the trunk and limb bones. Like the lesions in other bones jaw lesions appear as gradually increasing swellings consisting of fibrous tissue that replaces the normal bone structure. Trabeculae of new bone appear in the fibrous tissue, forming slender, arcuate and branched structures. Jaw lesions tend to be more heavily ossified than those in other bones, the trabeculae being thicker and blunter[50].

Ossifying fibroma is the term used for lesions that may be identical microscopically to fibrous dysplasia but which are clearly circumscribed, whereas the lesions of fibrous dysplasia have indefinite edges, merging into the adjacent tissues. In addition, ossifying fibroma tends to show persistence of growth and may in time attain large dimensions, whereas the lesions of fibrous dysplasia cease to grow when skeletal maturity has been reached. However, ossifying fibroma can be enucleated with excellent results. The lesions of fibrous dysplasia are not usually treated, unless causing an unacceptable degree of facial asymmetry, until general bodily growth has been completed, as earlier treatment can be followed by renewed growth or recurrence.[51]

TUMOURS OF CARTILAGE

Chondroma and chondrosarcoma are rare in the jaws, where they show the usual histological features. Cartilaginous growths, however, are rather more common in the mandibular condyle[52] and the coronoid process, where they may interfere with jaw opening and cause pain.[53] Most of these lesions are hyperplasias and not neoplasms.

Islets of cartilage are occasionally seen in various areas of the oral tissues, including the palate, tongue, buccal mucosa and gingivae. Sometimes they appear to be related to poorly-fitting dentures.

TUMOURS OF VASCULAR TISSUE

Haemangiomas are more common in the region of the head and neck than in other parts of the body. Most of them are in the skin. Their appearance in the soft tissues of the oral cavity, although less common than in the skin, is not rare; in the jaws, as in other bones except the vertebrae and calvarium, they are very uncommon, but they are important because very severe haemorrhage, difficult to control, may complicate surgery (including dental extraction) of the affected part.[54,55] Haemangiomas in the oral tissues appear in the usual capillary and cavernous forms and may affect any part of the mucosa. They range from very small, pedunculated, globular growths to extensive lesions similar to the 'port-wine stains' of the skin and involving large areas of mucosa; they may be single or multiple.

Haemangiomas may feature in several characteristic syndromes, and not infrequently the patient complains only of the more obvious lesions, such as an angioma of the skin or of the oral mucosa. The possibility of lesions elsewhere should therefore be kept in mind whenever a haemangioma is diagnosed in any situation. The most common syndromes in which oral haemangiomas or vascular anomalies feature include hereditary haemorrhagic telangiectasia (Rendu-Osler-Weber syndrome), Sturge-Kalischer-Weber syndrome and Maffucci's syndrome.[56]

The localized areas of capillary dilatation that constitute the lesions in *hereditary haemorrhagic telangiectasia* affect the skin, particularly of the face, and various mucosae. Lesions of the nasal mucosa are common, and frequently give rise to recurrent bleeding. Epistaxis is the commonest symptom, and often the first, since it can start in early life before the cutaneous lesions appear, usually in the third decade or later. Haemorrhage from oral lesions is also common but is rarely severe. These lesions appear especially in the tongue and lips. The *Sturge-Kalischer-Weber syndrome* is characterized by naevus flammeus in the distribution of the trigeminal nerve, intracerebral angioma and calcification on the same side as the naevus and epileptiform seizures affecting the opposite side. In addition, angiomas may be present in the skin, in the oral and other mucosae and in internal organs. The oral angiomas may be situated anywhere in the mucosa but are most prominent when in the gingiva, since they result, in time, in gross enlargements that can almost cover the teeth. In *Maffucci's syndrome* the multiple haemangiomas that accompany the multiple chondromas are usually present in the skin but lesions may, rarely, also be present in the oral mucosa.

Lymphangioma

Lymphangiomas may develop in the lips, cheek or palate. They are most frequent in the tongue, being among the more common causes of macroglossia (see p. 2).

Angiosarcoma

Malignant vascular tumours are very rare in the oral and oropharyngeal region.[57] Kaposi's sarcoma is described on page 18.

TUMOURS OF NEURAL TISSUE

Neurilemmomas (Schwannomas) and neurofibromas occasionally arise in the mouth.[58] When solitary and arising in the soft tissues they appear clinically like the common fibrous growths described on pages 81 and 82. Macroscopically and microscopically, they show no unusual features. When solitary and arising within bone they are usually in the mandible; in this situation they may sometimes produce a rather characteristic radiographic picture. The area of radiolucency caused by the tumour, which would otherwise hardly be distinguishable from that resulting from several other intra-osseous tumours, may be continuous on each side with the enlarged mandibular canal.

The oral tissues are involved in neurofibromatosis in up to 10% of cases.[59] There may be only one or two tumours in the region, or large numbers may be present. Neurofibromatosis is a cause of macroglossia, which is usually unilateral. The condition is generally present at birth or appears in the first few years of life.

Neurosarcoma is rare.

Multiple neural tumours are also seen in the multiple endocrine neoplasia syndrome (type II). They may appear anywhere in the oral mucosa, but the tip of the tongue and the central area of the upper lip are most frequently involved.[60]

Melanotic neuro-ectodermal tumour. This appears in infants, usually between 1 and 3 months of age and much more often in the maxilla than in the mandible.[61] The tumour forms a rather ill-defined mass in the bone, typically of blue-black appearance. Microscopically, clefts and spaces in a fibrous stroma are lined by cubical cells with large pale nuclei and numerous granules of melanin in the cytoplasm. These cells also form solid groups. A second type of cell, small and round, with a well-stained nucleus that almost fills the cytoplasm, is also present, usually in groups in the clefts. These cells, which are often separated by a fine fibrillar matrix, do not contain pigment (Fig. 2.32).

The tumour is believed to derive from the neural crest. High levels of urinary catecholamine derivatives have been found in some cases. Usually complete excision of the tumour is curative. However, there have been cases which appeared typical in every way when first seen, but which have repeatedly recurred and finally metastasized widely.

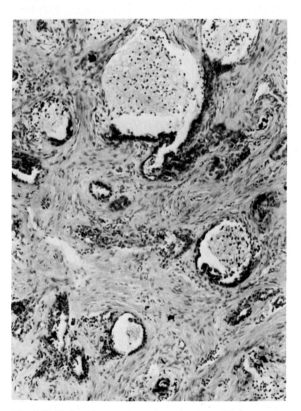

Fig. 2.32 Melanotic neuro-ectodermal tumour. The tumour consists of pigmented and non-pigmented cells in a fibrous stroma.

TUMOURS OF MUSCLE

These tumours are comparatively rare in the oral tissues. Leiomyoma is the commonest, the tongue being the usual site. Many of the tumours are of the angiomyomatous type.[62,63] Leiomyosarcoma is very rare.

Rhabdomyoma, a rare tumour in any site, is most often seen in the mouth, especially in the tongue or floor of mouth.[64] The tumour presents as a slowly growing swelling, consisting of large round or oval cells with eosinophilic granular cytoplasm. Cross-striations are prominent and easily seen in routine haematoxylin-eosin preparations. The tumour is readily excised; recurrence is very unusual. Rhabdomyosarcoma is more commonly encountered than rhabdomyoma, and in the case of oral tumours most patients are children. The usual histological types are seen.[65]

Granular cell myoblastoma, the histogenesis of which is still undecided, relatively frequently affects the mouth, the tongue being the most common site.[66] The pseudo-epitheliomatous hyperplasia that often affects the overlying epithelium can closely simulate squamous cell carcinoma.

Congenital epulis, seen in newborn infants as a pedunculated, or less often sessile, growth of the gingiva, is composed of cells very similar to those of granular cell myoblastoma. However, the overlying epithelium does not show pseudo-epitheliomatous hyperplasia. The lesion is much more common in females than in males. The incisor region of the maxilla is the usual site.[67]

GIANT CELL TUMOURS AND TUMOUR-LIKE LESIONS

Giant cell granuloma

Giant cell lesions may appear both within the jaws and in the oral soft tissues. Formerly, such lesions in the bone of the jaws were considered to be true giant cell tumours of bone, comparable to those in other parts of the skeleton; however, it is generally agreed that such growths are very rare in the jaws. Virtually all of the lesions that formerly were so designated were in fact fibromas or localized foci of fibrous dysplasia, or other lesions in which giant cells may be present. In particular, the lesion that

is now termed giant cell granuloma accounted for many of the cases.

The giant cell granuloma of the mouth and jaws affects children and young adults, mainly between the ages of 10 and 25; in contrast, true giant cell tumours are very rarely seen below the age of 20. The granuloma affects females oftener than males, and the mandible more often than the maxilla. It is always situated in the tooth-bearing area of the jaw, and nearly always anterior to the first permanent molar tooth.

Macroscopically, giant cell granulomas consist of friable, reddish-brown tissue; small cysts may be present. The general appearance is similar to that of giant cell tumour of bone; however, although the cortex is thinned and expanded, perforation is infrequent. Microscopically, the giant cells in most giant cell granulomas have a rather irregular and patchy distribution compared with that in the true giant cell tumours, in which the giant cells are more numerous and more evenly distributed throughout the lesion. The giant cells of the granuloma are not unlike osteoclasts and are distributed in a collagenous tissue that contains many spindle-shaped cells. However, unlike the spindle cells of the giant cell tumour, which may show irregularity in size and shape, with nuclear hyperchromatism and mitotic activity, those of the granuloma show no evidence of such features[68] (Fig. 2.33).

The true nature of the giant cell granuloma is unknown. It is benign, and it is readily cured by simple curettage.

Focal lesions of hyperparathyroidism

The skeletal changes in hyperparathyroidism comprise both generalized osteoporosis and focal lesions similar in structure to the giant cell granuloma described above. The focal lesions may form in any bone and are commonly multiple. Not infrequently, however, only a solitary lesion is present: in such cases the jaws are a favourite site. It is important, therefore, to consider the possibility of hyperparathyroidism when dealing with any giant cell lesion of the jaw.

Osseous lesions of primary hyperparathyroidism have become rare. However, because of the increased survival of patients in renal failure,

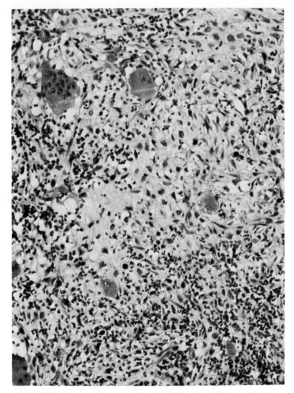

Fig. 2.33 Giant cell granuloma. The lesion consists of focal collections of giant cells in a fibrocellular matrix.

Haematoxylin-eosin   × 120

secondary hyperparathyroidism should be considered as a possible cause of osteolytic giant cell lesions and it may occasionally be a feature of kidney graft rejection.

Giant cell epulis (peripheral giant cell granuloma)

This lesion, which is more common in females than in males, appears most often between the ages of 30 and 40 years but is not infrequently seen in children and adolescents.[69] It takes the form of a rounded swelling, sessile or pedunculated, growing from the gingiva. It is more common in the mandible than in the maxilla and is characteristically deep red or maroon, and soft in consistency. Microscopically, the lesion consists of giant cells in a stroma of collagen fibres and spindle cells. The giant cells are often present in large numbers, but in some lesions they may be less numerous with a correspondingly greater prominence of the colla-

genous and spindle cell element. There is no capsule, but the lesion is benign. Like the giant cell granuloma of the jaws it is probably not a neoplasm but a granulomatous lesion resulting from local irritation, such as trauma from extraction of a tooth, the shedding of a deciduous tooth, calculus, or an ill-fitting denture.

OTHER PRIMARY TUMOURS

Lymphomas in the oral region are seen in the regional lymph nodes and more rarely in the extranodal lymphoid tissue of Waldeyer's ring and the small foci of lymphoid tissue associated with the minor salivary glands. Very often the patient has widespread disease but occasionally the oral lesions are the first to be noted. In most cases they are non-Hodgkin lymphomas, intra-oral Hodgkin lymphoma being rare.[70] Burkitt's lymphoma is a major cause of jaw tumours in endemic areas.

Oral lesions of *myeloma*, like those of lymphoma, are usually elements of widespread disease although again they may be the first to be detected.[71] Solitary lesions are occasionally seen, but like solitary lesions elsewhere disseminated disease is likely to follow sooner or later. Plasmacytoma most frequently affects the upper respiratory and alimentary tracts, with lesions in the mouth appearing as polypoid, pedunculated or more diffuse swellings. Microscopically, these lesions have to be differentiated from inflammatory collections of plasma cells, which are common in the oral tissues.[72]

Pigmented naevi and *malignant melanoma* are seen occasionally in the mouth.[73,74] *Ewing's tumour* and other uncommon neoplasms may rarely appear in the oral tissues.

METASTATIC TUMOURS

Metastatic tumours account for about 1% of the malignant tumours of the region. Deposits in the soft tissues are rare, but have been reported from a variety of primary sites. Metastatic tumours in the jaws are less uncommon; they appear in the mandible more often than in the maxilla, and they may give rise to symptoms while the primary growth remains silent.

The primary growths that most frequently metastasize to the jaws are carcinomas of breast. Bronchus, thyroid and prostate are the next most frequent primary sites; metastasis from a wide variety of other primary tumours has been recorded.[21]

REFERENCES

1. Scott JH, Symons NBB. Introduction to dental anatomy. 9th ed. London: Churchill Livingstone, 1982.
2. Sedano HO, Sauk JJ, Gorlin RJ. Oral manifestations of inherited disorders. Woburn, MA, USA: Butterworth, 1977.
3. Cawson RA. Essentials of dental surgery and pathology. 4th ed. Edinburgh: Churchill Livingstone, 1984.
4. Newbrun E. Cariology. 2nd ed. Baltimore: Williams & Wilkins, 1983.
5. Silverstone LM, Johnson NW, Hardie JM, Williams RAD. Dental caries: aetiology, pathology and prevention. London: Macmillan, 1981.
6. Clarke JK. Br J Pathol 1924; 5:141.
7. Murray JJ. Fluorides in caries prevention. 2nd ed. Bristol: Wright, 1982.
8. Cawson RA, Stocker IPD. Br Dent J 1984; 157:403.
9. English WJ II, Kaiser AB. Southern Med J 1979; 72:687.
10. Ryan ME, Hopkins K, Wilbur RB. Am J Child 1983; 137:592.
11. James L, McCaskey DL, Goris GB. Military Med 1978; 143:297.
12. Shear M. Cysts of the oral regions. 2nd ed. London: Wright, 1983.
13. Summers L. Arch Oral Biol 1974; 19:1177.
14. Pindborg JJ, Kramer IRH. Histological typing of odontogenic tumours, jaw cysts, and allied lesions. Geneva: World Health Organization, 1971.
15. Vedtofte P, Praetorius F. Int J Oral Surg 1979; 8:412.
16. Gundlach KKH, Kiehn M. J Maxfac Surg 1979; 7:299.
17. Rapidis AD, Angelopoulos AP, Scouteris C. Br J Oral Surg 1981; 19:43.
18. Buchner A, Hansen LS. Oral Surg 1980; 50:441.
19. Kuroi M. J Oral Surg 1980; 38:456.
20. El Deeb M, Sedano HO, Waite DE, Int J Oral Surg 1980; 9:301.
21. Lucas RB. Pathology of tumours of the oral tissues. 4th ed. Edinburgh: Churchill Livingstone, 1984.
22. Lucas RB, Pindborg JJ. In: Cohen B, Kramer IRH, eds. Scientific foundations of dentistry. London: Heinemann, 1976.
23. Pullon PA, Shafer WG, Elzay RP et al. Oral Surg 1975; 40:6160.
24. Slootweg PJ, Muller H. Oral Surg 1984; 57:168.
25. Robinson L, Martinez MG. Cancer 1977; 40:2278.
26. Courtney RM, Kerr DA. Oral Surg 1975; 39:424.
27. Franklin CD, Pindborg JJ. Oral Surg 1976; 42:753.
28. Praetorius F, Hjørting-Hansen H, Gorlin RJ et al. Acta Odont Scand 1981; 39:227.
29. Trodahl JN. Oral Surg 1972; 33:547.
30. Howell RH, Burkes EJ. Oral Surg 1977; 43:391.
31. Budnick S. Oral Surg 1976; 42:501.
32. Farman AG, Nortjé CJ, Grotepass FW et al. Br J Oral Surg 1977; 15:3.
33. Waldron CA, Giansanti JS, Browand BC. Oral Surg 1975; 39:590.
34. Larsson A, Forsberg O, Sjögren S. J Oral Surg 1978; 36:299.
35. Punniamoorthy A. Br J Oral Surg 1980; 18:221.
36. Abbey LM, Page DG, Sawyer DR. Oral Surg 1980; 49:419.
37. Bhaskar SN, Beasley JD, Cutright DE. J Am Dent Ass 1970; 81:949.
38. Pindborg JJ. Oral cancer and precancer. Bristol: Wright, 1980.
39. Jacobson S, Shear M. J Oral Path 1972; 1:66.
40. Ellis GL, Corio RL. Oral Surg 1980; 50:523.
41. Saito R, Nakajima T, Shingaki S et al. J Oral Maxillofac Surg 1982; 40:41.
42. Lee KW. Periodontics 1968; 6:277.
43. Angelopoulos AP. J Oral Surg 1971; 29:840.
44. Freedman PD, Cardo VA, Kerpel SM et al. Oral Surg 1978; 46:6386.
45. Eversole LR, Schwartz WD, Sabes WR. Oral Surg 1973; 36:49.
46. Van Hale HMMcM, Handlers JP, Abrams AM et al. Oral Surg 1981; 51:156.
47. Schneider LC, Dolinsky HB, Grodjesk JE. J Oral Surg 1980; 38:452.
48. Farman AG, Nortjé CJ, Grotepass F. Br J Oral Surg 1976; 14:12.
49. Roca AN, Smith LJ, Jing B-S. Am J Clin Path 1970;54:625.
50. Waldron CA, Giansanti JS. Oral Surg 1973; 35:190, 340.
51. Langdon JD, Rapidis AD, Patel MF. Br J Oral Surg 1976; 14:1.
52. Norman JdeB, Painter DM. J Maxfac Surg 1980; 8:161.
53. Hecker R, Corwin JO. J Oral Surg 1980; 38:6066.
54. Hayward JR. J Oral Surg 1981; 39:526.
55. Lamberg MA, Tasanen A, Jaaskelainen J. J Oral Surg 1979; 37:578.
56. Gorlin RJ, Pindborg JJ, Cohen MM. Syndromes of the head and neck. 2nd ed. New York: McGraw-Hill, 1976.
57. Wesley RK, Mintz SM, Wertheimer FW. Oral Surg 1975; 39:103.
58. Wright BA, Jackson D. Oral Surg 1980; 49:509.
59. Lorson EL, DeLong PE, Osbon DB et al. J Oral Surg 1977; 35:733.
60. Carney JA, Siezmore GW, Lovestedt SA. Oral Surg 1976; 41:739.
61. Cutler LS, Chaudhry AP, Topazian R. Cancer 1981; 48:257.
62. Farman AG, Kay S. Oral Surg 1977; 43:402.
63. Natiella JR, Weiders ME, Greene GW. J Oral Path 1982; 11:353.
64. Corio RL, Lewis DM. Oral Surg 1979; 48:525.
65. Sada VM. Int J Oral Surg 1978; 7:316.
66. Regezi JA, Batsakis JG, Courtney RM. J Oral Surg 1979; 37:402.
67. Welbury RR. Br J Oral Surg 1980; 18:238.
68. Franklin CD, Craig GT, Smith CJ. Histopath 1979;3:511.
69. Giansanti JS, Waldron CA. J Oral Surg 1969; 27:787.
70. Hashimoto N, Kurihara K. J Oral Path 1982; 11:214.
71. Epstein JB, Voss NJS, Stevenson-Moore P. Oral Surg 1984; 57:267.
72. Palmer RM, Eveson JW. Oral Surg 1981; 51:187.
73. Buchner A, Hansen LS. Oral Surg 1979; 48:131; 49:55.
74. Cochran AJ. Cancer 1969; 23:1190.

The salivary glands

ANATOMICAL CONSIDERATIONS

It is customary to consider the salivary glands in two main groups, major and minor. The major salivary glands are the paired parotid, submandibular and sublingual glands; the minor glands are small and multiple and are found in the mucosa and underlying tissues of the palate, the faucial region, the lips, the cheeks, the tongue (particularly at its base, deep to the lingual tonsil) and the floor of the mouth. The ducts of some of the faucial glands situated deep to the tonsil discharge into its crypts. The mucous glands of the soft palate and posterior third of the hard palate are very abundant; in the soft palate they form a thick mass, separated only by the palatal musculature from the mucous glands that open on to the floor of the nasopharynx.

Although the minor glands individually are small, in aggregate they represent a considerable volume of secretory tissue and contribute much mucus to the saliva. The contribution of the parotids is thinner, of the consistence of serum, and their secreting acini, accordingly called serous, are composed of large plump cells filled with prominent basiphile zymogen granules. A few isolated acini can be found in most parotids, but occasionally in part of the gland they may be numerous enough to mimic a submandibular lobule. Sebaceous glands are also occasionally found in the parotid, shedding fat-laden cells into the duct system (Fig. 3.1).

The secretion of the submandibular glands is intermediate in character; in addition to the mucus-secreting cells, their mixed acini contain serous cells, which are arranged peripherally as the

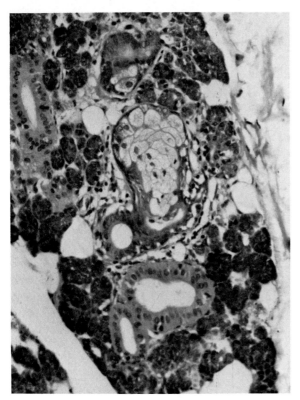

Fig. 3.1 A sebaceous gland in the parotid. Usually encountered only occasionally, they may very rarely, as in the gland from which this example was taken, be extremely numerous.

Haematoxylin-eosin   × 200

familiar demilunes or crescents of Giannuzzi. Ducts lined by low cuboidal epithelium—the intercalated ducts—lead from the secreting acini of both the parotid and submandibular glands and join with others to form intralobular ducts that are lined by tall eosinophilic epithelium with characteristic longitudinal striae—the striated ducts. These cells are active, considerably modifying the constitution of the secretion, much as the renal tubular epithelium modifies the glomerular filtrate. As these intralobular ducts unite, their lining epithelium changes to a simpler type and they emerge into the interlobular connective tissue, eventually converging to form the main secretory ducts which drain the glands. Many of the cells lining Wharton's duct, which carries the partly mucous secretion of the submandibular gland, are ciliate; the longer parotid duct, Stensen's, conveying a thinner serous secretion, is lined by cells which are normally not ciliate.

The sublingual glands are situated along the floor of the mouth forming a ridge between the tongue and the gums of the lower jaw. Each gland consists of a row of several distinct mucous lobules each with its own duct, of Rivinus, opening along the plica sublingualis. There is a separate posterior portion of the sublingual gland, not always present, which although mainly mucous, may contain occasional serous acini; the duct from this part of the sublingual may open into the terminal part of Wharton's duct. The precise relationships of the glandular masses and their ducts in the region where the anterior portion of the submandibular gland and the posterior part of the sublingual meet are complex and variable.[1] Between the acinar and ductal cells and the basement membrane there are flattened contractile myo-epithelial cells. These myo-epithelial cells, which have been known also as basket or basal cells, are inconspicuous in sections of normal salivary glands; they are a prominent feature of many salivary gland tumours.

The parotid glands enclose the branching facial nerves, a feature of great practical importance. They also enclose a number of small lymph nodes; there are glandular elements in the hilum and medulla of these nodes, as there may also be in lymph nodes in the upper part of the neck adjacent to, but not necessarily in contact with, the parotid.

CONGENITAL ANOMALIES

Congenital anomalies of the major salivary glands are rare. The rarest of all is complete absence of all the glands, a condition which results in xerostomia and severe dental caries. Agenesis of individual glands may occasionally be seen as an isolated phenomenon, or may be a feature of mandibulo-facial dysostosis. Hypoplasia of the corresponding glands is seen in hemi-atrophy of the face.

The accessory parotid gland, present in about a third of all subjects, is a small separate portion of the parotid situated near the anterior border of the masseter, with one or more ducts draining into Stensen's duct near its orifice.[2] Occasionally this is the only parotid tissue on one or both sides, in which case it is quite large, the normal site of the gland then being occupied by a pad of adipose tissue.

Congenital diverticula of the main ducts of the

major salivary glands, notably of the submandibular duct near its orifice, are not infrequent. Abnormal openings of the main ducts, or congenital fistulae, may be associated with various severe facial deformities. Atresia of the submandibular duct is an exceedingly rare anomaly.

Ectopic salivary tissue may be found in several sites in the head and neck, including the hypophysis, middle ear, mastoid, thyroid, anterior border of the sternomastoid and the region of the sterno-clavicular joint.[3,4] One such focus in the lower neck above the sterno-clavicular joint developed an opening on to the skin surface from which drops of clear fluid were discharged at meal times.[5] However, ectopic salivary tissue normally has no draining duct, and attention is drawn to it by cyst formation, inflammation, fistula formation or by the development of a tumour in it. Tumours of salivary gland type are occasionally seen within the body of the mandible, presumably arising in ectopic salivary tissue buried there.[6,7]

SIALOSIS

Bilateral, uniform, painless and non-inflammatory enlargement of the parotid glands, and less commonly of the submandibular glands, has been called sialosis or sialadenosis.[8]

The salivary gland enlargement seen in those rare individuals who are compulsively addicted to eating vast quantities of starch is understandable as a work hypertrophy,[9] whilst the prominent glands seen in some cases of acromegaly are clearly a part of the widespread organomegaly of that disease. There remain, however, a number of conditions in which enlargement of the salivary glands occurs, but in which the mechanisms involved are obscure. These include endocrine disorders, nutritional disturbances and adverse drug reactions.

Acromegaly has already been mentioned as one hormonal disturbance which understandably involves the salivary glands. The occurrence of parotid or submandibular gland enlargement in association with ovarian, thyroid or pancreatic endocrine disturbances is more difficult to account for. Sialosis has, for instance, been reported as occasionally occurring at puberty, during pregnancy, and particularly at the menopause, as well as after ovariectomy, whilst bilateral parotid swelling has sometimes been reported in patients with diabetes mellitus.

Severe malnutrition has long been recognized as a cause of bilateral parotid enlargement, the swelling being particularly obvious in emaciated subjects.[10] It has been reported from several parts of the world where there is widespread malnutrition, and was seen in survivors of wartime concentration camps. Although it is more frequent in those showing signs of pellagra and other vitamin deficiencies it seems probable that it results from a qualitative and quantitative deficiency of protein rather than a vitamin lack. Parotid enlargement of this sort has occasionally been reported as a presenting sign in anorexia nervosa.[11] The sialosis seen in some cases of cirrhosis of the liver seems also to have a nutritional basis, being most often seen in alcoholic cirrhosis where there is associated malnutrition.

A number of drugs have been reported as causing salivary gland enlargement in susceptible individuals. Iodides have long been known to do this, the resulting swelling of the parotids being known as 'iodide mumps'. Iodine is excreted and concentrated by the epithelial cells of the striated ducts of the salivary glands, its concentration in the saliva being many times that in the plasma. The effect is usually seen after prolonged administration of iodides, but occasionally follows intravenous urography with iodine-containing compounds. Another drug which may rarely cause parotid swelling is phenylbutazone,[12] as also may thiouracil, catecholamines and sulphonamides. Some drugs in susceptible individuals can produce glandular swelling either with or without signs of inflammation, so that there is some overlap between this drug-induced sialosis and allergic parotitis.

A great deal of experimental work has been carried out, mainly on rats and mice, in connection with the drug-induced sialosis which may follow the administration of various adrenergic and cholinergic drugs.[13] Isoprenaline given to rats, for example, leads to both hypertrophy and hyperplasia of the salivary glands, which subside when the treatment is stopped. There is a suggestion that excessive sympathetic stimulation may be one of the factors leading to sialosis in humans.

Whatever the cause of the sialosis, the histological abnormalities seen in biopsy specimens are remarkably similar, such differences as there are depending on the severity of the condition and its stage of evolution. The most obvious abnormality is marked enlargement of the individual cells of the acini. The cytoplasm of the enlarged cells may be packed with zymogen granules, larger and much more numerous than normal, or, at a later stage the cytoplasm may have a finely vacuolated appearance with no granules. In either case the nucleus is displaced to the base of the cell and the swollen acinar cells obliterate the tiny lumen normally seen at the centre of the acinus. The intralobular ducts are compressed by the greatly enlarged acini, and the sialogram often shows only the main branches of the duct system, the contrast medium failing to penetrate the terminal ducts. The interstitial tissue of the gland is usually somewhat oedematous. In the later stages of the condition the acinar tissue atrophies and there is infiltration of the gland by adipose tissue, so that it remains enlarged. A characteristic feature of the saliva in sialosis, particularly in the hormonal cases, is an increase in the potassium content of the saliva and a decrease in the sodium, this alteration being of diagnostic value.

CYSTS

Simple cysts, usually solitary, are occasionally found in the parotid. Clinically, they may be mistaken for tumours and removed as such, and since tumour tissue has sometimes been demonstrated in the wall of otherwise simple cysts this treatment is appropriate. If their true nature is suspected and the clear fluid contents are aspirated it is usual for the cavity to refill quite quickly. Microscopically, the cyst wall may show no more than a lining of cuboidal or flattened epithelium surrounded by a thin layer of fibrous tissue, but more often there is a layer of lymphoid tissue beneath the epithelial lining, and it seems probable that such cysts have developed from salivary tissue within an intraparotid lymph node. The lining epithelium may be oncocytic, and this, overlying lymphoid tissue, is reminiscent of adenolymphoma. Occasionally the cyst lining is found to be squamous and the cavity full of shed keratin scales, in which case the association with lymphoid tissue suggests the possibility of a branchial origin. However, the squamous epithelium could have resulted from metaplasia in a salivary duct, and although branchial cysts within the parotid are reported from time to time their branchial origin is difficult to prove, and such lesions are often non-committally called 'lympho-epithelial cysts'.[14]

The cause of parotid cysts is unknown. Obstruction is unlikely; ligation of the main parotid duct, as is sometimes done to prevent recurrent ascending infection, results in a short period of painful tension in the duct system, after which the gland gradually ceases to function and the acini atrophy. The same is true for smaller ducts within the gland blocked by microcalculi.

Although serous acini atrophy when there is obstruction to their outflow, mucous acini continue to function against pressure and mucous retention cysts of the minor salivary glands in the mouth are not uncommon. Microscopically, two distinct types of mucocele can be distinguished, retention and extravasation.[15] The retention mucocele is a cystic dilatation of the duct of a minor salivary gland and has an intact epithelial lining, whereas the extravasation mucocele is a false cyst resulting from rupture of the duct. The mucus in an extravasation mucocele is surrounded by a zone of histiocytes, many of them foamy and containing globules of mucus, and with a few often free in the cavity. There may be a few inflammatory cells also present, and the whole lesion develops a fibrous surround (Fig. 3.2). In large tense mucoceles the compressed innermost row of histiocytes may be misinterpreted as an epithelial lining. A small extravasation mucocele may become a solid granuloma, the mucus having all been phagocytosed.[16] The lower lip is far and away the commonest site for extravasation mucoceles, and most examples are from patients in the second or third decades of life. Retention mucoceles are much less common, and are almost always found elsewhere in the mouth, and usually in patients past middle age. Extravasation mucoceles are almost certainly traumatic in origin, though the actual injury, either a bite by the patient or an external wound, can rarely be remembered.

Mucous cysts of the minor salivary glands of the

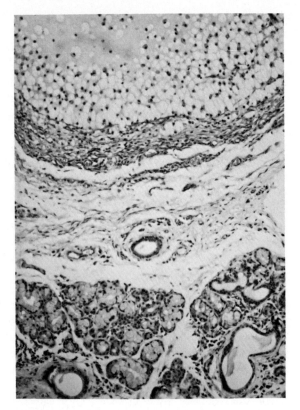

Fig. 3.2 Part of the wall of an extravasation mucocele of the lip, showing part of the gland below the mucus above. The mucus is being invaded by histiocytes from the zone of granulation tissue which surrounds it.

Haematoxylin-eosin   × 110

lips and cheek rarely exceed a centimetre in diameter, but cysts developing from the sublingual glands may reach a considerable size and interfere with speech, mastication and swallowing. Lying to one side of the frenulum of the tongue, such a cyst appears as a smooth, glistening, translucent bluish swelling which was long ago likened to the ventral aspect of a little frog, and accordingly called a ranula. Whereas the parotid ceases to function when obstructed, the sublingual gland continues secreting indefinitely. If the ranula is ruptured or incised it reforms, whilst removal of the roof of the cyst, though temporarily beneficial, is usually followed by recurrence. Sections of the cyst wall show it to be that of an extravasation mucocele, with no true epithelial lining. Rarely, after several unsuccessful attempts at cure, the mucus escapes through gaps in the mylohyoid muscle and burrows

widely in the loose tissues of the neck, the so-called plunging or burrowing ranula. This bulky swelling, normally unilateral, may reach as far down as the clavicle and up to the base of the skull. It has sometimes been suspected that the submandibular gland is responsible for ranulas, but its removal has not cured the condition; this is only achieved by removal of the sublingual gland, after which any neck swelling gradually disappears.[17,18] The submandibular gland is only very rarely implicated in a ranula, and then the swelling eventually subsides as the gland ceases to function.[19]

SALIVARY CALCULI

Salivary calculi or sialoliths are oftenest seen in adults. They are very rare before the age of 30 and most patients are between 40 and 60 years old, and are more often men than women, in a ratio of 3:2. The calculi, for some obscure reason, are more often on the right than on the left; in a recent series of 36 patients with parotid calculi, 28 were right-sided.[20] Salivary calculi are usually yellowish-tan in colour, with a smooth or slightly roughened surface. Multiple calculi, occasionally seen in the parotid, may be faceted. The stones are composed of calcium phosphate, with some calcium carbonate, and with small amounts of other constituents. The calcium phosphate is mainly in the form of hydroxyapatite, with some magnesium-substituted whitlockite, but there are some differences in crystal chemistry between parotid and submandibular stones.[21] Occasionally submandibular stones can be shown to have as their nucleus a toothbrush bristle or other foreign body, whilst sections of parotid glands which chance to cut across a very early calculus may show that it has inflammatory debris or a cluster of crystalloids as its core. There is no definite association with general disturbances of calcium metabolism.

Submandibular calculi, the commonest pathological condition of that gland, are two or three times as common as parotid calculi; stone in the sublingual or minor salivary glands is rare. It is most unusual for parotid and submandibular calculi to be seen in the same individual, or for the condition to be bilateral.

Submandibular calculi are usually much larger

than parotid ones. Wharton's duct is more elastic and distensible than Stensen's, and this, together with the mucus content of the submandibular saliva means that the calculus is less painful, and the patient tolerates it longer without consulting a doctor. The calculi are usually lodged at some point in the submandibular duct, quite often near its mouth. Only about 15% of submandibular calculi are in the intraglandular part of the duct system (Fig. 3.3). The calculus is commonly elongated, like a date stone, and causes corresponding dilatation of the duct around it. Its smooth surface is lubricated by the mucous secretion, and it may reach a considerable size before there is sufficient obstruction to cause the classical clinical picture of painful swelling of the gland on eating, with subsidence between meals. Mucus continues to be secreted in spite of the pressure caused within the duct by the obstruction. The stone may eventually become large and egg-shaped, even dwarfing the adjoining submandibular gland. Inflammation in the neighbourhood of the stone may lead to a local abscess, or the stone may eventually ulcerate into the adjacent tissues or into the mouth itself. The inflammation may extend along the duct to involve the gland, with the development of progressive fibrosis. The duct lining in contact with the stone usually shows squamous metaplasia.

Parotid calculi were at one time considered to be very much less common than submandibular ones, but with improved diagnostic methods they are increasingly being recognized as the commonest cause of recurrent unilateral swelling of the gland. Calculi that give rise to symptoms are nearly always in the parotid duct, and are particularly liable to become impacted where the duct turns inwards at the anterior border of the masseter, a site where they are difficult to visualize radiologically. They are usually small, but may occasionally be multiple. Inflammatory changes at the site of lodgement may lead to stricture. The secretion of serous glands, contrary to that of mucous glands, is diminished by obstruction, so that if a calculus is firmly lodged recurrent parotid swelling with meals is less common than in the case of submandibular stone; instead, there are likely to be recurrent painful attacks of inflammatory swelling of the gland, lasting some days at a time. The small calculi that are responsible for the recurrent parotitis in such cases may be difficult to demonstrate and are often overlooked.[22]

Microscopic calculi are not infrequently encountered, on histological examination, in the small ducts of the parotid, usually in association with atrophy of the corresponding lobules or acini.

Calculi in minor salivary glands have been considered extremely rare, but are being increasingly recognized and reported. In a recent series of 47 examples the great majority were in the upper lip, with the buccal mucosa as the next most common site.[23] There were rather more women than men in the series, and most cases were in the sixth, seventh or eighth decades, rather older than in the calculi previously considered. There is often squamous metaplasia or ulceration of the distended duct, with associated inflammation of the gland.

SALIVARY FISTULAE

Salivary fistulae are rare. They may be congenital, and then are usually associated with other, more serious, malformations of the face. Ectopic salivary tissue occasionally functions and drains on to the skin surface, above the sterno-clavicular joint or

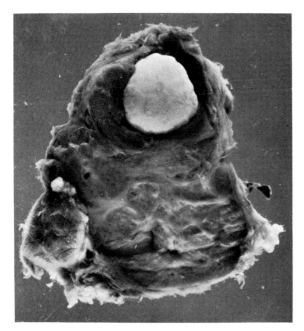

Fig. 3.3 Cross-section of a submandibular gland showing a rounded calculus (1.5 cm diameter) lodged in the main duct.

behind the ear in the mastoid region, and these openings may be described as fistulae; they have to be distinguished from branchial fistulae, which may be similarly situated.

Before antibiotics became generally available incision or spontaneous rupture of parotid abscesses was not infrequently followed by fistula formation. Injuries to, or operations on, the salivary glands or their ducts may heal leaving a fistula draining saliva on to the skin surface or into the mouth. Internal fistulae cause no inconvenience and require no treatment. The external fistulae almost always close spontaneously, provided there is no obstruction to the outflow along the duct of the gland concerned. Fistulae developing in association with stones in the duct, stenosis or tumour require re-establishment of a clear passage before they can be closed.

INFLAMMATORY CONDITIONS (SIALADENITIS)

Viral infections

Acute viral sialadenitis (mumps)

Mumps, by far the commonest cause of parotitis, is an acute infectious disease caused by a paramyxovirus. It occurs most frequently among children of school age. A survey of a large number of schoolboys showed that 60% had a clinical history of mumps by the age of 18, with serological evidence suggesting that a further 30% had had subclinical infections.[24] Those few individuals who escape in childhood may develop the disease as adults.

Typically, mumps has an acute onset with fever, headache and painful swelling of first one parotid and, usually quite soon, the other as well. The firm, elastic swelling of the glands, with reddening of the overlying skin, develops quite quickly after a relatively long incubation period of up to three weeks. The swelling, which is associated with greatly diminished secretion, persists for a week or 10 days and then gradually subsides. In about 10% of cases the submandibular glands are involved in addition or, exceptionally, alone. Although the salivary gland enlargement is the characteristic feature of the disease, other organs may be involved, particularly in adults: orchitis and pancreatitis are the most frequent extra-salivary manifestations; oophoritis and thyroiditis occur much more rarely. Involvement of the nervous system is not uncommon, particularly in the form of a so-called aseptic meningitis or of meningo-encephalitis; clinical involvement of the salivary glands may not be apparent in such cases.

The histological changes in the glands are known mainly from cases in which death occurred from other causes during the course of the disease;[25] death from mumps is very rare. Microscopically, the parotid is swollen from interstitial oedema and there is swelling and marked cytoplasmic vacuolation of the acinar cells, with similar but less marked degenerative changes in the ductal epithelium. The interlobular connective tissue is oedematous and may show fibrinoid degeneration of the collagen. There is a dense lymphocytic infiltrate, with some plasma cells and large mononuclear cells (Fig. 3.4). Although the changes are so marked, complete resolution is the rule. There is no definite evidence that any lasting structural or functional abnormalities of the salivary glands are attributable to mumps.

A clinical diagnosis of mumps, especially if only one parotid is affected, is only reliable during epidemics; at other times the diagnosis must be supported by laboratory investigations.

Cytomegalovirus infection

In sections of parotid glands of about 25% of all babies dying in early infancy there are present in the intralobular ducts occasional cells which are greatly enlarged and contain both intranuclear and cytoplasmic inclusions (Fig. 3.5). This finding is commoner in weakly or premature infants and is evidence of infection with the human strain of cytomegalovirus. The parotid involvement in the newborn is part of a generalized infection acquired from the mother. In the very rare cases in which the infection is fatal, affected cells are also found in many other tissues, particularly epithelial tissues, as in the liver, lungs, kidneys and pancreas, and there are grave effects on the nervous system. During life the affected cells are shed, and can be identified in the saliva, urine or sputum.

Infection may occur in later childhood and is

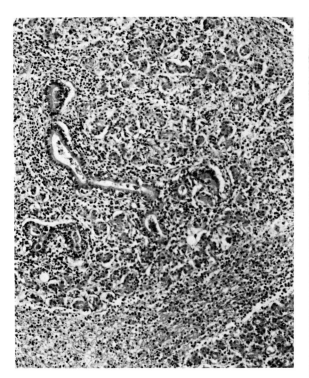

Fig. 3.4 Submandibular gland from a patient with mumps. The interlobular connective tissue in the lower left part of the figure is oedematous and heavily infiltrated by mononuclear cells. In the lobule above, the ducts are still recognizable but the acinar epithelium is hydropic and degenerate; the intralobular connective tissue is also oedematous and infiltrated by mononuclear cells.

Haematoxylin-eosin   × 100

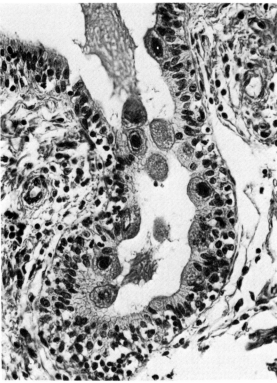

Fig. 3.5 Inclusion-body cytomegaly in an intralobular parotid duct of an infant. The affected cells are being extruded into the lumen of the duct.

Haematoxylin-eosin   × 350

then usually subclinical; very rarely an illness resembling glandular fever or hepatitis results. The illness has sometimes been called 'salivary gland inclusion disease', for although there are no particular signs or symptoms referable to involvement of the salivary glands it is in their ducts that the inclusions are most often seen. The mode of infection in older children is not known, but subclinical infection is so common that about 80% of adults in Britain have serological evidence of previous infection. There is evidence that endogenous virus can reactivate, despite pre-existing immunity, when that immunity is artificially suppressed. Therapeutic immunosuppression, as in transplant patients, and treatment with cytotoxic drugs or by whole body irradiation may all occasionally give rise to the disease in adults in this way. Disease due to the virus may also be a feature

of the acquired immune deficiency syndrome (AIDS)). The virus is, therefore, becoming increasingly important, and with the further demonstration that the infection can be sexually transmitted, the possibility of artificial immunization is being explored.[26]

Many animal species have their own species-specific strains of cytomegalovirus. For instance, sections of the salivary glands of most laboratory guinea-pigs show the striking and pathognomonic appearance of the infected cells.

Other viral infections

Parotitis is recognized as a feature of infections with other viruses, and as diagnosis becomes more exact the proportion of cases of sialadenitis considered to represent non-specific inflammation of the parotid and other salivary glands may well become smaller. Examples of parotitis due to Coxsackie A,[27] echoviruses, parainfluenza virus types 1 and 3,[28] and the virus of lymphocytic choriomeningitis[29] have been recorded.

Bacterial infections

Acute bacterial sialadenitis

The salivary glands are liable to infection by organisms that reach them from the mouth by way of their ducts. In the submandibular ducts this tends to be countered by the action of the ciliate epithelium and the mucoid nature of the secretion from the submandibular gland; the parotid gland, in contrast, is dependent on a free flow of its more watery saliva to oppose retrograde spread of bacteria along the duct. For these reasons, acute inflammation due to organisms from the mouth is much commoner in the parotid than in the other salivary glands. Apart from the rare cases where the organisms reach the glands by the bloodstream, the factors which predispose to parotitis are absence of an adequate flow of saliva down Stensen's duct, the presence of pyogenic organisms in the mouth, and lowered resistance.

Acute postoperative parotitis was a familiar complication after operations, usually abdominal or gynaecological, when fluids were withheld and the secretion of the gland was consequently suppressed. In recent years, improved oral hygiene and prevention or correction of postoperative dehydration have greatly reduced the incidence of this complication. If it does occur, treatment with antibiotics has reduced the risk of suppuration, though resistant strains may still occasionally lead to abscess formation. The organisms concerned are most often pyogenic staphylococci, though haemolytic streptococci, viridans streptococci or pneumococci are sometimes isolated from the purulent material expressed from the inflamed duct mouth.

Acute parotitis may similarly complicate acute infectious fevers. In some of these, particularly typhoid, the specific organism may be responsible for the parotitis also, possibly reaching it by way of the bloodstream. Acute parotitis occurs, too, in patients, often elderly, who are debilitated and dehydrated from other causes, such as in the terminal stages of malignant disease or mental illness, particularly if septic conditions are present in the mouth. Cases have been reported of parotitis in psychiatric patients on large doses of phenothiazine derivatives which, as a side-effect, suppress salivation in some people.[30] Young infants, dehydrated from any cause, such as gastro-enteritis, occasionally develop parotitis.[31]

Inflammatory swelling of the parotid is restricted by the fibrous capsule of the gland and the condition is therefore very painful. The glands—the condition is not infrequently bilateral—are enlarged and tender, and the overlying skin is stretched and shiny. Redness and swelling of the duct orifice in the mouth, with pus exuding from it on pressure, make the diagnosis clear and furnish material for bacteriological examination. The acute inflammatory changes are most marked in the duct system of the gland, the ducts being full of pus, but the inflammatory process soon extends out into the parenchyma of the gland with necrosis and abscess formation, if unchecked. If an abscess forms it may point spontaneously through the skin of the face or into the external acoustic meatus between its bony and cartilaginous parts. The infection may spread into the neck as a cellulitis or even into the mediastinum, and terminate with septicaemia and death. The mortality in debilitated patients may reach 30%.

Other causes of sialadenitis

Allergic parotitis is a rare condition in which acute inflammatory changes in the gland, usually with many eosinophils in the exudate, rapidly develop in response to a variety of allergens, including several drugs.[32] In a recently reported example of the condition, the patient presented a clinical picture closely resembling epidemic parotitis, with bilateral painful swelling of the parotid glands and fever, as a response to nitrofurantoin. The condition recurred each time she took the drug.[33]

An acute inflammatory reaction, with degenerative changes in the serous acini and focal necrosis, develops within 24 hours of irradiation of the salivary glands. This post-irradiation sialadenitis subsides without treatment within three days.[34]

Chronic and recurrent sialadenitis

Acute postoperative parotitis seldom recurs, and the other forms of acute parotitis are often terminal conditions. There are, however, patients who suffer repeated attacks of acute or subacute parotitis, or in whom parotitis becomes chronic.

Recurrent obstructive parotitis. Recurrent parotitis may be associated with some obvious abnormality impeding the flow of saliva and predisposing to ascending infection, such as a calculus or stricture. In the latter instance, the stricture may itself have formed at the site of lodgement of a calculus, subsequently passed, or it may be the outcome of a surgical or other injury, or have no apparent cause. The attacks of parotitis may be precipitated by any circumstances leading to temporary inhibition of salivation, and since each recurrence leads to further fibrosis and loss of secretory ability, a vicious circle develops (Fig. 3.6). As the glandular

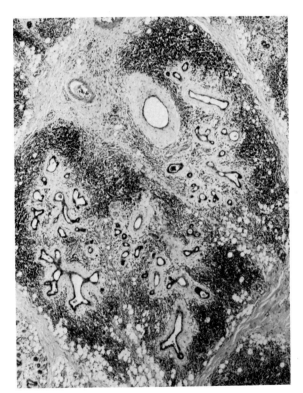

Fig. 3.6 Chronic atrophic parotitis. There is atrophy of the secretory elements, proliferation of small ducts, periductal and perilobular fibrosis, chronic inflammatory cell infiltration, and fatty infiltration

Haematoxylin-eosin ×35

tissue atrophies its place is taken by fibrous or adipose tissue. In addition to the cellular inflammatory infiltrate and newly-formed fibrous tissue in the gland, there may be squamous or goblet cell metaplasia in its ducts: mucus may then accumulate and distend the ducts, which may rupture, with interstitial extravasation of mucus and consequent aggravation of the sclerosing fibrous reaction. Comparable attacks of inflammation may be associated with calculi in a submandibular gland or its duct.

A rare form of *chronic sclerosing submandibular sialadenitis*, which may be bilateral, slowly leads to such firm fibrous swelling of the gland that the condition may be mistaken for a neoplasm. This form of pseudotumour is sometimes referred to as Küttner's tumour.

Recurrent non-obstructive parotitis. Recurrent bacterial parotitis may also occur in the absence of any demonstrable obstruction of the duct. The flow of saliva is normally sufficient to prevent invasion by mouth organisms along the duct, or to wash out any organisms that do get in while the gland is resting. If, however, there is any reduction in the amount or productivity of the glandular tissue, with consequently lowered secretion rate at the best of times, then organisms may be able to gain a foothold and set up inflammation in the gland. The organisms responsible are the usual mouth commensals, with *Streptococcus viridans* predominating, and the inflammation is less severe than the acute septic parotitis described above. With repeated attacks of subacute inflammation changes similar to those described for calculous obstruction, with progressive fibrosis and acinar atrophy, will follow. Since the inflammatory exudate in the ducts may act as a basis for stone formation, glands removed for severe recurrent swelling have often been found to contain small calculi, so that calculi can be an effect as well as a cause of recurrent inflammation.[22]

Most patients with recurrent subacute parotitis are adults, but there is an important group of children between the ages of 5 and 15. In these children, among whom boys are affected rather oftener than girls, the attacks of painful parotid swelling are usually thought to be due to mumps until their repetition makes it clear that this is not so. The attacks are generally precipitated by some other illness, or by teething, conditions in which the appetite is lost and salivation depressed. They tend to become less frequent and eventually to cease at about the time of puberty; rarely they are so numerous as to interfere seriously with schooling, and parotidectomy may then become necessary. Microscopy in these more severe cases shows that there has been increasing formation of lymphoid tissue around the interlobular and intralobular ducts, with progressive loss of secretory tissue, and, in the later stages, fibrosis. Microbiological investigations in the past have been disappointing, the commonest isolates being of *Strep. viridans*, without evidence that bacteria play any part in initiating the condition. There is some evidence that the disease is due to a viral infection, but the identity of the viruses remains uncertain.

That reduced salivation underlies the attacks in adults is strongly suggested by the facts that the flow of saliva from the opposite uninflamed gland is also significantly reduced, and that measures taken to stimulate salivation greatly reduce or abolish the attacks.[35] Occasionally there is a known cause for the xerostomia, such as involvement of the salivary glands in previous irradiation, Sjögren's syndrome or related condition, or the effects of drugs, a number of which reduce salivation as a side-effect. But the underlying cause is often not apparent; a constitutionally low rate of parotid secretion or the effects of a previous viral infection have been suggested.

Sialography in patients with chronic or recurrent parotitis, particularly in children, often shows the remarkable appearance that is referred to as *globular sialectasis*, or *punctate sialectasis*, globules of the opaque medium appearing in the system of branching ducts like clusters of currants on their stalks. This has been interpreted as a congenital malformation of the duct system and the suggestion has followed that it is the cause underlying the recurrent infection. However, serial sections of such glands have shown that the spherical opacities nearly always result from extravasation of contrast medium through weakened duct walls into adjoining lymphoid tissue, particularly into the follicles, with their sparse and distensible reticulin framework (Fig. 3.7). The extravasated medium provokes a granulomatous response, which increases the fibrous replacement of the gland.[36]

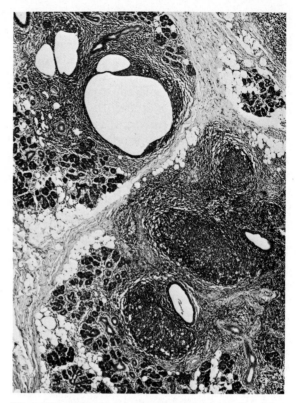

Fig. 3.7 Parotid from a boy, aged 9. A sialogram performed a few days previously had shown globular sialectasis. Parts of two lobules are shown. There is much lymphoid tissue, with follicle formation, in the neighbourhood of the larger ducts. Some atrophy of the acini is seen. The large clear areas of extravasation of the contrast medium—the largest has the remains of a lymphoid follicle stretched round it—can be distinguished from the smaller distended ducts with their intact epithelial linings.

Haematoxylin-eosin   × 40

Tuberculosis and other specific chronic infections

These are referred to on page 101.

Benign lympho-epithelial lesion and Sjögren's syndrome

Patients in whose parotid glands the changes described by Godwin in 1952 as the benign lympho-epithelial lesion[37] are present may show no other evidence of disease, or they may have the other pathological conditions present which go to make up Sjögren's syndrome.[38] The age and sex incidence, as well as the histological appearances of the affected gland, are the same in either case, but although patients with the isolated lesion some-times go on to develop the other features of Sjögren's syndrome this is by no means inevitable. The benign lympho-epithelial lesion usually affects middle-aged women, often at about the time of the menopause, though it is occasionally seen in men and at earlier ages. The patient may complain of a gradually increasing painless swelling of a parotid gland, either localized and tumour-like or more diffuse. The gradual enlargement may be inter-rupted by mildly painful episodes of increased swelling, and the condition may be bilateral, with the submandibular glands affected similarly, though distinctly less often. When more than one of the salivary glands are involved there will be dryness of the mouth (xerostomia), and patients quite often complain of this without there being appreciable swelling of the affected glands.

When the parotid is cut across, the affected lobules, though still distinct, are seen to be swollen, rounded and white, contrasting with the normal rhomboidal pale yellow lobules that may survive at the periphery of the gland.

Microscopically, affected glands show progres-sive lymphocytic infiltration of the lobules, at first round the intralobular ducts and later spreading to replace the acini. Germinal centres may form in the lymphoid tissue and sometimes become very large and conspicuous; occasionally, pseudofolli-cular aggregations of lymphocytes give a picture resembling that of a follicular lymphoma. There may also be small numbers of plasma cells in the infiltrate, and the intraparotid lymph nodes are hyperplastic. The lymphocytic infiltration, how-ever dense, generally ceases abruptly at the edge of the lobules. Whereas the acinar epithelium disap-pears, the ducts become converted into proliferat-ing masses of cells which on cross-section are referred to as epimyo-epithelial islands.[39] These islands are demarcated from the surrounding lymphoid tissue by a basement membrane, and foci of hyaline basement membrane material may be seen in among the cells of the island. The central lumen of the duct has often been obliterated, or it may be represented by one or more small rings of duct-lining epithelial cells, with or without a tiny lumen (Fig. 3.8). Occasional ducts, instead of being obliterated, are dilated to form small cysts, and these sometimes contain little calculi. The most

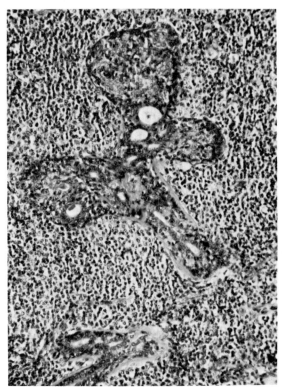

Fig. 3.8 An epimyo-epithelial island from a benign lympho-epithelial lesion of the parotid. The islands may be solid, with the duct lumen obliterated, but sometimes, as in this example, one or more tiny channels remain among the mass of proliferating cells. The island has a partial surround of hyaline basement material, foci of which are also present among the cells of the island.

Haematoxylin-eosin   × 125

numerous of the cells forming the island have been assumed to be myo-epithelial, as the name epimyo-epithelial suggests, but electron microscopists are reluctant to identify them as such; possibly they are undergoing squamous metaplasia. The extent of the involvement of the lobules is uneven: the more severely affected lobules tend to be in the neighbourhood of the main duct, and a few normal lobules are often to be seen at the periphery of the gland (Fig. 3.9).

The sialographic picture is similar to that described above as globular sialectasis (see p. 98), with extravasation of contrast medium into the lymphoid tissue, where, if oily, it will be sur-rounded by foreign-body giant cells and provoke a granulomatous reaction. It is of interest that many patients with symptoms and clinical findings

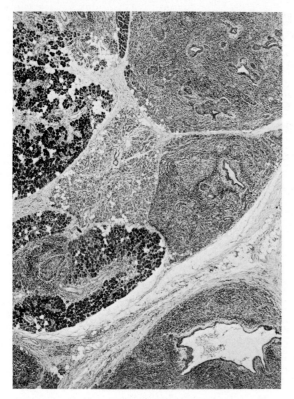

Fig. 3.9 Parotid from a patient with Sjögren's syndrome. There is part of a relatively normal lobule to the left, above. Part of a lobule at the bottom of the figure is completely replaced by lymphoid tissue and encloses a greatly dilated duct. The lobule to the right, above, shows the characteristic lymphoid infiltration almost completely replacing the acini, and also many epimyo-epithelial islands, many of them solid, resulting from proliferation of the cells of the ducts.

Haematoxylin-eosin   × 25

seemingly indicative of unilateral disease show diminished salivary secretion and a similar sialographic appearance on the other side as well.

There is a small but definite risk of the eventual development of some variety of malignant lymphoma in benign lympho-epithelial lesions, whether isolated or part of Sjögren's syndrome.[40-42] Patients with Sjögren's syndrome also have an increased liability to malignant lymphoma developing at sites other than the salivary glands.[43] This danger of malignant transformation, though not very great, has raised doubts whether it is wise to call lympho-epithelial lesions with no evidence of malignancy, benign. Some of the other terms in use for the condition, such as lympho-epithelial sialadenopathy, immunosialadenitis or chronic myo-epithelial sialadenitis, avoid the question of malignant potential.

Much rarer is the development of malignancy in the epithelial component of the benign lympho-epithelial lesion (see p. 122). The few reported examples of this have nearly always been in patients without evidence of Sjögren's syndrome.

Henrik Sjögren, a Swedish ophthalmologist, drew attention in 1932 to the association of a characteristic ocular lesion, keratoconjunctivitis sicca, with xerostomia due to changes in the salivary glands of the type described above, the eye condition resulting from similar changes in the lacrimal glands with loss of secretion.[44,45] The function of the minor mucous glands of the mouth and upper respiratory tract is often impaired also, so that rhinopharyngolaryngitis sicca develops as well as the dry mouth. In more than half the patients with these conditions there is also evidence of a collagen disease, usually rheumatoid arthritis; polymyositis, scleroderma, systemic lupus erythematosus and polyarteritis may be present, but less frequently. When all three conditions are present—keratoconjunctivitis sicca, xerostomia, and rheumatoid arthritis or other connective-tissue disorder—the term *Sjögren's syndrome* is applied; if only the first two are present the term *sicca syndrome* is used. There is an autoimmune basis for both syndromes which is discussed in connection with the lesions found in the mouth in Chapter 1 (see p. 41).

Mikulicz's syndrome

In 1892 von Mikulicz-Radecki described the case of a man of 42 with marked enlargement of his lacrimal, parotid, submandibular and palatal glands.[46] The lacrimal and submandibular swellings were removed during life and histologically examined; the parotid changes appear not to have been studied. The paper was illustrated by drawings of the microscopical appearances, but their interpretation is equivocal and an accurate diagnosis of the changes cannot be made. The patient died soon after from another condition. Subsequently, other cases characterized by swellings of both lacrimal and salivary glands were described and this association came to be known as Mikulicz's disease or Mikulicz's syndrome. Many of these subsequent cases proved to be manifestations of a variety of underlying conditions, such as leukaemia, lymphomas, tuberculosis and sarcoidosis. It was then suggested that Mikulicz's syndrome be used to cover cases with known causes, with Mikulicz's disease kept for those of unknown aetiology. It now appears probable that Mikulicz's disease and the lympho-epithelial lesion of Godwin are the same condition; but since the precise pathology of Mikulicz's original case cannot be determined it seems better to abandon the eponym and refer to all such cases by the diagnosis appropriate to the condition underlying the glandular enlargement.

Sarcoidosis

The parotids are involved in up to 6% of cases of sarcoidosis.[47] There may be lesions in the submandibular and minor salivary glands, and sometimes in the lacrimal glands also. The patient, of either sex, and usually between 30 and 45 years old, notices gradual firm, painless, nodular enlargement of the parotid gland, more often than not bilateral. When sarcoidosis involves the salivary glands some other manifestations of the disease, such as pulmonary infiltration, enlargement of mediastinal and other lymph nodes, and skin lesions, are always present. The volume and amylase content of the saliva from the affected gland are reduced, and the patient may complain of a dry mouth. There may be evidence of nerve involvement, especially of the cranial nerves, and this may include some facial weakness: the latter appears to be an essential affection of the facial nerve rather than its involvement or compression as it passes through the diseased parotid. Microscopically, the picture is that of the familiar sarcoid granuloma, made up of epithelioid histiocytes with occasional multinucleate giant cells, which runs its usual course with little or no necrosis, but with eventual fibrous scarring. The intraparotid lymph nodes may be involved, but most of the lesions are within the parenchyma of the gland. The granulomas tend to be near the intralobular ducts, which accordingly become obstructed, atrophy of the corresponding acini being the outcome. The sialogram has a stunted appearance, like a tree which has lost many of its terminal branchlets. The usual course is spontaneous disappearance of the symptoms within a year or so, recovery being greatly accelerated by steroid therapy.

Heerfordt's syndrome

Pathological changes similar to those of sarcoidosis are seen in the parotid in the syndrome described by Heerfordt as 'febris uveoparotidea subchronica'[48] (Fig. 3.10). This often starts with an acute pyrexial phase that is followed by enlargement of the salivary glands and various ocular manifestations, notably uveitis. There may also be cranial nerve involvement and skin lesions. The syndrome appears to be a particular manifestation of sarcoidosis.

Other chronic inflammatory diseases

Tuberculosis

Tuberculosis of the salivary glands is very rare. When it occurs it is usually confined to one parotid.

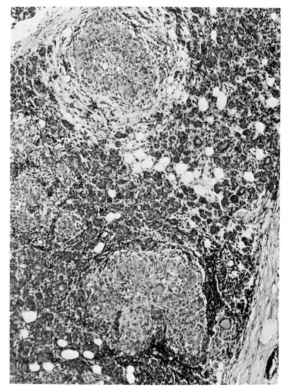

Fig. 3.10 Parotid from a patient with Heerfordt's syndrome. Part of a lobule showing granulomas of sarcoid type, the uppermost of which is becoming fibrotic.

Haematoxylin-eosin   × 75

It may involve the intraparotid lymph nodes as part of a regional lymphadenitis, or it may develop within the parenchyma of the gland.[49,50] Involvement of the lymph nodes is much the commoner form, and if there is no obvious tuberculous disease elsewhere the lump may be diagnosed as a tumour and removed as such. In the parenchymatous type the possibilities of haematogenous infection and of infection ascending the duct cannot be denied, but are unproven.

Actinomycosis

The parotid may be involved in cervico-facial actinomycosis, the chronic granulomatous process extending from the region of the angle of the mandible to invade the gland. Very rarely the disease may apparently be a primary affection of the parotid or submandibular glands.[51] The patient complains of a slowly increasing diffuse, firm, or even hard, swelling of the affected gland, not particularly painful, and unrelated to eating. The normal flow of saliva ceases, but it may be possible to express pus from the duct orifice, examination of which may establish the diagnosis. The gland is gradually destroyed and a chronic abscess cavity forms. If untreated, fistulas discharging the characteristic 'sulphur granule' pus either on to the skin surface or into the mouth may develop.

Other infections

Very occasionally other fungal infections, such as blastomycosis, may involve the salivary glands.

Syphilis in its later stages was formerly described as leading to either a diffuse chronic inflammatory fibrosis of the parotid or else to localized gummatous nodules, but with modern treatment of the disease this must be exceedingly rare.

TUMOURS OF THE SALIVARY GLANDS

Any of the salivary glands, major or minor, may be the seat of tumour formation, but the major glands, and in particular the parotids, are most commonly affected. As a rough approximation it can be stated that for every 100 parotid tumours there will be 10 tumours of the submandibular glands, 10 of the minor salivary glands and 1 of the sublingual.

Salivary gland tumours are rare, variously estimated as occurring in between 0.25 and 2.5 per 100 000 of the population,[52] and accounting for only 1 or 2% of all tumours. Various racial differences have been reported,[53–55] the most striking being the high incidence in Eskimos (see p. 122).[56] Although so uncommon, salivary tumours are of importance because they often occur in relatively young subjects and because correct treatment at an early stage can make the difference between cure and either death or years of misery. The parotid in particular is so situated that recurrent tumours and associated scarring or facial palsy are embarrassingly conspicuous.

Little is known about the causation of these tumours. The only definite aetiological factor seems to be previous irradiation. A recent study of large numbers of adults who had had radiotherapy for enlarged tonsils and adenoids when they were children showed a markedly increased incidence of salivary gland tumours, 26% of which were malignant. The first tumours began appearing five years after irradiation and new tumours were still appearing 30 years later.[57,58] An increased incidence of these and other tumours has also been reported in Japanese exposed to radiation from atom bombs.[59]

Many different names for the various types of salivary gland tumour and varied ways of classifying them have been in use, making comparison of published series from different centres difficult or impossible. The section headings that follow are based on the nomenclature and classification of epithelial tumours of the salivary glands recommended for international use by the World Health Organization.[60,61] Although the classification looks simple, it must be admitted that the tumours present so wide a range of histological patterns and behaviour that there is occasionally difficulty in fitting a tumour into the suggested histological categories.

1. Adenomas
   a. Pleomorphic adenoma (mixed tumour)
   b. Monomorphic adenomas
      (i) Adenolymphoma
      (ii) Oxyphilic adenoma
      (iii) Other types
2. Mucoepidermoid tumour

3. Acinic cell tumour
4. Carcinomas
   (i) Adenoid cystic carcinoma
   (ii) Adenocarcinoma
   (iii) Epidermoid carcinoma
   (iv) Undifferentiated carcinoma
   (v) Carcinoma in pleomorphic adenoma (malignant mixed tumour)

PLEOMORPHIC ADENOMAS

Pleomorphic adenomas are the commonest tumours of the major salivary glands, accounting for between 70 and 80% of parotid, and between 60 and 70% of submandibular neoplasms. These tumours have had many names in the past, the most popular being 'mixed parotid tumour', which reflected the presence of the cartilage-like areas. As similar growths occur in the submandibular and minor salivary glands, where the designation 'parotid' is inapplicable, the name became simply 'mixed tumour'. It is now generally accepted that the tumours are not in fact composed of different tissues but are essentially epithelial and, having regard to their very varied histological pattern, the term pleomorphic adenoma has come into general use.

Pleomorphic adenomas are commoner in women, in a ratio of about 5:4; they may appear at almost any time of life from childhood to old age, but perhaps oftenest in the fourth and fifth decades. They grow slowly, sometimes pausing in their growth for several years; if untreated they may in the course of time reach a great size. One of the largest parotid tumours on record weighed 60 lb (27 kg), and accounted for a third of the total weight of the woman who had carried it around for 30 years.[62] Parotid tumours usually protrude externally behind the angle of the jaw, below the ear. About 10% of parotid pleomorphic adenomas arise in that part of the gland deep to the facial nerve, and these may become quite large before any external swelling is noticed. Rarely, a deep lobe tumour grows through the gap between the mandible and the styloid process and stylomandibular ligament to enter the parapharyngeal space and displace the tonsil medially, the tumour then becoming dumb-bell or hour-glass-shaped.[63]

Pleomorphic adenomas are almost invariably solitary. Their surface is smooth, and though they may be rounded or ovoid they are more often nodular or bosselated. In most instances the cut surface is firm and white, but with scattered bluish areas of cartilage-like appearance; there may be occasional small cystic spaces, but distinctly cystic tumours are very unusual (Fig. 3.11). The consistence is sometimes soft, or even mucoid, so that during attempted removal the tumour may rupture and its substance be spilled.

Microscopically, there is considerable variation in structure both from tumour to tumour and in different parts of the same tumour; the designation pleomorphic is apt. Some areas have a straightforward adenomatous appearance, with duct-like structures lined by cubical or columnar epithelial cells and surrounded by an outer mantle of smaller, more darkly-staining cells of myo-epithelial type. The myo-epithelial cells may be polygonal, and they may then be arranged in few or many layers

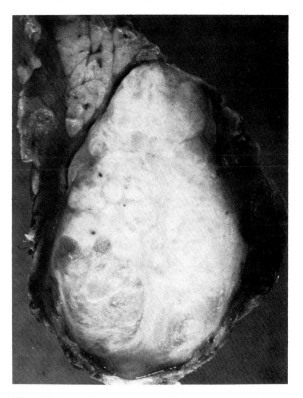

Fig. 3.11 Cut surface of a pleomorphic adenoma in the lower pole of the parotid. The tumour—its longest dimension is 3 cm—is solitary, circumscribed and characteristically nodular.

round the epithelium lining the ducts; or they may form solid compact masses, sometimes constituting the bulk of the tumour. They may be spindle-shaped and even markedly elongated—with their eosinophilic and often markedly striate cytoplasm they may give the tumour a strikingly myomatous appearance (Fig. 3.12). Characteristically, a basi-phile mucoid material accumulates among the myo-epithelial cells, which become more and more widely separated from one another and modified in appearance; ultimately, hydropic and embedded in the mucoid substance, they look uncommonly like cartilage cells (Fig. 3.13). Elsewhere, myo-epithelial cells, either solitary or in small groups or strands, scattered throughout a looser mucoid background give a myxoid appearance. Such myxoid tissue may make up the bulk of the tumour, the epithelial tubules being few and far between. This chondromyxoid tissue is a very characteristic feature of pleomorphic adenoma.

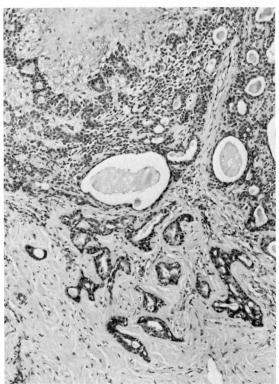

Fig. 3.13 Pleomorphic adenoma of the parotid showing ducts and surrounding myo-epithelial cells merging above into a cartilage-like area.

Haematoxylin-eosin   × 100

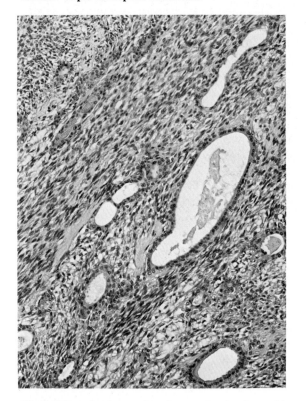

Fig. 3.12 Part of a pleomorphic adenoma showing ducts with a single layer of lining epithelium. Many of the surrounding myo-epithelial cells are plump and elongated and give a myomatous appearance to the growth.

Haematoxylin-eosin   × 120

In compact parts of the tumour, groups of myo-epithelial cells are sometimes seen which have become rounded or ovoid, less firmly attached to one another, and whose cytoplasm has taken on a hyaline or glassy appearance. With their nucleus to one side they look superficially like plasma cells. These hyaline or plasmacytoid cells, more often seen in tumours of the palate than of the major salivary glands, are, when present, considered to be a distinctive feature of pleomorphic adenomas (Fig. 3.14).[64]

Squamous epithelium may be found in pleo-morphic adenomas. The myo-epithelium appears to merge into foci of epidermoid cells and these cell groups may enlarge, keratinize and form epithelial pearls or even quite large cysts full of shed keratin scales (Fig. 3.15). Degeneration of the wall of such a cyst may release keratin into the tissues, where a foreign-body giant cell reaction develops. Rarely, sebaceous glands may be associated with the

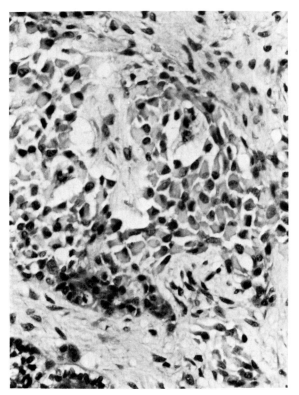

Fig. 3.14 A group of hyaline or plasmacytoid myo-epithelial cells in a pleomorphic adenoma of the palate.

Haematoxylin-eosin   × 250

squamous elements.[65] Other less common findings in pleomorphic adenomas are groups of oncocytes, and, particularly in Blacks, crystalline structures, arranged like the petals of a daisy, which are rich in tyrosine (Fig. 3.16).[66]

The tumours have a supporting fibrovascular stroma in which scattered fat cells are sometimes seen, whilst in some tumours elastic fibres form in the stroma.[67] Fibrous tissue also forms a capsule outside the tumour, of varying thickness and completeness. Degenerative changes may be seen in the central regions of long-standing tumours; the epithelial cells gradually fade away and the stroma becomes more hyaline, any elastic tissue present becoming more obvious in the clear background. As the tubules degenerate their basement membrane regions also take on the staining properties of elastic and may survive as collapsed wrinkled rings. Even after all nuclear staining has gone the ghostly outline of the chondroid tissue is readily recognizable. Calcification may occur in the degenerate tissue, and may go on to bone formation; bone is occasionally found in the living parts of pleomorphic adenomas.

Course and prognosis

The pleomorphic salivary adenomas are notorious for their tendency to recur after what has been considered by the surgeon to be adequate removal by enucleation or 'shelling out'. It seems clear that such recurrences represent the continued growth of tumour tissue left in situ or implanted in the operation field as a result of rupture of the tumour during removal. The familiar nodularity of the outer surface of the tumour may in places take the form of bulbous protrusions with relatively narrow necks which are liable to be divided during the operation, the excrescence then being left behind. It may be noted that when a tumour-containing salivary gland is sectioned these surface sprouts may appear as separate islands of tumour tissue because their necks are not in the plane examined: they are sometimes erroneously described as satellite nodules.[68] Pleomorphic adenomas removed intact with an adequate margin of parotid tissue do not recur.[69]

Recurrent tumours are sometimes solitary, but usually consist of multiple nodules (Fig. 3.17). If the original growth ruptured during removal, tumour tissue may be implanted anywhere in the surgical field: these implants are often outside the confines of the gland and develop with particular frequency in the cutaneous scar. Like the original tumour, the recurrent nodules grow slowly, sometimes not becoming apparent until many years after the first operation; they may then remain unchanged for quite a long time. Recurrent tumours are even more difficult to remove successfully than the original growth, for although there may appear to the surgeon to be only a single nodule, examination of the operative specimen usually shows other small deposits, disappointingly often at the limit of excision.

Although ordinarily benign, in the sense that they do not metastasize, pleomorphic adenomas have been known—very rarely—to give rise to a distant deposit, both the primary and the secondary growths showing a histological picture that differs little, if at all, from that of the typical pleomorphic adenoma described above.[70] In the few reported

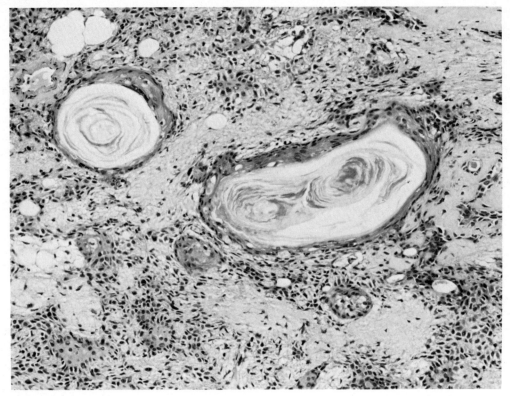

Fig. 3.15 Cysts lined by squamous epithelium and filled with layers of keratin in a parotid pleomorphic adenoma.

Haematoxylin-eosin   × 140

examples of this phenomenon the slowly growing secondaries have become apparent at such distant sites as the liver,[71] lungs or pelvic bones many years after the first operation on the parotid. There had usually been local recurrence of the parotid tumour, with further attempts at removal, in the course of which a minute fragment of tumour presumably got into a vascular channel, was carried to the distant site and slowly grew there. A much more real danger to the patient with a pleomorphic adenoma is the fact that at any stage in its life history a pleomorphic adenoma may start to grow rapidly and present unequivocal clinical and pathological evidence of frank malignancy. Occasionally, malignant characteristics are present when the tumour is first diagnosed and removed, but malignancy is likeliest to be seen as a change in the character of a tumour, primary or recurrent, that has been present for 15-20 years. The type of malignancy that develops is referred to later (see p. 123).

MONOMORPHIC ADENOMAS

Monomorphic adenomas differ from pleomorphic adenomas in having a more or less uniform pattern throughout, and particularly in lacking the mesenchyme-like chondroid or myxoid areas that are so common a feature of pleomorphic adenomas. Some, but not all, consist of a single cell type. Any of the various patterns which will be described in monomorphic adenomas may also be found in pleomorphic adenomas either in small foci, or occasionally forming the greater part of the tumour, so that before a tumour can be diagnosed as a monomorphic adenoma myxochondroid areas and other features peculiar to pleomorphic adenomas must have been sought, and not found. The first monomorphic adenoma to be described here, the adenolymphoma, is the commonest, accounting for over 70% of all monomorphic adenomas. The oxyphilic adenoma is another distinctive type of tumour. The rest of the monomorphic adeno-

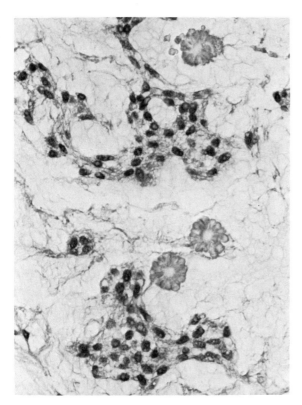

Fig. 3.16 Tyrosine-rich crystals arranged like daisy flowers in a pleomorphic adenoma from a Black woman.

Haematoxylin-eosin   × 250

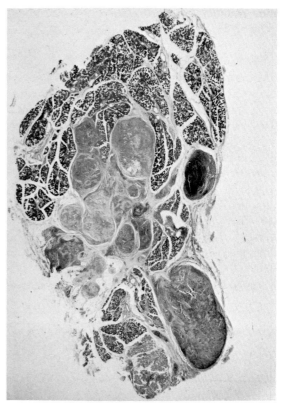

Fig. 3.17 Cross-section of a parotid gland excised because of recurrence of a pleomorphic adenoma, showing the multiple nodules of tumour so often found in such specimens.

Haematoxylin-eosin   × 5

mas, a varied collection, are grouped together in the WHO classification (see p. 102) as 'other types'.[60]

Adenolymphoma

The original account of this tumour by Albrecht & Arzt[72] in 1910 was followed by a detailed description by Warthin,[73] in 1929, under the title 'papillary cystadenoma lymphomatosum'. The tumour has also been called Warthin's tumour or cystadenolymphoma, but the usual name at present is adenolymphoma. It is not, of course, a lymphoma, and lymphadenoma would have been a better name had it not at one time been applied to Hodgkin's disease. It accounts for about 8% of tumours of the parotid, which is by far its commonest site. It occasionally arises in the submandibular gland, or in one of the lymph nodes adjacent to the parotid in which ectopic salivary tissue may occur. Rare examples have been reported

from the minor salivary glands, such as those of the palate, cheeks, lips and tongue.[74] The tumour is three or four times commoner in men than in women, and usually develops in the sixth or seventh decades; before middle age they are very rare. Published series of cases from America show them to be very uncommon in Blacks.[75]

Adenolymphomas grow slowly, and form soft, painless, rounded or ovoid swellings which are most often situated in the lower pole or posterior part of the parotid. They are usually fairly superficially placed in the gland. Adenolymphomas are well circumscribed and smooth, or only slightly lobulated, and can be shelled out easily if the surgeon favours that procedure. The cut surface is brownish in colour, as in most lesions rich in oncocytes, and, although occasionally solid, usually shows a number of cysts of various sizes. The cysts typically contain many plump papillary ingrowths from their walls, the remaining space being occupied by a brownish viscid fluid, which may be clear, or may be opaque and mistaken for pus or soft caseous material.

Microscopically, the adenolymphoma has a very characteristic structure, to which both epithelium and lymphoid tissue contribute. The epithelium is two-layered. The inner layer consists of a neat row of large, tall columnar cells with finely granular eosinophilic cytoplasm giving them a typically oncocytic appearance; beneath them there is a basal layer of smaller, cubical or pyramidal cells adjoining the basement membrane (Figs 3.18 and 3.19). Electron microscopy confirms the oncocytic nature of the cells of both layers, their cytoplasm being packed with large mitochondria, often of abnormal type, whilst other details of the fine structure relate them to the striated duct cells of the normal gland.

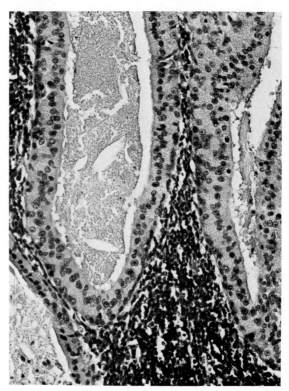

Fig. 3.19 Adenolymphoma. Higher magnification to show the characteristic appearance of the tall epithelial cells lining the spaces of the tumour. Note the regular position and orderly arrangement of the nuclei. It can also be seen that there is a definite, but less well defined, second layer of cells between the lumen and the stroma.

Haematoxylin-eosin   × 190

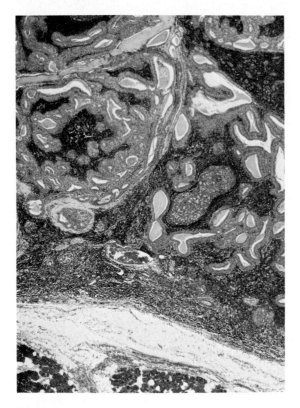

Fig. 3.18 An adenolymphoma showing clefts and tubules lined by tall eosinophilic epithelium in a lymphoid stroma. The tumour is clearly demarcated from the adjacent parotid glandular tissue below.

Haematoxylin-eosin   × 30

In over 50% of adenolymphomas mucous goblet cells in varying numbers can be found scattered here and there among the columnar epithelial cells; they are occasionally numerous and account for the mucoid consistence of the cyst fluid. Less often, localized patches of squamous metaplasia of the cyst lining are found. In the stroma of the tumour there are large accumulations of lymphocytes, with occasional plasma cells; lymphoid follicles with prominent germinal centres are usually conspicuously numerous.

The characteristic epithelium lines tubules and irregular clefts, as well as cysts. Cystic spaces, often of considerable size, are common, and papillary ingrowths from their walls have lymphoid tissue, often with follicles, for their cores. Occasionally the tumour is for the most part a single cyst with a layer of lymphoid tissue around it and with only an occasional papillary process protruding into it. The cyst fluid contains extruded eosinophilic epithelial cells, mucus, cholesterol crystals, corpora amylacea[76] and often some macrophages; the diagnosis has sometimes been made from the characteristic appearance of the aspirated fluid. Cyst contents occasionally escape into the stroma and provoke a granulomatous reaction there.

Rarely, adenolymphomas become infected and acutely inflamed.[77] If first seen by the surgeon in this condition they are likely to be diagnosed and treated as abscesses. As the inflammation subsides the stroma becomes increasingly fibrous and there is squamous metaplasia of much of the epithelium (Fig. 3.20). Areas of infarction are also occasionally seen in adenolymphomas. The necrotic area retains its structure, but all nuclear staining disappears; the living tumour tissue bordering the infarct shows squamous metaplasia. Squamous metaplasia has also been shown to follow the irradiation of

adenolymphomas. A histological subclassification of these tumours has recently been proposed based on the relative proportions of epithelial and lymphoid components and on the extent of metaplasia.[78]

In about 10% of cases the tumours are bilateral or multiple. This may be the case when the patient is first seen (Fig. 3.21), or further tumours may develop in the gland from which an adenolymphoma has been removed. Not infrequently, a similar tumour develops in the opposite parotid, perhaps several years later. This tendency to multiplicity accounts for supposed recurrences following removal of these otherwise simple tumours.

It is extremely rare for malignancy to develop in adenolymphomas. In the few convincing reports available the malignant tumour has always been a carcinoma of some sort, never a lymphoma, and in approximately 50% of the cases there has been previous irradiation.[78]

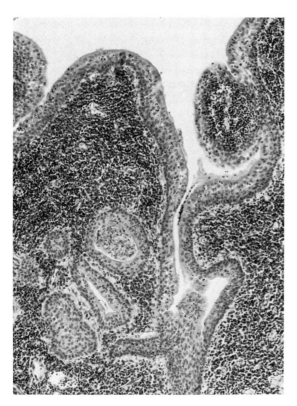

Fig. 3.20 Squamous metaplasia of the epithelium of an adenolymphoma.

Haematoxylin-eosin × 100

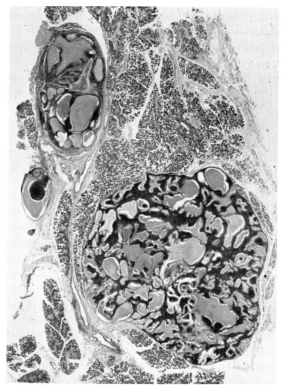

Fig. 3.21 Section showing three separate adenolymphomas in the same parotid. The tumours contain multiple cysts.

Haematoxylin-eosin × 5

The histogenesis of adenolymphoma has been much debated. The association of lymphoid tissue and epithelial elements was at one time thought to indicate that the tumours originated in branchial remnants, but the fine structure of the cells is against this. Another theory, that the lesion is akin to Hashimoto's disease and that the entire lymphoid stroma is an immunological reaction to the oncocytic cell proliferation does not cover all the facts.[79] The most likely explanation seems to be that adenolymphomas develop from salivary tissue enclosed within intraparotid and nearby lymph nodes. The acini of such salivary tissue usually atrophy or fail to develop, but the ducts remain and are liable to undergo oncocytic change and hyperplasia in later life. At the periphery of early adenolymphomas it may be possible to make out a peripheral sinus beneath a fibrous capsule, and the lymphoreticular tissue beneath shows the cellular composition of a normal lymph node. Further in, in the neighbourhood of the epithelium, plasma cells can be seen and there is evidence of an immunological reaction to the oncocytic epithelium, accounting for the lymphoid tissue of the tumour being much in excess of that in the original little lymph node.[78] The fact that adenolymphomas have been reported from sites where there are no lymph nodes, such as the palate, may seem to raise a difficulty, but many of these lesions are described as lacking lymphoid tissue or including at most a few lymphocytes, and so are not really comparable with parotid adenolymphomas. However, a recent report of two typical palatal adenolymphomas would seem to keep open the question whether the tumour can sometimes be a local lymphoid reaction to hyperplastic oncocytic epithelium not in a lymph node.[80]

Oxyphilic adenoma

Oxyphilic adenomas, or oncocytomas, are rare, accounting for no more than 1% of all tumours of the parotid glands. They are even rarer in the submandibular glands, and only occasional examples have been reported from the palate and other sites in the mouth. The tumour is a little commoner in women than in men, and is rarely seen before 50 years of age, with the highest incidence in the seventh decade.

The alternative name for the tumour indicates the likeness of the tumour cells to oncocytes, those greatly enlarged, strikingly eosinophilic, finely granular cells seen in various organs of the body, particularly in epithelial cells, in the later years of life. A few typical oncocytes can often be seen in the ducts of minor salivary glands of old people, for instance, where they may undergo hyperplasia to form microscopic nodules. The cytoplasm of oncocytes is seen ultramicroscopically to be packed with excessive numbers of apparently normal, and of unusually large and distorted, mitochondria.

Oxyphilic adenomas grow slowly to form firm, smooth, rounded or ovoid tumours, which are sometimes slightly lobulated. When cut across they are solid and uniform throughout, often with a brownish tinge to the pale-pink cut surface.

Microscopically, the tumour is composed of large, eosinophilic, finely granular cells (Fig. 3.22), with the nucleus round and usually centrally

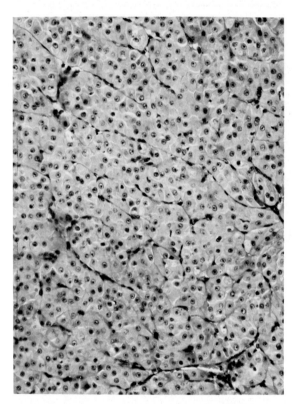

Fig. 3.22 Oxyphilic adenoma of the parotid (oncocytoma) composed of sheets of uniform cells with eosinophilic cytoplasm.

Haematoxylin-eosin   × 160

placed. The cells are arranged in solid acinar groups, broad bands or sheets, the type of arrangement and mutual pressure determining the shape of the cells. Tubules or tiny cysts are sometimes seen, but are not usual (Fig. 3.23). There is relatively little delicate fibrovascular supporting stroma among the cell groups. There may be a few lymphocytes here and there, but lymphoid follicles are only rarely present.

Oxyphilic adenomas are benign tumours and only rarely recur after removal. Serial sectioning of glands containing these tumours quite often shows focal collections of oncocytes away from the main tumour and these may be responsible for some reports of recurrence. Bilateral tumours are usually said to be very uncommon, though in one series a third of the patients had tumours in both parotids.[81]

Most varieties of salivary gland tumour may occasionally contain areas where their cells have been transformed into oncocytes. In pleomorphic adenomas this change may involve only small foci, but very rarely most of the tumour is oncocytic, with only a few areas left to indicate the correct diagnosis.[82] The same applies to mucoepidermoid tumours and even adenocarcinomas, the metastases of which may be partially or largely oncocytic. These possibilities have to be kept in mind before a tumour is accepted as a malignant oncocytoma, very few of which have been reported.

Oncocytosis. This rare condition may conveniently be mentioned here. In it, the acinar epithelium of the parotid is transformed in situ into oncocytes, either throughout the gland, or in multiple patches. The ducts are usually spared. The gland is enlarged and soft, and the condition is sometimes clinically misdiagnosed as a lipoma.

Other types of monomorphic adenoma

Some writers restrict the term monomorphic adenoma to the various tumours to be mentioned in this section, keeping adenolymphoma and oxyphilic adenoma as separate entities, though it would be difficult to word a definition of monomorphic adenoma that would exclude them.[83]

Monomorphic adenomas are rare, accounting for only 1 or 2% of all parotid tumours. Almost as many occur in the minor salivary glands, where, of course, they account for a distinctly higher percentage.[84] The upper lip is the commonest site of minor salivary gland monomorphic adenomas, with fewer in the cheek, palate and elsewhere.[83]

Monomorphic adenomas are found in rather older patients than are pleomorphic adenomas, most often between the ages of 50 and 70, and a little more often in women than in men.

They grow slowly and form firm, rounded or ovoid, smooth-surfaced tumours which are usually encapsulated or, at least, well demarcated from the surrounding glandular tissue. The cut surface is mainly solid, but one or more small cysts are not uncommonly present. A few tumours are predominantly cystic and multilocular; occasionally, particularly in the lip, the tumour may consist of a single cyst with one or more small nodules of tumour tissue in its wall.

Sporadic reports of salivary gland tumours, distinct from the familiar mixed tumour, had been appearing for many years,[85] but it was the account

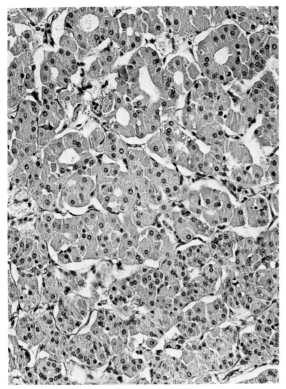

Fig. 3.23 An oxyphilic adenoma in which there are areas of tubule formation.

Haematoxylin-eosin   × 175

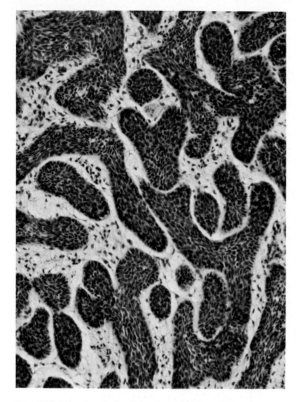

Fig. 3.24 A basal cell adenoma, showing the broad bands of smallish darkly-stained cells with uniform nuclei and relatively little cytoplasm.

Haematoxylin-eosin   × 175

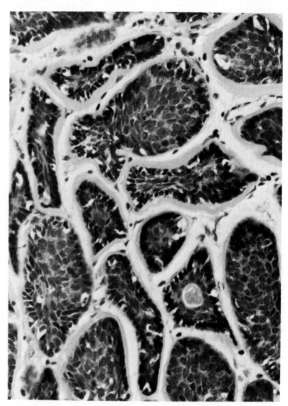

Fig. 3.25 Membranous basal cell adenoma, with hyaline bands surrounding the cell masses. Occasional small ducts are present.

Haematoxylin-eosin   × 250

of basal cell adenomas of the salivary glands by Kleinsasser & Klein in 1967[86] that stimulated interest in this group of tumours. Since then many more reports have appeared, and though some writers seem to regard basal cell adenoma as a convenient overall diagnostic label, others have chosen a variety of names for the different monomorphic patterns, and it is often difficult to decide which are synonyms and which refer to distinct entities.[87] Some of the terms used refer to the type of cell, such as basal, myo-epithelial, sebaceous or clear, whilst others indicate the arrangement, such as tubular, canalicular, trabecular or papillary cystadenoma. Although 'monomorphic' implies a uniform cytology and arrangement in individual tumours, there is a certain amount of overlap; basal cell adenomas may, for instance, contain occasional tubules.

The *basal cell adenoma*,[88] microscopically, consists of sheets and broad branching and interlacing bands of smallish cells having round to oval darkly-staining nuclei and relatively little cytoplasm (Fig. 3.24). The cell masses quite often have a palisade layer around them reminiscent of the basal cell carcinoma of the skin, and are sharply demarcated from the rather loose fibrous stroma. The tumour cells are uniform in size and staining, and the tumour has a fibrous capsule. In the compact cell masses there may be whorling of the parallel swathes of cells, and, as noted above, occasional small tubules may be seen.

A very rare variant of basal cell adenoma has prominent hyaline bands of basement membrane material surrounding the cell masses, giving an overall picture almost indistinguishable from a dermal cylindroma of sweat gland origin (Fig. 3.25). This tumour of the parotid may be multiple and occasionally bilateral, and some remarkable reports have appeared of the association of this tumour with multiple skin tumours of similar

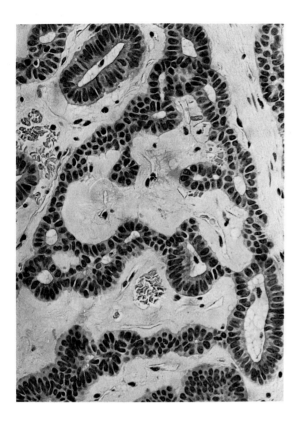

Fig. 3.26 Canalicular adenoma from the upper lip. The tumour is composed of epithelial cells of duct-lining type arranged as tubules or strands.

Haematoxylin-eosin   × 300

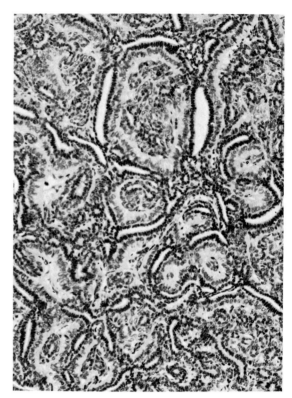

Fig. 3.27 Tubular type of monomorphic adenoma. The tubules, cut transversely or obliquely, are lined by a single layer of columnar or cubical cells surrounded by myo-epithelial cells.

Haematoxylin-eosin   × 150

appearance, or with a typical turban of scalp tumours, in the same patient. In one of the first descriptions of the tumour it was called a *membranous basal cell adenoma*,[89] but at least two other names have been proposed for it.[90,91]

The *canalicular adenoma*, a not uncommon tumour of the upper lip, is quite distinct from the basal cell adenoma. It consists of cubical or columnar epithelial cells forming duct-like structures, or arranged in interlacing cords and strands (Fig. 3.26). The ducts consist of a ring of epithelial cells only, with no outer mantle of myo-epithelial or basal cells. Electron microscopy shows similarities between these tumour cells and the excretory duct epithelium of the minor salivary glands.[92] Canalicular adenomas, which are much less often seen in the major salivary glands, may be largely cystic. Another tumour more often seen in minor salivary glands is the *papillary cystadenoma*, in which cystic

spaces are almost filled with papillary processes covered by the same cubical or columnar epithelium that lines the cysts.

Tubular adenomas have tubules lined by epithelial cells as their prominent feature, but these tubules usually have a mantle of cells of myo-epithelial type around them, bands of which cells often link neighbouring tubules together (Fig. 3.27). This appearance is quite often seen in parts of pleomorphic adenomas. Sometimes the strands of myo-epithelial cells linking up the tubules are so prominent, and the tubules are so small and sparse, that the overall picture is best described as trabecular. The cells of a *trabecular adenoma* may appear so featureless in routine sections that histochemical study is necessary to sort them out into duct-lining and myo-epithelial types[93] (Fig. 3.28). The tubular and trabecular adenomas overlap, and some writers combine them as *trabecular-*

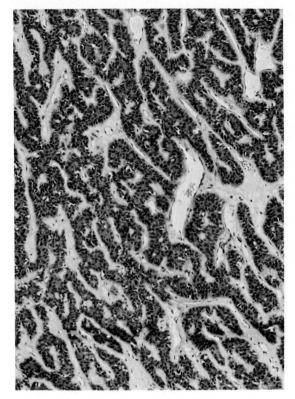

Fig. 3.28 Monomorphic adenoma, showing the trabecular pattern.

Haematoxylin-eosin   × 100

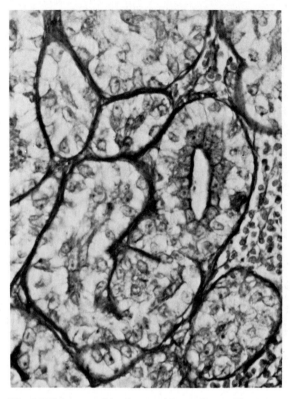

Fig. 3.29 Monomorphic adenoma, clear-cell type. The duct-lining cells are surrounded by a sheath of clear cells. Parts of the tumour may consist of clear cells only.

Periodic acid-Schiff   × 250

tubular adenomas.[94] In them there may sometimes be foci which mimic adenoid cystic carcinoma, and it is possible that such a carcinoma may occasionally develop from this type of adenoma. If there is doubt about the diagnosis the periphery of the tumour must be searched for evidence of infiltrative growth.

An early report entitled 'Glycogen-rich clear-cell adenoma of the parotid gland' described a tumour in which there were ducts lined by small cubical or low columnar cells surrounded by a zone of large clear cells.[95] In parts of the tumour there were few ducts, and the clear cells, which could be shown to contain glycogen, predominated. These *clear-cell adenomas* are uncommon, and need to be distinguished from other clear-celled salivary tumours (Fig. 3.29). A malignant tumour which has been called a salivary duct carcinoma usually contains areas resembling the clear-cell adenoma, and the distinction between the two may be so difficult that some writers regard all tumours of this sort with suspicion.[96]

Parts of a pleomorphic adenoma may be made up of compact masses of myo-epithelial cells; tumours entirely composed of such cells, variously arranged, have been called *myo-epitheliomas.* Opinions may differ as to whether a certain tumour is to be regarded as a myo-epithelioma or as a basal cell adenoma, depending on the interpretation of the electron microscopical appearances and histochemical evidence.

Final rare types of monomorphic adenoma to be mentioned are the *sebaceous lymphadenoma,*[97] characterized by sebaceous glands and squamous cysts in a lymphoid stroma (Fig. 3.30), and the even rarer *sebaceous adenoma*, a similar tumour without the lymphoid stroma.

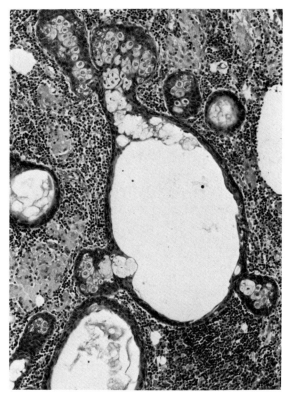

Fig. 3.30 Sebaceous lymphadenoma, showing sebaceous glands discharging into squamous-lined cysts. Groups of histiocytes are present in the lymphoid stroma.

Haematoxylin-eosin   × 100

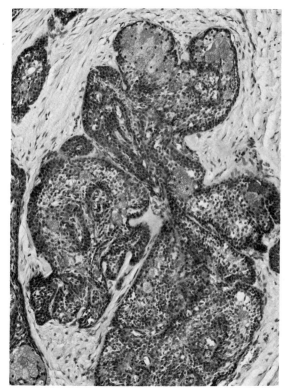

Fig. 3.31 An infiltrating well-differentiated mucoepidermoid tumour, showing solid collections of epidermoid cells and groups of large paler mucous cells at the top and lower left corner.

Haematoxylin-eosin   × 100

MUCOEPIDERMOID TUMOURS

The first description of the growths that are now known as mucoepidermoid tumours was given by Masson & Berger in 1924 under the name *épithélioma à double métaplasie*.[98] The first account with sufficient follow-up to indicate their clinical behaviour was published in 1945 by Stewart et al,[99] who called the tumours mucoepidermoid, and divided them into two groups, benign and malignant. As the name implies, they contain both mucus-producing cells and epithelial cells of epidermoid type, usually with demonstrable intercellular bridges. Electron microscopical studies indicate that both these varieties of cell may differentiate from intermediate cells of indeterminate type that are also a feature of the tumour. Myo-epithelial cells are not present. As a response to chronic inflammation or to the presence of calculi, the ducts of the salivary glands are liable both to squamous metaplasia and to the proliferation of mucus-secreting cells; such changes are often seen in the gland near a mucoepidermoid tumour.

Between 3 and 5% of parotid tumours are mucoepidermoid and a similar percentage of the much less numerous submandibular neoplasms. Mucoepidermoid tumours account for between 10 and 15% of minor salivary gland tumours, most of them being in the palate, the second most common site after the parotid. The tumours are rather more common in females, and cover a wide age range. A typical tumour has been reported in a 1-year-old child,[100] whilst tumours are also occasionally seen in old age. Most cases occur in the third and fourth decades, with an appreciable number in adolescents. The tumour may arise in the glands or their main ducts, and comparable tumours are seen in various other parts of the body, such as the nose and nasal sinuses, and the bronchi.

Both naked-eye and microscopical examination

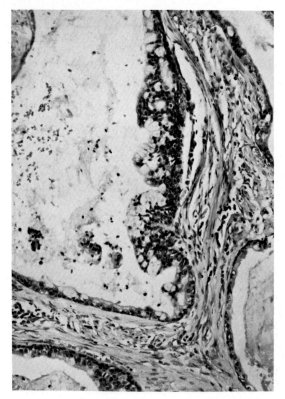

Fig. 3.32 A mucus-filled cyst in a well-differentiated mucoepidermoid tumour.

Haematoxylin-eosin   × 200

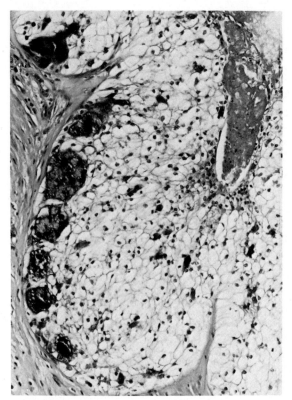

Fig. 3.33 Clear cells in a mucoepidermoid tumour. The mucous cells, if darkly stained with Ehrlich's haematoxylin, are easily distinguished from the clear epidermoid cells.

Haematoxylin-eosin   × 160

show a considerable range of structure, depending on the relative proportions of mucus-producing and epidermoid constituents (Fig. 3.31). If mucus production is plentiful many cysts, some of them large enough to be apparent on the cut surface, are likely to have formed, and from these mucus often escapes into the interstitial tissues, and even outside the apparent limits of the tumour (Fig. 3.32). Most mucoepidermoid tumours are well differentiated, though there is only sometimes actual keratin formation. In some tumours clear cells are present among the epidermoid cells, and may be a prominent feature of the microscopic picture (Fig. 3.33). These clear cells do not stain for fat or mucin, but glycogen may be present. The minority of mucoepidermoid tumours that are poorly differentiated are made up of epidermoid cells and the smaller intermediate cells, showing some pleomorphism and occasional mitoses, and with the

mucus cells much less in evidence, so that without special stains for mucus the tumour may be misinterpreted as a poorly-differentiated epidermoid carcinoma or even as an undifferentiated growth.

The well-differentiated growths are usually circumscribed, or even partially encapsulated, and are likely to be diagnosed as pleomorphic adenomas before operation. Microscopically, however, there is nearly always infiltrative growth somewhere at the periphery of the tumour, and unless it is removed with a good margin there is liable to be local recurrence. Mucus extravasated from the predominantly cystic growths may carry tumour cells with it into the surroundings, and such tumours are particularly liable to local recurrence, though still eventually curable. Well-differentiated mucoepidermoid tumours are unlikely to metastasize, though the possibility cannot be completely ruled out; the small percentage of tumours that are poorly differentiated are more liable to metastasize to local lymph nodes or spread to distant sites. Nevertheless, the overall prognosis for patients with mucoepidermoid tumours is very good, with 5-year survival rates of 88% and over being reported 20 years ago.[101] The few patients with these tumours who are going to die from them usually do so within two years of initial treatment, and a recent report quotes 96% determinate survival rates at both five and 10 years.[102] Although it is not now thought possible to make a clear-cut division into benign and malignant mucoepidermoid tumours the overall prognosis is so good that to call them all carcinomas, as is sometimes done, takes too pessimistic a view.

ACINIC CELL TUMOURS

Acinic cell tumours are rare and account for only 2 or 3% of tumours of the parotid, by far their commonest site of origin. Their occurrence in the submandibular or minor salivary glands, such as those of the palate and floor of mouth, is only very occasionally reported.[103,104] They may be found at almost any time of life, from about 10 years of age onwards, with most series showing the highest incidence in the fifth decade. Women are affected rather more often than men, and occasional bilateral tumours are on record.[105] It is of interest that the patients quite often complain of intermittent tenderness or even pain without any nerve involvement being subsequently demonstrable.[106]

Slow-growing acinic cell tumours are often well circumscribed or even encapsulated, though more rapidly growing examples with a short history may be less well defined. The tumour is only a little firmer than the normal gland, and the greyish-white cut surface, occasionally with yellowish areas, is usually solid. Small cysts are sometimes present or, rarely, the tumour may take the form of a single cyst with a nodule of growth in its wall.[107] Attempts at localized removal of the tumour are likely to be followed by recurrence, often as multiple nodules anywhere in the operative field.

The typical tumour cell, strikingly similar to the normal acinar cell of the parotid, is relatively large, with a basiphile cytoplasm in which there are granules staining dark blue in haematoxylin-eosin preparations (Fig. 3.34). The granules, which are PAS-positive, vary in size and may be as large and prominent as the zymogen granules of the normal gland. In parts of the tumour the cells may lack granules, and the bluish cytoplasm may appear finely vacuolated or even quite clear and empty. Another cell type, smaller and cubical, with weakly eosinophilic cytoplasm, may also be seen. These cells are sometimes arranged as tubules, resembling the intercalated ducts of the normal gland, from which it has been suggested the tumour arises.[103] These various cell types often co-exist in the same tumour and any type may predominate. The granular cells are often the most numerous, and some at least must be identified to justify the diagnosis.

The tumour cells, whether characteristically granular, or without granules, may be arranged in

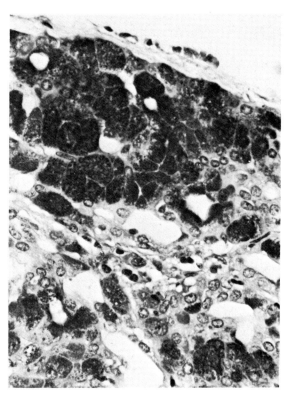

Fig. 3.34 Acinic cell tumour. Alveolar groups of tumour cells at the upper part of the figure are densely packed with darkly-stained granules; the tumour cells in the lower part are either sparsely granulated or devoid of granules.

Haematoxylin-eosin   × 300

neat acinar groups, or in cords, but are often in compact sheets, with little supporting stroma (Fig. 3.35). Here and there among the tumour cells apparently empty spaces probably represent trapped secretion, and if these are numerous a lattice-like pattern is produced (Fig. 3.36). With further fluid accumulation the spaces merge with one another until eventually the tumour tissue, broken up into coarsely papillary processes, comes to occupy quite large cysts. Much of the tumour may show only this so-called papillocystic pattern, and the diagnostic granular cells may be few and far between.

Rarely, the small spaces in the tumour referred to above contain, instead of clear fluid, an eosinophilic colloid-like material, the presence of which has sometimes led to confusion with a thyroid neoplasm, especially if seen in a cervical lymph node.[108] Another source of confusion is the predominantly clear-celled acinic cell tumour which may

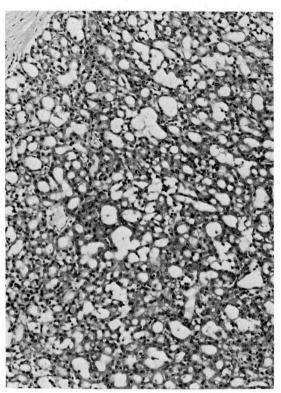

Fig. 3.36 An acinic cell tumour showing the lattice or lace-like pattern resulting from fluid accumulation.
Haematoxylin-eosin   × 100

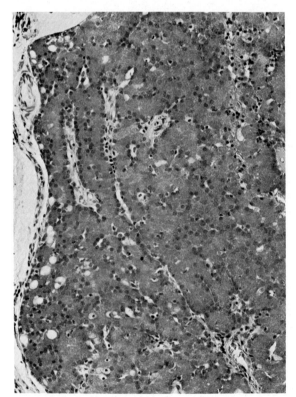

Fig. 3.35 A well-differentiated acinic cell tumour. The tumour cells, with their finely granular basiphile cytoplasm, are arranged in acinar groups or bands.
Haematoxylin-eosin   × 150

be mistaken for a metastasis of a clear-celled renal carcinoma, or vice versa.[109] Electron microscopy may help to determine the nature of the clear cells,[110] though their clarity is now regarded as a fixation artefact. Two other occasional histological features of acinic cell tumours worth noting are the presence of psammoma-like bodies among the tumour cells, and lymphoid tissue in the stroma.

In most acinic cell tumours the cells, whatever their type, show little pleomorphism or mitotic activity, though both these features may be marked in the few more malignant growths. Encapsulated acinic cell tumours removed with an ample margin of normal tissue rarely recur or metastasize. A recent review of a large series of these tumours, 92% of which were in the parotid, reported local recurrence in 12%, metastasis in 7.8% and death in 6.1%. The authors note that higher death rates have often been quoted—up to 50% at 15 years—but suggest that their own figures reflect an improvement in the early treatment of parotid tumours; they also found that biopsy of the tumour was associated with a markedly increased incidence of recurrence and metastasis. It is unusual for metastatic spread to local lymph nodes, or more distant sites, to occur before there has been at least one local recurrence. The metastases are often slow-growing and their removal may usefully prolong survival.[111]

Acinic cell tumours were originally described in two forms, adenoma and carcinoma, but it seems impossible to make a clear histological distinction between them, since even well-differentiated tumours very occasionally metastasize. Some writers call the whole group acinic cell carcinomas or adenocarcinomas, but others consider the non-committal term acinic cell tumours preferable.[103]

CARCINOMAS

Adenoid cystic carcinoma

Adenoid cystic carcinoma, which has been known also as adenocystic carcinoma, basalioma, cylindroma and cylindromatous carcinoma, accounts for only about 2% of all parotid tumours. It is the commonest malignant tumour of the submandibular gland, where about 15% of tumours are of this type.[112] Between 15 and 20% of minor salivary gland tumours are adenoid cystic carcinomas, the majority being in the palate. Identical growths arise in the mucous glands of the upper respiratory tract, and it was for one such, arising in the maxillary antrum and invading the orbit, that Billroth coined the name cylindroma.[113] The term cylindroma is now applied most often to a benign sweat gland tumour of comparable appearance but very different behaviour; potentially dangerous confusion would be avoided if the name were dropped from use altogether. There have been occasional reports of adenoid cystic carcinomas in children, but they are rare before the age of 20, and the majority of these tumours are seen between the ages of 40 and 60. They are slightly commoner in women than in men.

The tumours grow slowly and in their early stages may appear, clinically, to be circumscribed and benign. On examination after removal the cut surface is solid and pale, without cystic or mucoid areas and with no necrosis or haemorrhages. There may be apparent encapsulation at some part of the periphery, but there is nearly always obvious infiltrative growth which—particularly important if the surgeon thought he was dealing with an adenoma—all too often reaches the surface of the specimen.

Although so different from the pleomorphic adenoma in histological pattern and behaviour, the adenoid cystic carcinoma is made up of the same two cell types, duct epithelial cells and myoepithelial cells. The myo-epithelial cells are the more numerous. They do not disperse individually into a basiphile background, as in the pleomorphic adenoma, but remain as compact islands surrounded either by a hyaline sheath (the 'cylinder' of Billroth's term for the tumour) or by a mucoid substance. The hyaline and mucoid substances appear to be alternative forms of basement membrane material and a product of the myo-epithelial cells. The mucoid material in particular also accumulates here and there within the myo-epithelial cell masses to form round cyst-like collections, the 'adenoid cysts' that give the tumour its present name (Fig. 3.37). When these are large and numerous a cribriform pattern results: this is a feature very typical of certain of these tumours ('cribriform carcinomas') (Fig. 3.38). The epithelial component of the adenoid cystic carcinoma is made up of cells of duct-lining type which, with their eosinophilic cytoplasm, contrast with the myo-epithelial cells which have scanty pale cytoplasm. These duct epithelial cells usually play a minor part, appearing here or there in the cribriform islands as small groups, with or without a lumen. When a lumen is present it may be filled with a strongly eosinophilic PAS-positive substance. Rarely, these ducts may be dilated to form small cysts.

In parts of the tumour, instead of the cribriform arrangement, there may be a tubular pattern of growth, with ducts, often cut longitudinally or obliquely, each with a lining of epithelial cells and an outer mantle of myo-epithelial cells. A third possibility is a solid pattern of growth, with large irregular sheets of myo-epithelial cells without either type of cyst in them. These three main patterns—cribriform, tubular and solid—may all be seen in different parts of the same tumour, but

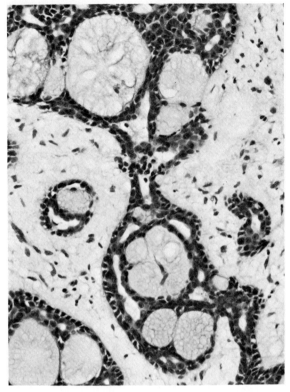

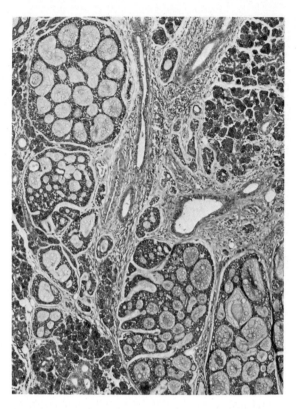

Fig. 3.37 Adenoid cystic carcinoma, showing ducts with a small narrow lumen and larger rounded collections of mucoid material in among the surrounding myo-epithelial cells.

Haematoxylin-eosin   × 250

Fig. 3.38 Adenoid cystic carcinoma of cribriform type in the submandibular gland. Note the absence of any clear line of demarcation. Such tumours usually extend well beyond the macroscopically apparent limits of the growth.

Haematoxylin-eosin   × 60

usually one or other predominates. Correlating the predominant histological pattern with the clinical course suggests that the solid pattern is the most sinister, the tubular pattern less malignant, and the cribriform in an intermediate position.[114] In addition to these three main growth patterns a number of other variants of the histological picture are possible.[115] Whatever the pattern, it is unusual to see many mitoses or much variation in cell size and staining in an adenoid cystic carcinoma.

It is important to note that both pleomorphic adenomas and certain monomorphic adenomas may contain small areas with a cribriform arrangement which have no ominous significance so long as the tumour is otherwise quite benign. There is, however, a strong suspicion that adenoid cystic carcinoma may sometimes originate in one variety of monomorphic adenoma, thus accounting for patients with adenoid cystic carcinomas who give

a long history of a very slowly enlarging smooth lump.

In its early stages an adenoid cystic carcinoma may be circumscribed, but it very soon infiltrates adjoining tissues, commonly sending out long finger-like columns, so that in sections foci of cribriform tumour, apparently isolated in the plane of sectioning, appear well outside the limits of the main growth. This makes it almost impossible for the pathologist to say whether removal of the tumour has been complete. The tumour has a special propensity for spreading along perineural spaces, though other tumours occasionally do likewise (Fig. 3.39). Bone is also insidiously permeated; palatal tumours extend through the Haversian systems of the underlying bone to reach the floor of the nose or antrum without at first producing any appreciable alteration in the radiological picture (Fig. 3.40). Although well differen-

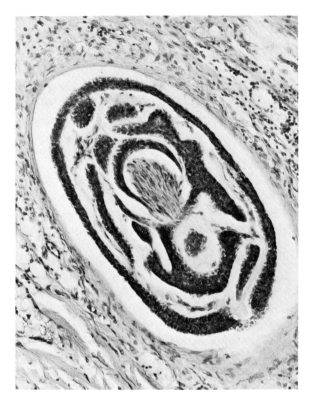

Fig. 3.39 Adenoid cystic carcinoma in the perineural space of a small nerve at the limit of removal of a parotid tumour.

Haematoxylin-eosin × 150

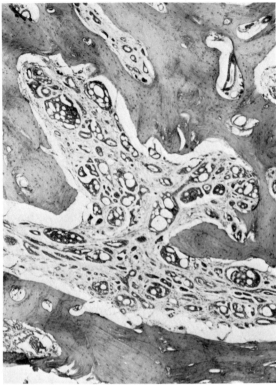

Fig. 3.40 Cribriform adenoid cystic carcinoma invading the maxilla from a tumour of the hard palate.

Haematoxylin-eosin × 60

tiated and slow growing, the adenoid cystic carcinoma is rarely completely eradicable surgically because of its insidious infiltration. Local recurrence is very common, and after several local attempts at eradication, distant metastases appear. Lymph node involvement is unusual, and when it does occur it is often by direct extension rather than by lymphatic metastasis.[116] The lungs are the commonest site of secondaries; it has often been remarked that patients with quite large pulmonary deposits of this tumour may still feel quite well for surprisingly long periods. Other secondaries may be found in the liver, bones and elsewhere. The tumour is radiosensitive but is rarely, if ever, curable by irradiation. Some recent reports suggest that chemotherapy may have something to offer in controlling the disease.[117] Usually it runs its inexorable course in 15 years or so, though one series quotes 13% still alive at 20 years.[118] At any stage in its progress the tumour may transform

into an anaplastic spindle-celled growth that is rapidly fatal.

Other carcinomas

Nearly all the carcinomas to be mentioned in this section can, on occasion, develop in a pleomorphic adenoma, the remains of which can be found somewhere in the tumour mass; the resulting malignant growth is then designated 'carcinoma in pleomorphic adenoma' without specifying the type of malignancy (see p. 123). The diagnostic labels in this section are only applied to tumours that are uniform throughout.

Adenocarcinomas

These are frankly malignant epithelial tumours made up of a single cell type and in which there is at least some tubule formation. Only 1 or 2% of major salivary gland tumours are adenocarcinomas, but they account for a higher percentage of minor salivary gland tumours. There is a wide range of malignancy; the well-differentiated tumours, commoner in the minor salivary glands, with well-formed tubules and few mitoses, grow slowly and may be cured by adequately wide excision. Tumours at the other end of the range grow fast, with many mitoses and areas of necrosis, infiltrate widely, metastasize, and are often rapidly fatal. Some adenocarcinomas produce mucus (*mucoid adenocarcinomas*), while others have a papillary arrangement (*papillary cystadenocarcinomas*) with or without mucus production.

There is one type of adenocarcinoma that is made up of two cell types, duct-lining cells and outer clear cells;[119,120] the latter are usually the more numerous and as they contain glycogen the tumour has been described as 'glycogen-rich adenocarcinoma'.[121] It has also been called a 'salivary duct carcinoma'[122] and appears to be the malignant counterpart of the clear-cell adenoma mentioned among the monomorphic adenomas.

Epidermoid or squamous cell carcinomas

These are rare in the salivary glands; they account for only about 2% of parotid tumours and for about the same number of tumours in the submandibular gland, where, of course, they form a higher percentage. They rarely, if ever, occur in the minor salivary glands, though necrotizing sialometaplasia may be misdiagnosed as epidermoid carcinoma. Necrotizing sialometaplasia is an uncommon benign lesion almost confined to minor salivary glands, most often those of the palate. It presents as a firm nodule which is usually ulcerated. Biopsy shows necrosis, possibly ischaemic, of the acinar tissue of the affected gland, with striking squamous metaplasia of the surviving ducts.[123]

In the parotid there is normally no squamous epithelium, but the ducts are prone to undergo squamous metaplasia in chronic inflammatory conditions, particularly when calculi are present, and this is presumed to be the source of such epidermoid carcinomas as do occur. Before a diagnosis of primary parotid epidermoid carcinoma is accepted, metastatic carcinoma in intraparotid lymph nodes, direct invasion of the parotid from a tumour outside it, and the possibility that the

carcinoma has developed in a long-standing pleomorphic adenoma, have to be excluded. Mucoepidermoid tumours with only occasional mucous areas must also be differentiated from epidermoid carcinomas; the former have a much better prognosis.

Epidermoid carcinomas occasionally contain sebaceous elements, and rarely these are so numerous that the tumour can be called a *sebaceous carcinoma*.[124]

Undifferentiated carcinoma

Occasional tumours of the salivary glands are so anaplastic that on light microscopy they can only be designated undifferentiated carcinomas. These account for between 3 and 4% of parotid tumours and double that percentage of submandibular growths. In one large series in which 3.2% of all parotid gland tumours were undifferentiated, they were divided into two groups on the basis of cell size.[125] Two-thirds of the tumours were classed as large-celled and the other third as small-celled. The large cells were either spheroidal or spindle-shaped with abundant cytoplasm, and on electron microscopy showed points of resemblance to either adenocarcinoma or epidermoid carcinoma cells (Fig. 3.41). When a carcinoma develops in a lympho-epithelial lesion it is usually of this sort, though occasionally it is possible on light microscopy to identify the tumour as either a very poorly-differentiated epidermoid or adenocarcinoma. These are the types of tumour that are particularly common in Eskimos[126] (Fig. 3.42).

The small-celled undifferentiated tumours, which superficially resemble oat cell bronchial carcinomas, also appear to be of two types. One has a fine structure suggesting it is of ductal origin, with both duct-lining and myo-epithelial cells, though these are scarcely distinguishable on light microscopy; it is possibly into a tumour of this type that adenoid cystic carcinoma occasionally transforms.[127] Electron microscopy of the other small-celled undifferentiated tumour shows it to have a neuroendocrine appearance, with neurosecretory granules present in the cells. This tumour would appear to be related to the tumour that arises from the Merkel cells of the basal layer of the epidermis.[128]

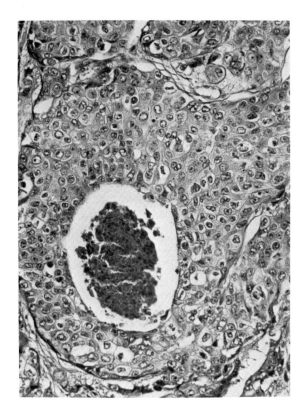

Fig. 3.41 Undifferentiated carcinoma of large cell type from a 50-year-old woman. The tumour had soon recurred after local removal, and in spite of radical parotidectomy and radiotherapy she died a year later.

Haematoxylin-eosin   × 160

Carcinoma in pleomorphic adenoma

The exceptionally rare occurence of metastasis of a pleomorphic adenoma has been mentioned above (see p. 105). Another and more frequent danger to which patients with this commonest of salivary gland tumours are liable is the development of frank carcinoma. It has long been recognized that any patient with a parotid tumour that has grown slowly, or that has been unchanged in size over a period of many years, may notice a sudden rapid increase in its size, often with pain and the development of facial weakness. Tumours that have recurred after attempted removal are equally liable to such an alteration in behaviour, which is a manifestation of malignant change. That this is a focal change in a benign tumour is shown by cases where the recurrent tumour has been multinodular and only one of the nodules has become carcino-

matous, the others remaining benign. The carcinoma that develops is often highly malignant, invading the rest of the gland, infiltrating adjacent muscle and overlying skin, and anchoring itself to bone. Lymphatic spread to the regional lymph nodes commonly occurs, and distant metastases—in one series, often in the spine[129]—may appear, so that most patients live only a very few years after the change in the character of the growth becomes evident.[130] Some longer survivals have followed radiotherapy and radical surgery.[131]

Microscopically, the element that metastasizes may take any of the forms of frank malignancy mentioned in the preceding account of carcinoma of the salivary glands. Adenocarcinoma, often poorly differentiated, and undifferentiated carcinoma are most often encountered, but epidermoid, mucoepidermoid or adenoid cystic carcinomas have been reported. Quite often more than one type of malignancy is present.

The development of malignancy in a pre-

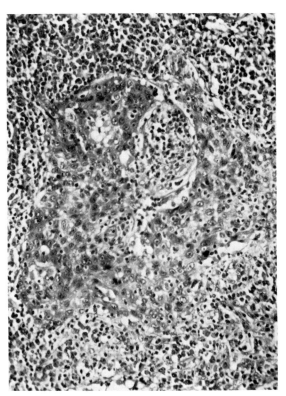

Fig. 3.42 Undifferentiated carcinoma with a lymphoid stroma, from a parotid tumour in an Eskimo woman.

Haematoxylin-eosin   × 175

existing pleomorphic adenoma is often suspected from the history, but confirmation should be based on histological examination of the operation specimen. There may be no difficulty in identifying both the invasive carcinoma and the remainder of the benign adenoma from which it developed (Fig. 3.43), but sometimes when the patient has given a long history of the presence of a lump the adenoma, buried in the carcinoma, is degenerate, perhaps even partly calcified. It may still, however, be possible to identify dead chondroid areas or the characteristic elastic fibres in the acellular hyaline background, and so confirm the diagnosis. Patients are not always aware of a slowly-growing pleomorphic adenoma, especially if deeply placed, and a malignant tumour with a short history may well be biopsied, diagnosed as, say, an undifferentiated carcinoma and treated other than surgically without the underlying adenoma being discovered. At

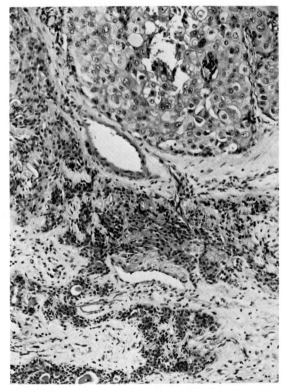

Fig. 3.43 Carcinoma arising in a pleomorphic adenoma of the palate which had been present for 30 years. The malignant tissue in the upper part of the field is quite distinct in appearance from the pleomorphic adenoma below.

Haematoxylin-eosin   × 120

the opposite end of the scale the diagnosis may be made on the recognition of a localized area of malignancy, perhaps with only early invasion through the capsule, in an adenoma clinically thought to be benign. Such cases should do well, if the initial operation is adequate, and will improve the overall survival figures of any series in which they are included.

There was a time when patients who were thought on clinical grounds to have a pleomorphic salivary adenoma of the parotid were occasionally advised to have no treatment, in view of the slowness of the growth of the tumour and of the danger of injury to the facial nerve during surgery. It is now recognized that if all pleomorphic adenomas were removed as soon as they are detected clinically, the occurrence of many highly malignant tumours would be avoided. In a series of 79 cases of carcinoma of the major salivary glands there was clear evidence that almost half had developed from pleomorphic adenomas or other tumours of restricted malignancy.[132] The interval between the initial recognition of a salivary tumour and the onset of rapid malignant growth is very variable; in the series just mentioned the average was 19 years, with 50 years as the longest interval.

The long interval which may elapse between the patient first noticing the tumour and the onset of malignancy makes it very difficult to estimate the chance of malignant transformation taking place. The relative numbers of benign and malignant pleomorphic adenomas in a series of salivary gland tumours give some indication, but as the great majority of the tumours in such series will have been present no more than a few years, the percentage of those with malignant change greatly underestimates the real liability to this occurrence. In one series 6% of parotid, 11% of submandibular, and 3% of all minor salivary gland tumours were carcinomatous pleomorphic adenomas.[133] In another series, from Japan, there were 282 pleomorphic adenomas and 48 carcinomas in pleomorphic adenoma, so that 14.5% of pleomorphic adenomas had become malignant.[130] Tumours in the deep part of the parotid, medial to the branching facial nerve, are likely to be present unnoticed for a much longer time than tumours more superficially placed; in one series already mentioned seven out of eight carcinomas from the deep part of the parotid has clearly originated in pleomorphic adenomas.[133] Apart from time, the only factor that may be concerned in the onset of malignancy is previous irradiation (Fig. 3.44).[134]

'Carcinoma in pleomorphic adenoma' was adopted as the diagnostic label for these tumours as a reminder of the danger of eventual malignancy in pleomorphic adenomas; it has been criticized by those who prefer the alternative term 'malignant mixed tumour' because it does not take into account the rare, but undoubted, examples of tumours of this sort which, with a short history, appear to have been malignant from the start.[133]

OTHER TUMOURS

Connective-tissue tumours of any type may be found in the salivary glands. Lipomas and vascular

tumours are perhaps the least rare. Fibrosarcomas and rhabdomyosarcomas are very occasionally seen in the parotid, and there have been reports of both benign[135] and malignant fibrous histiocytomas.[136] Malignant melanoma is an extremely rare primary salivary gland tumour; less rarely it is seen as a secondary tumour, usually in the parotid.[137]

A haemangioma is the commonest salivary gland tumour of children. The parotid is nearly always the site, though rarely the submandibular gland may be involved. Either at birth, or usually sometime in the first year of life, an ill-defined, rather soft, bluish swelling of the gland is noticed which increases in size when the infant cries or strains, and which may even pulsate. The condition is commoner in girls, and though occasionally the tumour may regress, surgical removal is usually necessary. Incomplete removal may be followed by local recurrence. Microscopically, the lobular ar-

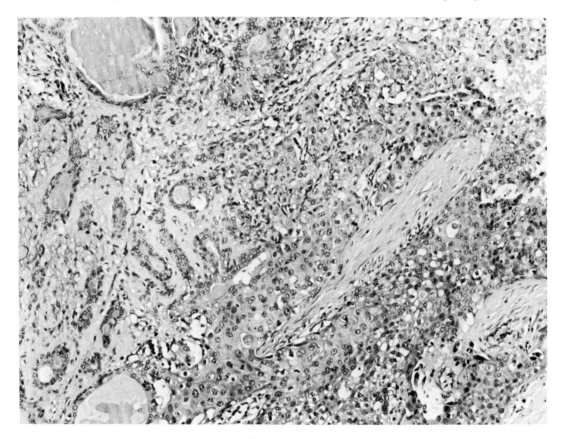

Fig. 3.44 Carcinoma in a pleomorphic adenoma of the deep part of the parotid of a man of 30 who, when 11 years old, had had radiotherapy for enlarged adenoids.

Haematoxylin-eosin   × 140

rangement of the gland can still be made out but much of the glandular tissue is replaced by closely packed vascular channels, which vary from capillary to cavernous in size. Scattered throughout the angiomatous tissue a few normal ducts and acini can be seen (Fig. 3.45). The condition appears to be a diffuse hamartomatous malformation of the vasculature of part of the gland rather than a true neoplasm. Haemangiomas are occasionally found in adults. Thrombosis may occur in small cavernous angiomas, and with subsequent calcification the lesion may be mistaken for a calculus radiologically.

Neurofibromas and neurolemmomas (neurinomas, schwannomas) may develop on the facial nerve within the confines of the parotid, either as a solitary lesion or as part of a more widespread neurofibromatosis. Long-standing neurolemmomas when bisected may show areas of cystic

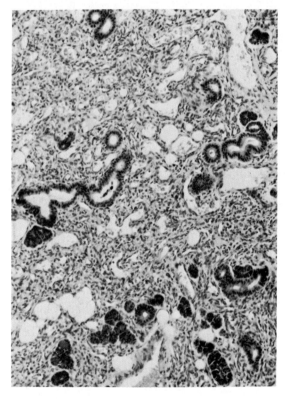

Fig. 3.45 Haemangioma of the parotid from a girl aged 6. Only a few scattered ducts and acini can be seen in the angiomatous tissue.

Haematoxylin-eosin   × 120

degeneration and golden patches of lipid accumulation in their otherwise uniform firm white substance. Microscopically, the neurolemmoma with its regimented or palisaded nuclei is quite characteristic, though a somewhat similar picture is occasionally seen in one type of monomorphic adenoma with a hyaline stroma in which the myoepithelial cells are compressed and elongated.

Lymphomas. The possibility of a malignant lymphoma developing on the basis of the lymphoepithelial lesion in patients with or without Sjögren's syndrome has already been mentioned (see p. 100), but lymphomas sometimes present as solitary lumps in otherwise normal parotid, or more rarely, submandibular glands. Since the parotid contains small lymph glands within its confines—an average of 20 has been quoted[41]—this is not surprising, and it is quite often possible to demonstrate that the tumour originated in such a node before infiltrating the salivary tissue around.[138] Microscopically, the picture may be that of Hodgkin's disease, though less often than in malignant lymphomas elsewhere, or it may be that of any of the non-Hodgkin lymphomas. Many of the tumours are nodular rather than diffuse and show fibrous banding, both of which features are associated with a better outlook, so that the prognosis of salivary gland lymphomas is usually reported to be a little better than at other sites. A condition histologically resembling follicular lymphoma, and even indistinguishable from it, is occasionally seen in this situation, usually in nodes that include salivary tissue, particularly salivary ducts: its prognosis appears usually to be good, following conservative excision, and its relation to true follicular lymphoma is debatable. A similar appearance may be seen in some cases of the benign lympho-epithelial lesion.

Secondary tumours are likely to develop in the intraparotid lymph nodes. Rarely, they develop in the substance of the gland proper, possibly even before the primary tumour is apparent. Renal carcinomas seem to be more liable than other cancers to metastasize to the parotids, where the metastatic tumour may be difficult to distinguish from the primary clear-cell tumours of the gland.[109] Other sites from which tumour has reached the parotid by the bloodstream are the lung, stomach and pancreas.[132]

TUMOURS OF THE MINOR SALIVARY GLANDS

In the preceding sections occasional mention has been made of tumours occurring in the minor salivary glands. Here the sites and types of minor salivary gland tumour will be briefly reviewed.

The overall incidence of tumours in the minor salivary glands is only about one tenth of that in the major glands. About 55% of minor salivary gland tumours are found in the palate, with 15%, the next largest group, in the upper lip. The remaining tumours are found in the floor of the mouth, in the cheeks, tongue and retromolar region and, rarely, within the mandible. The submandibular gland may abut on, and indent, the mandible,[139] and it is thought that during early development primordial salivary gland tissue may get trapped within the developing bone and subsequently give rise to a tumour of salivary gland type. The commonest intra-osseous epithelial tumour is a mucoepidermoid tumour, but some of these are thought to develop in odontogenic cysts.[140]

There are differences between the relative proportions of the various types of tumour in the major and minor glands. Only about 45% of minor salivary gland tumours are pleomorphic adenomas, whereas monomorphic adenomas, particularly in the lip, account for up to 10%. Mucoepidermoid tumours account for between 10 and 15% of the tumours, and adenoid cystic carcinomas, 15–20%, are also commoner than in the major glands. The percentage of adenocarcinomas in various published series varies widely from 3 to 18. Adenolymphomas and oxyphilic adenomas are very rarely seen, but small percentages of the other tumour types not already named make up the total.

The prognosis of minor salivary gland tumours is very good when they occur in the lip; nearly all lip tumours are benign, and in this situation there is little difficulty in removing them with a margin of normal tissue. Elsewhere in the mouth the tumours are more likely to be malignant, and the difficulties of complete removal, in the palate for instance, are considerable. There is therefore a considerable risk of local recurrence and of an eventual fatal outcome. Adenoid cystic carcinoma in particular is rarely if ever cured, though there may be repeated local recurrences over the course of the years before metastasis occurs.

SALIVARY GLAND TUMOURS IN CHILDREN

Less than 5% of all salivary gland tumours are seen in children under the age of 15. They differ from those in adults in that mesenchymal tumours are nearly as numerous as epithelial ones, and that only about two-thirds are benign. The commonest tumour in young children is the hamartomatous haemangioma, described above (see p. 125). Neural tumours may develop in children, and a diffuse swelling of the parotid or other salivary gland region is occasionally caused by a plexiform neurofibroma.[141] In such cases there are usually *café au lait* spots in the skin or other evidence of neurofibromatosis, but the salivary gland swelling is very occasionally the only abnormality.

Pleomorphic adenomas are the commonest epithelial tumours, as in adults; although occasionally

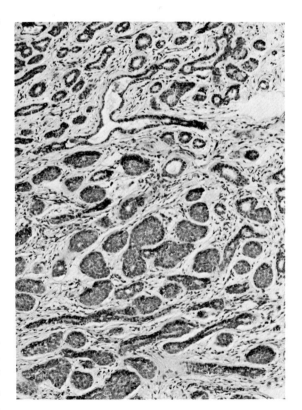

Fig. 3.46 Parotid tumour from an infant 6 weeks old. It is made up of branching columns of cells, some of which have a central lumen. The child was well and free from recurrence five years later.

Haematoxylin-eosin   × 100

reported in infancy it is not until the age of 9 or 10 that appreciable numbers of cases begin to occur. They are a little commoner in girls than in boys, and most are in the parotid, with a few in the submandibular gland, palate or elsewhere in the mouth. Mucoepidermoid tumours account for about 20% of salivary gland tumours in children; they have been reported in 1-year-olds, but most cases occur after the age of 6. Occasional acinic cell tumours have been recorded, but adenoid cystic carcinomas are very uncommon. A few, highly malignant tumours, sarcomas or anaplastic carcinomas, occur in children and these are almost invariably fatal.

An interesting, but very rare, parotid tumour that is present usually at birth is shown in Figure 3.46.[142] It is made up of broad columns or bands of epithelial cells of basal type, many of which develop central ducts, sometimes with quite a large lumen. The columns, with their rounded extremities, appear to be branching and pushing out into the normal part of the parotid or into surrounding tissues. There is no capsule, but the tumour has proved benign and has usually been called a basal cell adenoma, though occasionally mistaken for an adenoid cystic carcinoma. The appearance of the tumour, with its infiltrative edge, is reminiscent of the developing gland in the embryo, and the lesion is perhaps to be regarded as a hamartomatous developmental abnormality.

REFERENCES

1. Leppi TJ. J Dent Res 1967; 46: 359.
2. Polayes IM, Rankow RM. Plast Reconstr Surg 1979; 64: 17.
3. Micheau C. Arch Anat Pathol 1969; 17: 179.
4. Pesavento G, Ferlito A. J Laryngol Otol 1976; 90: 577.
5. Jernstrom P, Prietto CA. Arch Pathol 1962; 73: 473.
6. Stoch RB, Smith I. J Oral Surg 1980; 38: 56.
7. Seward GR. Br Dent J 1960; 108: 321.
8. Mason DK, Chisholm DM. Salivary glands in health and disease. London: Saunders, 1975: 213.
9. Silverman M, Perkins RL. Ann Intern Med 1966; 64: 842.
10. Banks P. Oral Surg 1968; 25: 732.
11. Hasler JF. Oral Surg 1982; 53: 567.
12. Cohen L, Banks P. Br Med J 1966; 5500: 1420.
13. Mason DK, Chisholm DM. Salivary glands in health and disease. London: Saunders, 1975: 219.
14. Weitzner S. Oral Surg 1973; 35: 85.
15. Harrison JD. Oral Surg 1975; 39: 268.
16. Hamperl H. Beitr path Anat 1931; 88: 193.
17. Roediger WEW, Lloyd P. Lawson HH. Br J Surg 1973; 60: 720.
18. Van den Akker HP, Bays RA, Becker AE. J Maxillofac Surg 1978; 6: 286.
19. Harrison JD, Sowray JH, Smith NJD. Br Dent J 1976; 140: 180.
20. Suleiman SI, Thomson JPS, Hobsley M. Gut 1979; 20: 1102.
21. Burstein LS, Boskey AL, Tannenbaum PJ, Posner AS, Mandel ID. J Oral Pathol 1979; 8: 284.
22. Beahrs OH, Devine KD, Woolner LB. Am J Surg 1961; 102: 760.
23. Jensen JL, Howell FV, Rick GM, Correll RW. Oral Surg 1979; 47: 44.
24. Babbott FL, Rodenberger BM, Ingalls TH. JAMA 1961; 178: 542.
25. Henson D, Siegel S, Strano AJ, Primack A, Fuccillo DA. Arch Pathol 1971; 92: 469.
26. Plotkin SA. J R Soc Med 1984; 77: 94.
27. Howlett JG, Somlo F, Katz F. Can Med Assoc J 1957; 77: 5.
28. Zollar LM, Mufson MA. Am J Dis Child 1970; 119: 147.
29. Lewis JM, Utz JP. N Engl J Med 1961; 265: 776.
30. Ragheb M. Geriatrics 1963; 18: 627.
31. Karlan MS, Snyder WH. Calif Med 1968; 108: 423.
32. Pearson RSB. Gut 1961; 2: 210.
33. Pellinen TJ, Kalske J. Br Med J 1982; 285: 344.
34. Kashima HK, Kirkham WR, Andrews JR. Am J Roent 1965; 114: 271.
35. Maynard J. J R Soc Med 1979; 72: 591.
36. Patey DH, Thackray AC. Br J Surg 1955; 43: 1.
37. Godwin JT. Cancer 1952; 5: 1089.
38. Bloch KJ, Buchanan WW, Wohl MJ, Bunim J. Medicine (Baltimore) 1965; 44: 187.
39. Morgan WS, Castleman B. Am J Pathol 1953; 29: 471.
40. Azzopardi JG, Evans DJ. J Clin Pathol 1971; 24: 744.
41. Hyman GA, Wolff M. Am J Clin Pathol 1976; 65: 421.
42. Schmid U, Helbron D, Lennert K. Virchows Arch Pathol Anat 1982; 395: 11.
43. Talal N, Sokoloff L, Barth WF. Am J Med 1967; 43: 50.
44. Sjögren H. Acta Ophthalmol (Copenhagen) 1932; 10: 405.
45. Sjögren H. Acta Ophthalmol (Copenhagen) 1933; 11 (suppl 2).
46. Mikulicz J von. Beitr Chir Festschrif Theodor Billroth 1892; 610.
47. Greenberg G, Anderson R, Sharpstone P, James DG. Br Med J 1964; 5413: 861.
48. Heerfordt CF. Albrecht v Graefes Arch Ophthal 1909; 70: 254.
49. Patey DH, Thackray AC. Arch Middlesex Hosp 1954; 4: 256.
50. Allen-Mersh MG, Forsyth DM. Tubercle 1958; 39: 108.
51. Hopkins R. Br J Oral Surg 1973; 11: 131.
52. Evans RW, Cruickshank AH. Epithelial tumours of the salivary glands. Philadelphia: Saunders, 1970: 11.
53. Davies JNP, Dodge OG, Burkitt DP. Cancer 1964; 17: 1310.
54. Loke YW. Br J Cancer 1967; 21: 665.
55. Thomas KM, Hutt MSR, Borgstein J. Cancer 1980; 46: 2328.
56. Wallace AC, MacDougal JT, Hildes JA, Lederman JM. Cancer 1963; 16: 1338.

57. Schneider AB, Favus MJ, Stachurn ME, Arnold J, Arnold MJ, Frohman LA. Am J Med 1978; 64: 243.
58. Shore-Freedman E, Abrahams C, Recant W, Schneider AB. Cancer 1983; 51: 2159.
59. Takeichi N, Hirose F, Yamamoto H. Cancer 1976; 38: 2462.
60. Thackray AC, Sobin LH. International classification of tumours: histological typing of salivary gland tumours. Geneva: World Health Organization, 1972.
61. Thackray AC, Lucas RB. Tumors of the major salivary glands (Atlas of tumor pathology, 2nd series, fasc. 10). Washington D.C. A.F.I.P., 1974.
62. Frylinck JR. S Afr Med J 1956; 30: 479.
63. Patey DH, Thackray AC. Br J Surg 1957; 44: 352.
64. Lomax-Smith JD, Azzopardi JG. Histopathol 1978; 2: 77.
65. Cameron WR, Stenram U. Cancer 1979; 43: 1429.
66. Chaplin AJ, Darke P, Patel S. J Oral Pathol 1983; 12: 342.
67. Azzopardi JG, Zayid I. J Pathol 1972; 107: 149.
68. Patey DH, Thackray AC. Br J Surg 1958; 45: 477.
69. Stevens KL, Hobsley M. Br J Surg 1982; 69: 1.
70. Chen KTK. Cancer 1978; 42: 2407.
71. Youngs GR, Scheuer PJ. J Pathol 1972; 109: 171.
72. Albrecht H, Arzt L. Frankfurt Z Path 1910; 4: 47.
73. Warthin AS. J Cancer Res 1929; 13: 116.
74. Baden E, Pierce M, Selman AJ, Roberts TW, Doyle JL. J Oral Surg 1976; 34: 533.
75. Dietert SE. Am J Clin Pathol 1975; 63: 866.
76. David R, Buchner A. Am J Clin Pathol 1978; 69: 173.
77. Patey DH, Thackray AC. Br J Surg 1970; 57: 569.
78. Seifert G, Bull HG, Donath K. Virchows Arch Pathol Anat 1980; 388: 13.
79. Allegra SR. Hum Pathol 1971; 2: 403.
80. Fantasia JE, Miller AS. Oral Surg 1981; 52: 411.
81. Blanck C, Eneroth C-M, Jakobsson PÅ. Cancer 1970; 25: 919.
82. Gray SR, Cornog JL, Seo IS. Cancer 1976; 38: 1306.
83. Mintz GA, Abrams AM, Melrose RJ. Oral Surg 1982; 53: 375.
84. Pogrel MA. Br J Oral Surg 1979; 17: 47.
85. Min BH, Miller AS, Leifer C, Putong PB. Arch Otolaryngol 1974; 99: 88.
86. Kleinsasser O, Klein HJ. Arch Klin Exper O, N & K 1967; 189: 302.
87. Gardner DG, Daley TD. Oral Surg 1983; 56: 608.
88. Evans RW, Cruickshank AH. Epithelial tumours of the salivary glands. Philadelphia: Saunders, 1970: 58.
89. Headington JT, Batsakis JG, Beals TF, Campbell TE, Simmons JL, Stone WD. Cancer 1977; 39: 2460.
90. Reingold IM, Keasbey LE, Graham JH. Cancer 1977; 40: 1702.
91. Batsakis JG, Brannon RB. J Laryngol Otol 1981; 95: 155.
92. Chen S-Y, Miller AS. Cancer 1980; 46: 552.
93. Harrison JD. J Pathol 1974; 144: 29.
94. Crumpler C, Scharfenberg JC, Reed RJ. Cancer 1976; 38: 193.
95. Corridan M. J Path Bact 1956; 72: 623.
96. Evans RW, Cruickshank AH. Epithelial tumours of the salivary glands. Philadelphia: Saunders, 1970: 265.
97. Tachen JA, McGavran MH. Cancer 1979; 44: 1388.
98. Masson P, Berger L. Bull Ass Franc Cancer 1924; 13: 366.
99. Stewart FW, Foote FW, Becker WF. Ann Surg 1945; 122: 820.
100. Hendrick JW. Am J Surg 1964; 108: 907.
101. Bhaskar SN, Bernier JL. Cancer 1962; 15: 801.
102. Fu KK, Leibel SA, Levine ML, Friedlander LM, Boles R, Phillips TL. Cancer 1977; 40: 2882.
103. Abrams AM, Melrose RJ. Oral Surg 1978; 46: 220.
104. Gardner DG, Bell MEA, Wesley RK, Wysocki GP. Oral Surg 1980; 50: 545.
105. Spiro RH, Huvos AG, Strong EW. Cancer 1978; 41: 924.
106. Ellis GL, Corio RL. Cancer 1983; 52: 542.
107. Hanson TAS. Cancer 1975; 36: 570.
108. Fisher ER, Hellstrom HR. Am J Clin Pathol 1962; 37: 633.
109. Sist TC, Marchetta FC, Milley PC. Oral Surg 1982; 53: 499.
110. Echevarria RA. Cancer 1977; 40: 563.
111. Sidhu GS, Forrester EM. Cancer 1977; 40: 756.
112. Eneroth C-M, Hjertman L, Moberger G. Acta Otolaryngol (Stockholm) 1967; 64: 514.
113. Billroth T. Virchows Arch Pathol Anat 1859; 17: 357.
114. Perzin KH, Gullane P, Clairmont AC. Cancer 1978; 42: 265.
115. Thackray AC, Lucas RB. Br J Cancer 1960; 14: 612.
116. Bosch A, Brandenburg JH, Gilchrist KW. Cancer 1980; 45: 2872.
117. Budd GT, Groppe CW. Cancer 1983; 51: 589.
118. Blanck C, Eneroth C-M, Jacobsson F, Jakobsson PÅ. Acta Radiol (Stockholm) 1967; 6: 177.
119. Donath K, Seifert G, Schmitz R. Virchows Arch Pathol Anat 1972; 356: 16.
120. Corio RL, Sciubba JJ, Brannon RB, Batsakis JG. Oral Surg 1982; 53: 280.
121. Mohamed AH, Cherrick HM. Cancer 1975; 36: 1057.
122. Evans RW, Cruickshank AH. Epithelial tumours of the salivary glands. Philadelphia: Sanders, 1970: 265.
123. Gad A, Willén H, Willén R, Thorstensson S, Ekman L. Histopathol 1980; 4: 111.
124. Gnepp DR, Brannon R. Cancer 1984; 53: 2155.
125. Nagao K, Matsuzaki O, Saiga H et al. Cancer 1982; 50: 1572.
126. Arthaud JB. Am J Clin Pathol 1972; 57: 275.
127. Wirman JA, Battifora HA. Cancer 1976; 37: 1840.
128. Kraemer BB, Mackay B, Batsakis JG. Cancer 1983; 52: 2115.
129. Thomas WH, Coppola ED. Am J Surg 1965; 109: 724.
130. Nagao K, Matsuzaki O, Saiga H et al. Cancer 1981; 48: 113.
131. Corcoran MO, Cook HP, Hobsley M. Br J Surg 1983; 70: 261.
132. Patey DH, Thackray AC, Keeling DH. Br J Cancer 1965; 19: 712.
133. Spiro RH, Huvos AG, Strong EW. Cancer 1977; 39: 388.
134. Saksela E, Tarkkanen J, Kohonen A. Acta Otolaryngol (Stockholm) 1970; 70: 62.
135. Shapshay SM, Wingert RH, Davis JS. Laryngoscope 1979; 89: 1808.
136. Benjamin E, Wells S, Fox H, Reeve NL, Knox F. J Clin Pathol 1982; 35: 946.
137. Greene GW, Bernier JL. Oral Surg 1961; 14: 108.
138. Schmid U, Helbron D, Lennert K. Histopathol 1982; 6: 673.
139. Uemura S, Fujishita M, Fuchihata H. Oral Surg 1976; 41: 120.
140. Fredrickson C, Cherrick HM. J Oral Med 1978; 33: 80.
141. Weitzner S. Oral Surg 1980; 50: 53.
142. Krolls SO, Trodahl JN, Boyers AC. Cancer 1972; 30: 459.

The oesophagus

ANATOMY

The oesophagus is a muscular tube about 25 cm long extending from the pharynx at the cricoid cartilage opposite the sixth cervical vertebra to the cardia about 2.5 cm to the left of the midline, opposite the tenth or eleventh thoracic vertebra. At the upper end is the cricopharyngeal sphincter. The distance from the incisor teeth to the upper end of the oesophagus is about 15 cm, and to the cardia about 40 cm. The oesophagus pierces the left crus of the diaphragm and has an intra-abdominal portion about 1.5 cm in length. The most easily recognized anatomical structures defining the lower oesophagus are the sling muscle fibres, transverse mucosal fold and internal and external cardiac notch or incisura.[1] The lower oesophageal sphincter is functional only. The principal relations are with the trachea, left main bronchus, the aortic arch and descending aorta, and the left atrium. It is supplied by the inferior thyroid, bronchial, left phrenic and left gastric arteries as well as by small twigs direct from the aorta, while its veins form a well-developed submucous plexus draining into thyroid, azygos, hemiazygos and left gastric veins, so providing an important link between systemic and portal systems.

Lymphatic channels from the pharyngeal region and upper third drain to the deep cervical nodes either directly or through paratracheal nodes; some also drain to the infrahyoid nodes. From the lower two-thirds they drain to the posterior mediastinal (para-oesophageal) nodes and thence to the thoracic duct, while from the infradiaphragmatic portion they drain to the left gastric nodes and to a ring of nodes around the cardia. Some lymph vessels may reach the thoracic duct directly. There are two sets of lymphatic channels in the oesophagus, one within the submucosa and one in the muscle coats.

With the exception of the intra-abdominal segment the oesophagus is lined by stratified, non-keratinizing squamous epithelium (Fig. 4.1) in which melanoblasts are present.[2] There is a recognizable basal cell layer which forms up to 15% of the total epithelial thickness and papillae of connective tissue which project upwards into the epithelium to a distance of 65% of the total epithelial thickness. These measurements have some significance in the detection of early reflux oesophagitis. Argyrophil cells are present in the basal cell layer but not in ducts or glands.[3] At its lower end the papillae and rete pegs are arranged longitudinally to form visible surface ridges and there is an abrupt change to columnar epithelium of cardiac type.[4] This change occurs at about

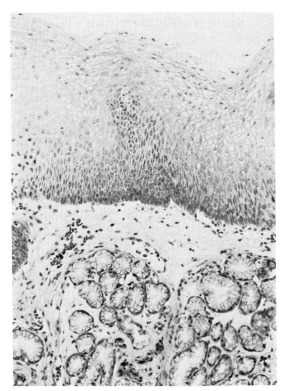

Fig. 4.1 Normal oesophagus showing non-keratinized squamous epithelium overlying submucosal seromucinous glands.

Haematoxylin-eosin   × 100

diaphragmatic level (about 1.5 cm above the lower end of the anatomical oesophagus) and shows as an irregular junctional line of grey and pink mucosa visible to the naked eye. Distally the simple cardiac glands gradually blend with those of normal fundic type. The muscularis mucosae has a variable pattern. Commonly, in the upper part it consists of isolated or irregularly arranged muscle bundles rather than a continuous sheet, but in the middle and lower thirds it forms a continuum of longitudinal and transverse fibres, often thicker than elsewhere in the gastrointestinal tract. It may become thinner again at the cardia.

The submucosa is wide. It contains the oesophageal mucous glands (Fig. 4.1) and a ramifying lymphatic plexus in a loose connective-tissue network, which accounts for the early and extensive submucosal spread of oesophageal carcinoma. The glands are arranged in rows parallel to the long axis.[5] They are acinar, tubular and mucus-secreting, and form lobules; from two to five lobules drain into a common duct lined by stratified columnar epithelium which passes obliquely through the muscularis mucosae into the lumen. Their number and position appear to be subject to wide variation. The glands secrete acidic mucins containing sulphate groups. Aggregates of lymphoid tissue, which are variable in number in the oesophageal submucosa, are found surrounding mucous gland ducts. Polymorphonuclear leukocytes are not normally present. The main muscle layer of the oesophagus is composed of well-developed circular and longitudinal coats. In the upper part these are striated, with a gradual change to smooth muscle in the middle part. In the lower third both coats are entirely smooth muscle and continue into gastric muscle with no anatomical sphincter.

The nerve supply to the oesophagus, as well as the rest of the gastrointestinal tract, may be divided into extrinsic and intrinsic components. The extrinsic innervation is through the autonomic nervous system, which is divided into the sympathetic and parasympathetic arms. The parasympathetic supply to the upper oesophagus is through the glossopharyngeal nerve, whereas the remainder is innervated through the vagus. The preganglionic fibres terminate in the myenteric plexus between the circular and longitudinal muscle coats. Fibres supplying striated muscle of the upper oesophagus terminate as motor end plates. The vagus also contains afferent nerves to complete reflex arcs. The sympathetic supply is through thoracic spinal nerves which end in prevertebral ganglia. The postganglionic fibres terminate in the myenteric plexus. Sympathetic nerves also contain afferent fibres whose cell bodies may reside either in the oesophageal wall (e.g. mechanoreceptors) or within the dorsal root ganglia. These will complete short and long reflex circuits respectively. The intrinsic innervation is through the myenteric plexus. The submucosal plexus is poorly developed in the oesophagus. The smooth muscle is supplied directly by two types of intrinsic neurons. These are excitatory, mainly cholinergic neurons and inhibitory, non-cholinergic neurons.[6]

Individual smooth muscle cells are not necessarily supplied by nerve terminals. Nerve processes with bead-like varicosities surround groups of muscle fibres and neurotransmitters are released into tissue spaces to reach the target cells by diffusion. The neurons supplying smooth muscle are driven not only by extrinsic parasympathetic fibres but by intrinsic interneurons. Excitatory intrinsic neurons supplying muscle are also inhibited, either directly by extrinsic sympathetic fibres or indirectly through presynaptic inhibition of excitatory interneurons.

It is now clear that noradrenaline and acetylcholine are not the only neurotransmitters released within the oesophagus, or gut in general, and a variety of alternatives have been proposed for the non-adrenergic, non-cholinergic neurons. Vasoactive intestinal polypeptide may act as the neurotransmitter for the inhibitory neurons supplying smooth muscle, whereas substance P may function as an excitatory neurotransmitter.[7] Formerly neurons of the myenteric plexus were classified according to whether they were argyrophil (with processes surrounding other neurons) or cholinesterase positive (and supplying muscle cells directly).[8] These classical light microscopic techniques show no clear correlation with more modern functional classifications in which neurotransmitter substances are characterized immunohistochemically and ultrastructurally.[9]

DEVELOPMENTAL ABNORMALITIES

Initially, in the developing oesophagus, the lining epithelium is columnar with ciliated cells developing by the 70 mm stage. The ciliated surface epithelium of the middle third then becomes stratified squamous, and this change extends upwards and downwards to form a complete squamous lining at term, though traces of ciliated epithelium may remain in postnatal life. The submucosal glands first appear during the final trimester of intrauterine development and much of their development is postnatal.

Duplications, diverticula and cysts

Duplications and congenital diverticula are extremely rare. Cysts are less rare and are found in the adjacent mediastinum or incorporated in the outer wall of the oesophagus at all levels. The majority are posterior in position, associated with vertebral abnormalities, and are lined by ciliated columnar or gastric type mucosa rather than squamous. They have a muscular or fibromuscular wall. The rarer anterior mediastinal cysts may be similar in structure or may have a more respiratory type epithelial lining with mucous glands resembling bronchial glands and sometimes cartilage, presumably of tracheal origin.[10]

Oesophageal atresia and stenosis

In atresia, a segment of the oesophagus is missing, leaving a proximal segment with a blind end either entirely separated from the distal segment or united by a solid fibrous cord. Stenosis implies narrowing of the lumen.

Isolated atresia or stenosis is relatively rare,[11] occurring in only 16% of cases.[12] It is commonly associated with hydramnios in the last three months of pregnancy.[13] Oesophageal atresia with tracheo-oesophageal fistula, however, is a relatively common congenital anomaly, with an incidence between 1:800 and 1:1500 live births.[13] It has occasionally been described in siblings,[14] but hereditary factors probably do not ordinarily play a part. Other congenital malformations are common and are described under the VATER syndrome which links together vertebral defects (hemi- or bifid vertebrae), anal atresia, tracheo-esophageal fistula and renal dysplasias.[15] Congenital heart defects also commonly occur[16] and when any one of these conditions is present in a neonate the others should be searched for. There is no significant difference in sex incidence. Maternal hydramnios may have been present, but is more common in association with pure atresia.

Several forms of atresia are described.[14,17] In the most common, the upper end of the oesophagus ends in a blind pouch; all coats of the bowel are present and the muscular wall is usually hypertrophied. The anterior wall of the pouch tends to fuse with the posterior wall of the trachea, but only rarely communicates with it. The lower oesophagus is normal at the cardia, but becomes progressively narrowed as it extends upward. It usually ends in the trachea at or within 2 cm of the bifurcation, but occasionally in one or other main bronchus. The opening is funnel or slit-shaped, and oesophageal and tracheal muscle are intimately blended. The gap between the blind pouch and the lower end varies from 1–5 cm, and there is sometimes a fibrous cord joining the two. Surgical operation is often feasible but subsequent apparent stenosis leading to recurrent respiratory infections is common; this may be due to stricture at the operation site.

The trachea normally develops as a gutter in the anterior wall of the primitive foregut. The lateral margins of the gutter fuse from below upwards to form a septum, from which the posterior wall of the trachea and the anterior wall of the oesophagus develop. In tracheo-oesophageal fistula the two lateral septa may meet on the posterior wall of the foregut instead of on its anterior wall. Alternatively the posterior wall may be drawn forwards leading to partial incorporation of the oesophagus in the trachea. The radiological finding of additional thoracic or lumbar vertebrae often with supernumerary ribs in many of these babies supports the idea of a growth disturbance during this period of development.[18] Occasional cases of fistula without atresia have been recorded and are compatible with survival to adult life.

Oesophagobronchial fistula with pulmonary sequestration

A small number of cases of oesophagobronchial fistula with bronchopulmonary sequestration have been reported. In these, the supernumary lung bud appears to arise from the lower part of the foregut in association with a congenital diaphragmatic hernia; its bronchus may or may not retain a patent communication with the oesophagus.[19,20]

Heterotopias in the oesophagus

The islands of ciliated epithelium sometimes found throughout the oesophagus in premature infants, more rarely in full-term babies and even occasionally in adults,[22] are remnants of the ciliated lining normally present at an early stage of development, and are not true heterotopias.

Patchy heterotopia of gastric epithelium occurs in the upper oesophagus.[23] The heterotopic mucosa appears as a pink, oval island, resembling a shallow ulcer.[24] The glandular elements may replace the squamous oesophageal epithelium or lie in the subepithelial tissue immediately beneath it.[25]

Congenital diaphragmatic hernia

Maldevelopment of the diaphragm may give rise to herniation of the abdominal contents into the thoracic cavity. In congenital hiatus hernia the oesophageal hiatus enlarges as the stomach herniates.

Congenitally short oesophagus

In this condition the squamous mucous membrane of the lower oesophagus is replaced by a mucosa lined by columnar epithelium. However, it is accepted that the columnar epithelial lining is nearly always acquired as a result of gastro-oesophageal reflux (see p. 139).

Anterior and posterior rachischisis

These conditions are anomalies of cervical and thoracic vertebrae characterized by their complete or partial division into halves. There may be anomalies of diaphragm formation with herniation of abdominal contents into the thorax.[26] Defects of the gastrointestinal tract may take the form of short oesophagus or of cysts lying between the tract and vertebrae, spinal cord or even dorsal skin.

MUSCULAR DISORDERS

Scleroderma and systemic sclerosis

Scleroderma in the oesophagus occurs as part of a generalized systemic disorder or as a more localized systemic sclerosis involving the alimentary tract. There is a vascular component consisting of elastosis and intimal fibrosis in the smaller arteries. This is accompanied by a gradual atrophy of smooth (but not striated) muscle with some fibrosis in the submucosa and non-specific inflammatory changes.[27] The amount and degree of fibrosis and collagenization vary markedly and may partly represent ischaemic change. The lower sphincter becomes incompetent and reflux oesophagitis may occur. Barrett's oesophagus with adenocarcinoma has been documented as a complication of scleroderma (see p. 139).[28]

Muscular dystrophies

Cases of progressive muscular dystrophy showing oedema and loss of smooth muscle fibres in the lower oesophagus have been described.[29] Those fibres which remained were disorientated, variable in size and vacuolated.

Diffuse muscular hypertrophy of the lower oesophagus

This condition differs in many respects from achalasia.[30] It is usually found at necropsy and does not produce symptoms during life. There is conspicuous thickening of all muscle coats (but especially the circular) of the lower end of the oesophagus, without narrowing of the lumen. There is a preponderence in males, and in some cases a coincident hypertrophy of the pylorus has suggested a congenital origin.

Acquired diverticula

Most oesophageal diverticula are acquired. They are divided into *pulsion diverticula* consequent on raised intraluminal pressure and *traction diverticula*, in which the oesophagus is secondarily involved from without in a chronic inflammatory process which heals by fibrosis producing consequent oesophageal distortion and diverticulum forma-

tion. Tuberculous lymphadenitis and 'cold abscess' of thoracic vertebrae are the most common causes of the latter (Fig. 4.2). Traction diverticula are therefore most common at or below the tracheal bifurcation. Complications include regurgitation, with the risk of aspiration pneumonia, and inflammation in the diverticulum, with the risk of haemorrhage and perforation. Carcinoma in a diverticulum has been reported.[31]

Recently a condition known as *intramural oesophageal diverticulosis* has been described, in which multiple small diverticula lined by squamous epithelium are present, particularly in the upper part of the oesophagus but sometimes throughout its length. The surface epithelium is normal.[32,33] Various suggestions have been made as to their pathogenesis. The most likely is that they are derived from the ducts of oesophageal mucous

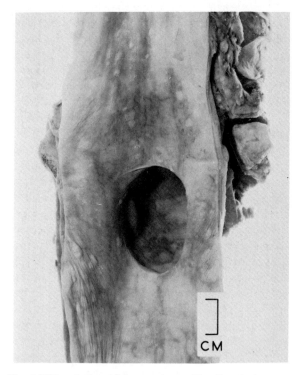

Fig. 4.2 Diverticulum of the oesophagus. The diverticulum which is just below the level of the bifurcation of the trachea, is of the traction type. It resulted from the shrinkage of scar tissue between the oesophagus and the inferior tracheobronchial lymph nodes, which had been the site of tuberculosis many years earlier.

Provided by Dr F. J. Paradinas, Curator of the Charing Cross Hospital Medical School Museum.

glands which have undergone squamous metaplasia in response to inflammation. Some examples may be secondary to strictures and webs (see p. 136).[34] The condition is also known as pseudo-diverticulosis.

Acquired hiatus hernia

Most diaphragmatic hernias are acquired. They are described from childhood onward, but the great majority occur in late adult life. A radiological study suggests that they are even more common than previously suspected, and that patients with them may present with symptoms suggestive of peptic ulcer or neoplasm.[35] There are three main types.[36]

In the sliding hernia, the lower oesophagus and stomach move through the oesophageal diaphragmatic hiatus, perhaps due to failure of the diaphragmatic muscle or stretching of the phreno-oesophageal ligament.[37] In para-oesophageal hernia part of the stomach herniates alongside the oesophagus. Traumatic hernia follows a breach in the diaphragm. The first type is thought to be predisposed to by chronic coughing, increased intra-abdominal pressure, kyphosis and obesity, but sometimes may be familial and dependent on an autosomal dominant gene.[38] Complications include reflux oesophagitis, though there is much dispute as to how often this occurs.[39]

Achalasia

In this condition food does not pass freely from oesophagus to stomach at the level of the cardia.[40] The physiological sphincter at the cardia fails to relax and the oesophagus proximal to the obstruction loses its normal peristaltic rhythm (though uncoordinated contractions may continue), becomes hypertrophied and often dilates, to contain a litre or more of food and fluid (megaoesophagus).[41] Clinically, patients suffer pain, regurgitation and dyspepsia over a long period, followed by episodes of respiratory infection and finally substernal oppression, regurgitation with choking and inhalation pneumonia. Radiological appearances may resemble those of Hirschsprung's disease (see p. 317) with a narrow, constricted, distal segment and gross dilatation of the oesophagus proximally.

Histopathological lesions have been described at various levels[41] and include degeneration and disappearance of nerve cells in the dorsal vagal nucleus, Wallerian degeneration of the vagus, destruction of the myenteric plexus (accompanied by chronic inflammatory cell infiltration and fibrosis)[8] and degenerative changes in the fibres of the muscularis externa. It is possible that non-cholinergic intrinsic neurons are the site of the primary injury. The motility disorder would therefore result from the loss of the inhibitory supply to the smooth muscle (vasoactive-intestinal-polypeptide-containing neurons—see p. 132) leading to a failure of relaxation. A neurotoxic virus or an autoimmune process has been offered as underlying causes.[41] Chagas' disease results in an identical clinical picture.

Secondary oesophagitis may, if severe, lead to ulceration and haemorrhage. Squamous carcinoma is an uncommon complication. Barrett's metaplasia (see p. 139) and dysplasia have been reported in postmyotomy patients, presumably in consequence of acquired reflux.[42]

MISCELLANEOUS CONDITIONS

Trauma

Perforation and rupture

The oesophagus is relatively well protected by surrounding structures in the neck, and traumatic lesions practically always arise from intraluminal causes. Among the more common are perforation or inflammation due to swallowed sharp foreign bodies, the impaction of foreign bodies with subsequent fistula formation, trauma during oesophagoscopy and the traumatic ulceration and inflammation which follows the ingestion of corrosive fluids.

Rupture of the oesophagus is rare and occurs as an abrupt longitudinal rent in the left lateral wall of the lower end of a previously normal oesophagus. It is much more common in males and is probably the result of a sudden rise in intra-oesophageal pressure due to sudden contraction or compression of the stomach following vomiting, over-distension due to food, or a blow on the abdomen.

Mallory-Weiss syndrome

Less traumatic procedures, including vomiting and severe retching, can produce partial oesophageal tears, usually just above the cardia. These usually involve the mucosa and can be associated with severe haemorrhage. They may fail to heal and progress to ulceration, with the risk of subsequent perforation. They are probably more common than has been supposed and should always be considered as a possible cause of unexplained upper gastrointestinal haemorrhage.

Varices

The normal venous drainage of the oesophagus includes a submucosal and an extramural plexus; both of these drain partly into the portal, partly into the systemic venous systems. In portal hypertension these venous plexuses dilate to form the so-called oesophageal varices, consisting of enormously dilated venous channels which lie immediately beneath the mucosa and are prone to rupture. There is some evidence that venous stasis and consequent anoxia produces degeneration and ulceration of the overlying oesophageal mucosa, which increases this risk. At autopsy the varices are collapsed and may be difficult to detect, but they can be shown by injection techniques if oesophagus and stomach are removed together. Intra-epithelial blood-filled channels have been described.[43] These may correspond to the cherry-red spots seen on endoscopy.

Webs and rings

Upper oesophageal webs are usually associated with the Paterson-Brown-Kelly syndrome and with postcricoid carcinomas. Lower oesophageal webs also occur and are separable from oesophageal rings. The webs have a variable location, usually occlude most of the lumen and consist of a thin layer of fibrous tissue covered on each surface by squamous epithelium to form a thin membrane. Oesophageal rings occur at the gastro-oesophageal junction; they produce a circular constriction of the lumen rather than occluding it, and consist of squamous or cardiac type mucosa, with or without muscle, which projects into the lumen.

OESOPHAGITIS

Non-specific bacterial oesophagitis

Non-specific bacterial infections may lead to an acute oesophagitis, which can simulate ischaemic heart disease clinically. Examples include diphtheria and streptococcal pharyngitis. There is congestion and dilatation of submucosal vessels with a variable polymorphonuclear infiltrate, progressing to ulceration of the squamous epithelium. A false membrane may form in diphtheria.

Herpes simplex oesophagitis

The oesophagus is the most common visceral site of infection with herpes simplex virus. Up to 25% of oesophageal ulcers detected postmortem have been ascribed to this virus.[44] When the diagnosis has been made during life, pain on swallowing is the usual symptom. The middle and distal thirds are the commonest sites. The earliest lesions are vesicles which break down to give shallow ulcers or erosions. The diagnosis is suggested histologically by the presence of intranuclear Cowdry type A viral inclusions and multinucleated giant cells (Fig. 4.3). Co-existent opportunistic infections due to cytomegalovirus, Candida, Mucor, Aspergillus or Torula should be excluded. Cytomegalic inclusions are usually found in endothelial cells and fibroblasts.[45] Cytomegalovirus oesophagitis has been reported in a patient with the acquired immunodeficiency syndrome.[46] Herpes oesophagitis in otherwise healthy patients has been described.[47]

Candidosis

Predisposing factors include the use of broad spectrum antibiotics as well as steroids and other immunosuppressant drugs employed in the treatment of malignant disease. Candida organisms may colonize pre-existing ulcers, e.g. herpetic or peptic. The mucosa of the middle and lower oesophagus either shows umbilicated warty lesions, sometimes with central ulceration or is studded with cream-coloured colonies of the fungus (Fig. 4.4). Necrosis, colonies of fungal hyphae, but little surrounding inflammatory reaction are seen on microscopy.[48-50]

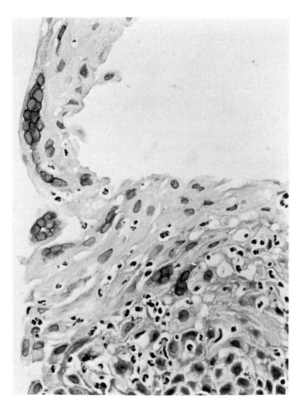

Fig. 4.3 Herpes simplex oesophagitis showing multinucleate giant cells with intranuclear viral inclusions.

Provided by Dr D. W. Day, Royal Liverpool Hospital

Haematoxylin-eosin   × 400

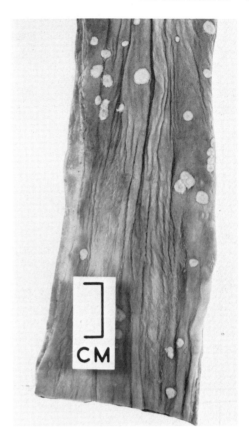

Fig. 4.4 Oesophageal candidosis. The oesophagus is studded with cream-coloured fungal colonies.

Specimen from the Gordon Museum, Guy's Hospital, London, reproduced by permission of the Curator, Mr J. D. Maynard. Photograph by Miss P. M. Turnbull, Charing Cross Hospital Medical School.

Tuberculous and granulomatous oesophagitis

Oesophageal tuberculosis is rare, and is almost always secondary to pulmonary disease.[58] It results either from the swallowing of infected sputum or from direct involvement of the oesophagus by a tuberculous hilar lymph node or infected lung. In either instance it is usually a terminal manifestation of advanced disease. Occasionally primary cases are reported in which there is ulceration with a typical caseating granulomatous reaction. Crohn's disease,[56] sarcoidosis[57] and syphilis have been documented, but are rare.

Chemical and drug-induced oesophagitis

Acute oesophagitis follows the ingestion of corrosive fluids such as phenol, lysol, acids, alkalies or lye.[51] It may also follow the consumption of hot food or fluid and a variety of drugs.[52]

Acute inflammation may in severe cases be followed by ulceration. Healing can be complicated by fibrosis and stricture formation. Occasionally complete separation of the squamous mucosa occurs, forming a mucosal cast which can be vomited.

Radiation oesophagitis

This may follow radiotherapy to the chest and severe cases may be complicated by ulceration, fibrosis and stricture formation. This is probably a consequence of ischaemia due to underlying arterial occlusion. Histological features include telangiectatic vessels lined by prominent endothelial cells and set within oedematous granulation tissue (Fig. 4.5). Bizarre fibroblasts may be present. The

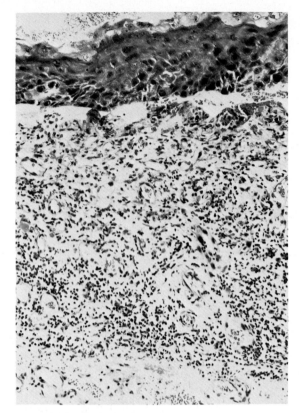

Fig. 4.5 Radiation oesophagitis. Biopsy appearance from a patient who had earlier received radiotherapy from a squamous carcinoma of the oesophagus. A sheet of degenerate squamous epithelium has separated from a layer of oedematous granulation tissue in which thin-walled vessels are lined by endothelial cells with prominent nuclei.

Haematoxylin-eosin   × 100

squamous epithelium may be ulcerated, degenerate or show features simulating dysplasia.[53] Radiation-associated carcinoma of the oesophagus has been described.[54]

Chagas' disease

Chagas' disease is caused by *Trypanosoma cruzi*, which is found in South and Central America, Mexico and part of Texas and possibly other states in the south of the United States. The main vector is the cone-nosed triatomine bug, *Panstrongylus megistus*. The trypanosomes develop in the bug's faeces. These are deposited on human skin at the time of biting, and penetrate it to enter the bloodstream and invade smooth muscle and myo-cardium. They multiply as the leishmania-like amastigote form which is ingested either by histiocytes adjacent to ganglion cells or taken up by by muscle and ganglion cells themselves, producing pseudocysts which rupture and liberate their contained parasites. Some of these probably release neurotoxins which in their turn produce ganglionic and preganglionic inflammatory changes while others appear in the bloodstream and repeat the cycle.

The disease progresses to a chronic phase, in which cardiomegaly, mega-oesophagus and mega-colon are the most conspicuous complications. The pseudocysts which develop in the circular and longitudinal muscle coats of the bowel in the acute phase rupture, releasing a neurotoxin which gives rise to an inflammatory reaction and destroys many of the ganglion cells. Microscopic examination of the oesophagus shows a striking reduction in the number of ganglion cells, but not necessarily a complete absence of them. The number of ganglion cells must be reduced by at least 50% to produce functional disturbance and by 90% to produce mega-oesophagus. Patients come to operation when the disease is chronic, inflammatory changes are minimal and the parasites are not demonstrable.[58,59]

Behçet's disease

Oesophageal involvement is rare in Behçet's disease (see p. 353) and is characterized by chronic, non-specific ulceration, spreading oesophagitis and stenosis. The middle third is the site of predilection.[60]

Peptic (reflux) oesophagitis

The terms peptic or reflux oesophagitis and gastro-oesophageal reflux indicate reflux of acid gastric contents into the lower oesophagus which may be symptomless or can present as heartburn and the sensation of refluxed acid content in the mouth. Reflux results from a failure of anti-reflux mechanism, which may be occasional, intermittent or continuous, and is commonly associated with hiatus hernia, pyloric stenosis and increased intra-abdominal pressure due to over-eating.[61]

The normal squamous epithelium which lines

the lower oesophagus is sensitive to the presence of acid gastric juice and regurgitated bile.[62] The initial response is a basal cell hyperplasia which can be followed by the return to normal, by ulceration and fibrosis or, in a significant number of patients, by a metaplasia of the squamous epithelium to a columnar type which is presumably more resistant to acid digestion.

The normal oesophageal squamous epithelium has a basal cell layer of up to 15% of the total thickness of the epithelium but not more, and connective-tissue papillae of lamina propria which never extend more than two-thirds of the way through the squamous epithelium. There are normally some plasma cells and lymphocytes but no polymorphs in the lamina propria. The earliest evidence of reflux is a hyperplasia of the basal cell layer, increasing its thickness beyond the normal 15%, with some nuclear pleomorphism, hyperchromatism, and an increased mitotic index (Fig. 4.6). Thinning of the epithelium over the papillae occurs so that they approach nearer to the surface.[63, 64] Intra-epithelial eosinophils may be a sensitive marker of reflux in children and young adults.[65] As with gastritis, however, there is no accurate correspondence of clinical symptoms with endoscopic, radiological or histological findings.[66]

This stage may regress, or it can go on to

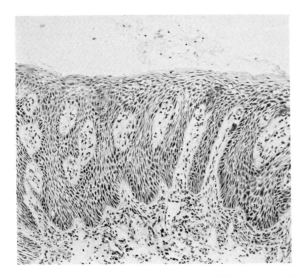

Fig. 4.6 Reflux oesophagitis showing basal cell hyperplasia and ingrowth of connective-tissue papillae which show oedema and vascular dilatation.

Haematoxylin-eosin   × 100

ulceration. When there has been any appreciable degree of ulceration longitudinal ridges can be seen, the crests representing thickened reparative mucosa while the troughs represent ulceration with surrounding congestion. Microscopically, the ridges consist of hyperplastic squamous epithelium with hyperkeratosis. This alternate ridging and ulceration ends abruptly at the cardia, but usually tails away gradually into the proximal mucosa. When ulceration has been severe, there is commonly extensive subsequent submucosal fibrosis which can produce thickening and shortening of the involved segment with narrowing of the lumen and can involve muscle coats and peri-oesophageal tissues. Sometimes squamous epithelial regeneration is incomplete and the lower oesophagus is lined by inflamed granulation or fibrous tissue which bleeds readily.

Peptic ulcer

A number of patients with reflux oesophagitis, and some without, develop peptic type ulcers in the lower oesophagus. These are usually small, partially healed and chronic. They occur either in islands of true gastric heterotopic epithelium without concomitant oesophagitis, or in zones of columnar cell metaplasia, or at the lower edge of zones of active oesophagitis when they can be surrounded by squamous or columnar cell epithelium. Like peptic ulcer in the stomach or duodenum they may be complicated by haemorrhage and perforation when acute, and by fibrosis and stricture when chronic. Microscopically, they resemble peptic ulcers elsewhere with a fibrous tissue base, destruction of muscle coats and replacement of the ulcerated mucosa by necrotic debris and granulation tissue.

Barrett's oesophagus[67]

There is now abundant evidence that the condition originally described as 'congenitally short oesophagus' and now sometimes known as 'the lower oesophagus lined by columnar epithelium', or Barrett's oesophagus, is rarely if ever congenital, but represents one form of reaction of the lower oesophageal epithelium to refluxed gastric contents. In some patients, instead of ulceration of the squamous epithelium, a columnar type epithelium develops to cover the lower oesophagus, usually as a continuous sheet but sometimes as scattered islands.[68] Sequential biopsies have shown that it can progressively replace squamous epithelium.[69] In patients who have had partial oesophagogastrectomy with anastomosis of oesophagus to fundus (after which reflux is common), the residual oesophagus is likely to become progressively lined by columnar epithelium.[70] On the other hand, antireflux surgery may lead to the regression of the lesion.[71] There are three possible epithelial patterns.[72] The first is the specialized form of columnar epithelium with a villiform surface containing intestinal goblet cells and columnar mucous cells (Fig. 4.7).[73,74] This is indistiguishable from incomplete intestinal metaplasia as described in the stomach.[75] The columnar mucous cells secrete either mainly neutral mucins or sulphomucins.[75,76] Paneth cells are rarely observed, but the presence

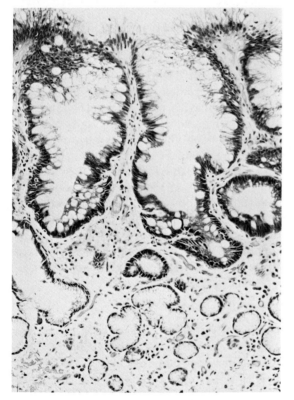

Fig. 4.7 Specialized or intestinalized columnar epithelium from lower oesophagus. The crypts and surface epithelium are lined by goblet cells and columnar mucous cells. Simple mucous glands of cardiac type occupy the lower field.

Haematoxylin-eosin   × 100

of endocrine cells has been noted.[73] The second epithelial pattern is the cardiac or junctional type. The third and rarest is the fundic type in which parietal and chief cells are represented. Superimposed inflammatory and atrophic changes are common in all three types.

At the upper edge of the metaplastic columnar epithelium there is often a zone of ulceration with fibrosis, active inflammation and sometimes stricture formation. Appearances suggest that this represents the proximal limit of a severe reflux oesophagitis in which a secondary protective epithelial metaplasia to a columnar cell lining has occurred more distally.

Any stricture of the oesophagus carries with it a liability to carcinomatous change in the associated epithelium. There is evidence that columnar metaplastic epithelium is liable to dysplastic and carcinomatous change.[77–79] This appears to be especially true for specialized mucosa in which the metaplastic columnar cells secrete sulphomucin.[75] However, Barrett's oesophagus can only be diagnosed in endoscopic biopsies in which columnar epithelium is detected at least 1.5 cm proximal to the lower oesophageal sphincter, preferably with manometric guidance.[79] Dysplasia in Barrett's oesophagus is similar to dysplasia described within intestinalized and non-intestinalized gastric mucosa. It has been observed in the mucosa bordering adenocarcinomas of the lower oesophagus, but is rarely discovered in the absence of carcinoma.[76,79]

TUMOURS OF THE OESOPHAGUS
BENIGN EPITHELIAL TUMOURS

Squamous papillomas are very rare and may be multiple. They are small, warty tumours composed of squamous epithelium showing little if any pleomorphism. They are thought to have no malignant potential.[80] Some papillomas show histological evidence of human papillomavirus infection.[81]

Glycogenic acanthosis presents as multiple white plaques and is commonly seen both at post mortem and on endoscopy. The epithelium is thickened and contains large glycogen-filled cells. The aetiology is unknown and the condition shows no relationship to cancer.[82]

Polyps. Dysplastic columnar epithelium has been observed within Barrett's oesophagus (see p. 139) but rarely forms a circumscribed polyp. Small polyps formed of glandular tissue resembling normal gastric epithelium arise in the lower oesophagus. They have been referred to as 'adenomas', but the associated oesophagitis indicates their probable inflammatory aetiology.[83]

Retention cysts are also likely to arise in a background of chronic inflammation.[82] These may be closely related to the lesions of intramural oesophageal diverticulosis (see p. 134).

MALIGNANT EPITHELIAL TUMOURS

Most malignant oesophageal tumours are squamous carcinomas (90%), but adenocarcinomas occur in the lower oesophagus and other types including carcinosarcoma, adenosquamous carcinoma, oat cell carcinoma, mucous gland carcinoma (e.g. adenoid cystic) and melanoma are encountered. In the USA and UK the overall incidence of all forms of oesophageal carcinoma varies from 5.2 to 10.4 per 100 000 people and accounts for 2–5% of deaths due to malignant disease. A higher incidence of squamous carcinoma is found in certain countries, notably China, Japan, South Africa and Iran (see below).[85]

Squamous carcinoma

Environmental factors are probably important in the aetiology of this neoplasm. Striking local variations within countries such as China and Iran may reflect peculiar dietary habits and argue against racial susceptibilities. Suggested dietary associations include the consumption of hot beverages, coarse vegetable fibres and pickled vegetables coupled to a deficiency of fresh vegetables and vitamins.[86] A heavy intake of alcohol and/or tobacco is more common in patients with oesophageal squamous carcinoma. The majority arise in the middle oesophagus. Those of middle and lower oesophagus are more common in males, whereas postcricoid carcinoma is far more common in women and is usually associated with the Plummer-

Vinson (Paterson-Brown-Kelly) syndrome. Most cases occur in the sixth and seventh decades.[87,88]

Precancerous conditions

Clinical settings associated with an increased risk of squamous carcinoma include strictures after swallowing lye,[89] achalasia (see p. 135), the Plummer-Vinson (Paterson-Brown-Kelly) syndrome,[90] coeliac disease[91] and tylosis[92,93] (keratosis palmaris and plantaris) and previous irradiation.[59,94]

Precancerous lesions

Particular histological abnormalities may predispose to squamous carcinoma. This is indicated by their increased prevalence in patients with precancerous conditions and their presence in the vicinity of frankly invasive carcinoma.

Chronic oesophagitis may either complicate diseases of the oesophagus such as hiatus hernia, diverticulum and achalasia or arise as a primary event. For example, a form of chronic oesophagitis affecting the mid-oesophagus is thought to reflect the dietary habits of high-risk Iranian communities (see above).[95]

The epithelium in chronic oesophagitis may either become hyperplastic (acanthotic) or atrophic. Neoplastic change has been observed in both epithelial alterations.[95]

Intra-epithelial neoplasia or dysplasia is regarded as the most important precancerous lesion. Most reports of oesophageal dysplasia are from countries with a high incidence of squamous carcinoma. The Chinese Co-ordinating Group carried out a mass survey on 21 581 inhabitants aged over 30 in the rural areas of Anyang, Hsinhsiung and Loyung.[96] The abrasive balloon technique was used to obtain cytological specimens. Smears from 2732 subjects (12.7%) showed mild dysplasia, 280 (1.2%) showed severe dysplasia and in 194 cases (0.9%) the appearances were consistent with invasive squamous carcinoma. A decade separated the maximum incidence of dysplasia and carcinoma, supporting a dysplasia-carcinoma sequence.

There is no evidence that white plaques arising within oesophageal epithelium are homologous with premalignant leukoplakia of other sites such as the mouth or vulva. White papules less than

1 cm in diameter are not uncommonly seen on oesophagoscopy, but such lesions, termed glycogenic acanthosis (see p. 140) are quite innocent.

Other causes of white plaques include chronic oesophagitis, lichen planus, candidosis and carcinoma-in-situ.

The neoplastic proliferation associated with oesophageal dysplasia results in the vertical compression of the underlying stroma. Highly vascularized finger-like processes thereby extend close to the surface. This abnormal vascularization may be appreciated in fresh specimens.

With the advent of severe or high-grade dysplasia (amounting to carcinoma-in-situ), more obvious macroscopic changes may be evident. The lesion may be circumscribed or annular, and elevated, flat or depressed. Examination usually reveals either a white plaque or a pink erosion.[97] Gross ulceration signifies advanced carcinoma. Dysplasia may be multifocal and sometimes involve large areas of mucosa.[98] The histology of oesophageal dysplasia is similar to its better-documented counterpart within the uterine cervix.[99] The neoplastic cells may be small (basaloid), large and non-keratinized or large and keratinized.[53] The first is conveniently graded in terms of the proportion of atypical basal cells occupying the mucosa. Atypical basal cells show a high nucleocytoplasmic ratio and

nuclei that are hyperchromatic, pleomorphic and mitotically active. In carcinoma-in-situ, the entire thickness of the mucosa is replaced by atypical basal cells (Fig. 4.8). Precise criteria for grading the large cell dysplasias have not been laid down. Difficulty may arise in distinguishing between true dysplasia and reactive basal cell hyperplasia associated with reflux oesophagitis. In some forms of dysplasia, the presence of koilocytotic change (cells with vacuolated cytoplasm) indicates an underlying human papillomavirus infection.[81]

Chronic inflammation and dysplasia have been described in the oesophageal mucosa of patients with the Plummer-Vinson (Paterson-Brown-Kelly) syndrome, though not in the epithelial web itself (see p. 136).[100]

Early oesophageal cancer

This term applies to carcinoma in which spread in continuity extends no further than the submucosa and disregards the presence or absence of lymph node metastases.[97]

Evidence from China suggests that the prognosis is good and progression to advanced carcinoma is slow.[101] It is probably unwise to employ this term when lymph nodes are involved. The lesion often presents as a shallow ulcer. Reactive epithelial

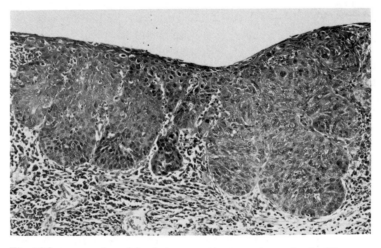

Fig. 4.8 Severe oesophageal dysplasia, amounting to carcinoma-in-situ. The normal epithelium is replaced by atypical basal cells showing nuclear enlargement, hyperchromatism and pleomorphism.

Haematoxylin-eosin   × 100

changes in the vicinity of acute peptic erosions must be carefully distinguished from early oesophageal carcinoma.

Advanced squamous carcinoma

This may be an ulcerating (Fig. 4.9), stricturing, or, less commonly, a protuberant tumour. Rarely, a diffuse infiltrative type of growth resembling the 'leather bottle stomach' (see p. 202) involves a length of oesophagus. There is a rare variety of verrucous squamous carcinoma of low malignancy.[102] Not uncommonly the main growth is surrounded by satellite tumours due to submucosal extension.

Squamous carcinomas show all grades of differentiation, from keratinizing squamous carcinomas with well-formed cell nests to undifferentiated growths without recognizable keratin or prickle cells, which are difficult to identify as squamous (Fig. 4.10). There is a marked tendency to variations in differentiation in different parts of the growth. Submucosal infiltration, not readily detectable by the naked eye, is often a conspicuous microscopic feature. Segmental resection is there-

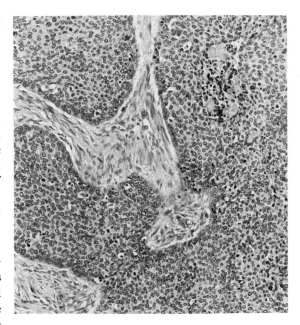

Fig. 4.10 Small cell, non-keratinizing variant of squamous cell carcinoma of oesophagus.

Haematoxylin-eosin   × 100

fore not often adequate, and in any surgically removed tumour a careful study should be made of the resected ends to ensure that removal has been complete. The tumour commonly infiltrates the muscle coats and often breaches them; local extension to surrounding structures is common. Estimations of the degree of differentiation of the growth are not very helpful in prognosis.

Adenocarcinoma

This may arise either at the gastro-oesophageal junction, within columnar epithelium lining the lower oesophagus (Barrett's oesophagus—see p. 139), or within squamous epithelium. In the latter instance the origin of the growth is likely to be from submucous oesophageal glands.[103] Adenocarcinoma arising at the junction could originate either within the stomach, within columnar epithelium lining the lower oesophagus (Fig. 4.11), or from submucous oesophageal glands. The microscopic appearances of junctional tumours may show a mixed adenosquamous pattern, a pattern reminiscent of some salivary gland tumours (Fig. 4.12) or any grade of adenocarcinomatous differentiation. It is interesting that adenocarcinomas arising in the stomach frequently spread up

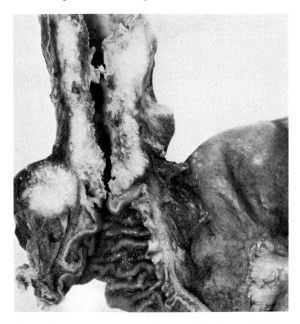

Fig. 4.9 Primary squamous carcinoma of the lower end of the oesophagus. All the coats of the wall of the oesophagus have been invaded. On the left, a lymph node in the vicinity of the left gastric artery is greatly enlarged as a result of metastatic involvement.

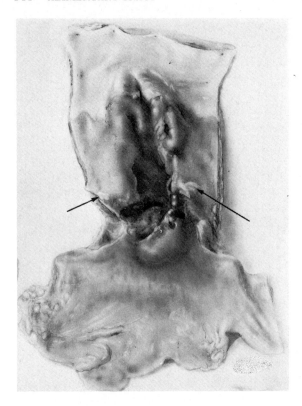

Fig. 4.11 Drawing of a specimen of oesophageal adenocarcinoma arising within columnar epithelium lining the lower oesophagus. The arrows point to surviving islands of squamous epithelium.

described as resembling sarcoma histologically but as having no malignant potential. Some authors have, therefore, cast doubt upon some of the reported cases of carcinosarcoma. Nearly all of the cases described have been polypoidal growths projecting into the lumen, a pattern which is very rare in other malignant oesophageal growths, except primary melanomas. These tumours are said to have a better prognosis than the ordinary squamous carcinoma. When metastases do occur they are almost always sarcomatous. The concept that the sarcomatous component in at least some of these tumours is derived from squamous epithelium is supported by electron microscopic studies.[106]

'Oat cell' carcinoma

These are described by a number of authors. Some are probably undifferentiated squamous carcinomas but others present a uniform oat cell type growth resembling the familiar 'oat cell' carcinoma of bronchus and involving submucosa and muscle coats. A secondary deposit from a primary bronchial carcinoma must be excluded, but some examples may originate within oesophageal glands. Neurosecretory granules have been demonstrated histochemically and at the ultrastructural level.[107]

into the oesophagus, whereas oesophageal squamous carcinomas rarely spread downwards into the stomach.

Carcinosarcoma and pseudosarcoma

A carcinosarcoma is a rare malignant tumour in which both epithelial and connective-tissue elements are mixed (Fig. 4.13). In assessing the nature of such a growth it should be remembered that squamous carcinomas may develop a spindle-cell pattern, either spontaneously or after irradiation.[109] Furthermore the squamous epithelium overlying a genuine malignant connective-tissue tumour, such as a leiomyosarcoma, can undergo secondary hyperplasia simulating cancer. There are also a number of reports of superficial squamous cell carcinoma or carcinoma-in-situ with an underlying so-called pseudosarcomatous reaction which is

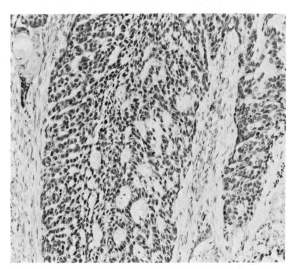

Fig. 4.12 Adenocarcinoma of oesophagus showing pattern reminiscent of a salivary gland tumour. The submucous oesophageal glands represent the likely site of origin.

Haematoxylin-eosin   × 100

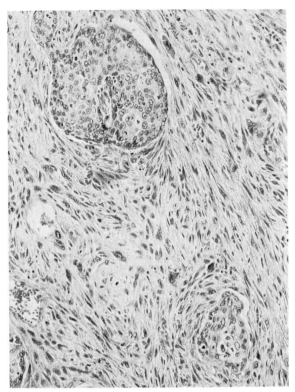

Fig. 4.13 Carcinosarcoma of the oesophagus showing malignant squamous epithelial islands within a sarcomatous stroma. The tumour was a polypoid growth projecting into the lumen of the oesophagus.

Haematoxylin-eosin   × 100

Malignant melanoma

Though it is now well recognized that melanoblasts can be found in normal oesophageal mucosa in about 4% of people, a melanoma presenting in the oesophagus is more likely to be secondary than primary. The criteria for a primary oesophageal melanoma are that it should be seen either to arise in or be surrounded by squamous epithelium showing junctional change. Most of the reported cases have also contained demonstrable melanin. Acceptable primary melanomas have affected elderly people and involved the middle or lower thirds of the oesophagus. The tumours are usually grey or black in colour and project as polypoid masses into the lumen. Microscopically, they have the characteristics of melanomas elsewhere, but pigmented cells are usually numerous and diagnosis is not difficult.[108]

Spread of oesophageal carcinoma

The most common and extensive form of direct spread is in the wall of the viscus, particularly in the submucosa and in submucosal lymphatics. In all resected specimens it is necessary to take transverse blocks from the entire circumference of the proximal and distal ends to ensure that the line of resection is clear of any submucosal extension of the growth, even though it may appear well clear to the naked eye. Downward extension of oesophageal carcinoma into the stomach is not common despite the continuity of the submucosa. Any extension may subsequently ulcerate through the mucosa producing satellite growths. Once the growth has breached the muscle coats it commonly involves the trachea or main bronchi, the lung parenchyma and the superior or posterior mediastinum. Less commonly, there is direct invasion of the aorta with perforation. More rarely, the pericardium, heart and laryngeal nerves are involved. By the time the diagnosis of oesophageal carcinoma is confirmed, metastases have occurred in 50–80% of cases. Adenocarcinomas seem to metastasize earlier, and more frequently, than the squamous type. The most common sites are the regional lymph nodes, probably because there are two separate sets of lymphatics, one draining mucosa and submucosa, the other the muscle coats. Nodes likely to be affected include paratracheal, parabronchial, para-oesophageal, posterior mediastinal, coeliac and upper deep cervical groups. Nodes below the diaphragm are frequently involved, including those in the splenic hilum.

Because there is a wide intercommunication between these groups, clinical involvement of the nodes palpable in the neck does not necessarily mean that the growth is in the upper or middle oesophagus.

Visceral metastases by the bloodstream occur most commonly to liver, lungs and adrenal glands; they are found in approximately 70% of all cases.[109]

Prognosis of oesophageal carcinoma

The prognosis of carcinoma of the oesophagus of all types is poor; in untreated cases the 1-year survival rate is low and the 5-year survival is rarely above 5%. In surgically-treated patients the prognosis depends partly on whether radical or palliative surgery is performed.[110] In most large series only 50–60% were suitable for radical operation and only about 7% of the original number diagnosed were alive after five years.[111] The prognosis appears to be better for squamous carcinoma of the lower third than for the same growth in the middle third, and worst of all for adenocarcinoma of the cardia. In studies on survival after radiotherapy, the 1-year survival of all treated cases was a little over 20%, but only 4% survived five years or more.[112]

Secondary tumours

Secondary tumours in the oesophagus are rare. Direct spread occurs most commonly from carcinoma of the stomach into the lower end of the oesophagus and less commonly from bronchus or thyroid. Lymphatic spread has been described from carcinoma of the breast[113] and bloodstream metastasis from primary tumours in the testis,[114] prostate[115] and pancreas.[116]

Leukaemias and lymphomas of all types may secondarily involve the oesophagus.[117] In their mildest form they present as subepithelial haemorrhages, which may induce secondary epithelial erosion; infiltration of leukaemic cells occurs in the submucosa either as microscopic deposits or macroscopic nodules which undergo necrosis and ulceration. These lesions are often complicated by secondary fungal infections, especially candidosis, particularly when irradiation or antimitotic drugs have been used. Occasional examples of apparently primary extramedullary plasmacytoma are described in the oesophagus.[118,119]

NON-EPITHELIAL TUMOURS

Smooth muscle tumours

Leiomyoma is the commonest benign tumour of the oesophagus.[120] It is more common in males and is seen in the lower more often than the upper part. Tumours are single or multiple. They originate from the smooth muscle either of muscularis mucosae or muscle coats, usually the latter. They present either as a large, polypoid mass projecting into the lumen or as a lobulated, intramural tumour, occasionally with crater-like ulceration of its mucosal surface; flat intramural growths are uncommon and usually undifferentiated. Occasionally the mass is mainly extra-oesophageal in position. The cut surface is greyish-white. Calcification is uncommon.

Although most smooth muscle tumours of the oesophagus are benign and many are discovered incidentally, the distinction between leiomyoma and leiomyosarcoma histologically can be difficult, if not impossible in some cases. The best guides to malignancy are the degree of cellularity, numerous mitotic figures, size of tumour and necrosis.

Benign smooth muscle tumours must be distinguished from the rare condition of diffuse leiomyomatosis[121] which occurs mainly in adolescents and young adults as an irregular thickening with narrowing of a segment of oesophagus and sometimes stomach. Histologically, there is a diffuse hyperplasia of smooth muscle, often with a whorled pattern and a considerable amount of intermingled fibrous tissue. Neural elements may also be hyperplastic and an infiltrate of lymphocytes and plasma cells is common. The condition is probably a malformation rather than a neoplasm.

The prognosis of smooth muscle tumours is good provided local excision is complete. Metastasis to regional lymph nodes is rare and only occurs in anaplastic types. Blood-borne metastasis occurs to lung and liver, but is usually a late manifestation.

Neurofibroma

This is a very rare submucosal tumour. It may be multiple as a manifestation of von Recklinghausen's disease.

Fibrous (fibrovascular) polyps

These polyps are occasionally seen at all levels of the oesophagus, but usually the upper third. They are composed of oedematous connective tissue containing a variable amount of fatty tissue and covered by intact stratified squamous mucosa. The latter often undergoes patchy ulceration from trauma and secondary infection. Sometimes, these polyps grow to a great size[122] and have long pedicles. When this occurs it is possible for the polyp to be regurgitated and hang outside the mouth.

MISCELLANEOUS TUMOURS AND TUMOUR-LIKE LESIONS

Lipomas and vascular malformations may be found in the oesophagus.

Miscellaneous rare tumours include granular cell myoblastoma,[122] ectopic pancreatic tissue, choriocarcinoma[123] and extremedullary plasmacytoma.[124]

REFERENCES

Anatomy

1. Melcher DH. Br J Surg 1969; 56: 904.
2. de la Pava S, Nigogosyan G, Pickren JW, Cabrera A. Cancer 1963; 16: 48.
3. Tateishi R, Taniguchi H, Wada A, Horai T, Tamaguchi K. Arch Pathol 1974; 98: 87.
4. Lendrum AC. Arch Intern Med 1937; 59: 474.
5. Atkinson A. Gut 1962; 3: 1.
6. Baumgarten HG. In: Bertaccini G, ed. Mediators and drugs in gastrointestinal motility. I. Morphological basis and neurophysiological control. Berlin: Springer, 1982.
7. Furness JB, Costa M. In: Bertaccini G, ed. Mediators and drugs in gastrointestinal motility. I. Morphological basis and neurophysiological control. Berlin: Springer, 1982.
8. Smith B. Gut 1970; 11: 271.
9. Burnstock G. Scand J Gastroenterol 1981; 16 (suppl 70): 1.

Developmental abnormalities

10. Arbona JL, Fazzi JG, Mayoral J. Am J Gastroenterol 1984; 79: 177
11. Guthrie KJ. J Path Bact 1945; 57: 363.
12. Rosenthal AH. Arch Path 1931; 12: 756.
13. Scott JS, Wilson JK. Lancet 1957; ii: 569.
14. Sloan H, Haight C. J Thorac Surg 1956; 32: 209.
15. Quan L, Smith DW, J Paediat 1973; 82: 104.
16. Barry JE, Auldist AW. Am J Dis Child 1974; 128: 769.
17. Willis RA. In: The borderland of embryology and pathology. London: Butterworth, 1962.
18. Stevenson RE. J Paediat 1972; 81: 1123.
19. Louw JH, Cywes S. Br J Surg 1962; 50: 102.
20. Halasz NA, Lindskog GE, Liebow AA. Ann Surg 1962; 155: 215.
21. Rector LA, Connerley ML. Arch Pathol 1941; 31: 285.
22. Raeburn C. J Path Bact 1951; 63: 157.
23. Morson BC, Belcher JR. Br J Cancer 1952; 6: 127.
24. Adler RH. J Thorac Cardiovasc Surg 1963; 45: 13.
25. de la Pava S, Pickren JW, Adler RH. NY St J Med 1964; 64: 1831.
26. Dodds GS. Am J Path 1941; 17: 861.

Muscular disorders

27 Treacy WL, Baggenstoss AH, Slocumb CH, Code CF. Ann Intern Med 1963; 59: 351.
28. McKinley M, Sherlock P. Am J Gastroenterol 1984; 79: 438.
29. Bevans M. Arch Pathol 1945; 40: 225.
30. Sloper JC. Thorax 1954; 9: 136.
31. Garlock JH, Dichter R. Ann Surg 1961; 154: 259.
32. Graham DY, Goyal RK, Sparkman J, Cagan ME, Pogonowska MJ. Gastroenterol 1975; 68: 781.

33. Wightman AJA, Wright EA. Br J Radiol 1974; 47: 496.
34. Patel RM, Mallaiah LR, Suster B. Am J Gastroenterol 1981; 76: 351.
35. Pride RB. Gut 1966; 7: 188.
36. Barrett NR. Br J Surg 1954; 42: 231.
37. Allison PR. Thorax 1948; 3: 20.
38. Carre IG, Froggatt P. Gut 1970; 11: 51.
39. Kramer P. Gastroenterol 1965; 49: 439.
40. Barrett NR. Br Med J 1964; i: 1135.
41. Vantrappen G, Hellemans J. In: Jewell DP, Selby WS, eds. Topics in gastroenterology, vol 10. Oxford: Blackwell Scientific, 1982.
42. Feczko PJ, Ma CK, Halpert RD, Batra SK. Am J Gastroenterol 1983; 78: 265.

Miscellaneous conditions

43. Spence RAJ, Sloan JM, Johnston GW, Grenfield A. Gut 1983; 24: 1024.

Oesophagitis

44. Nash G, Ross JS. Hum Pathol 1974; 5: 339.
45. McKay JS, Day DW. Histopathol 1983; 7: 409.
46. Balthazar EJ, Megibow AJ, Hulnick DH. Am J Roent 1985; 144: 1201.
47. Deshmukh M, Shah R, McCallum RW. Am J Gastroenterol 1984; 79: 173.
48. Kodsi BE, Wickremesinghe PC, Kozinn PG, Iswara K, Goldberg PK. Gastroenterol 1976; 71: 715.
49. Brown JW, McKee WM. Am J Dig Dis 1972; 17: 85.
50. Scott BB, Jenkins D. Gut 1982; 23: 137.
51. Kiviranta UK. Acta Otolaryngol 1952; 42: 89.
52. Mason SJ, O'Mera TF. J Clin Gastroenterol 1981; 3: 115.
53. Mandard AM, Marnay J, Gignoux M et al. Hum Pathol 1984; 15: 660.
54. Sherrill DJ, Grishkin BA, Galal FS, Zajtchuk R, Graeber GM. Cancer 1984; 54: 726.
55. Dow CJ. Gut 1981; 22: 234.
56. Ghahremani GG, Gore RM, Breuer RI, Larson RH. Gastrointest Radiol 1982; 7: 199.
57. Polachek AA, Matra WJ. Am J Dig Dis 1964; 9: 429.
58. Earlam RJ. Am J Dig Dis 1972; 17: 559.
59. Betarello A, Pinotti HW. Clinics in Gastroenterol 1976, 5: 27.
60. Mori S, Yoshihira A, Kawamura H, Takeuchi A, Hashimoto T, Inaba G. Am J Gastroenterol 1983; 78: 548.
61. Edwards DAW, Thompson H, Shaw DG, Misiewicz JJ, Bennett JR, Torrancet B. Gut 1973; 14: 233.
62. Sandry RJ. Gut 1962; 33: 16.
63. Bahar J, Sheahan DC. Arch Pathol 1975; 99: 387.

64. Thompson H. Clinics in Gastroenterol 1976; 5: 143.
65. Winter HS, Madara JC, Stafford RJ, Grand RJ, Quinlan J, Goldman H. Gastroenterol 1982; 83: 818.
66. Sladen GE, Riddell RH, Willoughby GMT. Br Med J 1975; i: 71.
67. Barrett NR. Surgery (St Louis) 1957; 41: 881.
68. Herlihy KJ, Orlando RC, Bryson JC, Bozymski EM, Carney CN, Powell DW. Gastroenterol 1984; 86: 436.
69. Mossberg SM. Gastroenterol 1966; 50: 671.
70. Hamilton SR, Yardley JH. Gastroenterol 1977; 72: 669.
71. Brand DL, Ylvisaker JT, Galfand M, Pope GE. N Engl J Med 1980; 302: 844.
72. Paull A, Trier JS, Dalton MD, Camp RC, Loeb P, Goyal RK. N Engl J Med 1976; 295: 476.
73. Trier JS. Gastroenterol 1970; 58: 444.
74. Thompson JJ, Zinsser KR, Enterline HT. Hum Pathol 1983; 14: 42.
75. Jass JR. J Clin Pathol 1981; 34: 866.
76. Peuchmaur M, Potet F, Goldfain D. J Clin Pathol 1984; 37: 607.
77. Haggitt RC, Tryzelaar J, Ellis FG, Colcher H. Am J Clin Pathol 1978; 70: 1.
78. Meuwissen SGM, Visser J, Leguit P, Wesdorp E. J Clin Gastroenterol 1983; 5: 71.
79. Skinner DB, Walther BC, Riddell RH, Schmidt H, Iascone C, DeMeester TR. Ann Surg 1984; 198: 554.

Tumours of the oesophagus

80. Waterfall WE, Somers S, Desa DJ. J Clin Pathol 1978; 31: 111.
81. Winkler B, Capo V, Reumann W, et al. Cancer 1985; 55: 149.
82. Bender MD, Allison J, Cuartos F, Montgomery C. Gastroenterol 1973; 65: 373.
83. Spin FP. Gastrointestinal endosc 1973; 20: 26.
84. Hover AR, Brady CE, Williams JR, Stewart DL, Christian C. J Clin Gastroenterol 1982; 4: 209.
85. Cook-Mozaffari P. In: Wright R, ed. Recent advances in gastrointestinal pathology. Philadelphia: Saunders, 1980: 267.
86. Munoz N, Crespi M, Grassi A, Qing WG, Qiong S, Cai LZ. Lancet 1982; i: 876.
87. Le Roux BT. Thorax 1961: 16: 226.
88. Miller C. Br J Surg 1962; 49: 507.
89. Bigelow NH. Cancer 1953; 6: 1159.
90. Wynder EI, Hultberg S, Jacobsson F, Bross IJ. Cancer 1957; 10: 470.
99. Wright JT, Richardson PC. Br Med J 1967; i: 540.
92. Howel-Evans W, McConnell RB, Clarke CA, Sheppard PM. Quart J Med 1958; 27: 413.
93. O'Mahoney MY, Ellis JP, Hellier M, Mann R, Huddy P. J Roy Soc Med 1984; 77: 514.
94. Goolden AWG. Br J Radiol 1957; 30: 626.
95. Crespi M, Munoz N, Grassi A et al. Lancet 1979; ii: 217.
96. Coordinating group for the research of oesophageal carcinoma. Chin Med J 1975; 1: 110.
97. Barge J, Molas G, Maillard JN, Fekete F, Bogolometz WW, Potet F. Histopathol 1981; 5: 499.
98. Ushigome S, Spjut HJ, Noon GP. Cancer 1967; 20: 1023.
99. Goran DA, Shields HM, Bates ML, Zuckerman GR, DeSchryver-Kecskemeti K. Gastroenterol 1984; 86: 39.
100. Jacobs A. J Clin Pathol 1960; 13: 463.
101. Yanjin M, Guangyi L, Xianzhi G, Wenheng C. J Roy Soc Med 1981; 74: 884.
102. Agha FP, Weatherbee L, Sams JS. Am J Gastroenterol 1984; 79: 844.
103. Azzopardi JG, Menzies T. Br J Surg 1962; 49: 497.
104. Scarpa FJ. Cancer 1966; 19: 861.
105. Takubo K, Tsuchiya S, Nakagawa H, Futatsuki K, Ishibashi I, Hirata F. Hum Pathol 1982; 13: 503.
106. Battifora H. Cancer 1976; 2275.
107. Briggs JC, Ibrahim NBN. Histopathol 1983; 7: 261.
108. Takubo K, Kanda Y, Ishi M et al. Hum Pathol 1983; 14: 727.
109. Morson BC, Dawson IMP. Gastrointestinal pathology. 2nd ed. Oxford: Blackwell Scientific, 1979: 48.
110. Garlock JH, Klein SH. Ann Surg 1954; 139: 19.
111. Tanner NC. In: Tanner NC, Smithers DW, eds. Tumours of the oesophagus. Edinburgh. Livingstone, 1961.
112. Dickinson RJ. Am J Med Sci 1961; 241: 662.
113. Polk HC, Camp FA, Walker AW. Cancer 1967; 20: 2002.
114. Willis RA. Spread of tumours in the human body. 2nd ed. London. Butterworth, 1952: 283.
115. Gross P, Freedman LJ. Arch Pathol 1942; 33: 361.
116. Toreson WE. Arch Pathol 1944; 38: 82.
117. Prolla JC, Kirsner JB. Ann Intern Med 1964; 61: 1084.
118. Morris WT, Read JL. J Clin Pathol 1972; 25: 537.
119. Ahmed N, Ramos S, Sika S, LeVeen HH, Piccone VA. Cancer 1976; 38: 943.
120. Skandalakis JE, Gray SW, Shepard D, Bourne GW. Smooth muscle tumours of the alimentary tract. 1st ed. Springfield: Thomas, 1962.
121. Fernandez JP, Mascarenhas MJ, Da Costa JC, Correia JP. Am J Dig Dis 1976; 20: 684.
122. Patel J, Kiefter RW, Martin M, Avant GR. Gastroenterol 1984; 87: 953.
123. Subramanyam K, Shannon CR, Paterson M, Davis M, Gourley WK. J Clin Gastroenterol 1984; 6: 113.
124. McKecknie JC, Fechner RC. Cancer 1971; 27: 694.

5

D. W. Day

The stomach

ANATOMY

The stomach is normally situated in the epigastric, umbilical and left hypochondriac regions but is fixed only at the gastro-oesophageal junction and at the first part of the duodenum. Its shape and position vary with body build in different individuals and in the same individual, depending on the nature and amount of the stomach contents and with the upright and recumbent position. Although in the living subject, especially when full, it is more or less tubular, it is described as having an anterior and a posterior wall, and the left convex and right concave margins are referred to respectively as the greater and lesser curvatures.

The stomach is divisible into four parts. The cardia is a small, macroscopically indistinct zone immediately distal to the oesophago-gastric junction; it can be distinguished from the fundal and body portions, into which it merges, only by the histological pattern of its epithelium. The fundus lies above a line drawn horizontally through the gastro-oesophageal junction. The body comprises roughly the proximal two-thirds of the remainder, and the pyloric antrum the distal third leading into the pyloric sphincter.

The wall of the stomach is made up of the following layers: the mucosa including the muscularis mucosae, the submucosa, the muscularis propria and the peritoneum.

The body mucosa is rugose and freely mobile on the muscle beneath, while the antral mucosa is flattened, less rugose and more firmly anchored. The boundary between them, however, is often not clearly visible to the naked eye, and the incisural notch, an indentation seen on barium studies some two-thirds of the way down the lesser curve, is not an accurate guide. The one distinguishing feature is the type of mucosa (see below), and antral type mucosa may extend far up the lesser curve, sometimes reaching the oesophagus. Gastric distension during a meal takes place at the expense of the greater curve, while the normal pathway for small amounts of food and for fluids and secretion is along the lesser curve or *Magenstrasse* ('stomach road').

The thickness of normal gastric mucosa varies and is largely dependent on the degree of distension of the stomach. In some individuals the rugae are thick enough to give a curious fine, cobblestone appearance, so-called *état mamelonné*, which is a variation of the normal and has to be distinguished from the pathological hypertrophy of the gastric mucosa seen in Menetrier's disease (see p. 219).

The submucous layer is composed of strong but loose areolar tissue in which the blood vessels and nerves break up before they enter the mucous membrane.

The muscular coat consists of smooth muscle arranged in three complete or almost complete layers: an external longitudinal, a middle circular and an inner oblique. The outer longitudinal layer is continuous with the longitudinal fibres of the oesophagus and duodenum and passes along and on each side of the curvatures, being thickest along the lesser curvature and towards the pylorus where the fibres take part in the formation of the pyloric sphincter. It is largely absent over the central parts of the anterior and posterior surfaces. The circular layer is more complete and is absent only from the fundus. It is continuous with the more superficial of the circular fibres of the oesophagus and is especially thickened in the wall of the pyloric canal where its fibres pass into the pyloric sphincter. The inner or oblique layer is continuous with the deepest circular fibres of the oesophagus. It forms an incomplete layer that encircles the fundus and passes obliquely and caudally around the body of the stomach towards the greater curvature.

The serous coat of the stomach is formed by the peritoneum which is closely attached to the muscular layer except near the curvatures where the connection is looser.

The stomach has a generous blood supply derived from branches of the coeliac, hepatic and splenic arteries, with abundant arterial anasto-

moses. The exceptions to this appear to be the lesser curve of the stomach and the first part of the duodenum which are relatively poorly vascularized and may contain as well areas of mucosa supplied by extramural end arteries alone, with no connection to submucosal plexuses.[1] This may be significant in the pathogenesis of peptic ulceration (see p. 184). The veins enter the portal system through the pyloric vein, the left gastro-epiploic and four or five short gastric veins which join the splenic vein, the right gastro-epiploic which joins the superior mesenteric vein, and the left gastric or coronary vein which runs along the lesser curve to join ultimately the portal vein and communicates with the oesophageal vein, thereby linking the portal and systemic systems.

There are numerous lymphatic channels which form a plexus in the submucosa from which many small vessels penetrate the muscularis mucosae and ramify in the lamina propria of the mucosa. These channels drain to the left gastric, right gastric and subpyloric lymph nodes, and also to paracardial, pancreatico-splenic and right gastro-epiploic nodes.

The nerve supply is from the terminal branches of both vagi, the right tending to supply the posterior surface and the left the anterior, and from numerous branches of the coeliac plexus of the sympathetic. Submucosal and myenteric nerve plexuses are both present.

Microscopic appearances of the gastric mucosa

The gastric mucosa is composed of tubular glands lying in a delicate stroma of connective tissue enclosing thin-walled blood vessels. The glands rest on the muscularis mucosae, which consists of smooth muscle fibres pierced by numerous lymphatics and small arteries and veins. With the light microscope the mucosa can be divided into two layers, superficial and deep. The superficial layer throughout the stomach is composed of a surface epithelium consisting of a single layer of tall, regular, mucin-secreting cells with basal nuclei, which dips down to form crypts (pits, foveolae) lined by similar cells. The deep layer comprises the glands which open into the bottom of the crypts, and it is on the structure of this glandular component that the mucosa can be divided into cardiac, body and pyloric types.

Cardiac mucosa extends distally from its sharp junction with the stratified squamous epithelium of the oesophagus for a variable distance of 0.5 cm up to 3–4 cm. Because it straddles the anatomical boundary of the oesophagus and stomach it has also been referred to as junctional mucosa. Approximately half the mucosal thickness is occupied by pits (Fig. 5.1). The underlying glands, which are simple tubular or compound tubulo-racemose in type, are lined by mucin-secreting cells, but occasional parietal and even chief cells can be present. Endocrine cells are frequent. The glands are often coiled and split up into groups or lobules by prolongations of the muscularis mucosae, and cystic dilatation is common.

Body mucosa forms the major part of the lining of the stomach. Under the dissecting microscope[2]

it has a honeycomb or Morocco leather appearance with a uniformly regular pattern of closely-packed papillae, with a circular gastric pit opening at the apex of each. Around groups of these papillae are crevices formed by fusion of pits which occurs near the surface at a very acute angle. However, many pits open directly on to the surface and pit fusion is much less marked than in the pyloric mucosa.[3]

Body mucosa is from 400–1500 μm (0.4–1.5 mm) thick of which approximately a quarter is the superficial zone and the remainder the deeper glandular zone (Fig. 5.2). The glands consist of simple, straight, tightly-packed tubules extending from the crypts to the muscularis mucosae where their blind ends are slightly thickened and coiled and rarely may be dilated. From one to four glands open through a slight constriction or neck into the

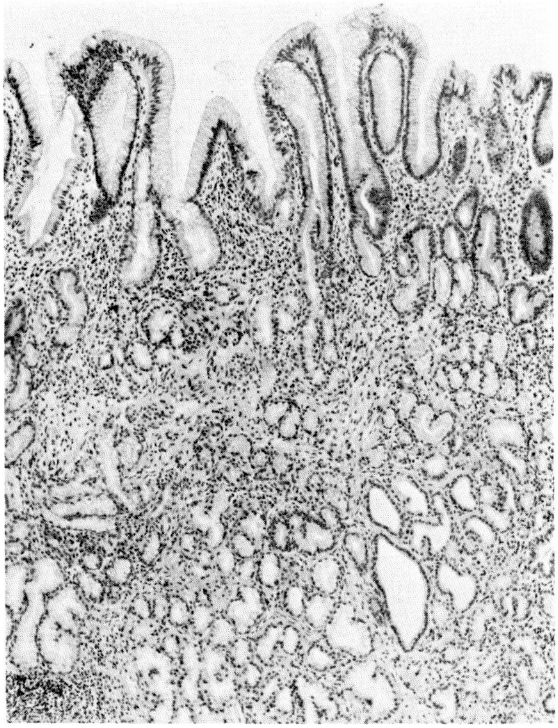

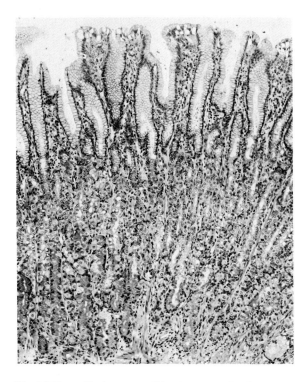

Fig. 5.1 Normal cardiac (junctional) mucosa. Simple tubular or compound tubulo-racemose glands are arranged in lobules by intersecting bands of smooth muscle derived from the muscularis mucosae. Glands, some of which show mild dilatation, are lined by mucin-secreting cells.

Haematoxylin-eosin   × 93

Fig. 5.2 Normal body mucosa. The pits account for about a third of the thickness of the mucosa. The middle third is occupied by the part of the glands in which the acid-producing oxyntic cells predominate, and the deepest third shows predominance of the more darkly-stained zymogenic cells (chief cells). There is a sparse scattering of lymphocytes in the lamina propria, especially in the region of the neck of the glands and between the pits.

Haematoxylin-eosin   × 117

bottom of each crypt. It has been estimated that there are approximately 35 million gastric body glands. The four types of cell present in the body glands are the mucous neck cells, parietal or oxyntic cells, chief or zymogenic cells, and endocrine cells.

The mucin-secreting neck cells are relatively few in number and are scattered amongst the parietal cells at the junction of the glands with the pits, although they may occur deeper in the glands, particularly near the pyloric region.[4] They are relatively small, approximately $7\,\mu m$ in width, irregular in shape, and appear to be deformed by neighbouring cells. They have a basal nucleus and finely granular cytoplasm, which stains positively with the periodic acid-Schiff reaction, although not as strongly as that of the surface and foveolar epithelial cells. Most of the cells lining the upper part of the glands are parietal cells, the source of hydrochloric acid, blood group substances and intrinsic factor. These are large ($20-35\,\mu m$), round or pyramidal cells with a central nucleus and an eosinophilic vacuolated cytoplasm corresponding to the extensive secretory canaliculus seen ultra-structurally. Their longest side is in apposition to the basement membrane and their apical end wedged between adjoining cells. Zymogen or chief cells, which secrete pepsinogen and other proteo-lytic pro-enzymes, predominate in the lower half of the gland and intermingle with parietal cells in the middle third (Fig. 5.3). In freshly-fixed material their cytoplasm contains refractile gran-ules which are variably basophilic. They have a large basal nucleus. The numbers of chief and parietal cells in individual glands varies in different parts of the body of the stomach, with a progressive increase in parietal cells and corresponding de-crease in chief cells as the pyloric region is approached.[5] Endocrine cells are described below.

Pyloric mucosa is present as a roughly triangular area in the lower third of the stomach, the boundary zone between it and body mucosa extending as an oblique line from a point about two-fifths of the way along the lesser curve to a point on the greater curve much nearer the pylorus. However, there is considerable individual variation especially in its extension along the lesser curve, so that it may reach almost to the cardia, particularly in women.[6,7] With the dissecting microscope it has a coarse

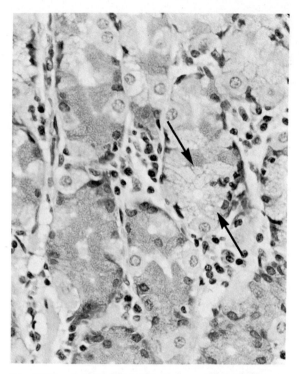

Fig. 5.3 Detail of Figure 5.2. The darker-staining granulated cells are chief cells. Parietal cells are pale-staining and show a central nucleus and apparent cytoplasmic vacuolation. Some mucous neck cells are also present (arrowed).

Haematoxylin-eosin   × 528

appearance than the body mucosa, with a uniform mosaic pattern with several papillae in each segment.[2] The mucosa is from $200-1000\,\mu m$ thick and the gastric pits are deeper and branch more than those in the body of the stomach. The glandular zone, composed of single or branched coiled tubules, surrounded at their bases by smooth muscle from the muscularis mucosae, occupies half or less of the total mucosal thickness (Fig. 5.4). The glands are less tightly packed than in body mucosa and intertubular reticulin is increased. They are lined by faintly granular mucin-secreting cells with a basal nucleus and are indistinguishable from mucous neck cells in sections stained with haematoxylin and eosin. Occasional parietal cells are present in all parts of the pyloric mucosa and may be more numerous close to the gastro-duodenal junction.[8] The most useful criteria for distinguishing body and pyloric mucosa in the normal stomach are the disappearance of chief cells

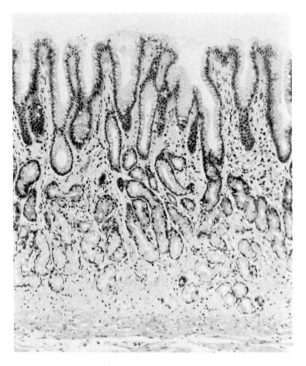

Fig. 5.4 Normal structure of the pyloric gland area of the mucosa of the stomach. The glands are simple branching tubules lined by mucin-secreting cells. The round clear cells with a central nucleus, and preferentially located in the upper half of the glands, are endocrine cells.

Haematoxylin-eosin   × 177

from the latter,[9] and the change from single tubular glands in the body to branched glands in the antrum.

The junction between the different types of gastric mucosa may be abrupt or there may be a transitional zone in which the pits occupy half the thickness of the mucosa and the glandular zone is composed of both body and pyloric or cardiac glands.

Endocrine cells, recognized in haematoxylin and eosin stained preparations as rounded clear or halo cells in the glandular layer, often wedged between the basement membrane of the glands and the epithelial cells, are widely and patchily distributed in the mucosa of all parts of the stomach.[10,11] A minority of these cells which contain serotonin (5-hydroxytryptamine), so-called enterochromaffin (EC) or argentaffin cells, may be demonstrated by their property of reducing silver salts without exposure to a reducing substance, and by a positive diazo reaction. The majority of endocrine cells are argyrophilic with the Grimelius technique on formalin-fixed tissue. Some endocrine cells fail to stain with either argentaffin or argyrophil methods. Recent work suggests that the enzyme neuron-specific enolase is present in all currently identifiable endocrine cells and in the nerves of the gastrointestinal tract.[12] Immunohistochemical staining techniques using antibodies specifically directed against biogenic amines or polypeptide hormones have identified in the body and antrum of the stomach D cells which produce somatostatin, EC_n cells which contain serotonin, D_1 cells which are VIP (vasoactive intestinal peptide) immunoreactive cells, P cells containing bombesin, and PP cells (pancreatic polypeptide). Enterochromaffin-like (ECL) cells are confined to the body of the stomach and are the most common endocrine cell at this site, occurring in the intermediate and deep portions of the fundic glands. These cells have distinctive ultrastructural granules but no cell product has been identified. The same applies to so-called X cells which are Grimelius positive and occur principally in the oxyntic mucosa. S cells containing secretin have been identified in the lower third of antro-pyloric mucosa. G cells, the source of gastrin, are present predominantly in the lower and middle thirds of the antro-pyloric mucosa, with relatively small numbers in the crypts and Brunner's glands of the proximal duodenum. They decrease in density from the pylorus to the gastric body.[13] The cells are argyrophilic with the Grimelius technique and lead haematoxyphilic, and on ultrastructural examination contain rounded secretory granules with a variably electron-dense core and with an average diameter of 150–250 nm (Figs 5.5 and 5.6).

FUNCTIONAL CONSIDERATIONS

The major functions of the stomach are motor and secretory, namely to act as a reservoir for ingested food and fluids which are acted upon by the various secretions of the mucosa, mixed, and propelled onwards at a controlled rate to the small intestine for further digestion and absorption.

Gastric juice is a mixture of secretions from the four types of gastric secretory cell, namely parietal,

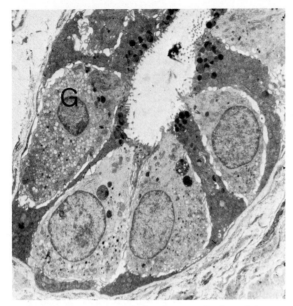

Fig. 5.5 Electron micrograph showing several pale-staining endocrine cells at the base of an antral gland. The apical surfaces of two of these cells are seen to communicate with the lumen of the gland. Dark neurosecretory granules are just visible at this magnification, mostly in the basal parts of the cells. The cell at the left (G) is a gastrin cell. Intervening cells with darker-staining cytoplasm and apical granules are mucous cells.

× 3200

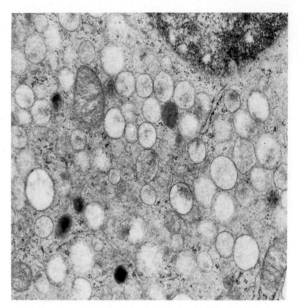

Fig. 5.6 Detail of the gastrin cell in Figure 5.5 shows numerous neurosecretory granules in the cytoplasm, most of which are electron lucent but a few of which have an electron-dense core. A few mitochondria are seen as well and part of the nucleus (top). Although morphology of neurosecretory granules is of some value in determining the type of endocrine cell, definitive identification is dependent on immunohistochemical techniques.

× 32 000

chief, mucous neck and surface epithelial cell. Mucus, produced by the latter two types of cell as well as by pyloric gland cells, forms a continuous thin layer of water-insoluble flexible gel, approximately 200 μm deep, which adheres to the surface of the gastric mucosa. Its gel-forming properties are due to glycoprotein of high molecular weight (about 2×10^6), each consisting of a polymer of four subunits joined by disulphide bonds. Complex carbohydrate side chains of the glycoproteins carry the determinants for A and H blood group substance activity.[14] The factors which stimulate mucus secretion are not known, but inhibition by ulcerogenic agents such as non-steroidal anti-inflammatory agents has been clearly demonstrated.[15,16] As well as mucus, the surface epithelial cells appear to be the main site of bicarbonate ion (HCO_3^-) secretion. The pH gradient between the surface of the mucosal cells and the lumen of the stomach resulting from the secretion of mucus and HCO_3^- is a major factor in the ability of the gastric mucosa to resist damage from high concentrations of intraluminal acid.[17]

Parietal cells secrete hydrochloric acid into the gastric lumen at a concentration up to about 160 mmol/l and against an ion gradient which is often several million to one. At the ultrastructural level this is reflected by the presence of numerous large mitochondria. The most typical and indeed unique feature of this cell is the invagination of its free apical surface to form an extensive secretory canaliculus which is lined by numerous microvilli, so that the apical surface area is enormously increased (Fig. 5.7). In the cytoplasm adjacent to the secretory canaliculus is an extensive system of tubules, vesicles or tubulo-vesicles (Fig. 5.8). Stimulation results in a marked hypertrophy of the canalicular system, whereas the tubulo-vesicles become less prominent, suggesting that eversion or fusion of their membranes with the plasma-lemma occurs with discharge of their contents into the canaliculi. Reconstitution of the tubulo-vesicles presumably results from pinocytosis of the plasmalemma.[18]

The regulation of acid secretion at the parietal cell level in man has been studied using isolated

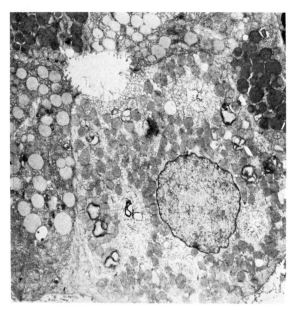

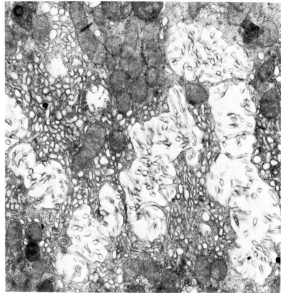

Fig. 5.7 An electron micrograph of a parietal cell showing the extensive secretory canaliculus and numerous mitochondria in the cytoplasm. The adjoining cells are chief cells (large pale granules) and mucous cells (dark granules).

× 4800

Fig. 5.8 Electron micrograph of parietal cell. Complicated and extensive system of tubules and vesicles adjacent to the secretory canaliculus. Numerous mitochondria can also be identified.

× 12 800

gastric glands from gastroscopic biopsies and determining the accumulation of ^{14}C-labelled aminopyrine as an indirect measurement of acid secretion. Histamine markedly stimulates aminopyrine accumulation, whereas gastrin is without any stimulatory action and the cholinergic drug carbachol has only a weak effect.[19] There is considerable variation between individuals in basal acid secretion, which also shows a circadian rhythm. Tonic vagal stimulation is probably the main factor in basal secretion, with spontaneous release of small amounts of gastrin making a minor contribution.

Seven pepsinogens have been identified in human gastric juice. On the basis of immunochemical characteristics they are separated into two groups. Group I pepsinogens are restricted to the chief cells and mucous neck cells, whereas group II pepsinogens are found in these cells and also in mucous cells of the pyloric and cardiac glands and in Brunner's glands.[20] Activation to the proteolytic enzyme pepsin occurs optimally at pH2 by the splitting off of peptide fragments from the N-terminal side of the polypeptide molecule. Irreversible inactivation occurs if the pH increases above 6, so that patients with achlorhydria may have no active pepsin in the presence of adequate pepsinogen secretion.

Intrinsic factor, a glycoprotein with a molecular weight of 60 000, is synthesized by the parietal cell in man.[21] Absence of this factor causes Addisonian anaemia ('pernicious anaemia') by interfering with the absorption of vitamin B_{12} from the small intestine, with the consequent failure of normal erythropoiesis. In general, substances which stimulate acid secretion stimulate the production of intrinsic factor,[22] although there is an earlier peak and a rapid fall to basal levels with the latter, suggesting release of preformed intrinsic factor.

The control of gastric secretion is the result of the integration of influences from the central and autonomic nervous system, and by paracrine and endocrine actions of hormones. The former subdivision of the digestive period of gastric secretion into cephalic, gastric and intestinal phases is an over-simplification since all phases proceed almost simultaneously and overlap in time.[23]

Muscle contraction in the stomach is regulated

by an intermittent electrical complex, termed the slow wave, which occurs at regular intervals of about 20 seconds and lasts about 4 seconds and originates near the mid greater curvature, from where it migrates around the stomach and towards the pylorus. Neural and hormonal influences facilitate or inhibit the occurrence of muscle contraction in association with the slow wave. The muscle of the upper body and fundus of the stomach does not show peristalsis, but its relaxation, principally through vagal reflexes, serves to accommodate ingested food.[24]

DEVELOPMENTAL ANOMALIES

Atresia and stenosis

Atresia of the stomach is a rare abnormality and presents as a complete pyloric obstruction with persistent vomiting from birth. In one reported case vascular connective tissue replaced the mucosa and muscularis over a 1 cm length at the pylorus.[25] In others there has been an imperforate septum, covered on each side by mucosa and often having smooth muscle in the septal wall. When perforate, a diaphragm of mucous membrane with a small central aperture is stretched across the pyloric canal. These perforate diaphragms have usually been incidental findings during surgical exploration of the stomach for peptic ulcer or suspected malignant disease,[26] but cases have been described in which the diaphragm caused symptoms of pyloric obstruction.[27,28] It is possible that some of these webs or diaphragms are acquired lesions resulting from healing of linear circumferential prepyloric and pyloric peptic ulcers.[29]

Congenital pyloric stenosis

Congenital pyloric stenosis occurs in 0.28–0.4% of all live births.[30,31] It is between four and five times more common in males than females and affects first-born children more commonly than those born subsequently. The pattern of inheritance is polygenic and there is an increased risk in siblings[32] and the offspring of affected children.[33] There is an association with other congenital gut obstructions, oesophageal atresia, anorectal anomalies, meconium ileus and duodenal atresia.[34] Environmental

factors may be important and experiments on pregnant bitches suggest that maternal excess of pentagastrin or gastrin can produce pyloric hypertrophy in the litters.[35]

The condition usually presents between the second and fourth weeks of life, but has been described in stillbirths. At operation, an elongated, smooth swelling of almost cartilaginous consistency and about two centimetres in length is found at the pylorus, and this terminates abruptly at the first part of the duodenum and markedly narrows the pyloric canal (Fig. 5.9). Microscopically, the circular muscle coat hypertrophies to between two and four times its normal thickness.[36] The primary

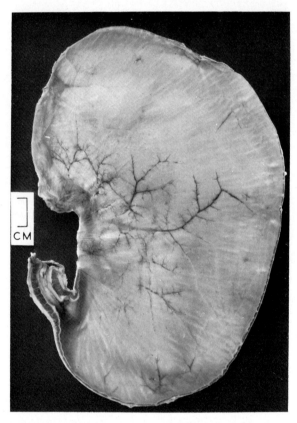

Fig. 5.9 Stomach of a child with congenital pyloric stenosis. The pyloric sphincter is greatly hypertrophied. In contrast, the rest of the stomach is enormously dilated and its wall is very thin.

Specimen from the Pathology Museum, Charing Cross Hospital Medical School, London, reproduced by permission of the Curator, Dr F. J. Paradinas. Photograph by Miss P. M. Turnbull, Charing Cross Hospital Medical School.

defect is probably in the myenteric plexus, and clumps of ganglion cells are present within the attenuated longitudinal muscle and only rarely extend into the circular coat. It has been suggested that one of the two distinct types of ganglion cell normally present is deficient in congenital stenoses.[37]

Duplications, diverticula and cysts

Developmental duplications, diverticula, and cysts which remain incorporated in, or attached to, the organ are all extremely rare in the stomach.[38-40] Many so-called duplications described in adults are probably an end-result of previous peptic ulceration with gastro-duodenal fistula and formation of a double channel.[41,42] In diverticula and cysts there is usually a well-formed mucosa of gastric type with muscularis mucosae and often submucosa; muscle coats are less constantly present and it is rare to see a well-formed circular and longitudinal coat.[43]

Detached cysts with a gastric epithelial lining and clearly of foregut origin may be found in the thoracic or abdominal cavities and are often associated with anomalies of the vertebral bodies.

Anomalies of position

Apart from the consequences of malrotation of the fetal gut, which is very rare, misplacement of the stomach is generally associated with a congenital defect in the diaphragm. The stomach may then lie partly or wholly within the thorax, and this condition may predispose to oesophagitis and to peptic ulceration in either the oesophagus or the stomach. Such anomalies are quite distinct from the columnar-lined (Barrett's) oesophagus (see p. 139), where no anatomical displacement of the true stomach occurs.

MISCELLANEOUS ACQUIRED CONDITIONS

Volvulus

Volvulus of the stomach is rare and may be acute or chronic. Often no cause is apparent. The condition is sometimes secondary to extragastric disease, such as a tumour adjoining the greater curvature, or it may occur in association with hiatus hernia. The greater curvature of the stomach rotates upward, forward and to the right on an axis corresponding to the lesser curvature. As it rotates it pulls the transverse colon and mesocolon up with it. Obstruction at the cardia and in the first part of the duodenum results, and this leads to distension of the stomach by its own secretions. Acute volvulus may result in gangrene from interference with the gastric blood supply.

Rupture

Rupture of the stomach is a rare condition mostly occurring in infants: in the majority of these cases the reason is not clear. Predisposing causes proposed include bacterial endotoxins, acute ulceration and congenital deficiencies of the gastric musculature, but the evidence for these is not convincing. Rupture of the adult stomach may result from blunt trauma, or following instrumentation, or occur spontaneously as a complication of vomiting. It is more common in women and usually occurs as a tear along the lesser curvature in the absence of any previous gastric disease.

Acute dilatation

This is an uncommon complication of abdominal operations, severe injury and acute diffuse peritonitis. It also occurs in those with respiratory difficulty, after over-eating,[44] and in association with acute pancreatitis.[45] It is caused by the presence of gas rather than fluid and the onset may be extremely rapid, leading to the regurgitation of small amounts of fluid, shock and collapse, but rarely to rupture.

Bezoars

Bezoars are foreign bodies in the stomach. They may be composed of hair (trichobezoar or hair ball), the commonest type in man, or of vegetable fibres, seeds or fruit skins (phytobezoar), or of a concretion derived from other ingested material, such as shellac, which may accumulate in the stomach of painters and French polishers. Bezoars containing both hair and vegetable matter (trichophytobezoars) have also been described. Tricho-bezoars may be found in young children, particularly girls, who are in the habit of chewing hair or blankets, but they occur most typically, and oftenest, in patients with chronic mental diseases.

Pyloric obstruction

There are a number of causes of narrowing of the pyloric outlet in adults. The most common are duodenal ulcer and prepyloric gastric ulcer, followed by carcinoma of the pylorus. In the case of peptic ulcers, oedema and submucosal fibrosis are the factors mainly responsible. Spasm of the sphincter contributes to the stenosis while the ulcer is active; later a permanent and unyielding narrowing of the pylorus results as the scar tissue in the region of the ulcer contracts.

Uncommon or rare causes are extrinsic adhesions,[46] infiltration by malignant lymphoma (see p. 216), involvement of the stomach in Crohn's disease (see p. 171) or eosinophilic gastro-enteritis (see p. 170), and the presence of a mucosal diaphragm usually at the pyloric ring. The diaphragm can be congenital (see p. 156), represent a prolapse of redundant gastric mucosa, or be the end-result of scarring of a superficial prepyloric ulcer, or of antral gastritis.

A primary form of *pyloric stenosis* occurs rarely in adults: it is associated with total or segmental hypertrophy of the circular muscle coat without obvious associated disease.[47,48] The aetiology is unknown and it has been suggested that it is a manifestation of a less severe form of the infantile disease (see p. 156) that has persisted without causing obstruction sufficient to interfere with gastrointestinal function early in life.

Diverticula

An acquired diverticulum of the stomach is very rare, with a reported prevalence of 0.02% at autopsy.[49] The usual site has been from the posterior wall of the stomach about 2 cm below the oesophago-gastric junction. Although usually symptomless there are occasional reports of bleeding from ulcers or erosions present within the diverticulum.[50]

GASTRITIS

The term 'gastritis' is often loosely used to cover any clinical condition in which there are conspicuous upper abdominal symptoms in the absence of clinical signs and radiological abnormalities. In such cases it is better to use the expression 'non-ulcerative dyspepsia' and to reserve the term gastritis for conditions in which histological changes are present.

In the past, histological studies of gastritis were made on necropsy material. These were unsatisfactory because postmortem autolysis is difficult to prevent even when formaldehyde is instilled into the stomach immediately after death, and may be difficult to distinguish from true antemortem pathological changes. The classification now generally used is based on biopsy studies[51] and the examination of gastrectomy specimens. The advent of fibreoptic endoscopy in particular, with the facility to remove samples of gastric mucosa under direct vision, has enabled a much clearer picture to be obtained of the distribution of inflammatory changes in the stomach, and by means of sequential examinations, to document their progression or regression.

Gastritis may be acute or chronic. It is primarily a disease of the mucous membrane of the stomach, although inflammatory changes in the submucosa and in the muscle coats are seen in certain types of acute gastritis.

ACUTE GASTRITIS

Aetiology

A variety of substances have been implicated in causing damage to the gastric mucosa including alcohol, aspirin, cortisone, phenylbutazone, indomethacin and a number of other non-steroidal anti-inflammatory drugs, although in man the evidence is largely circumstantial or anecdotal. Ingestion of corrosives such as caustic soda, phenol or lysol is associated with complete mucosal destruction in fatal cases. Acute mucosal damage accompanied by patchy coagulative necrosis has followed some two weeks after external radiation therapy for peptic ulcer disease.[52]

The gastric mucosa appears resistant to bacterial

infection although rarely a florid (phlegmonous) gastritis has occurred in patients with systemic illness or localized infection elsewhere, usually due to haemolytic streptococci. Symptoms of epigastric pain, nausea and vomiting, suggesting gastric involvement, are not uncommon in various viral illnesses but histological proof of gastritis is lacking. Transient acute gastritis with hypochlorhydria has been reported amongst a group of healthy volunteers participating in studies of acid secretion, but a putative organism was not identified.[53]

Clinical setting

In practice, acute gastritis is seen at endoscopy as a patchily or diffusely reddened mucosa, often with one or more erosions, in patients who have presented with haemetemesis and/or melaena. A similar clinical picture can occur following trauma, sepsis, major surgery, burns or hypothermia. Haemorrhagic or erosive gastritis is common therefore in patients in intensive therapy units and in those with malignant disease.[54] Because of this it is a frequent finding at postmortem in patients dying in hospital.

Pathogenesis

It is probable that aspirin and related drugs interfere with the gastric mucosal 'barrier' by reducing the amount of mucus produced and altering its biochemical characteristics as well as inhibiting the local production of cytoprotective prostaglandins.[55] Acid diffuses back into the mucosa with resultant histamine release and acute inflammation. In patients who are shocked and hypotensive, erosions probably develop on the basis of ischaemia due to a reduction in mucosal blood flow, again resulting in an increased permeability of the mucosa to hydrogen ions.

Pathological findings

Macroscopically, in cases coming to gastroscopy or necropsy, the mucosa is oedematous, red and is usually covered by large amounts of mucus. There may be well-defined petechial haemorrhages, larger zones of confluent mucosal or submucosal bleeding, small erosions or small, acute ulcers with sharp, well-defined edges and a greyish base. The distribution of erosions is related to the clinical circumstances. Following trauma or sepsis they are first observed in the fundus near the greater curve and with time develop distally, only involving the antrum when the lesions in the body are widespread and severe. Erosions caused by aspirin and ethanol, although most frequent in the antrum, can affect all segments of the stomach and the duodenum, and do not have a proximal to distal progression. They also tend to be smaller and to heal quicker.[56,57]

In acute phlegmonous gastritis, which usually occurs as a complication of generalized streptococcal infections, the stomach appears dark red and distended, with a fibrinopurulent exudate on the serosal surface. The submucosa is thickened and oedematous and the mucosa is haemorrhagic and often partly sloughed.

Histologically, there is oedema and haemorrhage into the interfoveolar subepithelial part of the lamina propria followed by necrosis of the surface epithelium and a variable amount of the underlying mucosa, with a surface slough consisting of degenerate epithelial cells, fibrin and some inflammatory cells (Fig. 5.10). These different stages correspond to the red and white-based erosions seen endoscopically. Withdrawal of the initiating stimulus results in glandular cell regeneration and the mucosa becomes normal in a few days.

It is unlikely that a single attack of haemorrhagic or erosive gastritis leads to chronic gastritis, but repeated insults by agents such as alcohol and aspirin may do so. Some studies have shown that an antecedent chronic gastritis is often associated with haemorrhagic gastritis.[58,59] The relationship of aspirin to chronic gastric ulcer is discussed elsewhere (see p. 166).

The main changes in phlegmonous gastritis are in the submucosa, and may be demonstrated in a snare biopsy.[60] There is thrombosis of submucosal vessels, with marked purulent inflammation and oedema and secondary mucosal sloughing.

CHRONIC GASTRITIS

Chronic non-specific gastritis is essentially a histological diagnosis and is the commonest change observed in gastric biopsies and resection speci-

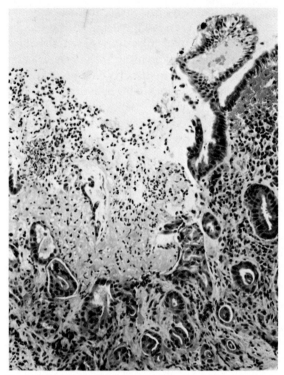

Fig. 5.10 Gastric erosion. There is disruption of the surface epithelium and necrosis of the superficial part of the mucosa which consists of degenerate epithelial cells, fibrin and some inflammatory cells.

Haematoxylin-eosin   × 165

mens. There is a poor correlation between microscopical appearances and clinical symptoms. At endoscopy, gastritis may be recognized with reasonable accuracy although its grading may not match the histological changes. As well as this, approximately 30% of biopsies from endoscopically normal mucosa show inflammation.[61] Chronic gastritis is often patchy, and multiple biopsies may be necessary to diagnose and evaluate it. In addition, individual biopsies have to be examined at different levels because of the frequently focal nature of the inflammation.

The diagnosis and classification of chronic gastritis is important because of its association with peptic ulcer and carcinoma.

Classification[51]

The classification of chronic non-specific gastritis takes into account (1) the type of mucosa, i.e.

cardiac, body, antral (pyloric), transitional or indeterminate; (2) the extent of inflammation within the mucosa, i.e. superficial or deep, the latter resulting in varying degrees of atrophy of the glandular compartment; (3) the activity of the gastritis, and (4) the presence and type of metaplasia. When this is done, three histological patterns emerge, namely chronic superficial gastritis, atrophic gastritis and gastric atrophy.

Chronic superficial gastritis. As the name implies, inflammation is confined to the superficial supraglandular layer of the mucosa (Figs. 5.11 and 5.12). There is an increase in plasma cells and lymphocytes, together with variable numbers of polymorphs, in the lamina propria between the foveolae and beneath the surface epithelium but not extending into the glandular layer. Although often focally distributed, polymorphs are invariably seen and often extend into foveolar and surface epithelium (Fig. 5.13). When inflammation is marked, the epithelium shows reactive changes, with a cuboidal appearance of the cells, associated with

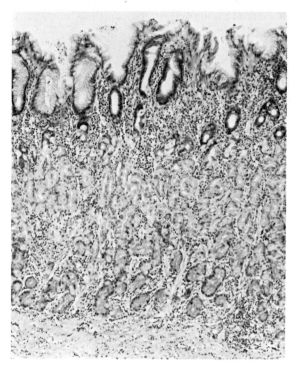

Fig. 5.11 Chronic superficial gastritis affecting body mucosa. Inflammation is confined to the supraglandular part of the mucosa and there is associated foveolar hyperplasia.

Haematoxylin-eosin   × 125

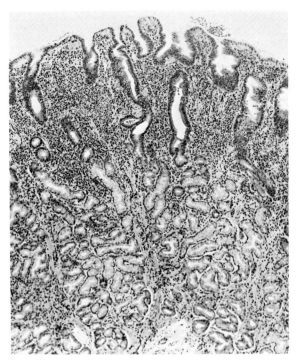

Fig. 5.12 Chronic superficial gastritis affecting the pyloric gland area of the mucosa. There is a dense inflammatory cell infiltrate in the lamina propria of the upper half of the mucosa and inflammatory cells have extended into the epithelium of the foveolae.

Haematoxylin-eosin × 108

diminished cytoplasm and mucin content, and enlargement and hyperchromatism of nuclei. Marked regeneration of the surface epithelium can give a syncytial appearance with sprouting bud-like masses of cells, some of which appear to be in the process of exfoliation (Fig. 5.14). Aggregates of polymorphs may be seen in the pit lumens forming crypt abscesses, and moderate or severe acute inflammation can be associated with adhesion of surface and foveolar epithelial cells. Oedema and vascular congestion may be conspicuous. Foveolar hyperplasia results in the formation of intrafoveolar papillae giving a corkscrew appearance and slight thickening of the mucosa overall.

Although the deep zone of the gastric mucosa in superficial gastritis is histologically normal there is a considerable fall in the secretion of acid and pepsinogen following histamine stimulation,[62] which appears to parallel the extent of mucosal involvement.[63]

Atrophic gastritis. In atrophic gastritis, inflammation involves the deeper layer of the mucosa and results in destruction of the glands. The inflammatory cell content and its nature can be very variable. Minor degrees of atrophy are difficult to assess, particularly in pyloric mucosa, and a stain for reticulin fibres to demonstrate their condensation around the glands can be helpful. In more advanced stages atrophy is readily apparent in routinely stained material as a widening and shortening of the glands. Accompanying this atrophic process two types of metaplasia can occur, pseudo-pyloric and intestinal. The former involves only body glands, whose specialized cells are replaced by mucous cells derived from proliferated mucous neck cells (Fig. 5.15). When widespread, the appearances in a biopsy from the body of the stomach may be indistinguishable from antral mucosa. However, parietal cells are not seen, whereas they are frequently present in small numbers in antral mucosa. As well as this, gastrin

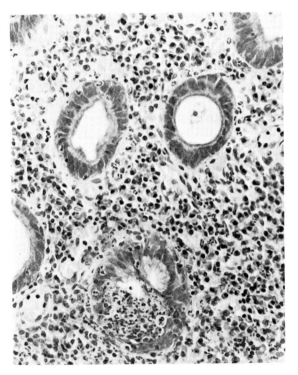

Fig. 5.13 Numerous polymorphonuclear leukocytes are present in the lamina propria and extend into the epithelium forming a small crypt abscess at one point.

Haematoxylin-eosin × 237

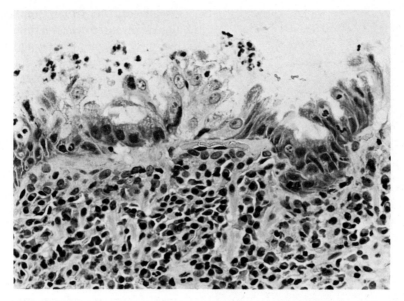

Fig. 5.14 Florid regenerative changes in actively inflamed gastric mucosa can result in a syncytial appearance of the surface epithelial cells.

Haematoxylin-eosin   × 375

cells are scanty or absent in pseudo-pyloric metaplasia and common, although patchily distributed, in antral mucosa.[64]

Intestinal metaplasia is common in atrophic gastritis and can affect any part of the gastric mucosa (Fig. 5.16), although most frequent in the antrum. It may be widespread and continuous, or in the form of scattered islands. It is a common change in the regenerative epithelium bordering peptic ulcers.[65] Its most characteristic feature is the presence of goblet cells which contain acidic mucins. These may be demonstrated with mucicarmine, or with the periodic acid-Schiff/alcian blue (PAS/AB) technique at pH 2.5 when they stain blue, in contrast to the PAS-positive neutral mucins present in surface and foveolar epithelium and mucous glands of the non-metaplastic gastric mucosa. In its fully developed or complete form (Fig. 5.17), intestinal metaplasia consists of cells which are normally present in the small intestine. Goblet cells are separated by non-mucin-secreting columnar cells which have a distinct striated border of microvilli. Goblet cells tend to be fewer in the deeper part of the mucosa. At the base of the metaplastic glands Paneth cells are present together with endocrine cells, many of which are argentaffin.

This complete form shares with small intestinal mucosa the same histochemical and ultrastructural characteristics,[66,67] although a villous architecture is only occasionally present. As well as this complete form (or type I), incomplete types of intestinal metaplasia also occur, although they are less common.[68,69] In one of these (type IIa), a mixture of gastric and small intestinal epithelium is seen, with goblet cells interspersed with columnar cells which secrete predominantly neutral mucins (Fig. 5.18). In another type (type IIb), intervening columnar cells are distended with mucus and thereby often difficult to distinguish from goblet cells. However, staining with the high iron diamine/alcian blue (HID/AB) technique at pH 2.5 shows them to contain abundant sulphomucins, in contrast to the non-sulphated sialomucins usually present in the goblet cells. In this respect they demonstrate characteristics of colonic rather than small intestinal epithelium although, unlike the former, no secretion of O-acylated sialic acid occurs.[69] Endocrine cells resemble those normally found in the small intestine.[70] In both types of incomplete metaplasia Paneth cells are uncommon. Individual cells tend to be taller in incomplete metaplasia, and in the 'colonic' variant, elongation,

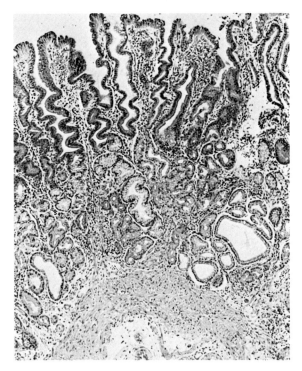

Fig. 5.15 In this biopsy, taken from the gastric body mucosa of a patient who had a partial gastrectomy for duodenal ulcer some 15 years earlier, there is extensive pseudo-pyloric metaplasia. Some of the mucous-lined glands are dilated and there is hyperplasia of the foveolae, some of which have a corkscrew appearance.

Haematoxylin-eosin   × 80

foveolar area can be marked. Mitotic counts reflect a high cell turnover in atrophic gastritis.[72]

A conspicuous feature in some patients with superficial and atrophic gastritis is the presence of aggregates and follicles of lymphoid tissue in the lamina propria, usually just above the muscularis mucosae, although they may occur in the submucosa as well (Fig. 5.19). This so-called *follicular gastritis* is not a distinct entity but represents a variant of chronic gastritis.

Gastric atrophy. In gastric atrophy the mucosa is markedly thinned with complete or near complete loss of glands and an absence of inflammation (Fig. 5.20), although lymphoid aggregates can be present. Tubules are lined by simple epithelium resembling that of normal superficial gastric epithelium, interspersed with goblet cells of intestinal type. Extensive cystic change in tubules, with bulging of cysts through the muscularis mucosae, is common.

tortuosity and branching of the metaplastic glands are prominent. There is indirect evidence that the type of intestinal metaplasia associated with sulphomucin secretion may be premalignant (see p. 167).

Morphological and autoradiographic studies indicate that intestinal metaplasia starts on the framework of an intact mucosa in the neck region of the gastric glands.[71] Thus in antral mucosa it is not infrequent to see partially intestinalized glandular tubules lined in their upper parts by intestinal cells and lower down by mucous gland cells. The latter are replaced by intestinal epithelium with a shift of the generative zone from the neck region to the base of one of the branched pyloric glands, and disappearance of the other glands.

The mucosa in atrophic gastritis is in general thinner than normal although hyperplasia of the

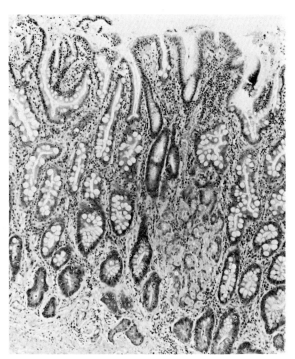

Fig. 5.16 Gastric body mucosa in which there is extensive intestinal metaplasia. A small residual focus of body glands is seen centrally.

Haematoxylin-eosin   × 150

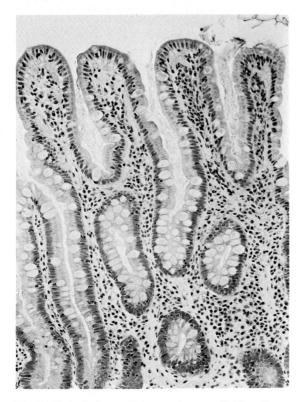

Fig. 5.17 Intestinal metaplasia, complete type. Goblet cells are interspersed amongst absorptive cells. In this example a villous architecture is also present.

Haematoxylin-eosin   × 180

Macroscopic appearances of gastritis

In resection specimens it is not usually possible to distinguish superficial chronic gastritis from normal mucosa macroscopically. In atrophic gastritis the mucosa may show some degree of flattening, with loss of rugose pattern, but frequently appears normal. It is easier to detect this abnormality when it is localized around an ulcer or carcinoma than when it is more generalized. In gastric atrophy, mucosal thinning and loss of rugae are usually, but by no means always, visible. In pernicious anaemia there is readily apparent associated thinning of muscle coats of the body, but this usually spares the antrum (see p. 167). Intestinal metaplasia cannot be recognized in unstained macroscopic specimens but may be detected by techniques for alkaline phosphatase or mucins applied to gross specimens.[73,74]

Topography of gastritis

Superficial gastritis and atrophic gastritis are more common in antral mucosa and along the *Magenstrasse* than in the body of the stomach. In patients with duodenal ulcer the gastritis has an almost exclusively antral distribution, but in gastric ulcer and cancer it tends to be much more widespread, although the antrum is nearly always involved. Atrophic gastritis, with or without gastric atrophy, affecting body mucosa with sparing of the antrum is the characteristic gastric lesion in patients with pernicious anaemia (but see p. 168).

Aetiological and predisposing factors

The lesions of chronic gastritis are likely to represent a common end-result of many different insults to the gastric mucosa. The frequency of the

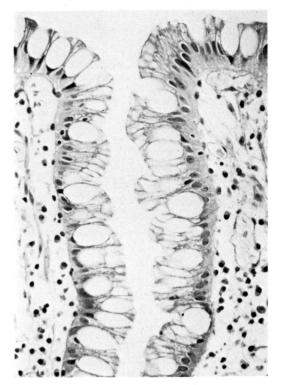

Fig. 5.18 Intestinal metaplasia, incomplete type. As well as goblet cells, tall columnar cells with apical mucin are present. Staining using the combined periodic acid-Schiff/alcian blue technique showed the latter cells to contain predominantly neutral mucin.

Haematoxylin-eosin   × 260

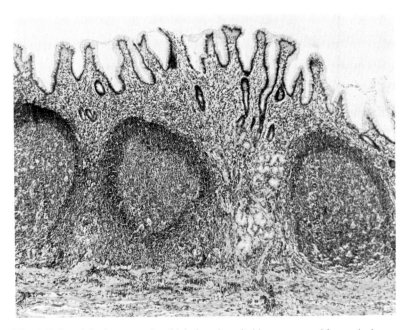

Fig. 5.19 Gastric body mucosa in which three lymphoid aggregates with germinal centres are seen. The group of glands between the lymphoid follicles are lined by mucous cells, i.e. pseudo-pyloric metaplasia is present.

Haematoxylin-eosin   × 77

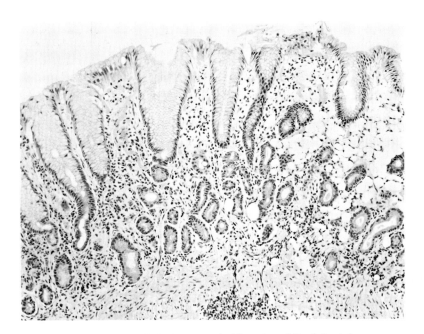

Fig. 5.20 Gastric atrophy. The body mucosa is thin and specialized glandular epithelium has been replaced by mucous cells. There is an absence of inflammation. Fat cells are seen to the right. Biopsy from patient with pernicious anaemia.

Haematoxylin-eosin   × 114

changes was shown in a recent biopsy study of asymptomatic volunteers with an average age of 33 years, where atrophic gastritis affecting antral and body mucosa was present in 34% and involved the antrum alone in a further 6%.[75] Epidemiological studies have shown variations in the prevalence of chronic gastritis. For example, it was detected in 78% of Japanese over the age of 50 compared to 30% of Americans.[76] Follow-up studies within populations have shown an increasing prevalence of gastritis with ageing which tends to progress from a superficial to an atrophic type,[77,78] although this may be a very gradual process taking many years.[79]

On the basis of differing clinical and pathological manifestations it has been proposed that there are two aetiologically distinct types of gastritis.[80]

In *type A gastritis* the body mucosa is predominantly affected with antral sparing. There is a high prevalence of antibodies to parietal cells,[81] somewhat lower to intrinsic factor antibodies,[82] and serum gastrin levels are usually elevated. Pepsinogen I levels in the serum are decreased, whereas those of pepsinogen II remain relatively normal. This is because the site of production of the former is the body glands alone, whereas pepsinogen II is derived from both fundic and pyloric glands.[83] In a proportion of individuals with these features, overt pernicious anaemia develops. Others have achlorhydria, low intrinsic factor secretion and may have low levels of vitamin B_{12} in the serum (latent pernicious anaemia) but do not have the clinical features of pernicious anaemia. Clinical and serological evidence of associated autoimmune diseases such as Hashimoto's thyroiditis and adrenal Addison's disease is not uncommon in patients with pernicious anaemia. Thus in one study, 47% of 100 pernicious anaemia patients had antibodies to the microsomal fraction of thyroid follicle cells and 29% had a positive tanned red cell test.[84] The finding of a considerably increased prevalence of severe atrophic gastritis affecting body mucosa, achlorhydria, parietal cell antibodies and raised fasting serum gastrin levels in first degree relatives of patients with pernicious anaemia[85] supports the view that genetic factors are implicated in type A gastritis.

Type B gastritis is much commoner than type A and inflammation predominantly affects antral mucosa, with or without body involvement. Parietal cell antibodies are usually absent, serum gastrin levels are low, and acid secretion is moderately to severely impaired. This type of gastritis spreads proximally with increasing age, extending more rapidly on the lesser than on the greater curvature.[86] Pseudo-pyloric metaplasia of body type mucosa may give the false impression of expansion of the pyloric gland area.[87] Dye-spraying techniques at endoscopy using Congo red to determine the extent of the acid-secreting area, and methylene blue to delineate areas of intestinal metaplasia, have shown that gastritis may occasionally extend distally from the cardiac region of the stomach, again preferentially involving the lesser curve.[88] The poor correlation of histological gastritis with symptoms, and the large number of ingested and endogenous agents which theoretically may damage the gastric mucosa have meant that no clear picture of the aetiological factors in this condition has emerged. Substances such as alcohol and salicylates, which are known to cause acute damage, might be expected to result in chronic gastritis when chronically administered but the evidence is conflicting. In one series, alcoholics over the age of 45 had a three times higher prevalence of chronic gastritis affecting the antrum when compared with non-alcoholics,[89] whereas another study of patients with alcoholic and other types of cirrhosis showed a similar prevalence of chronic gastritis as age-matched controls.[90] There is a strong positive correlation between excessive aspirin ingestion and chronic gastric ulcer,[91,92] but pathological examination in many of these cases has shown an absence of chronic gastritis in the surrounding gastric mucosa. The ulcers are also unusual in that they are frequently multiple and tend to be located along the greater curvature.[93,94]

Reflux of duodenal contents into the stomach has been implicated in the pathogenesis of chronic gastritis and gastric ulceration.[95,96] It is thought that the combination of bile acids, such as deoxycholic and chenodeoxycholic acid, and pancreatic juice cause stripping of the surface mucus and depletion of mucus from the epithelial cells, and allow hydrogen ions to diffuse back across the mucosa, initiating an inflammatory reaction subsequent to histamine release. The factors thought to predispose to reflux are poorly defined but probably include cigarette smoking.[97]

Alternative classification

A recent aetiopathogenetic classification of chronic gastritis[98] describes three main types: autoimmune, (which corresponds to type A gastritis described above), hypersecretory, and environmental chronic gastritis. Whilst recognizing that numerous aetiological factors may be involved in each type and that more than one type can be present in an individual, this classification helps to explain the relationship between chronic gastritis, peptic ulceration and gastric cancer.

In *hypersecretory gastritis* there is an excessive secretion of hydrochloric acid and pepsin. It is postulated that mucus production by the epithelial cells is inadequate in these circumstances to protect the mucosa and ulceration may result. Ulcers are usually duodenal or prepyloric, and chronic gastritis is limited to the antrum. In ulcers occurring higher up in the region of the angulus or midcorpus the gastritis is located in the immediate vicinity of the ulcer. This type is not accompanied by extensive intestinal metaplasia or dysplasia and has no malignant potential.

Environmental chronic gastritis shows marked variation in prevalence in different parts of the world and its geographical distribution coincides with areas of high gastric cancer risk. It is likely that dietary factors are important in this type and cause repeated injuries to the gastric mucosa over a long period.[99] Characteristically, the gastritis begins as multiple small foci at the junction between body and antral mucosa and spreads as new lesions appear on the lesser curvature above and below this junction. Confluence of neighbouring foci occurs so that large areas of the antrum, body and eventually fundus may be affected. This type of gastritis is usually accompanied by intestinal metaplasia. Peptic ulceration can occur, usually on the lesser curve and higher up in the stomach around the incisura than in hypersecretory gastritis. The higher up the lesser curve the ulcer is found, the more extensive the gastritis, with replacement of body glands by pyloric or intestinal metaplastic epithelium.[100] High-lying gastric ulcers

heal more readily but are more prone to recurrence than more distal ulcers with less extensive gastritis.[101] This, together with the fact that gastritis persists or worsens after ulcer healing,[102,103] implies that ulcers arise on the basis of a preceding gastritis rather than that the inflammation is a secondary event.

Chronic gastritis and gastric cancer

The relationship of chronic gastritis, and in particular intestinal metaplasia, to gastric cancer has been intensively studied. The prevalence of chronic atrophic gastritis is closely correlated with the death rate for gastric cancer in a population[76] and in follow-up studies it has preceded the development of gastric malignancy.[104,105] Intestinal metaplasia is commoner and more widespread in stomachs in which a cancer is present than in those with a benign lesion such as a peptic ulcer, and there is histological evidence that many gastric cancers, particularly those of intestinal type (see p. 203), arise from areas of intestinal metaplasia (Fig. 5.21).[106-108] Migrants moving from high-incidence areas for gastric cancer have shown a reduction in the prevalence of intestinal metaplasia.[109]

Because of the heterogeneous nature of intestinal metaplasia, recent interest has focused on the significance and inter-relationships of the different variants. Examination of resection specimens has shown a strong association between intestinal types of carcinoma and the presence in the adjacent mucosa of incomplete types of metaplasia with prominent sulphomucin secretion.[69,110,111] In an endoscopic biopsy study the prevalence and proportion of sulphomucin-positive intestinal metaplasia was higher in gastric cancer patients than in other groups,[112] suggesting that it may be a more specific marker of premalignancy.

THE STOMACH IN PERNICIOUS ANAEMIA

Characteristically, on gross examination, there is marked thinning of the upper two-thirds of the wall of the stomach, with atrophy involving the

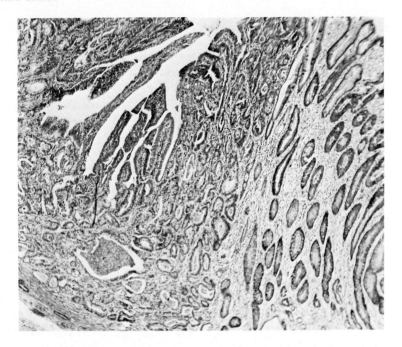

Fig. 5.21 Well-differentiated adenocarcinoma (intestinal type) arising from gastric mucosa that has undergone intestinal metaplasia (right of picture).

Haematoxylin-eosin   × 50

muscle layers as well as the mucosa. There is an abrupt transition to normal structure at the junction of the body with the pyloric antrum.

The main lesion histologically is an atrophic gastritis or gastric atrophy involving body mucosa.[113] When gastritis is present, there is a variable infiltrate of lymphocytes, plasma cells and eosinophils, but neutrophils are often absent or few in number. Immunohistochemical investigation has shown an increase in both T and particularly B lymphocytes,[114] and a reduction in the IgA/IgG ratio of immunoglobulin-containing cells.[115] There is metaplasia of body mucosa to small intestinal or more commonly pyloric type (Fig. 5.22), although some residual, irregularly distributed parietal cells may be present. Retention type cysts lined by simple mucin-secreting columnar epithelium are common in the mucosa, and are sometimes present in the submucosa also. The mucosa is usually markedly thinned but focal hyperplastic areas of intestinal metaplasia may be present and give the fundic mucosa a mamillated appearance. Antral mucosa can be normal or show varying degrees of gastritis, although usually this is less marked than

in the body. Antral gastritis is common in the general population and when present in patients with pernicious anaemia presumably represents the coincidence of type A and type B gastritis in the same individual (see p. 166).

Quantitation of gastrin cells has shown increased numbers and a raised serum gastrin in those with a normal antral mucosa, but a marked reduction in both cell numbers and gastrin levels in the presence of antral atrophic gastritis.[116]

In pernicious anaemia, and other conditions with a raised serum gastrin, hyperplasia of endocrine cells in the gastric body mucosa occurs, and this occasionally results in the development of single or multiple polypoid endocrine tumours. The endocrine cells have been characterized as enterochromaffin-like (ECL) cells.[117,118] Other types of polyp have been observed at endoscopy in from 20–37% of patients with pernicious anaemia.[119,120] These have been mostly sessile, below 2 cm in diameter and frequently multiple. Histologically, the majority have been hyperplastic in type, but some have shown dysplasia. In a recent biopsy study, dysplasia of moderate or severe degree was present in either the antrum or body in 11% of pernicious anaemia patients, and these changes were mostly observed in samples taken from endoscopically visible lesions.[120]

The risk of cancer in patients with pernicious anaemia is considered later (see p. 198).

OTHER INFLAMMATORY LESIONS OF THE STOMACH

A number of inflammatory processes may affect the stomach apart from chronic non-specific gastritis. They include varioliform gastritis, eosinophilic gastritis, and granulomatous gastritis. Because its acid secretion is protective, bacterial and fungal infections of the stomach are uncommon.

Varioliform (verrucous) gastritis

This condition gives rise to a characteristic endoscopic and radiological appearance. Multiple, small raised nodules with a central necrotic area are longitudinally arranged along folds of the greater curvature, and on the anterior and posterior walls of the antrum. Sometimes they have occurred in the fundus and cardiac regions. Occasionally the lesions are large and single and can resemble an early gastric cancer at endoscopy. Individual lesions have been termed complete erosions or aphthous ulcers.[121] Histologically, there is a central erosion with a necrotic base containing inflammatory debris associated with marked regenerative changes in the underlying and adjacent mucosa which contain sheets of closely-packed, variably distorted glands with swollen lining cells and hyperchromatic nuclei. These are set in an amorphous eosinophilic background matrix. These appearances, when florid, may be misinterpreted as malignant,[122] but mitoses are not prominent and there is a gradual transition to more obviously benign regenerating mucosa at the margin of the erosion, where there is foveolar hyperplasia and an infiltrate of plasma cells and lymphocytes.

The pathogenesis of this disorder is unclear. An allergic basis has been suggested because of the typical relapsing clinical course and high preva-

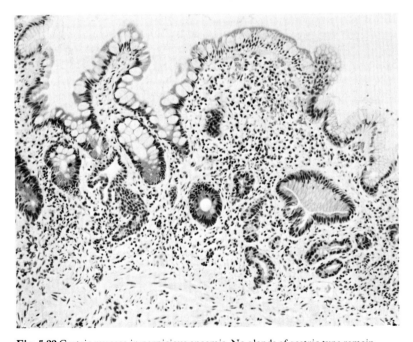

Fig. 5.22 Gastric mucosa in pernicious anaemia. No glands of gastric type remain. Simple mucous glands are present to the right and intestinal metaplastic epithelium to the left. There is low-grade inflammation.

Haematoxylin-eosin   × 150

lence of eosinophilia in the blood, and in one study increased numbers of IgE-containing plasma cells were demonstrated in the gastric mucosa adjacent to the erosions.[123] The lesions may persist for long periods, although healing has been reported following prednisolone therapy.[124]

Eosinophilic gastritis

The stomach is the commonest site of involvement in eosinophilic gastro-enteritis (also known as allergic gastro-enteropathy). This uncommon condition results in a diffuse thickening of one or more segments of the gastrointestinal tract and predominantly affects young adults, approximately 25% of whom have a history of asthma or allergy.[125] A peripheral blood eosinophilia is usually present at some stage in the disease and IgE levels may be elevated.[126] The antrum and pylorus are the usual areas affected in gastric disease and give rise to an appearance at endoscopy of thickening and deformity of this part of the stomach associated with diminished peristalsis, features indistinguishable from infiltrating carcinoma.[127] The mucosa may be reddened and swollen and contain erosions.

Pathological examination of resected specimens has shown a variable degree of oedema and infiltration by eosinophils, generally most marked in the submucosa but also affecting the muscle coats and subserosa. In mucosal biopsies there is an intense infiltration of the lamina propria by eosinophils which can extend into surface and glandular epithelium and give rise to focal necrosis and regenerative changes with nuclear enlargement, prominent nucleoli, decreased mucin content and increased numbers of mitoses of the epithelial cells. Gastric biopsy is of considerable value in diagnosis[128] since the changes are diffuse, although marked eosinophilic infiltrates may also occur in such conditions as Crohn's disease, tropical sprue, chronic granulomatous disease of childhood, and as a prominent component of the inflammation accompanying peptic ulcers and carcinoma. Occasional cases of localized disease, mostly of the small intestine, have been associated at the site of the lesion with the larvae of the ascarid parasite of fish, *Anisakis*.[129,130]

Granulomatous gastritis

Granulomatous lesions of the stomach are uncommon but may occur in sarcoidosis, in various infectious diseases including tuberculosis, syphilis and fungal diseases such as histoplasmosis, as a reaction to endogenous substances and to foreign material including indigestible food and sutures, and in Crohn's disease. Not uncommonly, however, no obvious predisposing factor is identified: so-called isolated granulomatous gastritis.

Sarcoidosis

Symptomatic involvement of the intestinal tract in sarcoidosis is rare although granulomas may be identified in up to 10% of gastric biopsies in patients with other evidence of sarcoid but without gastrointestinal symptoms.[131] When symptoms have been present, endoscopy has demonstrated features varying from a distal gastritis, with or without nodularity and mostly affecting the greater curve, to ulceration and narrowing of the antrum.[132,133]

Tuberculosis

Gastric tuberculosis is rare, even in parts of the world where intestinal tuberculosis is prevalent.[134] It is usually but not always associated with pulmonary tuberculosis.[135] The disease occurs in two forms, presenting either as an inflammatory mass, usually at the pylorus or on the lesser curvature, or as a large ulcer. Adhesions between the stomach and adjoining structures are generally a conspicuous feature, and there is enlargement and sometimes caseation of the regional lymph nodes, which are practically always involved.[136] Granulomas are necrotizing and often confluent but early forms may be indistinguishable from those in Crohn's disease or sarcoid. Stains for acid-fast bacilli are frequently negative and diagnosis may depend on culture or the presence of confirmed tuberculosis elsewhere.

Syphilis

Gastric involvement has always been a rare manifestation of syphilis. Rigid prominent gastric folds and multiple serpiginous erosions have been described in the secondary stage of the infection.[137] Granulomas may be present but the most common finding is a dense infiltrate of plasma cells accompanied by numerous neutrophils. The treponemes may be demonstrated using immunofluorescence or, less frequently, in a Warthin-Starry preparation. In the tertiary stage there may be ulceration, or diffuse fibrosis of the wall of the stomach, or a gummatous mass in the pyloric region. Involvement of the stomach in cases of congenital syphilis in childhood has been reported.[138]

Histoplasmosis

Disseminated infection by *Histoplasma capsulatum* affecting the stomach can result in the development of giant gastric folds, and biopsies show histoplasma-laden macrophages in the mucosa and submucosa.[139] Histoplasmosis is not a mycosis of worldwide occurrence. In those parts where it is not a naturally prevalent disease its presence in patients who have acquired the infection while travelling or living in endemic areas is often overlooked.

Foreign-body granulomas

These can result from a reaction to exogenous substances such as suture material which penetrates the mucosa,[140] and undigested food particles, particularly the insoluble coating of cereals which gain access to the stomach wall usually as a result of peptic ulceration. In these cases, palisaded histiocytes and foreign body giant cells surround recognizable foreign material (Fig. 5.23). In some circumstances, however, a similar reaction occurs around unidentifiable amorphous granular material which may be eosinophilic or basophilic and can be calcified and resemble in shape an ovum or worm. This probably represents a degenerative change of exposed smooth muscle or fibrous tissue in peptic ulcers produced by the digestive action of gastric juice (Fig. 5.24).[141] A foreign-body reaction may also result from cholesterol emboli, or from mucin in actively inflamed mucosa following glandular disruption.

Crohn's disease

Symptomatic involvement of the stomach often accompanied by contiguous duodenal disease has

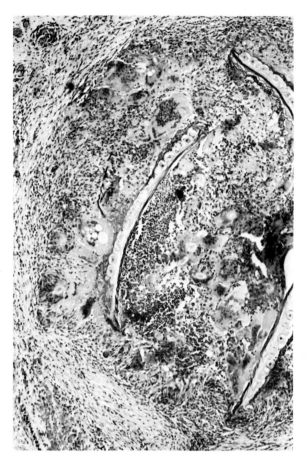

Fig. 5.23 Granuloma from vicinity of stomach, the result of perforation of a peptic ulcer. Fragments of vegetable matter (cereal) lie in a small chronic abscess, with macrophages and many foreign body giant cells about them.
Haematoxylin-eosin   × 40

been encountered in 1–2% of patients with Crohn's disease.[142,143] In the vast majority of cases, small or large intestinal disease has also been present at the time of diagnosis of upper gastrointestinal disease. The changes have predominated in the distal part of the stomach. Here the wall is thickened, with the mucosa consisting of enlarged rigid folds which may be nodular, the nodules often showing serpiginous erosion of their surface, or a typical cobblestone pattern may be seen with fissuring ulceration surrounding nodules. With severe disease, marked narrowing of the antrum and prepyloric region may result in organic pyloric stenosis. Microscopically, the mucosa is ulcerated, the characteristic deep fissures into muscle coats

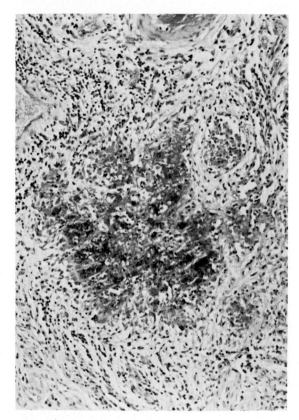

Fig. 5.24 Granulomatous reaction around amorphous eosinophilic material in the submucosa of the stomach. This is thought to be a degenerative change resulting from the action of gastric juice on exposed smooth muscle or fibrous tissue in peptic ulcers.

Haematoxylin-eosin   × 105

are usually present, the submucosal and serosal coats contain lymphoid aggregates and often non-caseating tuberculoid granulomas, and similar lesions may be present in lymph nodes along the lesser curve.

Isolated granulomatous gastritis

Isolated or idiopathic granulomatous gastritis refers to cases where non-caseating epithelioid cell granulomas have been present in the absence of recognized predisposing causes (Fig. 5.25).[144] In a majority of reported cases there has been thickening and narrowing of the antrum and prepyloric region and patients have presented with obstructive symptoms. In some there has been an associated

gastric ulcer or less commonly duodenal ulcer,[145] but examination of resection specimens has shown that the granulomas are not intimately related to these. Perigastric lymph nodes have also contained granulomas. It is probable that some cases are an atypical presentation of Crohn's disease, with small or large intestinal involvement developing subsequently.

Bacterial infections

Acute phlegmonous gastritis has been described on page 159. Anthrax may rarely involve the stomach.[146] It gives rise to a haemorrhagic gastritis, and regional lymph nodes may be enlarged and haemorrhagic also. The main histological features are oedema, mucosal ulceration and dilatation of lymphatics, and the bacilli are readily apparent in Gram-stained sections.

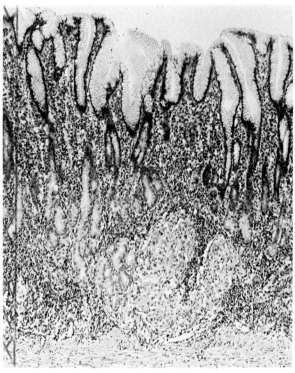

Fig. 5.25 Isolated granulomatous gastritis. Several non-caseating epithelioid cell granulomas which have coalesced are present in the lower part of the mucosa. This was an incidental finding in sections from blocks of an antrectomy specimen.

Haematoxylin-eosin   × 114

Mycoses

Primary gastric actinomycosis is very rare.[147] Endoscopy and radiological studies suggest a malignant tumour or ulcer, and the diagnosis is based on microscopic examination of the resected lesion, except when abdominal wall fistulae are present from which pus is available for culture.

Mycotic infection of the stomach is mostly due to *Candida albicans*, other strains of Candida, and *Torulopsis glabrata*.[148] Rarely, other fungi are responsible, particularly the zygomycetes (phycomycetes) (see below) and *Histoplasma capsulatum* (see p. 171).

Gastric candidosis usually occurs as an opportunistic infection in debilitated individuals, and is particularly associated with malignant neoplasms and the use of agents such as steroids, cytotoxic drugs and antibiotics. Occasional cases have been reported in uncompromised subjects.[149] Endoscopic appearances are of a white, yellow or greenish membrane of variable location and extension which can be easily removed to reveal an inflamed underlying mucosa, or there may be nodules a few millimetres in diameter which are mainly confined to the antrum. The former type is often associated with oropharyngeal or oesophageal involvement. As well as this, *Candida* infection of chronic peptic ulcers and ulcerated gastric cancers is common, and was demonstrated in one third of surgically resected peptic ulcer specimens in a recent study. The presence of numerous fungi in clusters, sometimes with invasion of deep layers of the exudate, was associated with a poor-risk group with a high postoperative mortality.[150]

Mucormycosis (phycomycosis, zygomycosis)[151] is notable because it takes the form of an acute necrotizing gastritis and because malnutrition appears to predispose to its development. The fungi responsible for mucormycotic gastritis (mainly species of *Rhizopus* or *Mucor*) have the affinity for the blood vessels that is characteristic of the 'opportunistic' zygomycetes. Extensive necrosis of the mucosa and other layers of the wall of the stomach develops and may result in perforation (Fig. 5.26).

Occasionally a massive growth of fungi (mycobezoar) can occur in the stomach and be misinterpreted as necrotic tumour at endoscopy.[152] Most

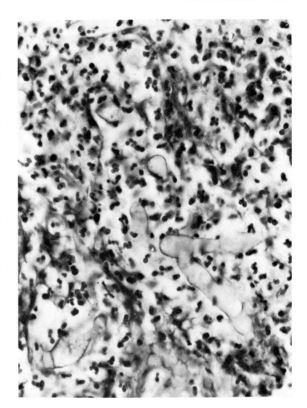

Fig. 5.26 Rhizopus species in submucosa of stomach in a case of acute perforating phycomycotic gastritis. The patient was a severely malnourished old-age pensioner in London. The characteristically broad and thin-walled hyphae are conspicuous in this field. The hyphae are not septate; the septum-like lines across some of them are folds produced by artefact during histological processing.

Haematoxylin-eosin   × 370

Provided by W. StC. Symmers.

examples have been in individuals who have had a gastric resection.

PEPTIC ULCER

The stomach and duodenum are the sites of the great majority of peptic ulcers. These lesions can occur also in any other part of the alimentary tract that is exposed to the action of pepsin and hydrochloric acid. Thus, a peptic ulcer may be found in the lower end of the oesophagus, in the jejunum at the site of a gastro-enterostomy (stomal ulcer), and in a Meckel's diverticulum containing acid-producing gastric mucosa (or in the ileum in the immediate vicinity of such a diverticulum).

They are also seen in the second, third or fourth parts of the duodenum or upper jejunum in the Zollinger-Ellison syndrome (see p. 184).

Peptic ulcers are usually classified as acute or chronic, based on the depth of penetration or degree of healing rather than duration, and it is generally assumed that all chronic ulcers originated in an acute ulcer, which failed to heal. Thus it is felt that chronic peptic ulcers must have two distinct sets of factors in their production, one group which initiates acute ulceration, and a second which prevents healing, though these are not readily separable.

In contrast to ulcers, where there is loss of the full thickness of the mucosa with a variable degree of penetration into underlying coats, erosions are shallow lesions which involve less than the full thickness of the mucosa so that some basal gland elements remain.

Gastric erosions

These commonly arise on the basis of severe physiological stress such as burns, trauma, uraemia, respiratory insufficiency and sepsis, and in these circumstances are usually multiple and affect the body and fundus of the stomach, at least initially (see p. 159). Intervening mucosa is commonly congested and can show petechial haemorrhages. Alternative names used in the literature are haemorrhagic gastritis, acute gastric mucosal lesions and acute stress ulcers. Erosions also arise following the ingestion of certain drugs (particularly non-steroidal anti-inflammatory agents) and alcohol. A third setting of acute gastric (or duodenal) erosions is in association with intracranial disease (Cushing's ulcers). Here they frequently progress to ulcers which may be full thickness and result in perforation,[153] a complication rarely encountered in the lesions resulting from stress or after drug ingestion. As well as this, hypersecretion of acid and pepsin is common in patients with intracranial disease,[154] but unusual in the other two groups.

Most erosions show complete mucosal regeneration as judged by endoscopy and there is no visible subsequent scarring. In some, full thickness mucosal erosion occurs and they become, by definition, acute ulcers.

Acute gastric and duodenal ulcers

These are larger than erosions, with congested slightly raised margins and greyish-yellow base (Fig. 5.27). Depth of penetration varies. Accompanying haemorrhage, which may be severe, is common, due to ulceration of submucosal vessel walls or congestion of the lamina propria.

Microscopically, there is an acute inflammatory reaction with fluid exudation in the involved underlying tissues; there may be an initial reparative fibroblastic response, but any appreciable degree of fibrosis puts the lesion into the chronic category.

Although erosions and acute ulcers commonly occur in the body of the stomach this is an uncommon site for chronic peptic ulcers. However, dye-spraying techniques at endoscopy using Congo

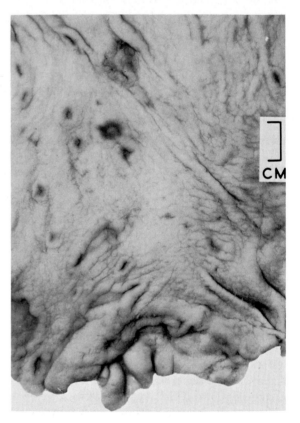

Fig. 5.27 Multiple acute peptic ulcers in the pyloric antrum. The size of the lesions varies considerably.

Specimen from the Gordon Museum, Guy's Hospital, London, reproduced by permission of the Curator, Mr J. D. Maynard. Photograph by Miss P. M. Turnbull, Charing Cross Hospital Medical School, London.

red, which allows macroscopic distinction between acid- and non-acid-secreting zones (Congo red turns blue on contact with acid), has shown that small scars, presumably the result of healing acute or early chronic ulcers, can be found in body mucosa, especially in patients below the age of 40.[155] This suggests that body type ulcers heal more readily than those in antral mucosa, and therefore do not become chronic.

Acute duodenal ulcers occur on the anterior or posterior walls of the first part of the duodenum. Haemorrhage and perforation are again recognized complications.

Chronic peptic ulcers

An ulcer may be regarded as chronic clinically when it has failed to heal over a reasonable period of time, and pathologically when attempts at repair have led to the formation of collagenous fibrohyaline tissue in the base of the ulcer, so that restoration to normal of the submucosa and muscularis propria is no longer possible; there is often concomitant failure of the mucosa to regenerate satisfactorily.

Chronic gastric ulcer

The majority of chronic gastric ulcers occur on the lesser curve, with a minority on the anterior and posterior walls, and approximately 5% on the greater curve. As mentioned above, they are very uncommon in body mucosa and careful histological examination shows that many have arisen at the junction of antral with body mucosa and are partially surrounded by mucosa of each type,[156] while others arise entirely in antral mucosa. The fact that they are commonly found higher up on the lesser curve in women than in men may reflect the greater extent of antral type mucosa in females, or the increase of antral over body mucosa which occurs with advancing age as a result of pseudopyloric metaplasia.[86]

Chronic gastric ulcers are usually single, although in about 5% of cases two or even more are present. Sometimes, when more than one ulcer is present, the individual lesions show different degrees of activity, and in some cases the scar of a healed ulcer is seen in the vicinity of an active chronic ulcer (Fig. 5.28). The majority of gastric peptic ulcers are less than 3 cm in diameter, often

smaller than 1 cm, and are round or oval. Lesser curve ulcers tend to enlarge in a saddle-shaped manner and on occasion may reach 10 cm or more in diameter.[157] The margin between a peptic ulcer and the adjacent mucosa is often quite sharp, and may be undermined to a slight extent producing a flask-like appearance on section. The floor of the ulcer is hard and covered with a white slough, and either blood clot or an eroded vessel can occasionally be seen within the crater (Fig. 5.29).

The induration in the base of a chronic ulcer involves all layers of the stomach wall and often extends into the adipose tissue in the root of the omentum and into the peritoneal covering, so that fibrous adhesions form between the outer aspect of the ulcerated part and neighbouring organs, particularly pancreas. The juxtagastric lymph nodes, and in particular those along the lesser curvature, are often enlarged and indurated as a result of chronic inflammatory changes: at operation this can add greatly to the difficulty in distinguishing

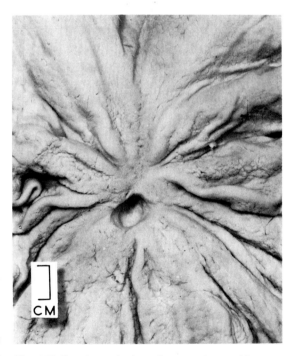

Fig. 5.28 Chronic peptic ulcer adjacent to the atrophic centre of a stellate scar typical of a healed peptic ulcer on the lesser curvature of the stomach.

Specimen from the Gordon Museum, Guy's Hospital, London, reproduced by permission of the Curator, Mr J. D. Maynard. Photograph by Miss P. M. Turnbull, Charing Cross Hospital Medical School, London.

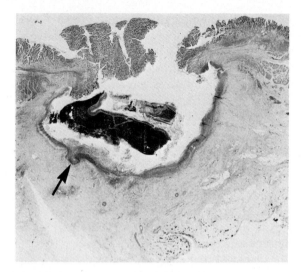

Fig. 5.29 Chronic gastric ulcer with blood clot in the ulcer crater associated with an eroded blood vessel (arrowed). Note the flask-shaped appearance of the ulcer with undermining of the mucosa at its margins.

Haematoxylin-eosin   × 3

between gastric carcinoma with lymph node involvement and a peptic ulcer. Surrounding mucosa appears flat and atrophic and the presence of gastritis, either local or more generalized, can be confirmed on microscopy.

Gastric peptic ulcers, particularly large ones, have to be distinguished from carcinomas. The distinction can usually be made by the clear-cut overhanging edges and absence of thickening in adjacent mucosa, but multiple biopsies should be taken from the circumference at endoscopy to exclude malignancy.

Microscopically, all chronic peptic ulcers have a characteristic structure in the stage of active necrosis. The base has four recognizable layers. On the luminal aspect there is a narrow layer of fibrinous exudate containing traces of tissue debris and occasional leukocytes. Deep to this exudative zone is a thin zone of necrosis in which the elements of the affected tissue have largely disintegrated and lost their identity in an amorphous, compact, eosinophilic meshwork in which a number of faintly haematoxyphile, smudge-like bodies represent the remains of the nuclei of dead tissue cells and leukocytes. The necrotic zone merges fairly abruptly into a thicker zone of surviving, moderately cellular granulation tissue: this, in its turn,

merges imperceptibly into the zone of fibrosis. These four histological zones—the superficial exudative zone, the necrotic zone, the granulation tissue zone, and the zone of cicatrization—are characteristic of chronic peptic ulcer. They are sometimes referred to as Askanazy's zones.[158] The fibrosis extends through the wall of the stomach, interrupting the muscle layers. The muscularis mucosae and the main muscle coat are drawn together round the margin of the ulcer and become fused at its edge. This is a sign characteristic of peptic ulceration, and is useful in the diagnosis of primarily carcinomatous ulceration ('cancer-ulcer') from carcinomatous change in the margin of a true peptic ulcer ('ulcer-cancer'). The arteries in the cicatricial zone often show very marked obliterative endarteritis. As the ulcerative process advances to the level of these vessels they may undergo obliteration by thrombosis and organization of the thrombus; if they are eroded before this protective occlusion has been completed, haemorrhage results.

The distinction between an active and a healing ulcer can be made by observing the margin of the mucosa, where signs of epithelial proliferation will be apparent (Fig. 5.30). If epithelium has grown over the ulcer for some distance, this may be regarded as a sign of attempted healing. Proliferative epithelial changes at the edge of a chronic ulcer are sometimes mistakenly interpreted as malignant change, particularly when the regenerating epithelium is partly buried in organizing granulation tissue. A healed ulcer is covered by a thin, simple, mucin-secreting epithelium (Fig. 5.31). Neither the muscularis mucosae nor the gastric or pyloric glands ever regenerate, and an old ulcer scar may be recognized as such by the submucosal and intramural fibrosis, the local covering of atrophic mucosa, and the absence of the muscularis mucosae. Occasionally inflammatory pseudo-polypoid proliferation takes place at an ulcer edge during healing.[159]

The mucosa surrounding a gastric ulcer invariably shows histological evidence of gastritis and this commonly involves the whole antral type mucosa. It may be of superficial or atrophic type and both intestinal and pseudo-pyloric metaplasia are common. The fact that the gastritis often worsens after an ulcer heals[103] suggests that it is a

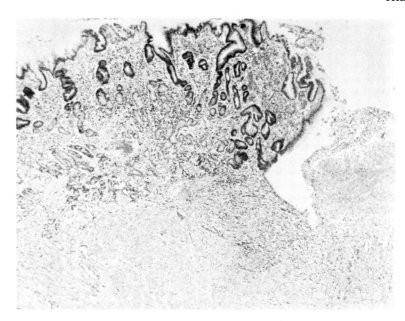

Fig. 5.30 Margin of an active peptic ulcer (ulcer slough is seen at the right). The deeply-staining epithelium of the foveolae and their architectural distortion is indicative of regenerative changes.

Haematoxylin-eosin   × 60

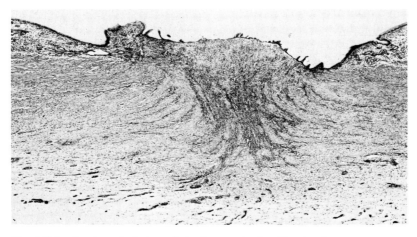

Fig. 5.31 Section through the base of a healing gastric ulcer. Simple columnar epithelium has grown in a single layer over the fibrous tissue.

Haematoxylin-eosin   × 14

Provided by W. StC. Symmers.

primary rather than a secondary phenomenon. Occasional ulcers, where chronic gastritis has not been a prominent feature in the surrounding mucosa, have arisen in individuals with a history of heavy aspirin intake (Fig. 5.32). In addition they have been characterized by a preferential location along the greater curvature of the stomach.[93,94]

Chronic duodenal ulcers

Most duodenal ulcers occur in the first part of the duodenum, and are usually immediately postpyloric in situation (Fig. 5.33); only occasionally is an ulcer found in the second part of the duodenum. Endoscopic studies have shown that in some 10–

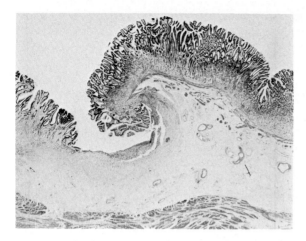

Fig. 5.32 Section of one of several shallow ulcers occurring on the greater curve of the stomach in a patient with rheumatoid arthritis who was taking large doses of aspirin and phenylbutazone. Note the absence of inflammation in the adjacent mucosa.

Haematoxylin-eosin   × 7

15% of cases the ulcers are multiple,[160] not uncommonly paired on the anterior and posterior walls. They are punched out in appearance, and scarring often produces considerable distortion.

Histologically, they show similar features to their gastric counterparts, although the tendency for fusion of the muscularis propria with the muscularis mucosae at the ulcer edge is not so marked. There is often some degree of surrounding duodenitis with some shortening and thickening of villi and an increased cellular infiltration in the lamina propria.

Complications of peptic ulcer

The complications of peptic ulcer are perforation, haemorrhage, involvement of adjacent organs, fibrosis and stenosis, and, very rarely, carcinoma.

Perforation. Acute and chronic gastric and duodenal ulcers, particularly those on the anterior wall which are not readily walled off by surrounding structures, are liable to perforate. In reported series duodenal and pyloro-duodenal perforations have been much commoner than perforation of gastric ulcers.[161,162]

The appearance of a perforated peptic ulcer is characteristic (Fig. 5.34). There is a neat, round hole in the floor of the ulcer, and the serosa around this perforation is hyperaemic and lustreless, and partly covered by white flakes of fibrinous exudate.

There are fine fibrinous adhesions between the region of the lesion and neighbouring organs, and commonly the hole is plugged by the greater omentum.

Any delay in surgical treatment of a perforated peptic ulcer will lead to diffuse peritonitis, at first the result of chemical irritation but from an early stage associated with secondary infection from bacterial contamination. Later complications include the formation of local abscesses at the site of perforation, and pelvic and subdiaphragmatic abscesses.

'*Food granulomas*' (see p. 171) are occasionally found in the tissues round the lower end of the stomach and the first part of the duodenum, usually in association with an active or healed peptic ulcer (Fig. 5.23).

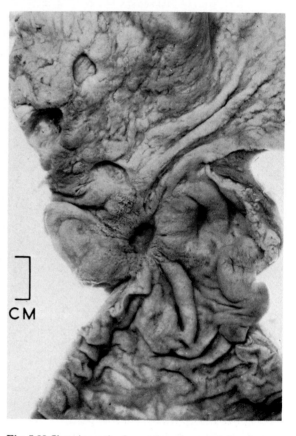

Fig. 5.33 Chronic peptic ulcer at the pylorus and three large acute peptic ulcers in the pyloric antrum (above).

Specimen from the Gordon Museum, Guy's Hospital, London, reproduced by permission of the Curator, Mr J. D. Maynard. Photograph by Miss P. M. Turnbull, Charing Cross Hospital Medical School, London.

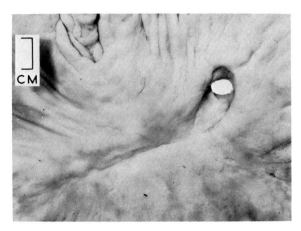

Fig. 5.34 Acute perforation of a chronic peptic ulcer on the lesser curvature of the stomach.

Specimen from the Gordon Museum, Guy's Hospital, London, reproduced by permission of the Curator, Mr J. D. Maynard. Photograph by Miss P. M. Turnbull, Charing Cross Hospital Medical School, London.

Haemorrhage. This is the commonest complication of chronic peptic ulcers and occurred in 16% of patients in a 15-year study in general practice.[163] Post-bulbar duodenal ulcers and stomal ulcers are particularly prone to bleed. Peptic ulcers in females, although less frequent than in males, may be more likely to undergo haemorrhage. The mortality rate for this complication has been of the order of 5–10%, being higher with gastric ulcers than duodenal ulcers.

Erosions and acute ulcers are also liable to be associated with extensive acute haemorrhage, since the lamina propria is extremely vascular, and gastric and duodenal submucosal vessels are thin walled, numerous, and of wide calibre (Fig. 5.35).

Involvement of adjacent organs. A peptic ulcer in the stomach or duodenum is liable to become adherent to the pancreas and may erode its substance. Localized pancreatitis develops at the site of the penetration but important complications are unusual: these include haemorrhage from erosion of the splenic artery and, very rarely, acute haemorrhagic pancreatic necrosis. If a peptic ulcer leads to adhesion between the stomach or duodenum and the transverse colon the ulcer may eventually perforate into the latter, giving rise to a gastrocolic or duodenocolic fistula. Occasionally, a peptic ulcer results in adherence of the stomach or duodenum to the liver: no special complications

result. However, endoscopic biopsies from the base of a deeply excavated peptic ulcer in which cords of liver cells are present may be misinterpreted as carcinoma unless this possibility is borne in mind.

Fibrosis and stenosis. Peptic ulceration in the region of the pyloric sphincter or cardia will lead to local fibrosis and stenosis, with signs of obstruction. If there is considerable submucosal fibrosis round an ulcer in the middle part of the stomach the deformity known as hour-glass stomach may develop (Figs. 5.36 and 5.37). When gastrectomy is performed for this condition it is often found that the ulcer has healed, leaving an area of intramural fibrosis radiating from its site on the lesser curvature and partially constricting the lumen.

Carcinoma. The term ulcer-cancer is used to denote a chronic gastric ulcer with carcinoma in its margin. Its prevalence has been debated for many years. The histological criteria essential for

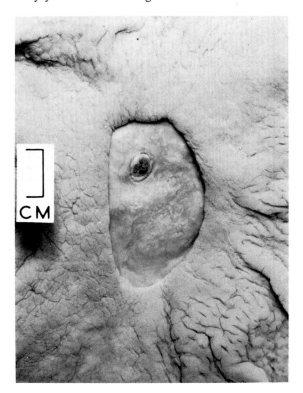

Fig. 5.35 A large artery, its lumen almost closed by fresh thrombus, is exposed in the floor of this acute gastric ulcer. The patient died after a massive haematemesis.

Specimen from the Gordon Museum, Guy's Hospital, London, reproduced by permission of the Curator, Mr J. D. Maynard. Photograph by Miss P. M. Turnbull, Charing Cross Hospital Medical School, London.

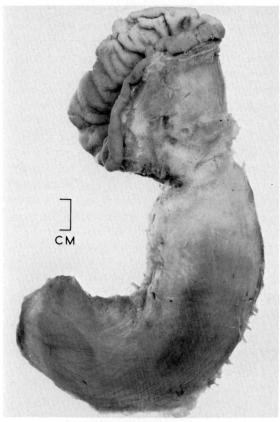

Fig. 5.36 'Hour-glass' stomach, the result of fibrosis accompanying a chronic peptic ulcer, with contraction of the scar. See also Figure 5.37.

Specimen from the Pathology Museum, Charing Cross Hospital Medical School, London, reproduced by permission of the Curator, Mr F. J. Paradinas. Photograph by Miss P. M. Turnbull, Charing Cross Hospital Medical School.

the diagnosis include (1) a cicatricial base to the ulcer, without malignant cells in this basal fibrous zone, which interrupts the muscle coat and extends out to the serosa; (2) fusion of the main muscle coat with the muscularis mucosae at the edge of the ulcer, and (3) the presence of unequivocal carcinomatous elements that invade the margin of the ulcer (Figs 5.38 and 5.39). Ulcer-cancers undoubtedly do occur, particularly when the ulcer is a large one, but the prevalence of cancer developing in a proven peptic ulcer and the presence of unequivocal evidence of previous peptic ulcer at the site of a proven carcinoma are both probably less than 1%. It has to be stressed that multiple sections through the base of an ulcer have to be examined and found to be free from cancer microscopically before excluding the presence of carcinoma in this area, which is so crucial in the differentiation between ulcer-cancer and cancer-ulcer. In an ulcerated scirrhous carcinoma the fibrous tissue and carcinoma cells are intimately intermingled, while in true ulcer-cancer the preexisting fibrous base is never invaded. Another source of error is to misdiagnose as malignant elements of regenerating epithelium at the edge of an ulcer which have grown down into submucosa and become secondarily entangled in, and often distorted by, reparative fibrous tissue. These do not have the nuclear hyperchromatism or show the multi-layering of cells of adenocarcinoma, and can usually be readily distinguished once the possibility of their presence is appreciated.

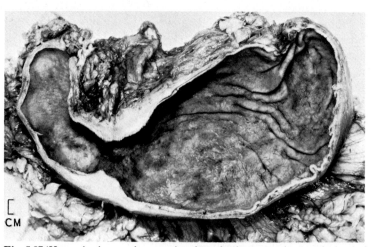

Fig. 5.37 'Hour-glass' stomach, opened to show the dense scar tissue at the level of the ulcer.

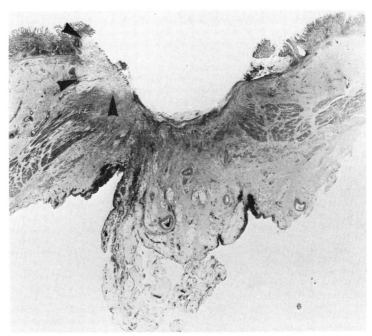

Fig. 5.38 Ulcer-cancer. In this section of a chronic peptic ulcer a clear area (arrowed) is present at one margin. This is illustrated in Figure 5.39. Note fusion of muscle coats on right.

Haematoxylin-eosin   × 4

Incidence, aetiology and pathogenesis of peptic ulcer

The aetiology and pathogenesis of peptic ulceration have generated much research and infinitely more hypothesis. On a pathophysiological level, a peptic ulcer, irrespective of where it arises, is thought to result from an imbalance in the aggressive forces of acid and pepsin and the defensive forces of mucosal resistance. The consensus of current opinion favours the idea that both gastric and duodenal ulcers are the common end-result of a heterogeneous group of disorders, and subgroups of patients have been identified on the basis of genetic, epidemiological, pathophysiological and immunological criteria.[164] However, it is conveni- ent to consider in general terms those factors which delineate duodenal and prepyloric ulcers on the one hand from gastric antral and lesser curve ulcers on the other. Before doing this the prevalence and incidence of peptic ulcer disease will be briefly discussed.

Prevalence and incidence. There are no wholly satisfactory estimates for the prevalence of peptic ulcer and the reasons for this have been well reviewed.[165, 166] The most reliable information has come from careful necropsy studies, which suggest that between 1 in 4 and 1 in 6 of all males in England over the age of 35 are likely to have had an active or a healed peptic ulcer which was duodenal, gastric, or duodenal followed by gastric, in a ratio of 7:2.5:1, with an increasing swing to gastric ulceration with advancing age. In women, sharp increases in ulcer frequency occurred before and after the menopause. Duodenal ulcer fre- quency was estimated in middle-aged and elderly women at about one in 13 and gastric ulcer frequency at one in 21. Combined lesions were observed in between one in 50 and one in 80 necropsies in postmenopausal women. The ratio of duodenal to gastric ulcers was only 1.7:1 in younger groups, decreasing to 0.5:1 by the menopause.[167]

The best estimate of peptic ulcer disease preva- lence assessed during life has come from a recent endoscopic study in Finland which demonstrated active duodenal ulcers and active gastric ulcers in 1.4% and 0.28% respectively of 358 control subjects participating in a study of gastric cancer and with a mean age of 46 (i.e. a 5:1 ratio of duodenal to

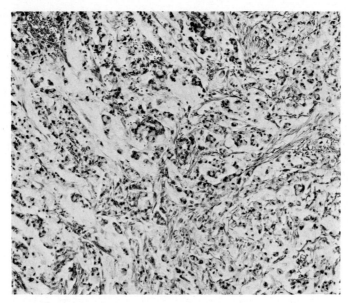

Fig. 5.39 Detail of Figure 5.38 shows the presence of groups of mucous-containing carcinoma cells of signet-ring type.

Haematoxylin-eosin   × 150

gastric ulcer). In a further 4.2% there was evidence of scarring of the duodenum or stomach, or a history of ulcer surgery, giving an estimated lifetime prevalence of at least 5.9%.[168]

In communities with a Western pattern of civilization there have been marked changes in ulcer disease type and frequency with time. Thus in Britain before 1900 gastric ulcer was predominant and particularly affected younger women. Considerable differences in ulcer prevalence and incidence have also been documented between countries and within countries. A reflection of the latter is that admission rates for perforated duodenal ulcer are considerably higher in northern than in southern parts of the United Kingdom.[169]

The marked fluctuation of peptic ulcer incidence from time to time and from place to place indicates the primary importance of environmental factors.

Duodenal and prepyloric ulceration

Hyperacidity. This is an important physiological abnormality in the majority of patients with duodenal ulcer and its role is reflected by the success of specific acid-reducing agents, such as H_2-receptor antagonists, in its treatment. The most commonly demonstrable abnormality is an in-creased meal-stimulated acid secretion, with an increased maximal acid output occurring in up to a half of the subjects, although the latter varies considerably in frequency in different countries, suggesting ethnic differences. Hypersecretion may theoretically occur in those with duodenal ulcer as a result of an abnormally large parietal cell mass, hyperfunction of gastrin (G) cells, increased stress-related cephalic stimulation and increased vagal drive. Postmortem studies[170] have shown an in-creased gastric mucosal area and increased numbers of parietal cells in duodenal ulcer subjects compared with controls, although there is a considerable overlap. The parietal cell mass correlates with the maximal acid output.[171,172] A subgroup of patients has been described with hypergastrinaemia and acid hypersecretion with normal antral gastrin concentrations and G-cell numbers, in which aggressive duodenal ulceration occurs that responds well to antrectomy.[173] A familial tendency has been observed in this group with G-cell hyperfunction. It is well known that in the Zollinger-Ellison syndrome (see p. 184) associated with pancreatic gastrin-secreting tumours, and consequent extreme hyperacidity, peptic ulceration occurs more distally in the duodenum or even in the jejunum. This syndrome has also been described in association with an antral G-cell hyperplasia without tumour[174] and can lead to an extension of body type mucosa almost up to the pylorus.[175]

Genetic factors. The association of blood group O and duodenal ulceration was first reported in 1954[176] and has been confirmed on numerous occasions since then. Those within that group who are in addition incapable of secreting their AB(O)H blood group substances in water-soluble form have a two to three times risk of developing a duodenal ulcer,[177] and an increased proneness to severe and recurrent bleeding from it.[178] Relatives of duodenal ulcer patients have two to three times the expected prevalence of ulcer in that site, but no increased risk of gastric ulcer.[179,180] More recent studies utilizing the radioimmunoassay of serum pepsinogen I have shown that about half of duodenal ulcer patients have raised levels, and the other half have normopepsinogenaemia, and that these for the most part show familial separation.[181] Other inherited tendencies associated with liability to duodenal ulcer which have been suggested include rapid gastric emptying and an exaggerated gastrin response to a protein meal.[182]

Rare, distinct genetic syndromes which predispose to duodenal ulceration include multiple endocrine adenomatosis syndrome, type I (MEA I, Werner's syndrome), an autosomal dominant disorder characterized by pituitary, parathyroid and pancreatic adenomas. The latter may secrete gastrin, resulting in a severe form of ulcer diathesis (Zollinger-Ellison syndrome). Systemic mastocytosis is another inherited multi-system syndrome complicated by duodenal ulceration, and results from excessive histamine production leading to gastric mucosal hypertrophy and acid hypersecretion.[183]

Stress. Although psychological stress has been proposed as an important factor to explain the occurrence or recurrence of duodenal ulcer, direct evidence for a causal role is lacking. A major problem has been the difficulty in scientifically defining and measuring an individual's stress. There is some evidence that foremen, business executives and doctors are more and farm labourers less liable to duodenal ulceration than the average person, but it is difficult to disentangle the effects of differing diets and economic factors from purely psychogenic ones. A study in air traffic controllers showed a similar ulcer incidence to that of the general population,[184] and in a case-control study of chronic duodenal ulcer patients in whom stressful life events were examined, no differences were found between cases and controls.[185]

In sum, stress probably plays an important role in the pathogenesis of duodenal ulcer, but the strength of this relationship has yet to be defined.

Gastric ulceration

Most antral or lesser curve ulcers are associated with normal or hypoacidity. In some there is a history of preceding duodenal ulcer. Although some degree of antral gastritis is common in patients with duodenal ulcer, inflammation is usually more severe and widespread with gastric ulcer,[186] particularly in those which occur high on the lesser curve. In such cases gastritis has resulted in replacement of body glands by mucous glands (pseudo-pyloric metaplasia), or by intestinal metaplastic epithelium.[100] These ulcers, whilst healing more readily than more distally sited lesions with less extensive associated gastritis, have a higher recurrence rate.[101] Biopsy studies have shown as well that gastritis persists or progresses following ulcer healing,[102,103] and suggest that gastritis precedes gastric ulcer rather than that the inflammation is secondary.

One of the main hypotheses proposed for the pathogenesis of gastric ulceration is that because of abnormal motility in the pyloro-duodenal region, there is reflux of duodenal contents into the stomach which gives rise to a chronic inflammatory reaction.[187,188] As a result the gastric mucosa is more susceptible to damage by acid or pepsin. There is evidence that bile acids, particularly deoxycholic and chenodeoxycholic acid, together with lysolecithin, formed by the action of pancreatic phospholipase A on the lecithin in bile, remove surface mucin and break the gastric mucosal barrier, causing back-diffusion of hydrogen ions. The advent of more physiological methods of studying reflux, using radiopharmaceuticals that are excreted by the liver into the bile, has shown, however, that the amount of bile reflux and the time it remains in the stomach are similar in normal controls and those with gastric ulceration, although it may be that the individual constituents of bile in the two groups are different.[189]

Alternative initiating theories have concentrated on antro-pyloric dysfunction giving rise to a delay in gastric emptying,[189,190] or on the role of stress in producing microvascular constrictive changes with resultant ischaemia and mucosal necrosis.[191] One interesting suggestion to explain the localization of gastric ulcers to the lesser curve of the stomach has been that this area is potentially more liable to ischaemia, deriving its blood supply from mucosal arteries which arise directly from the left gastric artery on the serosal surface, and not, as elsewhere, from submucosal plexuses.[192]

Other factors in the pathogenesis of peptic ulceration

A causal relationship between peptic ulceration and smoking has been strongly suspected but remains unproven.[97,193] However, the adverse effect of smoking on the healing of both gastric and duodenal ulcers appears well established.[194]

The fact that gastric ulcer is most commonly found in patients in the poorer economic grades has been regarded as evidence suggesting that dietary deficiencies may be an aetiological factor. Duodenal ulcer is very common in parts of southern India, and it has been supposed that this is the result of malnutrition.[195] However, it seems to be unlikely that malnutrition is of much importance in the causation of peptic ulceration in European and North American countries, where the disease is very common. One prospective study found that peptic ulcers were more common in individuals who had been habitual consumers of coffee and cola type soft drinks, whereas milk appeared to be protective.[196]

Drugs which have been implicated in the pathogenesis of peptic ulceration are non-steroidal anti-inflammatory agents and steroids, although a lot of the evidence is based on the results of retrospective case-control studies. There does, however, appear to be a positive association between chronic gastric ulcer and heavy intake of analgesics such as aspirin and paracetamol (acetaminophen),[91,92,197] and analysis of a large number of controlled studies where corticosteroids had been used showed little or no risk at low dosage,

but a two-fold increase in frequency of detected ulcers over control levels at higher dosage.[198]

Duodenal ulcer occurs with higher than expected prevalence in certain disease states. These include chronic lung disease,[199] where the association occurs even in the absence of smoking. The mechanism is unclear and there is no correlation between the occurrence of ulcer and the degree of carbon dioxide retention or the type of therapy used for the lung disease.[200] There is a high frequency of duodenal ulcer in patients with renal disease undergoing dialysis or transplantation,[201] and although such patients have hypergastrinaemia, available evidence suggests that removal of a circulating ulcer protector, possibly urogastrone, which is retained in renal failure, plays a role in the pathogenesis of ulceration in these circumstances.[202] Less well-established associated conditions include low blood pressure within the normal range,[203] and chronic pancreatic insufficiency,[204] suggesting a role for circulatory changes and inadequate alkalinization of the duodenum, respectively.

The stomach in Zollinger-Ellison syndrome

The majority of patients who develop the Zollinger-Ellison syndrome[205] have a primary gastrin-secreting tumour, usually in the pancreas, which stimulates the acid-secreting cells of the body of the stomach to maximal activity with consequent liability to duodenal or even jejunal ulceration. In approximately 10% of cases the tumours arise in the duodenum, most commonly the second part,[206] and on rare occasions occur in the stomach.[207] In about 20% of cases there are tumours in other endocrine organs, notably the parathyroids and the pituitary (multiple endocrine adenomatosis, type I).[208] In a minority of patients there is localized hyperplasia of antral gastrin-secreting (G) cells which results in an identical clinical picture.[209]

Grossly, the stomach shows very prominent folds in the body not unlike the appearance in Menetrier's disease (see p. 219). Histologically, a number of abnormalities can be present. Full-thickness biopsy of body mucosa shows marked thickening due to glandular hyperplasia resulting from a proliferation of parietal cells, and there may be extension of specialized glandular epithelium into the antrum so that virtually the entire gastric mucosa is of fundal type.[210] Foveolae are normal and there is no associated inflammation. Proliferation of enterochromaffin-like (ECL) cells in the stomach has been described,[211] and occurs in other conditions where there is a raised serum gastrin (see p. 188). The duodenal mucosa shows features of non-specific duodenitis in which gastric metaplasia of the surface epithelium is a prominent feature.[212] In antral G-cell hyperplasia the endocrine cells are larger than normal and greatly increased, sometimes forming small clusters or micro-adenomas,[213] whereas in the Zollinger-Ellison syndrome associated with a gastrinoma there are normal or decreased numbers of gastrin cells.[214]

GASTRIC POLYPS

The word polyp is a non-specific clinical term used to describe any focal lesion which projects above the surface of surrounding mucosa. In common usage it implies a substantive process occurring in the mucosa or less commonly the submucosa. Gastric polyps have been detected in only about 0.4% of autopsies[215] but have been reported in up to 5% of routine endoscopic examinations, although in the latter situation many of them were of small size.[216]

The classification of gastric polyps is a matter of debate, but from a clinical point of view, the most important distinction is between the neoplastic and non-neoplastic groups. Here they will be considered under five headings—regenerative (hyperplastic), neoplastic, hamartomas, heterotopias and a miscellaneous group.

Regenerative polyps

These are the commonest type of gastric polyp, comprising 50–90% of the total.[217,218] They are smooth-surfaced or only slightly lobulated, oval or hemispherical in shape, and rarely greater than 1.5 cm in diameter. Their surface is frequently eroded. The majority are sessile but larger polyps may be pedunculated. They can be single or multiple and may occur anywhere in the stomach although commonest in the antrum. When multiple, they may be widely scattered, or confined to one area, sometimes being concentrated at the junction of body and antral mucosa (Fig. 5.40).

Microscopically, the surface is composed of elongated crypts in which intraluminal infolding and branching is frequent and cystic dilatation almost invariable in the deeper parts of the polyp (Fig. 5.41). The lining cells consist of a single layer of regularly arranged hypertrophied superficial (foveolar) type epithelium containing abundant neutral mucin (Fig. 5.42). Small groups of pyloric type glands are present beneath the proliferating foveolae and connect with some of them. Parietal and chief cells are uncommon even when the polyp occurs in body mucosa. Intestinal metaplasia can occur but is rarely a conspicuous feature and when present is usually focal. Bundles of smooth muscle fibres growing into the polyp from the muscularis mucosae are frequently seen and the lamina propria is variably oedematous and infiltrated by plasma cells and lymphocytes, and lymphoid aggregates with germinal centres can sometimes be conspicuous. At sites of erosion there is a fibrinopurulent exudate associated with the presence of numerous acute inflammatory cells and proliferated capillaries in the subjacent tissues. In such areas, bizarre-appearing, pleomorphic cells with hyperchromatic nuclei and prominent nucleoli may be seen scattered or in small groups in the stroma. Some of them show mitoses. These are regenerative and not

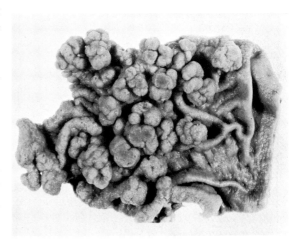

Fig. 5.40 Regenerative polyps. Numerous, slightly lobulated polyps up to 1 cm in diameter are present in the antrum.

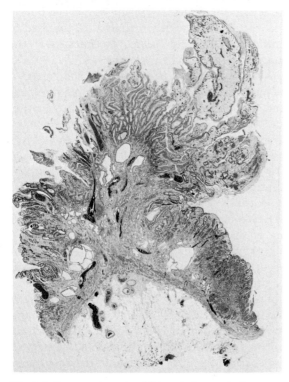

Fig. 5.41 Regenerative polyp. This typical example shows erosion of the surface and cystic change. The appearances merge with those of the surrounding mucosa.

Haematoxylin-eosin   × 9

malignant cells, although the cell type from which they are derived is uncertain.[219] The mucosa adjacent to a hyperplastic polyp usually shows similar though less marked changes of hypertrophy and hyperplasia of foveolar cells, and mild to moderate inflammation with or without focal intestinal metaplasia and cyst formation, so that there is no clear demarcation between the two.

Because of their histological features, and the fact that they can develop at the site of, or bordering, ulcers and erosions[220] and at gastro-enterostomy stomas (see p. 198), it seems that these polyps arise on the basis of excessive regeneration following mucosal damage.

A distinctive feature of a minority of hyperplastic polyps has been an onion skin infolding of the papillary surface epithelium which macroscopically corresponds to a central dimple. These polyps, which have been separately categorized,[221] are usually multiple and arranged in a band in the fundic mucosa adjacent to the pyloric antrum. They probably result from over-exuberant healing of gastric erosions. Another classification separates polyps with foveolar hyperplasia only, and which tend to be small, from larger polyps in which there is also stromal and glandular hyperplasia (so-called hyperplasiogenous polyps).[222] The essential change, however, in all of them appears similar, varying only in degree.

Although there is general agreement that the malignant potential of hyperplastic polyps is low, occasional examples of malignant change have been reported.[221,223,224] The polyps are often associated, however, with an independent carcinoma elsewhere in the stomach. Thus they were found in 10% of cases of advanced gastric cancer and in 18% of cases of early gastric carcinoma in one report.[216]

Neoplastic polyps

These are uncommon and consist of adenomas and of polypoid carcinomas (types I, IIa and IIa + IIc early gastric cancers; see p. 208). Occasionally carcinoid tumours arise in the stomach and then often take the form of a polyp.

Various mesenchymal tumours may also present as a hemispherical or occasionally as a pedunculated gastric polyp covered by smooth stretched mucosa in which central ulceration is frequent. The commonest types are smooth muscle tumours (see p. 213), followed by neurogenic tumours (see p. 219). Metastatic tumours, which are frequently multiple, may have a similar appearance at endoscopy.[225]

Adenomas

These are uncommon lesions in the stomach. They are sessile or broad-based, mostly single and predominate in the antrum. In surgical series they have frequently been large with an average diameter of 4 cm and sometimes reach enormous proportions. They have an irregular surface with papillary projections separated by deep fissures (Fig. 5.43). Increasing use of endoscopy, however, has resulted in recognition of smaller, flatter, usually lobulated adenomas, often with a slightly depressed centre, which protrude into the lumen

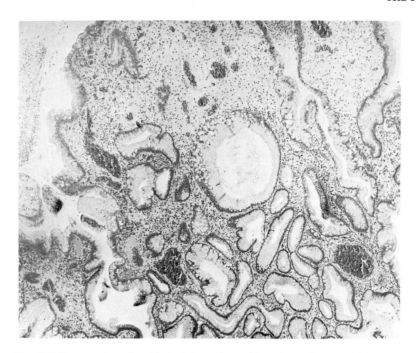

Fig. 5.42 Regenerative polyp. Marked elongation and branching of crypts which are lined by hypertrophied mucous cells. There is oedema and low-grade inflammation in the stroma of this polyp.

Haematoxylin-eosin   × 60

by only a few millimetres; these have been referred to rather confusingly as borderline lesions or as lesions with atypical epithelium.[226] Microscopically, larger adenomas have a villous or tubulovillous architecture (Fig. 5.44); the small flat lesions have a tubular pattern. Their epithelium consists of crowded, columnar cells with large, hyperchromatic, elongated nuclei and amphophilic to slightly basophilic cytoplasm. Mucin is either absent or scanty. Pseudostratification of nuclei and frequent mitoses are seen. Occasional goblet cells can be present along with Paneth and argentaffin cells. Within the polyp, small islands of uninvolved but usually metaplastic epithelium occur, and occasional pyloric glands are present at the base. In the sessile tubular adenomas (borderline lesion) cystic dilatation of glands is common beneath the dysplastic epithelium. There is a sharp transition between adenomatous epithelium and that of the adjacent mucosa, which often shows atrophic gastritis with intestinal metaplasia (Fig. 5.45). This, and the features of the adenomas themselves, suggest that they have originated from metaplastic

glands.[227] There is a significant association with the development of adenomas in patients with pernicious anaemia, where intestinal metaplasia is invariable. Unlike hyperplastic polyps, adenomas have a significant potential for malignant change which, in reported series, has averaged 40%.[228] On the other hand, it is probable that only a small minority of gastric cancers arise from previously benign adenomas. Gastric adenomas show varying degrees of epithelial atypia or dysplasia and examination of multiple sections is essential, particularly when more marked degrees of dysplasia are present, to detect any areas of invasion of neoplastic cells through the basal membrane of the glands and pits. The distinction on histological grounds between highly-differentiated intramucosal adenocarcinoma and severe dysplasia in an adenoma is often particularly difficult.

Endocrine cell tumours

These tumours, often referred to as carcinoid tumours when distinctive morphological patterns

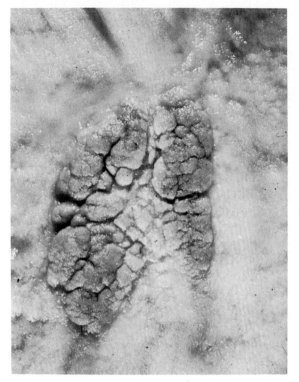

Fig. 5.43 Gastric adenoma. This 3 cm diameter sessile lobulated tumour was present on the anterior wall of the mid-stomach.

only be demonstrable when fixatives such as Bouin's solution have been used. They are only rarely argentaffin positive.[229,230]

There is an interesting association between the presence of endocrine cell tumours, which may be multiple, or of diffuse hyperplasia of endocrine cells in the body of the stomach, and conditions in which there is a raised serum gastrin. These include pernicious anaemia,[117] atrophic gastritis,[231] following gastrojejunostomy,[232] and the Zollinger-Ellison syndrome.[211] It is presumed that the raised gastrin levels result in proliferation of endocrine cells, which have been characterized as enterochromaffin-like cells.

Gastric endocrine cell tumours have only rarely been associated with systemic effects of the carcinoid syndrome.[233] They may elaborate 5-hydroxytryptophan and histamine, but only rarely serotonin.[234,235] Very occasional tumours have produced adrenocorticotrophic hormone (ACTH) and resulted in Cushing's syndrome.[236]

In general these tumours are slow-growing and, even when metastases to regional lymph nodes have occurred, may be compatible with long-term survival.[237] Recent studies have shown that a

are seen microscopically, are not common in the stomach, where they make up about 5% of the total of such tumours occurring in the gastrointestinal tract. They are commonly polypoid and mostly arise in the antrum. Multiple tumours occur in 6–7% of cases. They may be covered by intact mucosa or show central ulceration, and larger tumours may be indistinguishable grossly from ulcerated adenocarcinoma. The cut surface may be yellow but is more often grey.

Histologically, they are composed of small uniform cells which are arranged in nests and infiltrating strands, or have an anastomosing ribbon-like pattern. Occasionally a tubular or acinar arrangement is seen (Fig. 5.46). There is a loose, vascular, connective-tissue stroma, which rarely may be hyalinized, and tumour cells may be aggregated around sinusoids to form rosettes. There is often associated hyperplasia of gastric glands and pits. Most tumours are argyrophilic with the Grimelius technique, although this may

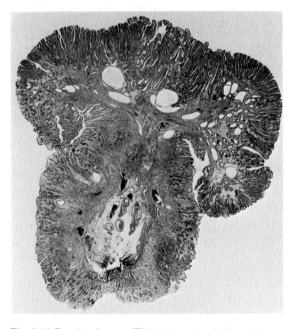

Fig. 5.44 Gastric adenoma. This 1.5 cm polyp had a tubulovillous growth pattern. It differed from the typical lesion in this site by being pedunculated, and was readily amenable therefore to endoscopic snare polypectomy.

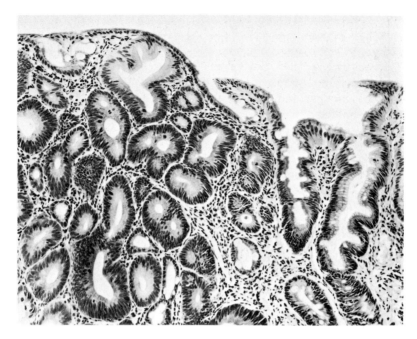

Fig. 5.45 Junction of sessile tubular adenoma, in which there is mild epithelial dysplasia, and adjacent mucosa where intestinal metaplasia is present.

Haematoxylin-eosin   × 150

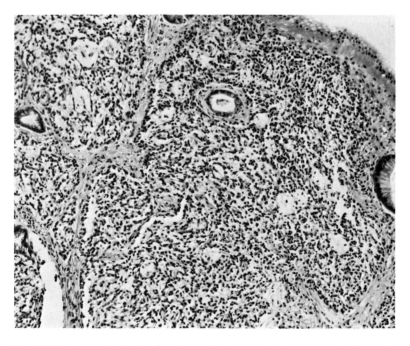

Fig. 5.46 Gastric carcinoid. Small uniform cells in a pseudo-acinar pattern infiltrate the mucosa between separated but intact foveolae.

Haematoxylin-eosin   × 150

significant proportion of resected gastric tumours, initially considered to be adenocarcinomas, represent atypical or poorly-differentiated endocrine cell tumours.[238,239] Histologically, they may take the form of sheets of cells without a recognizable pattern, or even consist in part of spindle cells in a very vascular stroma resembling a sarcoma.

Hamartomas

Peutz-Jeghers polyps

Although polyps are most common in the upper small bowel in this dominantly inherited condition, they have been noted at endoscopy in the stomach in nearly half of affected individuals.[240] In this site they are lobulated, rarely pedunculated, and mostly number less than 10. Although usually found incidentally, gastric polyps may bleed, and there is a low but definite risk of malignant change.[241]

Histologically, the characteristic feature is the tree-like branching of the muscularis mucosae with overlying mucosa being of normal or hyperplastic antral or fundal type, depending on the site of the polyp. As well as the typical polyp, hyperplastic polyps may also occur in the stomach in this condition.

Juvenile polyps

The predominant site for this type of polyp is the large bowel, particularly the lower rectum (see p. 363) but in individuals where numerous polyps are present, the upper gastrointestinal tract is frequently involved. Familial and non-familial cases of juvenile polyposis have been described, and in one recent report of the former type, multiple polyps were restricted to the stomach.[242] When numerous gastric polyps are present, this may lead to chronic and severe loss of blood and protein.

In the stomach, juvenile polyps have been more numerous in the antrum or restricted to that site, and larger lesions have been pedunculated. Typically they are rounded with a smooth surface and may show evidence of haemorrhage. Similar histological appearances to those of the large bowel are present, with cystically dilated glands lying in an abundant lamina propria (Fig. 5.47).

In some cases of juvenile polyposis, the gastric

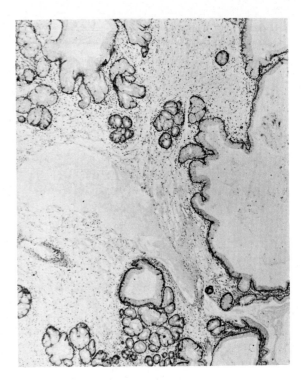

Fig. 5.47 Juvenile polyp. Mucous glands, some of which are cystically dilated, lie in an oedematous lamina propria which is devoid of smooth muscle fibres.

Haematoxylin-eosin   ×37

Histological preparation provided for photography by Dr B. C. Morson, St Mark's Hospital, London.

lesions have been indistinguishable histologically from hyperplastic polyps.[243]

Heterotopias

Islands of heterotopic or aberrant pancreatic tissue, usually single and with or without a considerable smooth muscle element, may occur within 3–4 cm of either side of the pylorus.[244] They are usually submucosal, but occasional examples are seen in muscle coats and on the serosal surface. They vary from a few millimetres to several centimetres in diameter and have the appearance of a hemispherical sessile polyp, often with an umbilicated centre (Fig. 5.48). A distinctive feature of some has been the presence of a ductal opening visible as a dimple on the surface. Histological examination shows pancreatic acini and ducts in which cystic change is common (Figs 5.49 and 5.50). Sectioning may

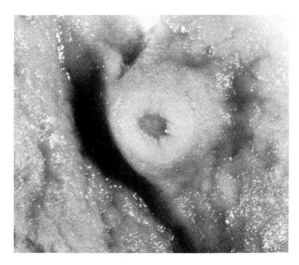

Fig. 5.48 Ectopic pancreas. This 5 mm diameter hemispherical polyp with a central dimple was an incidental postmortem finding in the antrum of the stomach.

glands, or the latter elements without pancreatic tissue may be found alone, when the term adenomyoma or 'myo-epithelial hamartoma' has been applied.[245] Larger lesions near the pylorus produce symptoms of gastric outlet obstruction, and ulceration and bleeding may occur. Lesions near the ampulla can cause obstruction of the common bile duct.[246] The majority, however, are incidental findings either at endoscopy or at postmortem.

Miscellaneous polyps

Cronkhite-Canada syndrome

In this rare disorder of unknown aetiology and without any familial tendency there is generalized gastrointestinal polyposis associated with skin pigmentation, alopecia and atrophy of the nails.[247] The major symptom is watery diarrhoea which can precede or follow the ectodermal changes and which can give rise to marked electrolyte disturbances and hypoproteinaemia. The majority of patients have been middle-aged or elderly and there is a slight male predominance.

Macroscopically, the polyps have a glistening, glassy appearance due to the presence of mucous

disclose ducts leading to the lumen. Islets of Langerhans are present in approximately one third of cases. This pancreatic tissue may be accompanied by bundles of hypertrophied smooth muscle surrounding ducts lined by tall columnar or cuboidal epithelium along with collections of Brunner's

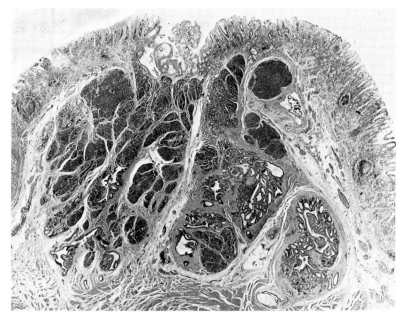

Fig. 5.49 Ectopic pancreas in wall of stomach. The characteristic dimple in the mucosa over the ectopic tissue is well seen. See also Figure 5.50.
Haematoxylin-eosin   × 8
Provided by W. StC. Symmers.

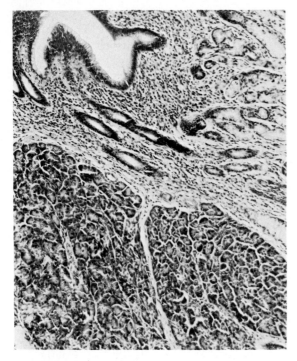

Fig. 5.50 Higher magnification of part of the field of Figure 5.49, showing typical acinar pancreatic tissue. No islets were found in this specimen.

Haematoxylin-eosin   × 150

cysts and may be sessile or finger-like in appearance or result in irregular, polypoid, nodular folds. Histologically, there is intense oedema of the lamina propria associated usually with increased cellularity, and elongation and tortuosity of the foveolae with marked cystic change in the pits and glands (Figs 5.51 and 5.52). Cysts may rupture and result in inflammation and the presence of muciphages in the lamina propria. The histological appearances are not specific and may be indistinguishable from those of juvenile polyps.[248]

Fundic glandular cyst

Although only described recently, this type of polyp has been observed in up to 1.5% of routine gastroscopies.[249] Most cases have occurred in middle-aged women and no specific association with other gastric diseases has been noted. Together with adenomas and hyperplastic polyps[250,251] this lesion has also been reported in the stomachs of patients with adenomatosis (familial polyposis) of the colon (see p. 36).[252]

They appear at endoscopy as clusters, often numbering in the order of 15 to 30, of small, mostly sessile lesions (up to about 5 mm in diameter) with a glassy transparent appearance, that are restricted to the body and fundus of the stomach, i.e. within the acid-secreting area.[253] Histologically, cysts of variable size are present at different levels of the gastric glands, admixed with normal glands (Fig. 5.53). These cysts are often interconnected and are lined by mucin-secreting cells, rather atrophic parietal cells and some chief cells, although the latter are not conspicuous. There is usually no associated inflammation.

The histogenesis of this type of polyp is unclear. Follow-up has shown that the number and size of polyps tend to remain unchanged, but in some cases spontaneous disappearance over a period of several months or a few years has been observed.[254]

Inflammatory fibroid polyp

The stomach is the most frequent site in the gastrointestinal tract for this uncommon lesion.[255,256] Alternative names which have been used to describe it have been eosinophil granuloma, gastric fibroma with eosinophil infiltration, gastric submucosal granuloma, polypoid eosinophilic gastritis and inflammatory pseudotumour. In most cases a single, smooth-surfaced oval polyp with a short pedicle and which often shows surface erosion has been present in the pyloric antrum. Histologically, inflammatory fibroid polyps consist of non-encapsulated, extremely vascular and usually loose connective tissue in the submucosa infiltrated by variable numbers of inflammatory cells. Blood vessels range from capillaries to larger thin- or thick-walled channels which are often surrounded by a zone of loose connective tissue giving a characteristic whorled pattern (Fig. 5.54).

The precise nature and aetiology of this polyp is unknown. Occasional examples have arisen at the edge of a peptic ulcer or carcinoma (Fig. 5.55), and a jejunal polyp has been described following mucosal damage after a saline emetic[257] suggesting an over-reactive healing process. A proposed neurogenic origin[258] appears unlikely and is not substantiated by ultrastructural examination.[259]

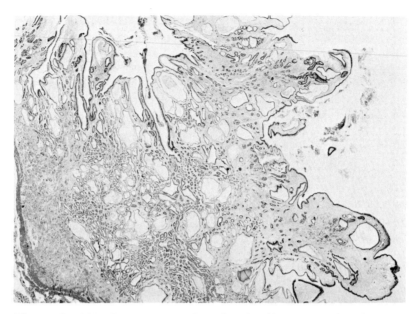

Fig. 5.51 Cronkhite-Canada syndrome. Irregular polypoid appearance of gastric mucosa. Part of muscularis mucosae is seen (bottom left). See also Figure 5.52.

Haematoxylin-eosin   × 4.5

Histological preparation provided for photography by Dr B. C. Morson, St Mark's Hospital, London.

MALIGNANT EPITHELIAL TUMOURS

ADENOCARCINOMA

Gastric adenocarcinoma is of major importance worldwide as a cause of death from malignant disease. In the United Kingdom it results in approximately 12 500 deaths/year making it the third commonest fatal malignancy after carcinoma of the bronchus and large bowel. The facts which have emerged from epidemiological studies and which provide the clues to the aetiology of this important disease will now be considered.

Epidemiology

Age and sex incidence

Stomach cancer incidence and mortality rates rise steeply with age, showing a constant rate of increase. Men are more often affected by the disease than women, the ratio varying from approximately one in young adults to a maximum of two or more

around the age of 60 and falling thereafter to approach unity again at advanced ages. It has been proposed that allowing for a latent interval this relates to differences in total calorie consumption between the sexes.[260]

This sex ratio shows little variation in different countries. When malignant tumours are subdivided according to their location within the stomach, however, there is more variation in the sex ratio, and adenocarcinoma occurring at the cardia appears to have a higher male to female predominance than tumours at other sites.[261]

Geographical variation

There are large differences in the incidence of cancer in different countries. Thus there is an approximately 30-fold greater incidence of the disease in Japan and several Asian republics of the USSR compared to large parts of rural Africa south of the Sahara. Even inside countries where reporting and classification of gastric cancer incidence and mortality can be assumed to be uniform,

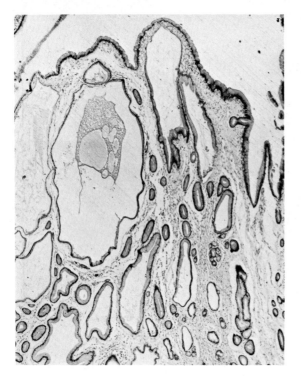

Fig. 5.52 Higher magnification of part of the field of Figure 5.51, showing elongated and cystically dilated foveolae and oedema of the lamina propria.

Haematoxylin-eosin   × 37

Histological preparation provided for photography by Dr B. C. Morson, St Mark's Hospital, London.

wide variations occur from area to area. For example, there are considerable differences in age-adjusted death rates within Japan,[262] and in the countries of Latin America there is a tendency for populations in the central Andean region to be at higher risk than residents of the tropical zones.

Variations of incidence and mortality with time

Striking reductions in the incidence and mortality of the disease with time have occurred in many developed countries,[263,264] apparently unaccounted for by such factors as more precise diagnosis, changes in age distribution of the population or in the ratio of foreign-born to indigenous groups. The decline has been most marked in the USA, where gastric cancer was the major cancer 45 years ago and where the age-adjusted mortality rate in males dropped from 28 per 100 000 in 1930 to 9.7

per 100 000 in 1967. In Japan the decline has occurred more recently, the decrease in stomach cancer in males varying from 19–35% in age-specific death rates between the years 1955 and 1973. Some, but not all, of this reduction can be attributed to the nationwide programme of early detection of stomach cancer.[265]

Studies in migrants

Studies of Japanese who have moved to the USA have shown a relatively slow fall in mortality from gastric cancer in the first generation, but the rate drops sharply in their offspring born in the USA.[266] In first-generation Japanese living in Hawaii those born in high-risk prefectures in Japan had a significantly higher risk of gastric cancer than those born in low-risk prefectures. This difference was not apparent in the next generation.[267] On the other hand, the risks for large bowel cancer among these same migrants rose during their lifetime to approach the risk characteristic of the United States' white host population. These findings highlight the importance of environmental factors in determining the incidence of gastric cancer. The fact that the migrants continue to have the high rates of their country of origin suggests either that they are exposed in young life to an exogenous agent which determines the later development of gastric cancer, or that they retain their former way of life and in particular their dietary habits in the new country, whereas their offspring adopt the life-style of their birth place. It appears from analysis of these groups and from studies in Colombia, where migrants from high- to low-risk areas retain a high risk of gastric cancer,[268] that factors acting in early life are important in determining the onset of disease later.

Variation with social class

A number of epidemiological investigations from different countries have shown a relationship of socio-economic factors to gastric cancer mortality. In general, the lower the income, social class or living standard the higher the mortality from gastric cancer.[269] Studies have shown an increased number of deaths from gastric cancer associated with specific occupations. These include coal-

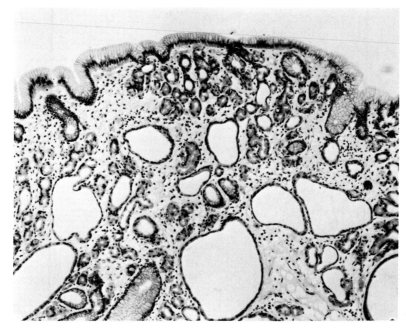

Fig. 5.53 Fundic glandular cyst. Cystic change in body glands. The flattened epithelium of the cysts includes parietal and chief cells.

Haematoxylin-eosin   × 111

Histological preparation provided for photography by Dr A. B. Price, Northwick Park Hospital, Harrow, Middlesex.

mining,[270] working with asbestos fibres[271] and working in the rubber industry.[272] However, it is probable that socio-economic status is more important than specific occupational risk factors in accounting for the extra risk of cancer in these groups.

Dietary influences

An obvious environmental influence and one subject to worldwide variation is food, and numerous epidemiological studies have been carried out to assess the possible significance of dietary factors on the incidence of gastric cancer. The possible effects of diet in the causation of gastric cancer are:

1. The presence of carcinogens occurring naturally in food or of precursors which in vivo are converted into carcinogens
2. The introduction of carcinogens in the preparation of food
3. The absence of a protective factor or factors.

Dietary studies have tended to give confusing results since the long interval between exposure and onset of disease complicates the collection of reliable and relevant histories of food practices. It is known that the total calorie intake does not account for differences between countries with low and high gastric cancer mortalities. General conclusions which have been reached show an association of gastric cancer with a high consumption of starches and a reduced consumption of fat, fresh fruits and green, leafy vegetables. In Hawaii, Japanese stomach cancer patients drank significantly less milk than matched controls and ate a greater amount of pickled vegetables and dried, salted fish, the elevated risk being roughly proportional to the quantity of these foods eaten.[267]

The way in which food is prepared is also relevant. In Iceland, where stomach cancer accounts for 35–45% of all malignant tumours, high levels of various polycyclic hydrocarbons have been found in smoked mutton and trout, eaten in large quantities by segments of the population most at risk of developing carcinoma.[273,274] It has been proposed that the high incidence of stomach cancer

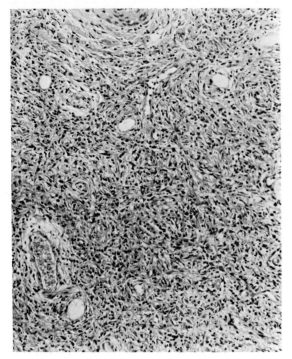

Fig. 5.54 Inflammatory fibroid polyp. Fibroblastic tissue with a sprinkling of inflammatory cells and numerous blood vessels are seen.

Haematoxylin-eosin   × 150

in Japanese could be explained by their consumption of rice to which commercial talc has been added to improve its flavour, the latter contaminated by asbestos. Talc crystals, but not asbestos fibres, have been demonstrated in the tumour cells of Japanese gastric cancer patients.[275]

Despite these associations between certain foods and increased risk, no single item has been identified which is common to all high-risk areas. More consistent results have been obtained for foods associated with a decreased risk, such as lettuce or celery. It therefore seems likely that it is the interplay of dietary factors which is important, with protective as well as antagonistic effects.

The role of N-nitrosamines, a potent group of carcinogens, in the pathogenesis of gastric cancer, has recently been emphasized.[276] N-nitroso compounds may be formed in vivo by the interaction of nitrites and secondary amines or amides. Nitrosatable compounds occur naturally in many foods, particularly in fish and meat, or may be ingested as drugs.[277] The nitrosating nitrite and more import-

antly nitrate are present in vegetables, drinking water, and cured meat products to which nitrate or nitrite has been added as a preservative. The N-nitrosation reaction is acid catalysed, but can be catalysed by bacteria at neutral pH values. Bacterial colonization of the stomach may occur in chronic gastritis or following partial gastrectomy and gastro-enterostomy.[278] There are several reports of carcinoma developing in the gastric stump many years after gastric resection (see p. 198), and increased nitrite levels in the gastric juice have been found in post-gastrectomy patients.[279] Urinary tract infections also result in the production of N-nitrosamines in the bladder and these could act secondarily on the stomach.[280] Epidemiological studies have shown an increased incidence of gastric cancer in areas where the water supply contained high concentrations of nitrate.[276,281] The significance of these findings awaits precise measurements of the levels of exposure to nitrate and total nitrate intake in such populations.

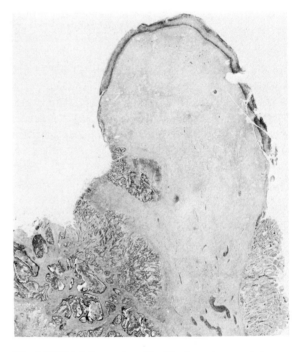

Fig. 5.55 This inflammatory fibroid polyp was present at one margin of an ulcerated gastric cancer in the antrum. The surface of the polyp is covered with a fibrinopurulent exudate. Invasive carcinoma is seen on the left and antral mucosa at bottom right.

Haematoxylin-eosin   × 4.3

Endogenous factors

Numerous studies have been carried out on the hereditary aspects of gastric carcinoma and a hereditary influence has been clearly demonstrated in the approximately 20% increased liability of people of blood group A to have the disease compared with people of other blood groups.[282] There have been several reports of family aggregations of gastric cancer, although most can be criticized on the basis of incomplete or inaccurate collection of the family data or the lack of suitable controls. Woolf (1961)[283] studied both the blood relatives and the spouses of propositi with gastric cancer and found that there was a two-fold increase in gastric cancer in blood relatives compared with controls, but no increase in spouses over their controls. Although this suggests that genetic factors are operating it does not exclude the possibility of environmental influences, since cancer patients and their spouses share a similar environment only during their married lives. The increased risk of gastric cancer in patients with pernicious anaemia is well established, as is the importance of heredity in pernicious anaemia.

Epidemiology-pathology studies

Interesting results have come from studies in which the histology of gastric cancer has been compared in high- and low-risk populations. Lauren (1965)[284] (see p. 203) divided gastric cancer into two main types: diffuse carcinoma, which tends to occur in younger people, and so-called intestinal type, which occurs in an older age group and is associated with a higher incidence of intestinal metaplasia in the mucosa away from the tumour. Using this classification it was found that in high-risk areas the predominant type of tumour was the intestinal type and that when the gastric cancer risk is reduced in a population it is this type that accounts for most of the reduction.[281] Thus comparison of the pathology of stomach cancer in Japan and in Japanese Hawaiians showed that the estimated incidence rates for diffuse carcinomas were the same in both localities, but the corresponding rates for intestinal, mixed intestinal and diffuse, and other types were much reduced in

Hawaii.[285,286] The age incidence slopes of the two main types were different and an association with blood group A was limited to diffuse type carcinomas, thus suggesting that the two types may be caused by different aetiological factors. Conflicting results have come from a study of material from the low-incidence areas of Minnesota, USA and New Zealand and from the high-incidence areas of Korea and Kyushu, Japan, where it was found that the age-sex specific proportions of diffuse type gastric cancer in these different populations did not vary.[287]

In summary, although epidemiological studies have provided many clues, the principal causes of gastric cancer remain unknown. This is largely related to the fact that environmental influences which initiate carcinogenesis in a susceptible individual occur many years prior to diagnosis or death from the disease, at which time detection or measurement of exposure to such influences may not be possible. The link between cause and effect becomes less tenuous if precursor lesions can be identified.

Precancerous lesions and conditions

A precancerous condition is best regarded as a clinical state associated with a significantly increased risk of cancer, whereas a precancerous lesion is a histopathological abnormality in which cancer is more likely to occur than in its apparently normal counterpart. In many clinical conditions with an increased risk of cancer, there is also an identifiable precancerous lesion, but this is not invariably so. In the stomach, precancerous conditions include pernicious anaemia, the presence of a gastric stump, and possibly Menetrier's disease (see p. 219). The relationship of gastric ulcer and gastric cancer is discussed on page 179. However, only a tiny proportion of the total number of gastric carcinomas arise in this way, the vast majority occurring without any predisposing condition.

Precancerous lesions in the stomach are atrophic gastritis with intestinal metaplasia (see p. 167), and epithelial dysplasia, which can occur in ordinary (foveolar) gastric epithelium as well as in intestinal metaplasia.

Pernicious anaemia

Adenomatous polyps and carcinoma of the stomach are both stated to be three to four times more common in patients with pernicious anaemia than in the general population.[288-290] Interestingly, a proportion of patients who present with gastric cancer without a previous history of pernicious anaemia have positive intrinsic factor antibodies and malabsorption of vitamin B_{12} reversed by administration of intrinsic factor, and appear therefore to be in a 'pre-pernicious anaemia stage'.[291] The cancers arising in patients with pernicious anaemia predominate in the fundus and cardia, are often polypoid, and frequently multiple (Fig. 5.56).[292]

The operated stomach

The relative risk of adenocarcinoma arising in the stomach of patients operated on more than five

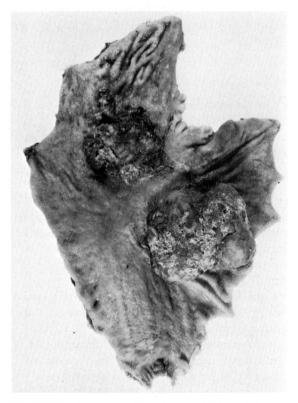

Fig. 5.56 Two large polypoid carcinomas with irregularly ulcerated surfaces are arising from the anterior and posterior walls respectively of the body of the stomach. The specimen was resected from a man of 68 who was diagnosed as having pernicious anaemia 10 years before.

years before for benign conditions appears to be increased compared to the general population.[293,294] The mean interval in most series between the time of operation and the diagnosis of malignancy has been from 20-30 years.[295-297] No consistent difference in frequency has been found between patients operated on for gastric ulcer as compared with duodenal ulcer, or relating to the type of operation carried out (Billroth I and Billroth II resection or gastrojejunostomy alone). The majority of cancers have occurred close to the site of anastomosis (Fig. 5.57).[298,299]

Atrophic gastritis develops rapidly after operation and in one study was present in 54% of patients at two years, affecting 81% of those operated on for antral or pyloric canal ulcers.[300] Atrophic changes are particularly marked in the gastric mucosa close to the stoma, whereas inflammation can be more conspicuous, although often patchy, in the remnant mucosa away from the anastomotic site. Single or multiple polypoid lesions are common at or close to the stoma.[301] Many of these are hyperplastic or regenerative, others are pseudo-polyps resulting from the construction of the anastomosis. The terms gastritis cystica polyposa[302] and stomal polypoid hypertrophic gastritis[303] have been used to describe these lesions (Fig. 5.57).

Epithelial dysplasia has been reported in 7-21% of patients.[297,304-307] It can take the form of a focal sessile adenoma but more often has been described in a flat mucosa. It may be widespread or multifocal, and its detection has frequently been in asymptomatic individuals. Its prevalence may be related to a number of factors including the interval since operation, type of operation, number of biopsies taken and their site in the stomach, and the variable cancer risks in the different geographical populations studied. As well as this, a major factor is in the subjective assessment and interpretation of dysplasia.

Epithelial dysplasia

The main histological and cytological features of epithelial dysplasia are cellular atypia, abnormal differentiation, and disorganized mucosal architecture. These can occur in ordinary gastric (foveolar) epithelium as well as in intestinal metaplasia. The

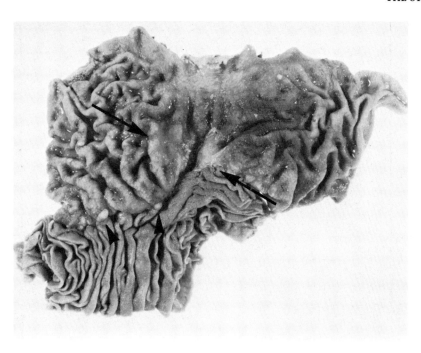

Fig. 5.57 Cancer in the operated stomach. An ulcerated plaque-like cancer (arrowed) is present in the stomach at the site of anastomosis with the small bowel. In addition several small polypoid lesions (arrowheads) are seen at the junction of small bowel and stomach; so-called stomal polypoid hypertrophic gastritis.

difficulty in recognizing and categorizing these changes is reflected in the number of classifications of gastric epithelial dysplasia which have been proposed.[308-314] These show points of similarity but also significant differences, notably the inclusion in some, as low-grade dysplasia, of epithelial changes associated with regeneration, and commonly seen in active gastritis or related to benign peptic ulcers. The latter are best termed inflammatory or regenerative epithelial change and distinguished from dysplasia although this is not always straightforward, particularly in small biopsy samples.

Gastric epithelial dysplasia has been most clearly characterized in adenomas (see p. 186). These uncommon lesions consist of deeply-stained glands often with a regular tubular pattern and lined by epithelium composed of tall columnar cells with basal rod-shaped nuclei crowded together (Fig. 5.58). Small amounts of mucin, usually sulphated, are often present at the apex of the cell, and Paneth cells and goblet cells may also be seen. With increasing degrees of dysplasia the nuclei become oval or rounded, vary in size, are often not so deeply stained, and contain prominent nucleoli. Nuclear stratification and loss of polarity develop and increased numbers of mitoses are present. Mucin secretion is minimal or absent and Paneth cells disappear. Associated with these cytological changes and abnormalities of differentiation there is increasing disorganization of the architecture of the glands with bunching and a back-to-back arrangement. Carcinoma is diagnosed when dysplastic cells are seen to have penetrated the basal membrane of the pits or glands and spilled into the lamina propria (Fig. 5.59). This may be obvious, but there are circumstances where the distinction between severe degrees of dysplasia and a well-differentiated tubular or papillary carcinoma is impossible. The expression carcinoma-in-situ is not a suitable one in this situation since the distinctive criteria for this diagnosis in a multi-layered squamous epithelium such as that of the skin or cervix cannot be applied to the single layered epithelium of the stomach, where focal invasion may occur unpredictably. Follow-up of

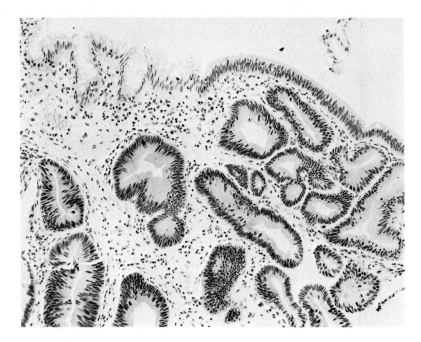

Fig. 5.58 Mildly dysplastic epithelium of a sessile tubular adenoma contrasts with adjacent normal gastric surface epithelium.

Haematoxylin-eosin   × 135

From D. W. Day, Biopsy Pathology of the Oesophagus, Stomach and Duodenum, 1986, courtesy of the publishers, Chapman & Hall.

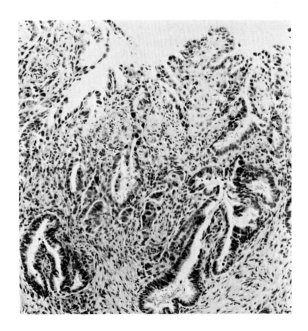

Fig. 5.59 Severely dysplastic glands are present which show irregular branching. There is obvious invasion of the lamina propria in several areas by noeplastic cells.

Haematoxylin-eosin   × 162

adenomas has demonstrated their malignant potential with carcinomas mostly occurring in tumours over 2 cm in diameter.[315]

Similar changes to those in adenomas have been described in a flat mucosa and these appearances have been associated with the development of, or accompany intestinal type gastric cancers. Dysplasia does not appear to play a prominent role, or may be a more subtle change, in the development of diffuse type carcinoma. However, some authors have described proliferation and rounding up of mucin-containing cells with loss of polarity of the nuclei in the neck region of the gastric glands and a change in the nature of their mucin which becomes alcianophilic.[316,317]

It is important to realize that the degree of risk associated with epithelial dysplasia is not yet established. Severe dysplasia on its own is not an indication for surgical intervention. However, experience of epithelial dysplasia in other organs suggests the importance of close follow-up for individual patients (including endoscopy and biopsy). Documentation must be adequate to provide an increasing body of knowledge about dysplasia and its significance. Patients with gastric stumps and pernicious anaemia appear to be the most promising clinical groups in which to study the subject further.

Macroscopic features and topography of gastric cancer

Carcinomas of the stomach are most common in the prepyloric region, pyloric antrum and on the lesser curve. They are less common at the cardia and in the body of the stomach, thus following the distribution of pyloric type mucosa. Carcinoma confined to the fundus is rare.

Grossly, they may be ulcerating, nodular, fungating or infiltrative in type. Ulcerated gastric cancers are commonest and usually occur in the antrum or in the region of the lesser curve. They differ from benign peptic ulcers in a number of ways. They have an irregular margin with raised edges, and surrounding tissue is firm and appears thickened, uneven and infiltrated. The ulcer has a necrotic, shaggy, often nodular base. Mucosal folds radiating from the ulcer crater do not have a regular appearance as with benign ulcers and frequently show club-like thickening and fusion (Fig. 5.60). Malignant ulcers tend to be larger than their benign counterparts. However, a significant proportion of malignant ulcers lack these appearances.[318,319] Because of this it is particularly important that all ulcerated lesions seen at endoscopy, even when appearing to be healing (like benign ulcers, malignant ulcers can heal on medical therapy),[320] should be systematically biopsied.

Fungating and nodular tumours typically consist of friable masses which project from a broad base into the cavity of the stomach. They tend to occur in the body of the stomach, in the region of the greater curve, posterior wall or fundus, and at the time of diagnosis are usually large, when surface ulceration and bleeding may be prominent features (Fig. 5.61).

Infiltrative cancers may spread superficially in the mucosa and submucosa giving rise to plaque-like lesions with flattening of the rugal folds and an opaque appearance of the mucosa. Superficial ulceration may supervene. More frequently, infiltration involves the entire thickness of the stomach wall usually over a limited area in the region of the

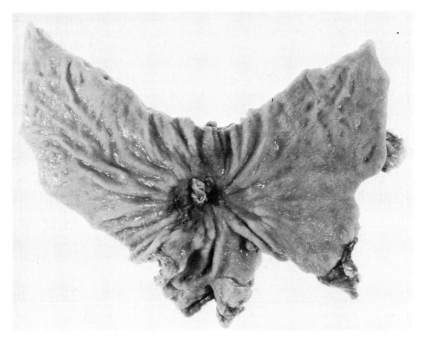

Fig. 5.60 Ulcerated gastric cancer centred on the lesser curve. The border of the ulcer is irregular and radiating mucosal folds are thickened and indurated.

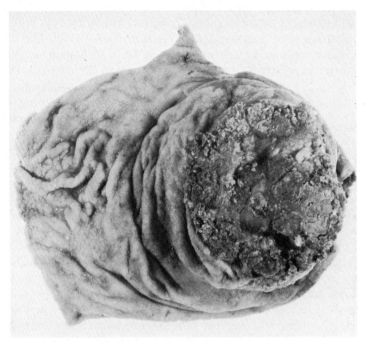

Fig. 5.61 This large fungating carcinoma with irregular ulceration of its surface is arising from the body of the stomach.

pylorus, but rarely extensively to produce the so-called linitis plastica* or 'leather-bottle' stomach. In these cases the wall is markedly thickened and assumes a cartilaginous consistency due to an extensive fibrotic response to tumour cells in the submucosa, muscle coats and subserosa (Fig. 5.62).

Many gastric carcinomas, irrespective of type, secrete mucin, which gives the tumour, or parts of it, a gelatinous appearance to the naked eye; these are called colloid carcinomas.

Microscopic features

Microscopical examination of gastric adenocarcinomas shows a marked variation in their structure. This diversity is apparent not only between different tumours but not infrequently in different areas of an individual tumour. Perhaps this is not

surprising when one considers the complex nature of the normal gastric mucosa with its varied cell types as well as its proneness to undergo metaplasia to an intestinal type of epithelium. Because of this variability, a complicated nomenclature arose in an attempt to describe the appearances of the tumour and any products of secretion, as well as the nature of the stroma. This inevitably gave rise to confusion and together with the lack of clear correlation between microscopic grading and gross patterns of the tumours led the American pathologist Stout (1953)[321] to state that histological classification was valueless and that a knowledge of the gross appearance of the tumours was more valuable in diagnosis and assessment of prognosis. This notwithstanding, a brief consideration of the classifications in current use will be given, together with an opinion of their relative merits.

World Health Organization (WHO) classification[322]

This divides adenocarcinoma of the stomach into papillary, tubular, mucinous and signet-ring cell types, the typing of any particular tumour being

---

* The name linitis plastica was introduced by William Brinton, who believed the disease to be an inflammatory condition of the 'filamentous network of areolar tissue' round the blood vessels of the stomach wall. He coined the term linitis because of the supposed resemblance of the fibrous tissue on the cut surface of the lesion to glistening threads of woven linen (W. Brinton, *The Diseases of the Stomach*, London, 1859, p. 310).

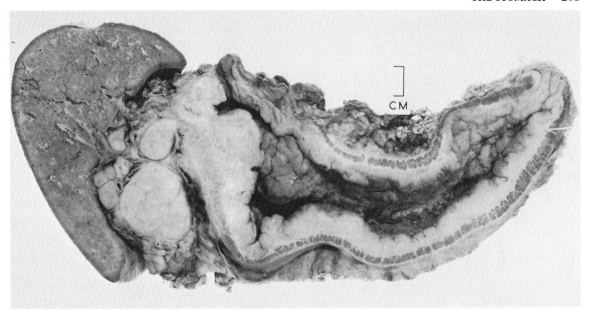

Fig. 5.62 Diffuse scirrhous carcinoma of the stomach ('leather-bottle' stomach). The marked thickening of the wall of the stomach is characteristic, involving mainly the mucosa and submucosa, but with penetration of the muscular coats leading to unusually clear delineation of the muscle bundles. There is heavy involvement of the tissues between the stomach and the spleen, including lymph nodes and the tail of the pancreas.
Specimen from the Gordon Museum, Guy's Hospital, London, reproduced by permission of the Curator, Mr J. D. Maynard.
Photograph by Miss P. M. Turnbull, Charing Cross Hospital Medical School, London.

based on its predominant component. Papillary adenocarcinomas are composed of pointed or blunt finger-like epithelial processes with fibrous cores. Some tubular formation may be present but the papillary pattern predominates, particularly in cystic structures. Typically this tumour grows as a polypoid mass into the lumen of the stomach. Tubular adenocarcinomas consist of branching glands embedded in or surrounded by a fibrous stroma. Large amounts of mucin are present in the mucinous adenocarcinoma which may be visible in the gross specimen. In some tumours dilated glands contain mucin which may be present as well in the interstitium, whereas in other varieties disintegrated epithelial components are seen as ribbons or groups of cells floating in lakes of mucin (Fig. 5.63). Signet-ring cell carcinomas (Fig. 5.64) are composed mainly of isolated tumour cells with large amounts of intracellular mucin and often associated with considerable fibrosis. All these types of tumour may be graded as well, moderately, or poorly differentiated. In this classification undifferentiated carcinomas and 'unclassified' carcinomas are separate groups.

Lauren classification[284]

This classification, which has been widely used in epidemiological studies, was based on a pathological examination of operative specimens of gastric cancer collected at the University of Turku, Finland, between 1945 and 1964. It cuts across the classical descriptions and allocates gastric carcinomas to two main groups, intestinal type and diffuse type. These differ not only in their general and cellular structure, secretion of mucus and mode of growth but in their clinical correlations also.

In general, intestinal type carcinomas (Fig. 5.65) have a glandular structure often with papillary or solid areas, and are made up of large, clearly defined pleomorphic cells with large, variably-shaped and hyperchromatic nuclei often in mitosis. Well-polarized, columnar cells with a well-developed brush border are usually observed lining glandular lumina, and secretion, if present, tends to be extracellular or to occur focally in the cytoplasm in a minority of cells. Diffuse type carcinomas are composed of separated single cells or small clusters of cells (Fig. 5.66). Occasionally a

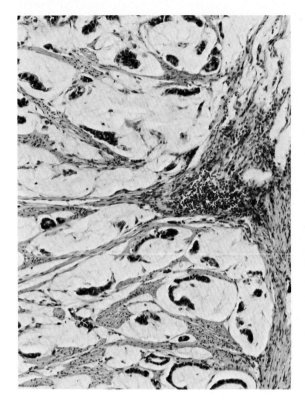

Fig. 5.63 Mucinous carcinoma of stomach. The muscle fibres of the wall are compressed between accumulations of mucus (the pale structureless material occupying most of the field). Surviving carcinoma cells are conspicuous, but they account for relatively very little of the bulk of such growths, which consist largely of the mucus secreted by the tumour or left free in the interstices of the tissues after death of the cells.

Haematoxylin-eosin × 100

Provided by W. StC. Symmers.

more solid or aggregated appearance is present but even then the cells are only loosely attached to each other. A glandular structure is uncommon and when present the lumina are small and poorly defined. Individual cells are small and uniform with indistinct cytoplasm and regular, often pyknotic nuclei in which mitoses are infrequent. In the few tumours with gland formation the lining cells are unpolarized, and when a surface brush border is present, it is sparse and uneven. Mucin secretion is always present and usually extensive throughout the tumour, being evenly distributed in the cytoplasm of the majority of cells. If extracellular, secreted mucin is dispersed in the stroma.

The mode of growth in the two types of tumour varies. Thus intestinal carcinomas are mostly well

defined and show considerable variation in structure in different parts. Inflammatory cell infiltration is usually profuse. Diffuse carcinomas have a more uniform structure, are not so well defined, and are characterized by a wider spread in the mucosa. As a rule, connective-tissue proliferation is more marked and inflammatory cell infiltration less prominent than in intestinal type carcinomas.

Solid and mucinous tumours can occur in both groups but are distinguishable on structural grounds.

Grossly in Lauren's series, 60% of the intestinal

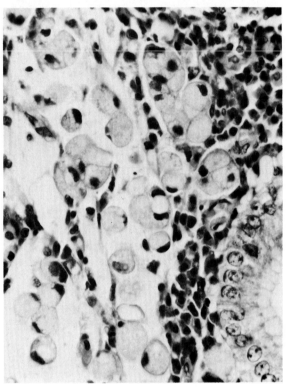

Fig. 5.64 The pale rounded cells in the lamina propria of the gastric mucosa contain globules of mucus that have displaced the nucleus to the periphery of the cytoplasm. The globules differ widely in size; in some cells they have coalesced to occupy most or all of the cytoplasm, in the form of a single vacuole. This illustrates the development of 'signet-ring' cells, so called from the likeness of the peripheral nucleus and single thin-walled vacuole to the outline of such a ring. It can be impossible sometimes to distinguish between mucin-containing tumour cells and macrophages that have taken globules of mucin into their cytoplasm, as may happen not only in simple mucous cysts but also in the stroma of mucinous carcinomas. Part of a normal gastric gland is seen to the right of the picture.

Haematoxylin-eosin × 400

Provided by W. StC. Symmers.

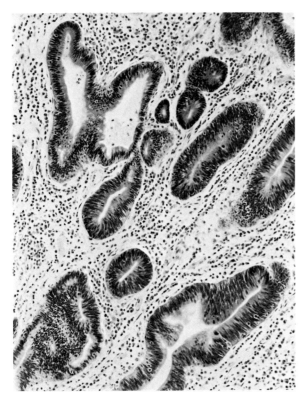

Fig. 5.65 Intestinal type carcinoma. Varying-sized glands are lined by columnar cells which have a prominent brush border. Scattered inflammatory cells are present in the stroma.

Haematoxylin-eosin   × 132

type tumours were polypoid or fungating, 25% excavated and 15% infiltrating whereas the corresponding figures for diffuse carcinomas were 31, 26 and 43% respectively.

An important difference was the increased frequency and extent of intestinal metaplasia in non-tumorous mucosa in the intestinal group compared with the diffuse type carcinomas. Overall, 53% of the tumours were classed as intestinal, 33% diffuse and 14% unclassified because of their atypical or poorly-differentiated structure. When the histology was correlated with clinical features it was found that the mean age of patients with intestinal tumours was 55.4 years and there was a 2:1 male:female ratio. With diffuse carcinomas the sex ratio was approximately one and the mean age of the patients 47.7 years. The 3-year survival rate in the 153 patients with 'curative' treatment was 43% in those with intestinal type tumours, and 35% in the group with diffuse tumours.

The structural and clinical characteristics of the two types of tumour led Lauren to suggest that their aetiology and pathogenesis might be different.

Classification of Mulligan & Rember[323]

The main difference between this classification and that of Lauren is the recognition of the pylorocardiac gland cell carcinoma as a distinct group. These tumours are well demarcated and fungate into the lumen of the stomach or are sometimes widely ulcerated and fibrosed. Microscopically, varying-sized glands are lined by stratified or singly orientated low to tall cylindrical cells. When singly orientated there is often striking vacuolation, giving rise to clear cells (Fig. 5.67) which stain brilliantly with periodic acid-Schiff. Papillary infolding of the glands is sometimes conspicuous or the lining cells may be flattened by inspissated secretion so that a mesothelial appearance results. Tumours have a tendency to be sited in the antrum or at the cardia and as their name suggests are

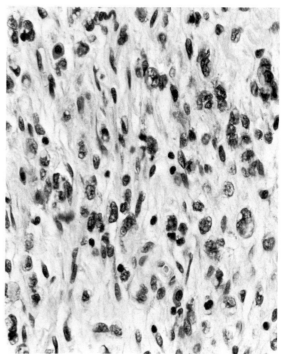

Fig. 5.66 Diffuse type carcinoma. Individual and small groups of tumour cells are present with an intervening fibrous stroma. Inflammatory cells are sparse.

Haematoxylin-eosin   × 600

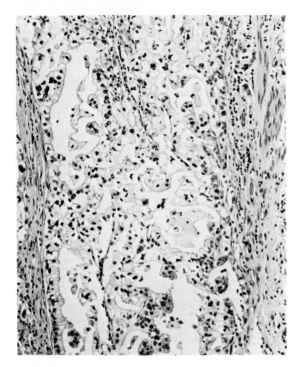

Fig. 5.67 Pyloro-cardiac gland cell carcinoma. Glands show prominent papillary infolding and are lined by cells with a clear cytoplasm.

Haematoxylin-eosin   × 150

presumed to arise from the epithelial cells of the pyloric and cardiac glands deep in the gastric mucosa. The male:female ratio for this type of tumour in Mulligan & Rember's material was 4.13 compared with 2.81 for the whole series.

Classification of Ming[324]

This classification divides tumours into an expanding type (67%) and an infiltrative type (33%). In the former case tumour cells grow *en masse* and by expansion, and result in the formation of discrete tumour nodules, whereas tumour cells of the infiltrative type penetrate individually and widely, eventually resulting in diffuse involvement of the stomach. The primary emphasis in this classification is not the architectural structure of the tumours but their biological behaviour as manifest by their growth patterns. There was some correlation of the two types with their gross appearance.

Thus among the expanding type the tumour was fungating in 63%, ulcerated in 20%, polypoid in 10%, superficial in 4% and diffuse in 3%. With the infiltrative type the carcinoma was diffuse in 68%, ulcerated in 27% and fungating in 5%. The two types of tumour appeared to have a different histogenesis. In the case of expanding tumours there was intestinal metaplasia in the adjacent mucosa of the vast majority which was extensive in half of the cases, and dysplasia of the metaplastic glands was frequent. However, intestinal metaplasia was much less common with infiltrative carcinoma and dysplasia was not seen.

Expanding carcinomas, whatever their degree of differentiation, tended to be surrounded by small amounts of fibrous tissue often associated with varying numbers of lymphocytes and plasma cells, whereas the tumour cells of infiltrative carcinoma were mostly embedded in a densely collagenous and relatively acellular connective tissue. Expanding carcinomas were twice as common in males as in females. Infiltrative carcinomas were equally distributed between the sexes. Both types of cancer occurred predominantly in patients older than 50 years of age but infiltrative carcinoma was more common under the age of 50, particularly in females.

Relative merits of the different classifications

To be of maximum benefit a histological classification of tumours should fulfil three criteria: it should be easy to apply by different pathologists and be reproducible, it should aid in the assessment of the prognosis of the different types of tumour, and it should relate to the histogenesis and if possible the aetiology of the several types of tumour.

The WHO classification fulfils the first criterion if not the latter two, although a considerable proportion of tumours fall into the undifferentiated and unclassified groups, and tumours of mixed appearance are classified according to the predominant component. However, it is of undoubted value as a standard descriptive classification in routine work and serves as a base for achieving international uniformity.

The Lauren classification has been widely used in epidemiological investigations, and most studies in this context have shown that the proportion of intestinal type tumours is greater in high gastric cancer incidence areas than in low-incidence areas, and that when the gastric cancer risk is reduced in a population it is the intestinal type of tumour that accounts for most of the reduction. There have been two main drawbacks to the use of the Lauren classification for routine purposes. The first is that in a considerable proportion of cases both types of pattern are seen, especially when extensive sampling of the tumour is carried out. Secondly, when applied to a series of cases, the 5-year survival rate for both types is approximately the same.[325]

The classification of Mulligan & Rember has not been widely used in practice. This is because of difficulty in distinguishing the pyloro-cardiac gland cell carcinoma from the intestinal type, except when obvious clear cells are present.[326] The high male to female sex ratio of the pyloro-cardiac gland cell carcinoma is of interest in that this has been reported in other studies of tumours, particularly at the cardia but also at the pylorus.[327,328]

The classification of Ming, although based on biological rather than purely structural patterns, in practice is similar to Lauren's but has the advantage that it can be applied to those cases which remain unclassified by the latter system.

EARLY GASTRIC CANCER

Early gastric cancer is defined as a carcinoma which is limited to the mucosa or to the mucosa and submucosa only (Fig. 5.68), irrespective of whether or not metastasis to lymph nodes has occurred. It can be subdivided therefore after histological examination into two groups, intramucosal and submucosal carcinoma, both with potential for lymph node metastasis. The term 'early' is not meant to imply a stage in the genesis of the cancer but is used to mean gastric cancer which can be cured.[329] In fact study of these cancers has shown that some may remain confined to the superficial layers for several years, although expanding laterally to a considerable degree, whereas others penetrate the gastric wall rapidly and can invade into the submucosa when they are of the order of 3–5 mm in diameter.[330,331]

Cases of early gastric cancer as defined above have been reported for many years from several countries under a variety of terms such as superficial spreading carcinoma,[332] surface carcinoma[333] and *cancer gastrique au début*.[334] However, it was as a result of a massive screening programme in Japan in the early 1960s that increasing numbers of early cancers were detected utilizing radiology, partic-

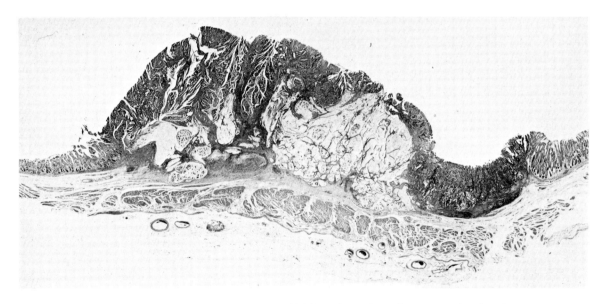

Fig. 5.68 Early gastric cancer. In this example the tumour, which is partly mucinous, has penetrated to the submucosa over much of its extent.

Haematoxylin-eosin   × 5

ularly the double contrast technique, and endoscopy.

Classification

With this very large experience, and on the basis of macroscopic appearances at endoscopy and in gastrectomy specimens, early gastric cancers were classified by the Japan Gastroenterological Endoscopic Society into three main types and three subtypes as follows:

Type I: the *protruded* type. The tumour projects clearly into the lumen and includes all polypoid, nodular and villous tumours.

Type II: the *superficial* type, where unevenness of the surface is inconspicuous. This is further subdivided into three subgroups:

    Type IIa: elevated. This is seen as a flat, plaque-like lesion, well circumscribed and only slightly raised above the surrounding mucosa.

    Type IIb: flat. No abnormality is macroscopically visible apart from some colour change at endoscopy. These lesions are usually found incidentally in carefully examined resection specimens.

    Type IIc: depressed. There is slight depression below the adjacent mucosa. Surface erosion may be apparent from a thin covering of exudate.

Type III: the *excavated* type. There is ulceration of variable depth into the gastric wall. It is rarely seen in pure form and is almost always combined with one or more of the other types.

Combinations of types are commoner than single types and all possible combinations of the five varieties have been documented. When describing a particular lesion the dominant macroscopic feature is placed first, e.g. III + IIc, IIc + III, IIa + IIc. Whereas there is a good correlation between the endoscopic recognition of early gastric cancer by an experienced observer and its subsequent confirmation as such on microscopical examination of the resected specimen, it should be remembered that a similar appearance can result from early and advanced cancers in fixed specimens (Fig. 5.69).

Some clinicians have found this classification cumbersome to use and have suggested that division of early gastric cancers into excavated and

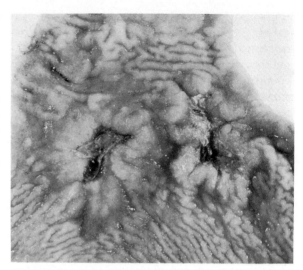

Fig. 5.69 Histological examination of these similar-appearing ulcerated cancers showed the one on the right to have tumour cells infiltrating the whole thickness of the muscularis propria, whereas in the left-hand lesion tumour extended only as far as the submucosa, i.e. by definition it was an early gastric cancer (type IIc + IIa).

protruded forms is as informative.[335] However, there is no doubt that the Japanese classification is more valuable particularly for the description of combinations of types. It has also resulted in a much more careful appraisal of the gastric mucosa by endoscopists looking for the variable, and often extremely subtle, appearances of early gastric cancer, and this has resulted in an increasing proportion of such cancers being diagnosed in countries outside Japan.

Johansen[336] has modified the classification in a helpful way for the pathologist and describes *elevated* (types I and IIa), *depressed* (IIc, IIc + IIa, IIa + IIc), *ulcer-associated* (III, III + IIc, IIc + III) and *imperceptible* (IIb) types. In a study of 90 cases from Denmark, 20 were elevated, 23 depressed, 35 ulcer-associated and 12 imperceptible. Differences have emerged regarding the relative disposition of these various types in different countries, with combination forms of type III making up about 70% of all early gastric cancers in Japan and between 40 and 50% in the main European publications.[336–338]

The location of early gastric cancers is similar to that of advanced gastric cancer with the majority of tumours occurring in pyloric type mucosa and centred on the lesser curve. Despite being limited in their extension through the wall of the stomach they can reach a large size, so that in one series they averaged 30 mm in diameter (range 3–90 mm).[336] Elevated and ulcer-associated cancers tend to be the largest, and imperceptible tumours the smallest. About 10% of gastrectomy specimens in cases of early gastric cancers will show multifocal lesions, and of course early gastric cancer can be associated with advanced tumours also.

Histology

Using the WHO classification[322] early gastric cancers may be grouped into papillary, tubular, mucinous and signet-ring cell carcinomas. The majority have been of tubular or signet-ring cell type with a minority of papillary and mucinous forms. Occasionally a mixed pattern is present. When the histological appearance is compared with the different macroscopic types it is found that elevated early gastric cancers (types I and IIa) are almost invariably well differentiated (Fig. 5.70),[336,339] and imperceptible tumours (type IIb) poorly differentiated (Fig. 5.71). The histology of ulcer-associated lesions has varied in different series with some showing a majority of poorly-differentiated tumours[336] and others a predominance of well- and moderately well-differentiated tumours.[339] A more even distribution of differentiation is seen in depressed early gastric cancers. One study showed that well-differentiated tumours were more likely to have extended to the submucosa whereas poorly-differentiated forms were intramucosal.[336]

The diagnosis of carcinoma from biopsies taken from a lesion suspected of being early gastric cancer by the endoscopist may not be straightforward. The presence of small numbers of undifferentiated or signet-ring cells in the lamina propria (Fig. 5.64) can easily be missed and their detection is facilitated if stains for mucin are routinely employed. As well as this, carcinoma has to be distinguished from regenerating epithelium and from the cellular and architectural abnormalities which make up epithelial dysplasia (see p. 198). The distinction between severe degrees of the latter and highly-differentiated tubular carcinomas such as those comprising many of the type I and IIa

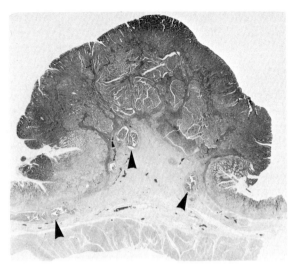

Fig. 5.70 In this polypoid early gastric cancer (type I) well-differentiated adenocarcinoma cells have spread into the submucosa where they have invaded lymphatics (arrowed).
Haematoxylin-eosin   × 4

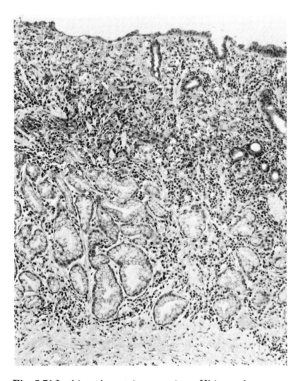

Fig. 5.71 In this early gastric cancer (type IIb), poorly-differentiated carcinoma cells of signet-ring type are present in the lamina propria of the superficial half of the mucosa.
Haematoxylin-eosin   × 153

early gastric cancers, may be very difficult in biopsy material. The term carcinoma-in-situ is best avoided in connection with the gastric mucosa as it has had different connotations when applied by various authors. The expression 'border-line lesion' or 'atypical epithelium'[226] has been employed by the Japanese to describe the histology of macroscopically round, elevated or protruded lesions of the gastric mucosa which resemble a type IIa early gastric cancer. They comprise well-demarcated, slightly atypical but regularly arranged glands of the superficial layer of the mucosa made up of tall, columnar cells with elongated rod-shaped nuclei. Paneth and goblet cells are often seen and in the deeper part of the mucosa normal gastric glands remain, often accompanied by numerous microcysts. It is now generally agreed that these represent slightly elevated or even flat adenomas which progress only slowly, or in some cases possibly not at all, to invasive carcinoma. There is good evidence that a sizeable proportion of type I and IIa early gastric cancers result from malignant change in an adenoma. Thus residual adenomatous components may be seen on histological examination of such lesions,[340] and associated adenomas may be present elsewhere in the stomach.

Considerable disagreement exists regarding the frequency of ulcer-cancer but, if strict criteria are adhered to, the incidence is low. That the ulceration is usually a secondary phenomenon was suggested from a study of early gastric cancers grouped according to their largest diameter, where it was shown that the tendency to undergo erosion or ulceration was directly correlated with increasing size.[341]

Histogenesis

It might be expected that increased availability of cancers limited to the mucosa and submucosa should improve knowledge regarding the histogenesis of carcinoma of the stomach. However, no major advance has resulted from recent research. Many of the tumours have arisen on the basis of chronic atrophic gastritis with intestinal metaplasia. Even tumours where intestinal metaplasia is minimal or absent in the adjacent mucosa can often show metaplastic features. Study of very small signet-ring cell tumours has shown cells in intimate

association with the germinal zone of the glands, suggesting an origin from undifferentiated cells at the base of the gastric crypts. An origin from glandular cells of the pylorus and cardia has been postulated[323] but not convincingly demonstrated.

Whether early gastric cancer represents an incipient stage in all types of advanced gastric cancer is not clear. Typing of early gastric cancers into intestinal and diffuse varieties using Lauren's classification showed a higher mean age and male to female ratio in the intestinal group,[336] which corresponds to the situation in advanced gastric cancers.

Prognosis

The 5-year survival rate of advanced gastric cancer, when a potentially curative operation has been carried out, is of the order of 20%. Early gastric cancer has a much more favourable prognosis. In one Japanese survey based on 2364 operated cases of early gastric cancer the 5-year survival was calculated to be 93.4% for intramucosal carcinomas without lymph node metastasis and 91.5% when these were present. The corresponding figures for submucosal carcinomas were 89.0 and 80.5% respectively. Metastatic tumour in lymph nodes was present in 5.3% of the intramucosal carcinoma patients and in 19.6% of the submucosal carcinoma group.[342]

The high incidence of gastric cancer in Japan and the widespread use of upper gastrointestinal endoscopy has resulted in a situation where approximately 30% of gastrectomies for carcinoma are for early disease. The rate is considerably less outside Japan, but in specialist centres the diagnosis of early gastric cancer is being made much more frequently, and this has been brought about by the close co-operation of radiologist, endoscopist and pathologist.

Spread of gastric carcinoma

Direct. Gastric carcinomas are highly infiltrative tumours and in resection specimens the majority have extended into the subserosa. According to the site of the primary growth, penetration of the serosa may result in direct spread to pancreas, liver, spleen, transverse colon and omentum, and often leads to early transperitoneal dissemination. Adhesions between the primary growth and neighbouring structures, particularly transverse colon, are common, and tumour cells grow along them to reach the diaphragm or abdominal wall. Tumours at the cardiac end of the stomach infiltrate freely into the oesophagus both along the mucosal surface and within the wall (Fig. 5.72), and at the distal end extension into the duodenum, observed microscopically, is not uncommon,[343] particularly with carcinomas located less than 1 cm from the pyloric ring. There are a number of interesting reports of cases of linitis plastica where cancer cells have extended along the wall of long segments of the intestinal tract, producing an induration rather like that found in the stomach itself,[344] or more commonly have given rise to single or multiple strictures of the small or large intestine. Poorly-differentiated carcinoma cells are present in tissue spaces and lymphatics, and it is possible that peristalsis has played a part in their onward propulsion.

Macroscopical observation and palpation cannot be relied upon to define the margins of either early or advanced gastric cancer at operation and frozen section examinations of resected margins, particularly where the margin of excision is less than 4 cm, are desirable to ensure that recurrence does not occur in the gastric remnant.

Lymphatic. Lymph node metastases are present in 90% of autopsies on gastric carcinomas and in 70% of surgical resections. Their distribution varies according to the location of the tumour. Involvement of nodes along the lesser and greater curves is common and extension to the next zone, namely the para-aortic nodes and those of the coeliac axis, is often seen. Tumours of the mid-portion of the stomach may give rise to metastasis in pancreatic and splenic nodes, and lesions high in the stomach can metastasize to mediastinal lymph nodes. Spread by way of the thoracic duct to the left supraclavicular nodes (the 'sentinel' or 'signal' nodes of Troisier and of Virchow), though well recognized clinically, is not common. It is important for the surgeon to remove, and the pathologist to examine, all nodes, however small, since even the smallest apparently uninvolved node may contain secondary growth, and there is evidence that prognosis depends on the number of nodes involved.

Occasionally there is generalized involvement of serosal lymphatics by tumour, leading to a 'sugar icing' effect.

Bloodstream. Spread via the bloodstream results

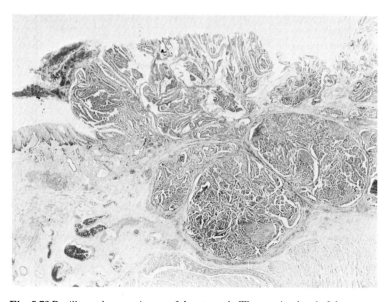

Fig. 5.72 Papillary adenocarcinoma of the stomach. The proximal end of the tumour is undermining oesophageal epithelium.

Haematoxylin-eosin ×10

from invasion of tributaries of the portal venous system and may occur even in the absence of lymph node involvement. Metastases can occur in almost any organ but are most commonly seen in the liver, followed by lung, skin and ovaries: the latter are also involved by transperitoneal spread.

Transperitoneal. Secondary deposits of tumour from carcinoma of the stomach are common in omentum, peritoneum and mesentery but are rare over the spleen; it is almost impossible to determine whether these are blood-borne, or due to transperitoneal spread of cancer cells. The same applies to secondary ovarian deposits, well known as one form of Krukenberg tumour.

Prognosis of gastric carcinoma

The dismal overall prognosis of gastric carcinoma, with 5-year survival rates of between 20–30% for advanced cancer after gastrectomy, has led to much endeavour towards earlier diagnosis. The experience of the Japanese has shown that diagnosis and surgery of early gastric cancer results in 5-year survival rates of the order of 90%.[345]

Prognosis bears no relationship to macroscopic type of growth, location of tumour or duration of symptoms prior to surgical treatment.[346-348] It depends mostly on the presence or absence of involved lymph nodes.

Lymph node involvement. The prognosis is markedly better when no lymph nodes are involved, and better than average when only one or two nodes are affected.[349] As mentioned above, a careful search for, and histological examination of, all lymph nodes must be made, as absence of enlargement is no criterion of freedom from metastasis.

Size of tumour. There is some evidence that the prognosis is better for tumours less than 2 cm in diameter.[350]

Histological features related to prognosis. Study of the pathology of gastric cancer in long-term survivors has shown an association with particular characteristics of tumours or particular types of tumour. Thus circumscribed growths with a smooth or scalloped border which advance through the gastric wall en bloc were present in 25 of 30 patients who survived five years after gastric resection.[351] A 'pushing' margin or a combination of a 'pushing' and infiltrating margin was associated with a 52.6% 5-year survival in a group of 19 patients (12 with tumour in local lymph nodes) compared with a 12.8% survival in 86 patients where the tumour margin was entirely infiltrating.[352]

The inflammatory reaction in the stroma of tumours has been investigated in several studies[325,353,354] which have shown that as a general rule the prognosis is better in tumours with a pronounced lymphocytic and plasma cell infiltrate. In one large series of surgically removed tumours, 4% had distinctive gross and microscopic features. They were well circumscribed with a homogeneous cut surface and a rather soft consistency, similar to a malignant lymphoma. Histologically, uniformly distributed groups of polygonal, small to medium-sized cells with little pleomorphism and only occasional mitoses were separated by a dense infiltrate of lymphocytes and plasma cells. The margin of the tumour was sharply defined. Even with invasion of the serosa the prognosis in this group of patients was good.[355] The same type of tumour has been referred to as a 'blue cell carcinoma'[351] because of its appearance at low magnification, and as 'medullary carcinoma with lymphoid infiltration'.[356]

Another type of tumour which, although uncommon, appears to have a good prognosis is composed of lakes of extracellular mucus in which tumour cells float either singly or in groups often arranged as tubules or ribbons (Fig. 5.63).[357] Here again the tumour has a rounded or 'pushing' margin.

SQUAMOUS CELL AND ADENOSQUAMOUS CARCINOMA

A pure squamous carcinoma at the cardia is likely to be of primary oesophageal origin. Pure squamous cell carcinoma of the stomach does occur but is exceedingly rare, and a glandular component is often present when such tumours are extensively sampled following resection.[358] They have been described as a complication of gastric involvement in tertiary syphilis[359] and were observed in two patients following long-term cyclophosphamide therapy.[360]

Occasional cases of adenosquamous carcinoma

have been reported in the stomach,[358,361] mostly in the distal half. They comprise varying proportions of glandular and squamous neoplastic tissue (Fig. 5.73).

NON-EPITHELIAL TUMOURS

The overall prevalence of non-epithelial neoplasms of the stomach is low, and apart from smooth muscle tumours and primary neoplasms of lymphoid tissue, other types are rare.

Lipomas

Gastric lipomas are rare, and important only because they may give rise to severe haemorrhage or chronic anaemia, which is curable by excision of the tumour.[362,363] They are single, often large, and lobulated. They arise from the normal adipose tissue of the submucosa, usually in the antrum, and project into the lumen; rarely, they become pedunculated. Microscopically, they consist of normal adipose tissue and many would consider them as hamartomas rather than neoplasms.

Smooth muscle tumours

Although smooth muscle tumours of the stomach are often found at autopsy,[364] and the stomach is the commonest site in the gastrointestinal tract for such tumours, symptomatic lesions are uncommon, occurring in approximately 0.2% of examinations in one endoscopic series.[365] Presentation in such cases is usually with bleeding as a result of mucosal ulceration over the tumour, iron-deficiency anaemia, or abdominal pain. Males are more likely to be affected than females and most patients are between 30 and 70 years old. Macroscopically, the tumours are tan, grey or pink in colour and are usually well circumscribed. Larger tumours, particularly those that are malignant, may show areas of haemorrhage, necrosis and cystic degeneration. When small they occupy an intramural position but with increasing size project either into the lumen of the stomach (endogastric—Fig. 5.74), or on to the serosal aspect (exogastric). A few project in both directions giving a 'dumb-bell' appearance. Occasional endogastric tumours are pedunculated.

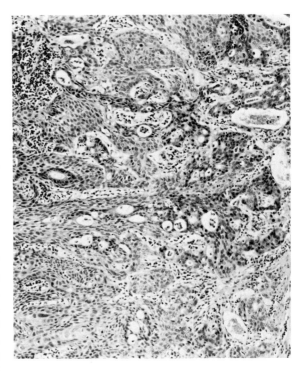

Fig. 5.73 Adenosquamous carcinoma. An admixture of glandular and squamous carcinoma is present. The tumour grossly was a plaque-like lesion on the anterior wall of the mid-stomach.

Haematoxylin-eosin   × 150

Distribution is fairly uniform throughout the cardia, fundus and pylorus.

Microscopically, a very wide range of appearances may be present even in sections from different parts of the same tumour and this can make classification of individual tumours as benign or malignant difficult. The commonest basic pattern is of easily recognizable bundles of spindle-shaped smooth muscle cells with elongated nuclei and abundant cytoplasm interspersed with varying amounts of collagen fibres and arranged in whorls and interlacing bundles. A palisade arrangement of nuclei is frequent and has led to many of these tumours being misdiagnosed as schwannomas. Individual nuclei sometimes show bizarre changes, including irregular distribution of chromatin. Giant cell forms, which are probably degenerative and certainly do not necessarily indicate malignancy, are common. In the more slowly growing tumours a pseudocapsule of compressed surrounding muscle is present, but more rapidly growing

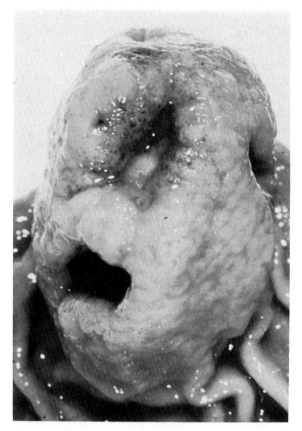

Fig. 5.74 Smooth muscle tumour. This 6 cm diameter tumour was present in the body of the stomach. Several crateriform areas of ulceration interrupt the overlying mucosa.

tumours appear to infiltrate the surrounding tissues diffusely.

A well-characterized variant[366,367] consists of large, rounded and polygonal cells with a centrally located nucleus and abundant slightly acidophilic cytoplasm. Perinuclear cytoplasmic vacuolation is common but has been shown to be a fixation artefact (Fig. 5.75).[368] Tumours of this pattern have been variously referred to as leiomyoblastomas and bizarre smooth muscle tumours but the terms epithelioid leiomyoma and epithelioid leiomyosarcoma are preferred to describe this variant of benign and malignant smooth muscle tumours. Examination of smooth muscle tumours predominantly of ordinary type will not infrequently reveal focal areas with an epithelioid pattern.

It can be difficult, and sometimes impossible, to say whether a smooth muscle neoplasm will behave as a benign or malignant tumour. Those features, taken together, which are most helpful are the gross size, the number of mitotic figures present, and infiltration of surrounding tissues. Cellular pleomorphism and hyperchromasia are less reliable indicators of malignancy.[367,369]

The prognosis of malignant tumours is adversely affected by high histopathological grade of malignancy, a size of more than 5 cm in diameter, and by invasion of adjacent organs such as the liver, pancreas or retroperitoneal soft tissues.[370] Metastasis to regional lymph nodes is uncommon, occurring only in the most anaplastic patterns of tumour.

Tumours and tumour-like conditions of lymphoid tissue

Benign lymphoid hyperplasia (pseudolymphoma)

This uncommon lesion most frequently presents as an ulcer with overhanging margins, but nodularity and an infiltrative appearance of surrounding

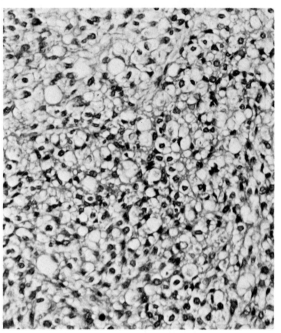

Fig. 5.75 Smooth muscle tumour. This tumour is composed of round and polygonal cells with variably-sized nuclei and abundant cytoplasm containing clear spaces. The term epithelioid leiomyoma is given to this variant.

Haematoxylin-eosin   × 600

tissue may be present. Sometimes there is a mass or plaque without gross ulceration. Although usually single, multiple lesions can occur. The antrum is the usual site.[371] In general they have a smaller diameter and present in a younger age group than malignant lymphomas, but there is considerable overlap. The diagnosis of benign lymphoid hyperplasia has frequently only been made after re-analysis of resection specimens or surgical biopsies originally diagnosed as malignant lymphoma, but associated with long-term survival.

Histologically, the predominant cells are lymphocytes although other cell types including eosinophils, polymorphs and plasma cells may be encountered. Prominent reactive follicle centres are seen amidst the lymphoid infiltrate, and the latter is frequently dissected and separated by bands of fibrous tissue. Although the changes are most marked and may be confined to the mucosa and submucosa (Fig. 5.76), it is not uncommon for

transmural and serosal involvement to occur. In the latter case muscle fibres are separated and not destroyed by the infiltrate. Ulceration of overlying mucosa is common and there may be evidence of previous peptic ulceration, in the form of dense scar tissue replacing muscle. The lesions are not clearly demarcated and tend to fade gradually into adjacent fibromuscular tissue. Chronic follicular gastritis is frequently present in adjacent mucosa (see p. 163).

Benign lymphoid hyperplasia (pseudolymphoma) is considered to be an exaggerated response to peptic ulceration, but the changes may persist following healing of the ulcer. Although generally considered to be benign, recent reports of focal lymphoma associated with a pseudolymphomatous reaction,[372] of transitional zones between benign reactive follicles and lymphomatous nodules[373] and of monotypic cytoplasmic immunoglobulin in the infiltrate of some cases of morphologically typical

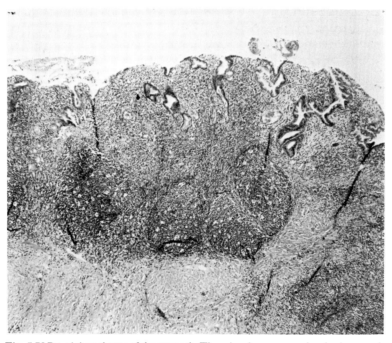

Fig. 5.76 Pseudolymphoma of the stomach. There is a dense mucosal and submucosal cellular infiltrate with underlying fibrous tissue. Associated glandular distortion and focal erosion of the surface epithelium is present. Several lymphoid follicles are present at the junction of mucosa and submucosa.

Haematoxylin-eosin   × 37

Histological preparation provided for photography by Dr A. J. Blackshaw, Bedford General Hospital, Bedford.

pseudolymphomas,[374] suggest that this lesion has malignant potential. A similar progression from a benign lymphoproliferative lesion has been proposed for some malignant lymphomas developing in other extranodal sites such as the thyroid and the salivary glands.

Malignant lymphoma

Primary lymphomas represent some 1.5–3.5% of malignant tumours of the stomach and are the commonest non-epithelial malignancy. The stomach is the major extranodal site for these tumours. The clinical presentation and macroscopic appearances are often indistinguishable from gastric carcinoma but their behaviour and prognosis differ. The age at diagnosis of gastric lymphoma varies widely but in most cases is over 50 with a peak prevalence in the seventh decade. The sex distribution is approximately equal. The common presenting symptoms are abdominal pain, nausea and vomiting, weight loss, loss of appetite and melaena. In a minority a mass is palpable.

Macroscopically, the tumours are most common in the body, are sometimes seen in the antrum and pylorus, and are rare at the cardia. They can be multiple or widely diffused, and are then difficult to distinguish from superficial spreading or 'leather-bottle' carcinomas. They originate in lymphoid tissue in the lamina propria and submucosa, and infiltrate beneath the mucosa, forming nodular or polypoid masses which project into the lumen. Sometimes, a more diffuse plaque-like or generalized thickening of the mucosa and submucosa occurs. The overlying mucosa often shows a cobblestone pattern and may ulcerate, to produce one or more wide, shallow ulcers with overhanging edges and a greyish-yellow base (Fig. 5.77). These resemble carcinomatous ulcers but can be distinguished by a curious thickening of the adjacent mucosa, which forms a type of giant rugose hypertrophy.

Histologically, gastric lymphomas show a range of appearances. It is generally agreed that primary Hodgkin's disease of the stomach is exceptionally rare. Most of the non-Hodgkin's lymphomas are diffuse but approximately one-fifth have a nodular component. Using the Rappaport classification[375] the majority have been of diffuse 'histiocytic' type, with poorly-differentiated lymphocytic lymphomas forming the next commonest group. Newer classifications are based not only on morphological

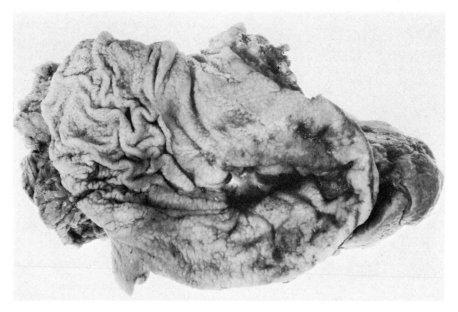

Fig. 5.77 Primary malignant lymphoma of the stomach. This large ulcerated lesion was present in the body of the stomach. It had infiltrated through the wall of the stomach although regional lymph nodes were not involved.

characteristics but take into account as well the functional properties of the cells,[373,376,377] and immunological techniques used to determine surface antigens[378] and the presence of intracytoplasmic immunoglobulin[379,380] have suggested that many of these tumours are of B-cell origin. Most can be categorized as follicle centre cell lymphomas and consist of variable proportions of centrocytes and centroblasts. In some high-grade tumours, immunoblasts have been the predominant cell type. It is probable, however, that a minority are non-B-cell tumours and represent true histiocytic lymphomas,[379,381] but the prevalence of this subgroup is disputed and may reflect geographical and perhaps ethnic differences in the material studied.

Independent of the constituent cells which comprise a malignant lymphoma, the overall appearances are of a diffusely infiltrative pattern which often leaves mucosal glands intact. Although some variation in cell size is usually present the infiltrate is essentially monomorphous (Fig. 5.78),

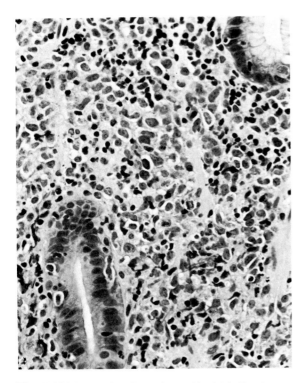

Fig. 5.78 Malignant lymphoma (centroblastic) infiltrating mucosa of stomach with preservation of the gastric foveolae.
Haematoxylin-eosin × 375

contrasting with the polymorphous nature of the infiltrate in pseudolymphoma. Nuclear size and mitotic rate are also useful features enabling delineation from benign lesions in the majority of cases.[382] Focal invasion of glandular epithelium by centrocytes and centroblasts may be seen and, when present, these so-called lympho-epithelial lesions are considered to be pathognomonic of follicle centre cell lymphoma.[383] The spread of lymphoma through the gastric wall is variable, but low-grade tumours showing plasmacytic differentiation tend to be more superficial than high-grade lesions such as diffuse centroblastic lymphomas, where full thickness invasion is more frequent.[384]

The prognosis of gastric lymphomas is better overall than for other gastrointestinal lymphomas and carcinomas, and relates best to the stage of the disease.[382,385,386] In one series after surgical resection for cure the overall 5-year disease-free survival was 47%. In those without spread to perigastric lymph nodes the survival rate was 78% decreasing to 29% where local nodal involvement was present.[386] Large tumours,[382,386] and those where ulceration has occurred,[379] have also been associated with a poorer prognosis in some reports.

Plasmacytoma

Primary solitary or multiple plasmacytomas confined to the stomach are rare,[387] although one report considered that almost one-third of gastric lymphomas were of this type.[388] This was probably because of the inclusion of tumours showing plasmacytoid differentiation such as lymphoplasmacytic lymphomas (immunocytomas) and follicle centre cell lymphomas. If the term is restricted to tumours in which there is a monotonous proliferation of plasma cells and in which there is monotypic staining using immunohistochemical techniques,[389] the prevalence seems to be low. Most lesions have been in the distal part of the stomach and macroscopically are indistinguishable from carcinoma or other lymphoid neoplasms. Paraproteins are seldom present in the serum and urine. Occasionally the stomach is involved secondarily in myelomatosis and this may result in multiple polyps.[390]

So-called *plasma cell granuloma* is an inflammatory condition of unknown cause which has to be differentiated from plasmacytoma. It may mimic a carcinoma at endoscopy and histologically consists of large numbers of mature plasma cells scattered in vascular granulation tissue. Intra- or extracellular hyaline globules of immunoglobulin are often conspicuous. The polyclonal immunoglobulin pattern, demonstrable immunohistochemically, confirms the reactive nature of this lesion.[391,392]

Vascular tumours

Glomus tumour

These rare lesions arise from glomus bodies near arteriovenous anastomoses and present as solid or occasionally cystic submucosal tumours in the distal part of the stomach.[393,394] Extension into the muscularis propria may occur and ulceration of overlying mucosa results in bleeding, the major clinical symptom. Microscopically, they consist of lobules of very uniform cells containing round nuclei with coarsely clumped chromatin and with a moderate amount of eosinophilic cytoplasm. A clear zone partly or completely surrounding the nucleus may be present. Between and within tumour lobules are tortuous and branched, thin-walled and generally empty vascular channels lined by normal endothelium. On ultrastructural examination the tumour cells have shown features of smooth muscle or characteristics of pericytes.[395]

Kaposi's sarcoma

Kaposi's sarcoma is a rare neoplasm of primitive vasoformative mesenchyme[396] which in Europe and North America has typically involved the skin of the legs of elderly males and run an indolent course. Visceral involvement is uncommon. Recently, however, there have been increasing reports of an uncommonly severe form of the disease with a widespread distribution of skin lesions, generalized lymphadenopathy and visceral involvement, and often associated with unusual opportunistic pathogens, affecting young homosexual males in the USA and elsewhere.[397,398] These individuals have all had an acquired severe defect in cell-mediated immunity, referred to as the acquired immunodeficiency syndrome (AIDS). Kaposi's sarcomas have also arisen in patients with induced immune deficiency, e.g. following renal transplantation.[399] In these groups involvement of the gastrointestinal tract is common although often asymptomatic and at endoscopy of the upper gastrointestinal tract the stomach has shown a range of appearances from multiple, purple, maculo-papular lesions up to 5 mm in diameter to larger nodular or polypoid areas, or nodules with central umbilication.[400] Histologically, intertwining bundles of atypical spindle-shaped cells are interspersed with endothelium-lined vascular spaces. Extravasated red blood cells, lymphocytes and histiocytes are present (Fig. 5.79). The visceral lesions have responded to chemotherapy, whereas local irradiation is the preferred treatment for the lesions of the skin.

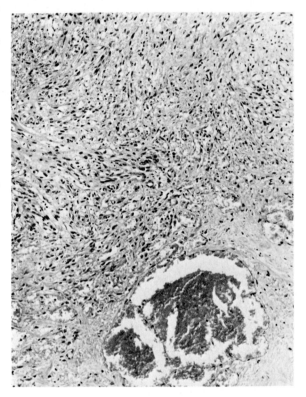

Fig. 5.79 Kaposi's sarcoma involving the stomach. Vascular spaces with interlacing spindle cells are present in the submucosa. The section was taken from one of several haemorrhagic lesions found in the stomach at postmortem in a young woman dying from acquired immune deficiency syndrome (AIDS).

Haematoxylin-eosin   × 150

Histological preparation provided for photography by Dr T. R. Helliwell, Department of Pathology, University of Liverpool.

Tumours of nervous tissue

These include small traumatic neuromas, which may be in the base of an ulcer or ulcer scar, and neurofibromas and neurilemmomas (schwannomas) both of which are uncommon symptomatic lesions. The latter may occur in neurofibromatosis when the tumours are multiple and usually grouped closely together. Tumours of nervous tissue containing ganglion cells are rare.[401,402]

Occasional examples of *granular cell tumours* have occurred in the stomach.[403] These have been well circumscribed, submucosal tumours up to 4 cm in diameter. Some have been associated with ulceration of the overlying mucosa. Ultrastructural studies[404] have shown features similar to those of Schwann cells.

Other tumours

Occasional examples of primary choriocarcinoma of the stomach have been reported, with a mixture of trophoblastic and carcinoma cells in either the primary tumour or its metastases. In some, chorionic gonadotrophin activity was present in the serum or demonstrated immunohistochemically in the tumour cells.[405,406]

Other rare tumours include rhabdomyosarcoma,[407] xanthofibroma,[408] and haemangiopericytoma.[409]

Metastatic tumours are uncommon in the stomach. Most are asymptomatic but they can cause haematemesis, pyloric obstruction or perforation.[410,411] The primary tumour has usually been a carcinoma of breast,[412] lung, pancreas, thyroid or prostate or a malignant melanoma.[413] The secondary deposits may be single or multiple and frequently show central ulceration or umbilication. Diffuse infiltration of the gastric wall by metastatic lobular carcinoma of the breast may simulate linitis plastica.[414] Leukaemic involvement of the stomach[415,416] occurs in approximately 5% of cases and takes the form of nodules, plaques, or diffuse infiltrations of the mucosa and submucosa. Overlying mucosal ulceration is common.

OTHER CONDITIONS

Menetrier's disease

Approximately 300 cases of this enigmatic disorder have been reported since its original description.[417] Grossly the stomach is characterized by enormous thickening of gastric folds which may additionally have a nodular or polypoid appearance. Body mucosa is affected particularly along the greater curve, and the antrum is usually spared (Fig. 5.80).[418] The involved areas typically resemble cerebral convolutions. The common clinical symptoms associated with these changes are epigastric pain, which is often food-related, weight loss, vomiting and diarrhoea. Occasionally presentation is with haematemesis or melaena. Acid-secretion studies show that the majority of patients have hypo- or achlorhydria,[419] and there is a non-selective loss of plasma proteins into the gastric lumen, often resulting in a low serum albumin and sometimes associated with peripheral oedema.

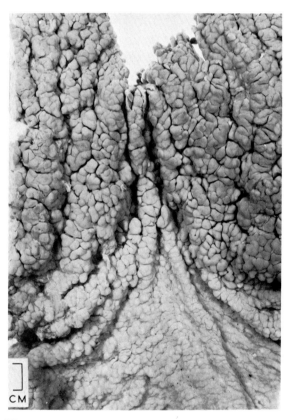

Fig. 5.80 The stomach in Menetrier's disease. The nodular, furrowed appearance predominantly affecting the body mucosa is typical of this rare condition.

Specimen from the Pathology Museum, Charing Cross Hospital Medical School, London, by permission of the Curator, Dr F. J. Paradinas. Photograph by Miss P. M. Turnbull, Charing Cross Hospital Medical School.

Microscopically, the mucosa is markedly thickened due to extreme elongation and tortuosity of the gastric pits and to a lesser extent to elongation of the glands (Fig. 5.81). This is most prominent in the apical regions of the gastric folds, and between the folds the mucosa may be of normal thickness. The body glands may contain a relatively normal distribution of specialized cells but usually there is a variable replacement by mucin-secreting cells. In the deeper part, cystic dilatations containing mucin develop; these are lined by superficial type epithelium and sometimes push down through the muscularis mucosae, which also grows up between the tubules. There may be pseudo-pyloric, but rarely intestinal, mucosal metaplasia, and the lamina propria is oedematous and infiltrated by lymphocytes, plasma cells and polymorphs. Lymphoid follicles can be prominent.

The nature of Menetrier's disease is unknown

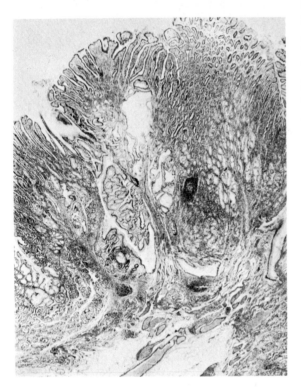

Fig. 5.81 Gastric body mucosa in Menetrier's disease. The mucosa is markedly thickened. Many of the glands are lined by mucous cells and similar cells line cystic spaces deep in the mucosa.

Haematoxylin-eosin   × 15

and its aetiology may be multifactorial. The few cases reported in children have been of a self-limited illness, and the presence of a peripheral eosinophilia in the majority has suggested the possibility of an allergic reaction in this age group.[420] The natural history of the disease in adults is unclear since in most reported cases a gastric resection has been carried out soon after diagnosis. There have been occasional examples of spontaneous remission in which protein loss from the stomach has stopped, and this has been accompanied by histological transition to an atrophic gastritis.[421,422]

A major point of controversy has related to the cancer risk in Menetrier's disease.[423] In several cases the finding of thickened gastric folds at endoscopy, or after radiological examination at the time of diagnosis of gastric cancer, has been attributed to Menetrier's disease, but adequate histological confirmation has been lacking and it is more likely that an infiltrating carcinoma has given rise to this appearance secondarily. As well as this, gastric resection soon after the diagnosis of Menetrier's disease has been the usual method of treatment in the past so that in these instances any possible cancer risk could not be assessed. There are, however, a few bona fide cases[423–425] where gastric cancer has been detected several years after the diagnosis of Menetrier's disease and which lend support therefore to its being a premalignant condition.

Gastric xanthelasma

These lesions, also known as lipid islands, have been noted at endoscopy in 0.4–6.3% of non-operated patients[426,427] but their prevalence is higher in patients with a gastric stump, increasing with the length of follow-up.[426]

Macroscopically (Fig. 5.82), they appear as yellow or orange, clearly demarcated macules with a somewhat irregular outline, mostly 1–2 mm in diameter and rarely exceeding 5 mm. They occur preferentially in the antrum and related to the lesser curve in non-operated subjects, and close to the stoma, on the posterior wall, or along the greater curvature in operated patients. Xanthelasma may be single or multiple but rarely exceed 10 in number.

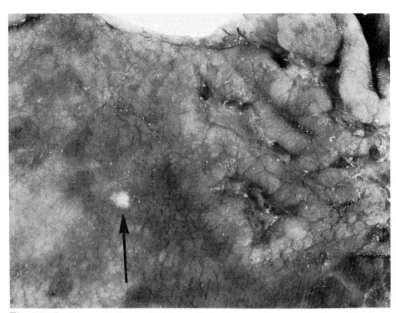

Fig. 5.82 Gastric xanthelasma. This 2 mm lesion (arrowed) was an incidental finding in a gastrectomy specimen resected for gastric carcinoma (seen at right).

Histologically, a focal group of foam cells is present in the lamina propria (Fig. 5.83) predominantly in the superficial parts of the mucosa. Individual cells are polygonal or rounded with distinct cell outlines and are from 10–30 µm in diameter. The cytoplasm has a distinctive fine mesh-like network and the nucleus is small, round or oval, and central, or slightly eccentric. No mitoses or atypia are present.

The most important distinction in practice is from infiltrating carcinoma of signet-ring and other mucus-secreting varieties,[428,429] particularly in the setting of the postoperative stomach where there is an increased risk of malignancy. Apart from the endoscopic appearances when present, and the cytological features described above, the use of a periodic acid-Schiff/alcian blue (PAS/AB) stain is very helpful in differentiating the two, as carcinoma cells will stain strongly due to their content of either PAS or alcian blue positive mucin (not infrequently a mixture), whereas foam cells are unstained or only faintly PAS positive. Foam cells are also sudanophilic.

The pathogenesis of these lesions is unclear. Chemical analysis has shown the presence of cholesterol in all and of neutral fat in one-third.[430] The association with chronic gastritis and intestinal metaplasia and their frequency in the operated stomach suggests that biliary reflux is an important aetiological factor. Ultrastructural studies suggest that the foam cells originate from two sources, histiocytes and smooth muscle cells.[431]

Vascular abnormalities

Haemangiomas and hereditary or acquired telangiectasias are rare vascular malformations in the stomach. Most haemangiomas are small although occasional large lesions have been reported.[432] Sometimes they are polypoid. In hereditary haemorrhagic telangiectasia (Osler-Weber-Rendu syndrome) gastrointestinal bleeding, often recurrent, occurs in some 20% of cases.[433] Multiple lesions may be observed at gastroscopy.[434] Acquired telangiectasias (also referred to as angiodysplasia) of the stomach have been reported in a number of clinical settings including systemic sclerosis,[435] following irradiation therapy,[436] and in patients undergoing long-term haemodialysis.[437] As with angiodysplasia of the large bowel (see p. 354) a significant proportion of reported cases have been in elderly individuals with aortic valve disease,[436] particularly aortic stenosis. The pathogenesis of acquired telangiectases in these disparate circumstances is not clear, although it is likely that multiple factors are involved. Mechanisms which

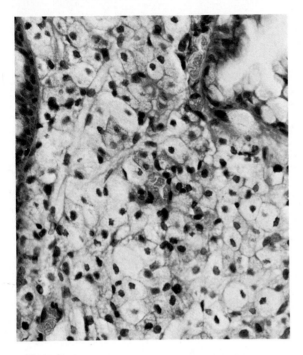

Fig. 5.83 Gastric xanthelasma. Foamy macrophages fill the lamina propria between epithelial crypts.

Haematoxylin-eosin   × 600

have been proposed include weakening of vessel walls due to degenerative disease, ischaemia resulting from low flow states, or low-grade venous obstruction as a result of muscle contraction and organ distension. Cholesterol embolization has also been suggested as one cause of angiodysplastic lesions in the gastrointestinal tract.[438] Microscopically, there is dilatation of veins, venules and capillaries in the submucosa and lamina propria. These lesions may be very difficult to identify in resection specimens unless specific vascular injection techniques are carried out.[439,440]

Ectasia of mucosal capillaries associated with fibromuscular hyperplasia of the lamina propria and thickening of the mucosa has been described in individuals with chronic iron deficiency anaemia and who have a distinctive appearance at endoscopy consisting of parallel longitudinal rugal folds traversing the gastric antrum and each containing a visible convoluted and sacculated column of blood vessels.[441] These changes probably result from mucosal prolapse, and the pathological features are analogous to those seen in so-called solitary ulcer of the rectum (see p. 352).

REFERENCES

Anatomy

1. Piasecki C. J Anat 1974; 118: 295.
2. Salem SN, Truelove SC. Br Med J 1964; ii: 1503.
3. Goldstein AMB, Brothers MR, Davis EA jr. J Anat 1969; 104: 539.
4. Rubin W, Ross LL, Sleisenger MH, Jeffries GH. Lab Invest 1968; 19: 598.
5. Hogben CAM, Kent TH, Woodward PA, Sill AJ. Gastroenterol 1974; 67: 1143.
6. Landboe-Christensen E. Acta Pathol Microbiol Scand 1944; 54 (suppl): 671.
7. Oi M, Oshida K, Sugimura S. Gastroenterol 1959; 36: 45.
8. Tominaga K. Gastroenterol 1975; 69: 1201.
9. Grossman MI. Gastroenterol 1960; 38: 1.
10. Lechago J. In: Sommers SC, Rosen PP, eds. Pathology annual, vol 13, part 2. New York: Appleton-Century Crofts, 1978: 329.
11. O'Briain DS, Dayal Y. In: De Lellis RA, ed. Diagnostic immunocytochemistry. New York: Masson, 1981: 75.
12. Bishop AE, Polak JM, Facer P, Ferri G-L, Marangos PJ, Pearse AGE. Gastroenterol 1982; 83: 902.
13. Voillemot N, Potet F, Mary JY, Lewin MJM. Gastroenterol 1978; 75: 61.

Functional considerations

14. Watkins WM. Science 1977; 152: 172.

15. Menguy R, Masters BS. Surg Gynec Obstet 1965; 120: 92.
16. Bickel M, Kauffman GL. Gastroenterol 1981; 80: 770.
17. Flemström G, Turnberg LA. Clin Gastroenterol 1984; 13: 327.
18. Helander HF, Hirschowitz BI. Gastroenterol 1972; 63: 951.
19. Haglund U, Elander B, Fellenius E, Leth R, Rehnberg O, Olbe L. Scand J Gastroenterol 1982; 17: 455.
20. Samloff M. In: Berk JE, ed. Developments in digestive diseases, vol 2. Philadelphia: Lea & Febiger, 1979: 1.
21. Levine JS, Nakane PK, Allen RH. Gastroenterol 1980; 79: 493.
22. Chanarin I. Gut 1968; 9: 373.
23. Konturek SJ. In: Duthie HL, Wormsley KG, eds. Scientific basis of gastroenterology. Edinburgh: Churchill Livingstone, 1979: 133.
24. Heading RC. In: Reis Lvd, ed. Frontiers of gastrointestinal research, vol 6. Basel: Karger, 1980: 35.

Developmental anomalies

25. Burnett HA, Halpert B. Arch Pathol 1947; 44: 318.
26. Sames CP. Br J Surg 1949–50; 37: 244.
27. Rota AN. Arch Pathol 1953; 55: 223.
28. Bjorgvinsson E, Rudzki C, Lewicki AM. Am J Gastroenterol 1984; 79: 663.

29. Rhind JA. Br Med J 1965; 1: 1309.
30. Davison G. Arch Dis Child 1946; 21: 113.
31. MacMahon B, Record RG, McKeown T. Br J Soc Med 1951; 5: 185.
32. McKeown T, MacMahon B, Record RG. Ann Eugen 1951; 16: 260.
33. Carter CO, Powell BW. Lancet 1954; i: 746.
34. Dodge JA. In: Apley J, ed. Modern trends in paediatrics. London: Butterworth, 1974: 229.
35. Dodge JA, Karim AA. Gut 1976; 17: 280.
36. Belding HH, Kernohan JW. Surg Gynec Obstet 1953; 97: 322.
37. Rintoul JR, Kirkman NF. Arch Dis Child 1961; 36: 474.
38. Bremer JL. Arch Pathol 1944; 38: 132.
39. McLetchie NGB, Purves JK, Saunders RL de CH. Surg Gynec Obstet 1954; 99: 135.
40. Wieczorek RL, Seidman I, Ranson JHC, Ruoff M. Am J Gastroenterol 1984; 79: 597.
41. Farack UM, Goresky CA, Jabbari M, Kinnear DG. Gastroenterol 1974; 66: 596.
42. Sufian S, Ominsky S, Matsumoto T. Gastroenterol 1977; 73: 154.
43. Tabusky J, Szalay G, Meade WS. Am J Gastroenterol 1973; 59: 327.

Miscellaneous acquired conditions

44. Devitt PG, Stamp GWH. Gut 1983; 24: 678.
45. Murray WJG. Postgrad Med J 1984; 60: 631.
46. Ger R. Br Med J 1964; ii: 294.
47. McLaughlin RT, Madding GF. Am J Surg 1962; 104: 874.
48. Wellmann KF, Kagan A, Fang H. Gastroenterol 1964; 46: 601.
49. Palmer ED. Int Abstr Surg 1951; 92: 417.
50. Gibbons CP, Harvey L. Postgrad Med J 1984; 60: 693.

Gastritis

51. Whitehead R, Truelove SC, Gear MW. J Clin Pathol 1972; 25: 1.
52. Goldgraber MB, Rubin CE, Palmer WL, Dobson RL, Massey BW. Gastroenterol 1954; 27: 1.
53. Ramsey EJ, Carey KV, Peterson WL et al. Gastroenterol 1979; 76: 1449.
54. Klein MS, Ennis F, Sherlock P, Winawer SJ. Dig Dis 1973; 18: 167.
55. Rees WDW, Turnberg LA. Lancet 1980; 2: 410.
56. Sugawa C, Lucas CE, Rosenberg BF, Riddle JM, Walt AJ. Gastrointest Endosc 1973; 19: 127.
57. Hoftiezer JW, O'Laughlin JC, Ivey KJ. Gut 1982; 23: 692.
58. Langman MJS, Hansky JH, Drury RAB, Jones FA. Gut 1964; 5: 550.
59. Winawer SJ, Begar J, McCray RS, Zamcheck N. Arch Intern Med 1971; 127: 129.
60. Bron BA, Deyhle P, Pelloni S, Krejs G, Siebenmann RE, Blum AL. Dig Dis 1977; 22: 729.
61. Taor RE, Fox B, Ware J, Johnson AG. Endosc 1975; 7: 209.
62. Bock OAA, Richards WCD, Witts LJ. Gut 1963; 4: 112.
63. Rohrer GV, Welsh JD. Gastroenterol 1967; 52: 185.
64. Sloan JM, Buchanan KD, McFarland RJ, Titterington P, Sandford JC. J Clin Pathol 1979; 32: 201.

65. Oohara T, Tohma H, Aono G, Ukawa S, Kondo Y. Hum Pathol 1983; 14: 1066.
66. Lev R. Lab Invest 1966; 14: 2080.
67. Goldman H, Ming S-C. Lab Invest 1968; 18: 203.
68. Iida F, Murata F, Nagata T. Histochem 1978; 56: 229.
69. Jass JR. J Clin Pathol 1980; 33: 801.
70. Mingazzini P, Carlei F, Malchiodi-Albedi F et al. J Pathol 1984; 144: 171.
71. Hattori R, Fujita S. Pathol Res Pract 1979; 164: 224.
72. Croft DN, Pollock DJ, Coghill NF. Gut 1966; 7: 333.
73. Graham RI, Schade ROK. Acta Pathol Microbiol Scand 1965; 65: 53.
74. Stemmermann GN, Hayashi T. J Nat Cancer Inst 1968; 41: 627.
75. Kreuning J, Bosman FT, Kuiper G, van der Waal AM, Lindeman J. J Clin Pathol 1978; 31: 69.
76. Imai T, Kubo T, Watanabe H. J Nat Cancer Inst 1971; 47: 179.
77. Siurala M, Isokoski M, Varis K, Kekki M. Scand J Gastroenterol 1968; 3: 211.
78. Cheli R, Santi L, Ciancamerla G, Canciani G. Dig Dis 1973; 18: 1061.
79. Ormiston MC, Gear MWL, Codling BW. J Clin Pathol 1982; 35: 757.
80. Strickland RG, Mackay IR. Dig Dis 1973; 18: 426.
81. Taylor KB, Roitt IM, Doniach D, Couchman KG, Shapland C. Br Med J 1962; ii: 1347.
82. Ardeman S, Chanarin I. Gut 1966; 7: 99.
83. Samloff IM, Varis K, Ihamaki T, Siurala M, Rotter JI. Gastroenterol 1982; 83: 204.
84. Doniach D, Roitt IM, Taylor KB. Br Med J 1963; i: 1374.
85. Varis K, Ihamaki T, Harkonen M, Samloff IM, Siurala M. Scand J Gastroenterol 1979; 14: 129.
86. Kimura K. Gastroenterol 1972; 63: 584.
87. du Plessis DJ. S Afr J Surg 1963; 1: 3.
88. Tatsuta M, Saegusa T, Okuda S. Endosc 1974; 6: 20.
89. Parl FF, Lev R, Thomas E, Pitchumoni CS. Hum Pathol 1979; 10: 45.
90. Brown RC, Hardy GJ, Temperley JM, Miloszewski KJA, Gowland G, Losowsky MS. J Clin Pathol 1981; 34: 744.
91. Cameron AJ. Mayo Clin Proc 1975; 50: 565.
92. Piper DW, McIntosh JH, Ariotti DE, Fenton BH, MacLennan R. Gastroenterol 1981; 80: 427.
93. MacDonald WC. Gastroenterol 1973; 65: 381.
94. Hamilton SR, Yardley JH. Gastroenterol 1980; 78: 1178 (abstract).
95. du Plessis DJ. S Afr Med J 1960; 34: 101.
96. Rhodes J, Barnardo DE, Phillips SF, Rovelstad RA, Hofmann AF. Gastroenterol 1969; 57: 241.
97. Taylor WH, Walker V. J Roy Soc Med 1980; 73: 159.
98. Correa P. Cancer Surveys 1983; 2: 437.
99. Correa P, Haenszel W, Cuello C, Tannenbaum S, Archer M. Lancet 1975; ii: 58.
100. Ball PAJ, James AH. Lancet 1961; i: 1365.
101. Tatsuta M, Okuda S. Gastroenterol 1975; 69: 897.
102. Mackay IR, Hislop IG. Gut 1966; 7: 228.
103. Gear MWL, Truelove SC, Whitehead R. Gut 1971; 12: 639.
104. Siurala M, Varis K, Wiljasalo M. Scand J Gastroenterol 1966; 1: 40.
105. Walker IR, Strickland RG, Ungar B, Mackay IR. Gut 1971; 12: 906.
106. Morson BC. Br J Cancer 1955; 9: 377.

107. Nakamura K, Sugano H, Takagi K. Gann 1968; 59 : 251.
108. Sipponen P, Kekki M, Siurala M. Cancer 1983; 52 : 1062.
109. Correa P, Cuello C, Duque E et al. J Nat Cancer Inst 1976; 57 : 1027.
110. Heilmann KL, Hopker WW. Pathol Res Pract 1979; 164 : 249.
111. Segura DI, Montero C. Cancer 1983; 52 : 498.
112. Sipponen P, Seppala K, Varis K et al. Acta Pathol Microbiol Scand 1980; 88 : 217.
113. Magnus HA. J Clin Pathol 1958; 11 : 289.
114. Kaye MD, Whorwell PJ, Wright R. Gastroenterol 1982; 82 : 1097 (abstract).
115. Odgers RJ, Wangel AG. Lancet 1968; ii : 846.
116. Stockbrugger R, Larsson L-T, Lundqvist G, Angervall L. Scand J Gastroenterol 1977; 12 : 209.
117. Hodges JR, Isaacson P, Wright R. Gut 1981; 22 : 237.
118. Borch K, Renvall H, Leidberg G. Gastroenterol 1985; 88 : 638.
119. Elsborg L, Andersen D, Myhre-Jensen O, Bastrup-Madsen P. Scand J Gastroenterol 1977; 12 : 49.
120. Stockbrugger RW, Menon GG, Beilby JOW, Mason RR, Cotton PB. Gut 1983; 24 : 1141.

Other inflammatory lesions of the stomach

121. Morgan AG, McAdam WAF, Pyrah RD, Tinsley EGF. Gut 1976; 17 : 633.
122. Isaacson P. Histopathol 1982; 6 : 377.
123. Lambert R, Andre C, Moulinier B, Bugnon B. Digestion 1978; 17 : 159.
124. Farthing MJG, Fairclough PD, Hegarty JE, Swarbrick ET, Dawson AM. Gut 1981; 22 : 759.
125. Johnstone JM, Morson BC. Histopathol 1978; 2 : 335.
126. Caldwell JH, Sharma HM, Hurtubise PE, Colwell DL. Gastroenterol 1979; 77 : 560.
127. Navab F, Kleinman MS, Algazy K, Schenk E, Turner MD. Gastrointest Endosc 1972; 19 : 67.
128. Leinbach GE, Rubin CE. Gastroenterol 1970; 59 : 874.
129. Kuipers FC, van Thiel PH, Rodenburg W, Wielinga WJ, Roskam RTh. Lancet 1960; ii : 1171.
130. Watt IA, McLean NR, Girdwood RWA, Kissen LH, Fyfe AHB. Lancet 1979; ii : 893.
131. Palmer ED. J Lab Clin Med 1958; 52 : 231.
132. Sirak HD. Arch Surg 1954; 69 : 769.
133. Gould SR, Handley AJ, Barnardo DE. Gut 1973; 14 : 971.
134. Misra RC, Agarwal SK, Prakash P, Saha MM, Gupta PS. Endosc 1982; 14 : 235.
135. Guirguis MM, Ghaly AF, Abadir L. Bristol Med Chir J 1983; 98 : 73.
136. Gaines W, Steinbach HL, Lowenhaupt E. Radiol 1952; 58 : 808.
137. Reisman TN, Leverett FL, Hudson JR, Kaiser MH. Dig Dis 1975; 20 : 588.
138. Willeford G, Childers JH, Hepner WR Jr. Pediat 1952; 10 : 162.
139. Fisher JR, Sanowski RA. Dig Dis 1978; 23 : 282.
140. Sanders I, Woesner ME. Am J Gastroenterol 1972; 57 : 558.
141. Sherman FE, Moran TJ. Am J Clin Pathol 1954; 24 : 415.
142. Fielding JF, Toye DKM, Beton DC, Cooke WT. Gut 1970; 11 : 1001.
143. Rutgeerts P, Onette E, Vantrappen G, Geboes K, Broeckaert L, Talloen L. Endosc 1980; 12 : 288.
144. Fahimi HD, Deren JJ, Gottlieb LS, Zamcheck N. Gastroenterol 1963; 45 : 161.
145. Schinella RA, Ackert J. Am J Gastroenterol 1979; 72 : 30.
146. Dutz W, Saidl F, Kohout E. Gut 1970; 11 : 352.
147. Van Olmen G, Larmuseau MF, Geboes K, Rutgeerts P, Penninckx F, Vantrappen G. Am J Gastroenterol 1984; 79 : 512.
148. Ahnlund HO, Pallin B, Peterhoff R, Schonebeck J. Acta Chir Scand 1967; 133 : 555.
149. Nelson RS, Bruni HC, Goldstein HM. Gastrointest Endosc 1975; 22 : 92.
150. Katzenstein A-LA, Maksem J. Am J Clin Pathol 1979; 71 : 137.
151. Deal WB, Johnson JE III. Gastroenterol 1969; 57 : 579.
152. Gabrielsson N. Endosc 1971; 2 : 66.

Peptic ulcer

153. Bowen JC, Fleming WH, Thompson JC. Surg 1974; 75 : 720.
154. Gordon MJ, Skillman JJ, Zervas NT, Silen W. Ann Surg 1973; 178 : 285.
155. Tatsuta M, Okuda S. Gastroenterol 1976; 71 : 16.
156. Oi M, Oshida K, Sugimura S. Gastroenterol 1959; 36 : 45.
157. Jennings DA, Richardson JE. Lancet 1954; ii : 343.
158. Askanazy M. Virchows Arch Pathol Anat 1924; 250 : 370.
159. Mori K, Shinya H, Wolff WI. Gastroenterol 1971; 61 : 523.
160. Classen M. Clin Gastroenterol 1973; 2 : 315.
161. Dean ACB, Clark CG, Sinclair-Gieben AH. Gut 1962; 3 : 60.
162. Cohen MM. Can Med Assoc J 1971; 105 : 263.
163. Fry J. Br Med J 1964; 2 : 809.
164. Rotter JI. Dig Dis Sci 1981; 26 : 154.
165. Langman MJS. In : Carter DC, ed. Peptic ulcer. Edinburgh : Churchill Livingstone, 1983 : 1.
166. Kurata JH, Haile BM. Clin Gastroenterol 1984; 13 : 289.
167. Watkinson G. Gut 1960; 1 : 14.
168. Ihamaki T, Varis K, Siurala M. Scand J Gastroenterol 1979; 14 : 801.
169. Brown RC, Langman MJS, Lambert PM. Br Med J 1976; 1 : 35.
170. Cox AJ. Arch Pathol 1952; 54 : 407.
171. Card WI, Marks IN. Clin Sci 1960; 19 : 47.
172. Cheng FCY, Lam SK, Ong GB. Gut 1977; 18 : 827.
173. Taylor IL, Calam J, Rotter JI et al. Ann Intern Med 1981; 95 : 421.
174. Cowley DJ, Dymock IW, Boyes BE et al. Gut 1973; 14 : 25.
175. Levy Th, Dufougeray F, Neuberger Ph. Am J Dig Dis 1972; 17 : 767.
176. Aird I, Bentall HH, Mehigan JA, Roberts JAF. Br Med J 1954; 2 : 315.
177. Clarke CA, Edwards JW, Haddock DRW, Howel-Evans AW, McConnell RB, Sheppard P. Br Med J 1956; 2 : 725.
178. Lam SK, Ong GB. Gut 1976; 17 : 169.
179. Doll R, Kellock TD. Ann Eugen 1951; 16 : 231.
180. Monson RR. Am J Epidemiol 1970; 91 : 453.
181. Rotter JI, Petersen GM, Samloff IM et al. Ann Intern Med 1979; 91 : 372.
182. Rotter JI. Dig Dis Sci 1981; 26 : 154.
183. Ammann RW, Vetter D, Deyhle P, Tschen H, Sulser H, Schmid M. Gut 1976; 17 : 107.
184. Feldman EJ, Elashoff JD, Samloff IM, Grossman MI. N Engl J Med 1980; 302 : 1206.

185. Piper DW, McIntosh JH, Ariotti DE, Calogiuri JV, Brown RW, Shy CM. Gut 1981; 22: 1011.
186. Morson BC. Br J Cancer 1955; 9: 365.
187. du Plessis DJ. Lancet 1965; i: 974.
188. Ritchie WP jr, Delaney JP. Surg Forum 1968; 19: 312.
189. Alexander-Williams J, Wolverson RL. Clin Gastroenterol 1984; 13: 601.
190. Rhodes J, Calcraft B. Clin Gastroenterol 1973; 2: 227.
191. Hase T, Moss BJ. Gastroenterol 1973; 65: 224.
192. Barlow TE, Bentley FH, Walder DN. Surg Gynec Obstet 1951; 93: 657.
193. Wormsley KG. Gastroenterol 1978; 75: 139 (editorial).
194. Piper DW, Greig M, Coupland GAE, Hobbin E, Shinners J. Gut 1975; 16: 714.
195. Somervell TH, Orr IM. Br J Surg 1936–37; 24: 227.
196. Paffenbarger RS, Wing AL, Hyde RT. Am J Epidemiol 1974; 100: 307.
197. Levy M. N Engl J Med 1974; 290: 1158.
198. Conn HO, Blitzer BL. N Engl J Med 1976; 294: 473.
199. Bonnevie O. Gastroenterol 1977; 73: 1000.
200. Glick DL, Kern F jr. Gastroenterol 1964; 47: 153.
201. Shepherd AMM, Stewart WK, Wormsley KG. Lancet 1973; i: 1357.
202. Lam S-K. Clin Gastroenterol 1984; 13: 447.
203. Medalie JH, Neufeld HN, Goldbourt U, Kahn HA, Riss E, Oron D. Lancet 1970; ii: 1225.
204. Langman MJS, Cooke AR. Lancet 1976; i: 680.
205. Zollinger RM, Ellison EH. Ann Surg 1955; 142; 709.
206. Oberhelman HA jr. Arch Surg 1972; 104: 447.
207. Larsson L-I, Rehfeld JF, Stockbrugger R et al. Virchows Arch Pathol 1973; 360: 305.
208. Newsome HH. Surg Clin N Amer 1974; 54: 387.
209. Friesen SR, Tomita T. Ann Surg 1981; 194: 481.
210. Neuburger P, Lewin M, Bonfils S. Gastroenterol 1972; 63: 937.
211. Bordi C, Cocconi G, Togni R, Vezzadini P, Missale G. Arch Pathol 1974; 98: 274.
212. James AH. Gut 1964; 5: 285.
213. Polak JM, Stagg B, Pearse AGE. Gut 1972; 13: 501.
214. Arnold R, Hulst MV, Neuhof C, Schwarting H, Becker HD, Creutzfeldt W. Gut 1982; 23: 285.

Gastric polyps

215. Plachta A, Speer FD. Am J Gastroenterol 1957; 28: 160.
216. Rosch W. Front Gastrointest Res 1980; 6: 167.
217. Ming S-C, Goldman H. Cancer 1965; 18: 721.
218. Tomasulo J. Cancer 1971; 27: 1346.
219. Dirschmid K, Walser J, Hugel H. Cancer 1984; 54: 2290.
220. Mori K, Shinya H, Wolff WI. Gastroenterol 1971; 61: 523.
221. Nakamura T. Chirurg 1970; 41: 122.
222. Elster K. Endosc 1974; 6: 44.
223. Kozuka S, Masamoto K, Suzuki S, Kubota K, Yokoyama Y. Gann 1977; 68: 267.
224. Remmele W, Kolb EF. Endosc 1978; 10: 63.
225. Dutta SK, Costa BS. Am J Gastroenterol 1979; 71: 598.
226. Sugano H, Nakamura K, Takagi K. In: Murakami T, ed. Early gastric cancer. Tokyo: University of Tokyo Press, 1971: 257.
227. Morson BC. Br J Cancer 1955; 9: 550.
228. Ming S-C. In: Yardley JH, Morson BC, Abell MR, eds. The gastrointestinal tract. Baltimore: Williams & Wilkins, 1977: 149.
229. Jones RA, Dawson IMP. Histopathol 1977; 1: 137.

230. Wilander E, Portela-Gomes G, Grimelius L, Westermark P. Gastroenterol 1977; 73: 733.
231. Russo A, Buffa R, Grasso G et al. Digestion 1980; 20: 416.
232. Bordi C, Senatore S, Missale G. Dig Dis 1976; 21: 667.
233. Christodoulopoulos JB, Klotz AP. Gastroenterol 1961; 40: 429.
234. Chejfec G, Gould VE. Hum Pathol 1977; 8: 443.
235. Wilander E, Grimelius L, Lundqvist G, Skoog V. Am J Pathol 1979; 96: 519.
236. Marcus FS, Friedman MA, Callen PW, Churg A, Harbour J. Cancer 1980; 46: 1263.
237. Lattes R, Grossi C. Cancer 1956; 9: 698.
238. Rogers LW, Murphy RC. Am J Surg Pathol 1979; 3: 195.
239. Sweeney EC, McDonnell L. Histopathol 1980; 4: 215.
240. Utsunomiya J, Gocho H, Miyanaga T et al. Johns Hopkins Med J 1975; 136: 71.
241. Cochet B, Carrel J, Desbaillets L, Widgren S. Gut 1979; 20: 169.
242. Watanabe A, Nagashima H, Motoi M, Ogawa K. Gastroenterol 1979; 77: 148.
243. Goodman ZD, Yardley JH, Milligan FD. Cancer 1979; 43: 1906.
244. Zarling EJ. Gastrointest Endosc 1981; 27: 175.
245. Lasser A, Koufman WB. Dig Dis 1977; 22: 965.
246. Bill K, Belber JP, Carson JW. Gastrointest Endosc 1982; 28: 182.
247. Cronkhite LW jr, Canada WJ. N Engl J Med 1955; 252: 1011.
248. Kindbloom L, Angervall L, Santesson B, Selander S. Cancer 1977; 39: 2651.
249. Sipponen P, Laxen F, Seppala K. Histopathol 1983; 7: 729.
250. Utsunomiya J, Maki T, Iwama T et al. Cancer 1974; 34: 745.
251. Ranzi T, Castagnone D, Velio P, Bianchi P, Polli EE. Gut 1981; 22: 363.
252. Burt RW, Berenson MM, Lee RG, Tolman KG, Freston JW, Gardner EJ. Gastroenterol 1984; 86: 295.
253. Tatsuta M, Okuda S, Tamura H, Taniguchi H. Gastrointest Endosc 1981; 27: 145.
254. Iida M, Yao T, Watanabe H, Imamura K, Fuyuno S, Omae T. Gastroenterol 1980; 79: 725.
255. Helwig EB, Ranier A. Am J Pathol 1952; 28: 535.
256. Johnstone JM, Morson BC. Histopathol 1978; 2: 349.
257. Calam J, Krasner N, Haqqani M. Dig Dis Sci 1982; 27: 936.
258. Goldman RL, Friedman NB. Cancer 1967; 20: 134.
259. Williams RM. Histopathol 1981; 5: 193.

Malignant epithelial tumours

260. Griffith GW. Br J Cancer 1968; 22: 163.
261. MacDonald WC. Cancer 1972; 29: 724.
262. Hirayama T. In: Murakami T, ed. Early gastric cancer. Tokyo: University of Tokyo Press, 1971: 3.
263. Hakama M. Ann Clin Res 1972; 4: 300.
264. Clemmesen J. Acta Pathol Microbiol Scand 1977; 261: 1.
265. Hirayama T. Cancer Res 1975; 35: 3460.
266. Buell P, Dunn JE jr. Cancer 1965; 18: 656.
267. Haenszel W, Kurihara M, Segi M, Lee RKC. J Nat Cancer Inst 1972; 49: 969.
268. Correa P, Cuello C, Duque E et al. J Nat Cancer Inst 1976; 57: 1027.

269. Stukonis M, Doll R. Int J Cancer 1969; 4: 248.
270. Matolo NM, Klauber MR, Gorishek WM, Dixon JA. Cancer 1972; 29: 733.
271. Enterline P, De Coufle P, Henderson V. J Occ Med 1972; 14: 897.
272. McMichael AJ, Andjelkovic DA, Tyroler HA. Ann NY Acad Sci 1976; 271: 125.
273. Dungal N. JAMA 1961; 178: 789.
274. Sigurjonsson J. Br J Cancer 1967; 21: 651.
275. Matsudo H, Hodgkin NM, Tanaka A. Arch Pathol 1974; 97: 366.
276. Hill MJ, Hawksworth G, Tattersall G. Br J Cancer 1973; 28: 562.
277. Lijinsky W. Cancer Res 1974; 34: 255.
278. Drasar BS, Shiner M. Gut 1969; 10: 812.
279. Jones SM, Davies PW, Savage A. Lancet 1978; i: 1355.
280. Hicks RM, Walters CL, Elsebai I, El Aasser A-B, El Merzabani M, Gough TA. Proc Roy Soc Med 1977; 70: 413.
281. Correa P, Cuello C, Duque E. J Nat Cancer Inst 1970; 44: 297.
282. Aird I, Bentall HH. Br Med J 1953; i: 799.
283. Woolf CM. Cancer 1961; 14: 199.
284. Lauren P. Acta Pathol Microbiol Scand 1965; 64: 31.
285. Munoz N, Asvall J. Int J Cancer 1971; 8: 144.
286. Correa P, Sasano N, Stemmermann GN, Haenszel W. J Natl Cancer Inst 1973; 51: 1449.
287. Kubo T. Cancer 1973; 31: 1498.
288. Mosbech J, Videbaek A. Br Med J 1950; 2: 390.
289. Jorgensen J. Acta Med Scand 1951; 139: 472.
290. Magnus HA. J Clin Pathol 1958; 11: 289.
291. Shearman DJC, Finlayson NDC, Wilson R, Samson RR. Lancet 1966; ii: 403.
292. Schell RF, Dockerty MB, Comfort MW. Surg Gynec Obstet 1954; 98: 710.
293. Stalsberg H, Taksdal S. Lancet 1971; ii: 1175.
294. Domellof L, Janunger K-G. Am J Surg 1977; 134: 581.
295. Terjesen T, Erichsen HG. Acta Chir Scand 1976; 142: 256.
296. Domellof L, Eriksson S, Janunger K-G. Gastroenterol 1977; 73: 462.
297. Schrumpf E, Serck-Hanssen A, Stadaas J, Aune S, Myren J, Osnes M. Lancet 1977; ii: 467.
298. Kobayashi S, Prolla JC, Kirsner JB. Dig Dis 1970; 15: 905.
299. Hammar E. Acta Pathol Microbiol Scand 1976; 84: 495.
300. Pulimood BM, Knudsen A, Coghill NF. Gut 1976; 17: 463.
301. Janunger K-G, Domellof L. Acta Chir Scand 1978; 144: 293.
302. Littler ER, Gleibermann E. Cancer 1972; 29: 205.
303. Koga S, Watanabe H, Enjoji M. Cancer 1979; 43: 647.
304. Borchard F, Mittelstaedt A, Kieker R. Pathol Res Pract 1979; 164: 282.
305. Savage A, Jones S. J Clin Pathol 1979; 32: 179.
306. Farrands PA, Blake JRS, Ansell ID, Cotton RE, Hardcastle JD. Br Med J 1983; 286: 755.
307. Watt PCH, Sloan JM, Kennedy TL. Br Med J 1983; 297: 1407.
308. Grundmann E. Beitr Pathol 1975; 154: 256.
309. Ming S-C. Front Gastrointest Res 1979; 4: 164.
310. Cuello C, Correa P, Zarama G, Lopez J, Murray J, Gordillo G. Am J Surg Pathol 1979; 3: 491.
311. Oehlert W, Keller P, Henke M, Strauch M. Front Gastrointest Res 1979; 4: 173.
312. Morson BC, Sobin LH, Grundmann E, Johansen A, Nagayo T, Serck-Hanssen A. J Clin Pathol 1980; 33: 711.
313. Jass JR. Histopathol 1983; 7: 181.
314. Ming S-C, Bajtai A, Correa P et al. Cancer 1984; 54: 1794.
315. Kamiya T, Morishita T, Asakura H, Miura S, Munakata Y, Tsuchiya M. Cancer 1982; 50: 2496.
316. Schlake W, Grundmann E. Pathol Res Pract 1979; 164: 331.
317. Oehlert W. In: Ming S-C ed. Precursors of gastric cancer. New York: Praeger, 1984: 73.
318. Dekker W, Tytgat GN. Gastroenterol 1977; 73: 710.
319. Graham DY, Schwartz JT, Cain GD, Gyorkey F. Gastroenterol 1982; 82: 228.
320. Sakita T, Oguro Y, Takosu S, Fukutomi H, Miwa T, Yoshimori M. Gastroenterol 1971; 60: 835.
321. Stout AP. Washington DC: Armed Forces Institute of Pathology, 1953; F 65 (Tumors of the stomach; fascicle 21).
322. Oota K, Sobin LH. Geneva: WHO, 1977; International Histological Classification of Tumours, No 18 (Histological typing of gastric and oesophageal tumours).
323. Mulligan RM, Rember RR. Arch Pathol 1954; 58: 1.
324. Ming S-C. Cancer 1977; 39: 2475.
325. Hawley PR, Westerholm P, Morson BC. Br J Surg 1970; 57: 877.
326. Teglbjaerg PS, Vetner M. Acta Pathol Microbiol Scand 1977; 85: 519.
327. MacDonald WC. Cancer 1972; 29: 724.
328. McPeak E, Warren S. Am J Pathol 1948; 24: 971.
329. Murakami T. In: Murakami T, ed. Early gastric cancer. Tokyo: University of Tokyo Press, 1971: 53.
330. Oohara T, Tohma H, Takezoe K et al. Cancer 1982; 50: 801.
331. Kodama Y, Inokuchi K, Soejima K, Matsusaka T, Okamura T. Cancer 1983; 51: 320.
332. Stout AP. Arch Surg 1942; 44: 651.
333. Mason MK. Gut 1965; 6: 185.
334. Gutmann RA. Bull Soc Radiol Med France 1933; 21: 347.
335. Hermanek P, Rosch W. Endosc 1973; 5: 220.
336. Johansen A. Early gastric cancer: a contribution to the pathology and to gastric cancer histogenesis. Copenhagen: Poul Petri, 1981.
337. Elster K, Kolaczek F, Shimamoto K, Freitag H. Endosc 1975; 7: 5.
338. Kinosita R, Nagayo T, Tanaka T, eds. Epidemiological, experimental and clinical studies on gastric cancer. Tokyo: Maruzen, 1968: 113.
339. Nagayo T, Yokoyama H. Int J Cancer 1978; 21: 407.
340. Johansen A. Pathol Res Pract 1979; 164: 316.
341. Nakamura K, Sugano H, Takagi K, Fuchigami A. Gann 1967; 58: 377.
342. Hayashida T, Kidokoro T. Stomach Intestine 1969; 4: 1077.
343. Menuck L. Dig Dis 1978; 23: 269.
344. Fernet P, Azar HA, Stout AP. Gastroenterol 1965; 48: 419.
345. Kidokoro T. In: Murakami T, ed. Early gastric cancer. Tokyo: University of Tokyo Press, 1971: 45.
346. Brooks VS, Waterhouse JAH, Powell DJ. Br Med J 1965; 1: 1577.
347. Urban CH, McNeer G. Cancer 1959; 12: 1158.
348. Brown CH, Merlo M, Hazard JB. Gastroenterol 1961; 40: 188.

349. Harvey HD, Titherington JB, Stout AP, St John FB. Cancer 1951; 4: 717.
350. Comfort MW, Gray HK, Dockerty MB et al. Arch Intern Med 1954; 94: 513.
351. Steiner PD, Maimon SN, Palmer WL, Kirsner JB. Am J Path 1948; 24: 947.
352. Martin C, Kay S. Surg Gynec Obstet 1964; 119: 319.
353. Inokuchi K, Inutsuka S, Furusawa M, Soejima K, Ikeda T. Cancer 1967; 20: 1924.
354. Inberg MV, Lauren P, Vuori J, Viikari SJ. Acta Chir Scand 1973; 139: 273.
355. Watanabe HM, Enjoji M, Imai T. Cancer 1976; 38: 232.
356. Hamazaki M, Sawayama K, Kuriya T. J Karyopathol 1968; 12: 115.
357. Brander WL, Needham PRG, Morgan AD. J Clin Pathol 1974; 27: 536.
358. Straus R, Heschel S, Fortmann DJ. Cancer 1969; 24: 985.
359. Vaughan WP, Straus FH II, Paloyan D. Gastroenterol 1977; 72: 945.
360. McLoughlin GA, Cave-Bigley DJ, Tagore V, Kirkham N. Br Med J 1980; 1: 524.
361. Mingazzini PL, Barsotti P, Malchiodi Albedi F. Histopathol 1983; 7: 433.

Non-epithelial tumours

362. Yoon IL, Luddecke HF. Am J Surg 1958; 96: 453.
363. Fiddian RV, Parish JA. Br J Surg 1960; 48: 98.
364. Meissner WA. Arch Pathol 1944; 38: 207.
365. Lee FI. Postgrad Med J 1979; 55: 575.
366. Martin JF, Bazin P, Feroldi J, Cabanne F. Ann Anat Pathol 1960; 5: 484.
367. Stout AP. Cancer 1962; 15: 400.
368. Cornog JL jr. Cancer 1974; 34: 711.
369. Berg J, McNeer G. Cancer 1960; 13: 25.
370. Shiu MH, Farr GH, Papachristou DN, Hajdu SI. Cancer 1982; 49: 177.
371. Hyjek E, Kelenyi G. Histopathol 1982; 6: 61.
372. Brooks JJ, Enterline HT. Cancer 1983; 51: 476.
373. Heule BV, van Kerkem C, Heimann R. Histopathol 1979; 3: 309.
374. Eimoto T, Futami K, Naito H, Takeshita M, Kikuchi M. Cancer 1985; 55: 788.
375. Rappaport H. Washington DC: Armed Forces Institute of Pathology, 1966; F8–97 (Tumors of the haematopoietic system; section 3, fascicle 8).
376. Lukes RJ, Collins RD. Cancer Treat Rep 1977; 61: 971.
377. Lennert K, Mohri N, Stein H, Kaiserling E, Muller-Hermelink HK. Malignant lymphomas other than Hodgkin's disease. Berlin: Springer, 1978.
378. Yamanaka N, Ischii Y, Koshiba H et al. Gastroenterol 1980; 79: 673.
379. Seo IS, Binkley WB, Warner TFCS, Warfel KA. Cancer 1982; 49: 493.
380. Papadimitriou CS, Papacharalmpous NX, Kittas C. Cancer 1985; 55: 870.
381. Isaacson P, Wright DH, Judd MA, Mepham BL. Cancer 1979; 43: 1805.
382. Brooks JJ, Enterline HT. Cancer 1983; 51: 701.
383. Wright DH, Isaacson PG. Biopsy pathology of the lymphoreticular system. London: Chapman & Hall, 1983: 270.
384. Moore I, Wright DH. Histopathol 1984; 8: 1025.
385. Lewin KJ, Ranchod M, Dorfman RF. Cancer 1978; 42: 693.
386. Dworkin B, Lightdale CJ, Weingrad DN et al. Dig Dis Sci 1982; 27: 986.
387. Remigio PA, Klaum A. Cancer 1971; 27: 562.
388. Henry K, Farrer-Brown G. Histopathol 1977; 1: 53.
389. Scott FET, Dupont PA, Webb J. Cancer 1978; 41: 675.
390. Goeggel-Lamping C, Kahn SB. JAMA 1978; 239: 1786.
391. Isaacson P, Buchanan R, Mepham BL. Hum Pathol 1978; 9: 355.
392. Domenichini E, Martiarena HM, Rubio HH. Endosc 1982; 14: 148.
393. Kay S, Callahan WP jr, Murray MR, Randall HT, Stout AP. Cancer 1951; 4: 726.
394. Almagro UA, Schulte WJ, Norback DH, Turcotte JK. Am J Clin Pathol 1981; 75: 415.
395. Osamura RY, Watanabe K, Yoneyama K, Hayashi T. Acta Pathol Jpn 1977; 27: 533.
396. Akhtar M, Bunuan H, Ali MA, Godwin JT. Cancer 1984; 53: 258.
397. Gottlieb MS, Schroff R, Schanker HM et al. N Engl J Med 1981; 305; 1425.
398. Hymes KB, Cheung T, Greene JB et al. Lancet 1981; ii: 598.
399. Penn I. Transplantation 1977; 27: 8.
400. Ahmed N, Nelson RS, Goldstein HM, Sinkovics JG. Gastrointest Endosc 1975; 21: 149.
401. Pack GT. Ann NY Acad Sci 1964; 114; 985.
402. Tapp E. J Path Bact 1964; 88: 79.
403. Abdelwahab IF, Klein MJ. Am J Gastroenterol 1983; 78: 71.
404. Goodman MD, Cooper PH. Am J Dig Dis 1972; 17: 1117.
405. Jindrak K, Bochetto JF, Alpert LI. Hum Pathol 1976; 7: 595.
406. Smith FR, Barkin JS, Hensley G. Am J Gastroenterol 1980; 73; 45.
407. Templeton AW, Heslin DJ. Am J Roent 1961; 86: 896.
408. Berger L, Shenoy YMV, Ames S. NY State J Med 1962; 62: 2032.
409. Vauclin P, Thau FP. Mem Acad Chir 1966; 92: 368.
410. Menuck LS, Amberg JR. Am J Dig Dis 1975; 20: 903.
411. Adams HW, Adkins JR, Rehak EM. Am J Gastroenterol 1983; 78: 212.
412. Choi SH, Sheehan FR, Pickren JW. Cancer 1964; 17: 791.
413. Nelson RS, Lanza F. Gastrointest Endosc 1978; 24: 156.
414. Cormier WJ, Gaffey TA, Welch JM, Welch JS, Edmonson JH. Mayo Clinic Proc 1980; 55: 747.
415. Cornes JS, Jones TG. J Clin Pathol 1962; 15: 305.
416. Prolla JC, Kirsner JB. Ann Intern Med 1964; 61: 1084.

Other conditions

417. Menetrier P. Arch Physiol Norm Pathol 1888; 1: 32, 236.
418. Kenney FD, Dockerty MB, Waugh JM. Cancer 1954; 7: 671.
419. Scharschmidt BF. Am J Med 1977; 63: 644.
420. Chouraqui JP, Roy CC, Brochu P, Gregoire H, Morin CL, Weber AM. Gastroenterol 1981; 80: 1042.
421. Frank BW, Kern F jr. Gastroenterol 1967; 53: 953.
422. Berenson MM, Sannella J, Freston JW. Gastroenterol 1976; 70: 257.
423. Chusid EL, Hirsch RL, Colcher H. Gastroenterol 1961; 40: 429.

424. Van Loewenthal M, Steinitz H, Friedlander E. Gastroenterologia 1960; 93: 133.

425. Wood GM, Bates C, Brown RC, Losowsky MS. J Clin Pathol 1983; 36: 1071.

426. Domellof L, Eriksson S, Helander HF, Janunger K-G. Gastroenterol 1977; 72: 14.

427. Terruzzi V, Minoli G, Butti GC, Rossini A. Endosc 1980; 12: 58.

428. Heilmann K. Beitr Pathol 1973; 149: 411.

429. Drude RB jr, Balart LA, Herrington JP, Beckman EN, Burns TW. J Clin Gastroenterol 1982; 4: 217.

430. Kimura K, Hiramoto T, Buncher CR. Arch Pathol 1969; 87: 110.

431. Böger A, Hort W. Virchows Arch Pathol Anat 1977; 372: 287.

432. Kerekes ES. Radiol 1964; 82: 468.

433. Driscoll JE, Rabe MA. Am Surgeon 1954; 20: 1281.

434. Owen WJ, McColl I. J Roy Soc Med 1979; 72: 937.

435. Rosekrans PCM, de Rooy DJ, Bosman FT, Eulderink F, Cats A. Endosc 1980; 12: 200.

436. Weaver GA, Alpern HD, Davis JS, Ramsey WH, Reichelderfer M. Gastroenterol 1979; 77: 1.

437. Cunningham JT. Gastroenterol 1981; 81: 1131.

438. Bank S, Aftalion B, Anfang C, Altman H, Wise L. Am J Gastroenterol 1983; 78: 206.

439. Mitsudo SM, Boley SJ, Brant LJ, Montefusco CM, Sammartano RJ. Hum Pathol 1979; 10: 585.

440. Quintero E, Pique JM, Bombi JA. Hum Pathol 1984; 15: 1003 (letter).

441. Jabbari M, Cherry R, Lough JO, Daly DS, Kinnear DG, Goresky CA. Gastroenterol 1984; 87: 1165.

The small intestine

PHYSIOLOGICAL AND ANATOMICAL CONSIDERATIONS

Digestion of food is completed in the small intestine, and the breakdown products of protein,[1] fat[2] and carbohydrate[3] are transferred across the epithelial lining to the blood capillaries and the lacteals in the lamina propria. The transfer is effected in part by passive diffusion and in part is an active process associated with enzyme systems that are present in the absorptive cells and their microvilli; these systems may be deficient or absent in congenital and acquired diseases. Different substances are preferentially absorbed in particular sites: in general, the lower part of the ileum can assume the absorptive functions of the more proximal parts of the small bowel but the converse is not true, especially for substances such as vitamin B_{12}.

There has been increasing appreciation that many disorders of the small intestine lead to mucosal flattening and malabsorption.[4] The use of endoscopic duodenal biopsy, though it presents its own problems in interpretation,[5] as well as the established jejunal capsular biopsies together with more sophisticated techniques which include histochemistry,[6] immunocytochemistry,[7] scanning and transmission electron microscopy[8] and morphometry,[9] have greatly enlarged our knowledge of small intestinal function and disease. Although intestinal mucosal damage from whatever cause tends to follow an overall common pattern,[10] there are variations within the pattern which often allow a differential diagnosis to be made. A thorough knowledge of normal small bowel histology and of the value of specialized techniques in biopsy interpretation is essential.

MACROSCOPIC AND FUNCTIONAL ANATOMY

The adult duodenum is 20–25 cm in length. It is almost entirely retroperitoneal and forms a fixed C-shaped organ around the head of the pancreas; the pancreatic and bile ducts open into its second part. The upper two-fifths of the remaining small bowel are arbitrarily defined as jejunum, the lower three-fifths as ileum. Their combined length measured at necropsy varies from 3–9 m, with a mean of a little under 6 m;[11] when measured during life the length is only some 2.8 m,[12] presumably because of the tone present in the longitudinal muscle coat. They are suspended by a mesentery.

From within outward there is a mucosal lining with a connective-tissue lamina propria, which rests on a thin muscularis mucosae. Underlying this is a submucosa in which lie lymphatics, blood vessels, lymphoid tissue and a submucosal plexus of ganglion cells and nerve fibres. There is then a well-developed inner circular muscle coat and a thinner outer longitudinal muscle coat which completely surrounds the bowel and is not aggregated into taeniae. A second, myenteric, plexus of ganglia and nerve fibres lies between the two coats. External to the muscle is a thin serosa containing fibrous and elastic tissue and covered by mesothelial cells.

The mucosa and submucosa and, to a lesser extent, the serosa are freely movable upon the muscle coats. The inner mucosal layer presents an enormous absorptive surface, not only because of its length but because the mucous membrane is thrown into crescentic folds or plicae, the valvulae conniventes. These plicae are most prominent in the upper jejunum and become smaller towards the lower ileum; they are apparently dependent on smooth muscle tone in the muscularis mucosae, since relaxation of this coat causes them to disappear while its contraction emphasizes their presence. This is important in biopsy interpretation; a biopsy which does not include muscularis mucosae may give a false impression of partial mucosal flattening. Contraction and dilatation of the intestine are possible only when the elasticity of the submucosa is normal; when there is submucosal fibrosis the muscularis can be immobilized and atrophy of the plicae can then result.[13]

The ileum terminates in an 'ileocaecal valve'; this term, though in common use, is probably a misnomer since the 'valve' is not a valve proper but a sphincter.

The blood supply of virtually the whole of the small bowel is derived from the superior mesenteric artery; the upper duodenum also receives branches from the coeliac axis. Within the mesentery the superior mesenteric artery branches to form anastomosing arcades which allow a wide collateral circulation at this level. From these arcades, short straight arteries pierce the bowel wall and reach the submucosa, supplying muscle coats *en route*. There is a good detailed description of the villous microcirculation[14] which is further described below. Returning blood drains through the superior mesenteric vein to the portal vein and liver.

The intrinsic nervous system of the small bowel has a greater degree of independence than is often appreciated.[15] It has its own afferent receptor and efferent motor pathways and a complex system of integration between them, and is linked with the sympathetic system through the coeliac and superior mesenteric ganglia and plexuses and with the cranial and sacral parasympathetic plexus through the vagus nerve and the sacral plexuses. Within the gut are two main plexuses. The myenteric has numerous ganglion cells in small groups while the submucosal has single scattered ganglion cells. All are histologically similar but there are three main neural transmitters which can be partially identified using special techniques. Noradrenergic fibres are postganglionic, sympathetic and inhibitory and are usually argyrophilic. Fibres liberating vasoactive intestinal polypeptide (VIP) are intrinsic, multiaxonal and communicating rather than direct suppliers of muscle and are usually also inhibitory; they can be recognized using immunocytochemical techniques. Cholinergic fibres liberate acetylcholine; some are excitatory and preganglionic; others are intrinsic. They are not argyrophilic but their demonstration is complicated by the fact that acetylcholinesterase, readily demonstrable histochemically, is not a reliable indication that a fibre is cholinergic since it is also found in adrenergic fibres including those in the mucosa.[16,17]

The gut-associated lymphoid tissue (GALT) and immunity

Potentially antigenic material is continually ingested from birth onward. The small bowel is adapted to recognizing it and mounting an appropriate immune response which may be suppressive or stimulatory.[18,19] The majority of antigenic material is transferred to underlying immune competent cells through the specially modified enterocytes (M cells) which overlie lymphoid follicles and Peyer's patches; some is sampled by intra-epithelial lymphocytes, which are thymus-dependent and have the same surface antigen (OKT 8) as the cytotoxic T cells in peripheral blood.[20] Lymphoid follicles, with or without germinal centres, lie single astride the mucosa and submucosa in the duodenum and jejunum; in the ileum, while some remain single, there is a tendency to aggregate and form Peyer's patches. They contain both B and T lymphocytes and macrophages are present in the adjacent connective tissue. Antigenic material ingested by the M cells can thus be readily processed by macrophages and T-helper cells and then presented to B cells, which can then develop via immunoblasts into mature plasma cells which secrete appropriate antibodies. Alternatively, T-suppressor cells can prevent an immune response.

Antibody-producing plasma cells are normally present in a ratio of $IgA:IgM:IgG = 20:10:1$.[21] They can be distinguished immunocytochemically. IgA and IgM, but not IgG, are transported across the mucosal surface by combination of their contained J chain with secretory component within surface enterocytes and form a protective 'paint' on the enterocyte surface.

MICROSCOPY

The mucosa consists of glandular epithelium and a supporting framework of fine connective tissue (the lamina propria). These rest on the muscularis mucosae. The latter consists of smooth muscle fibres associated with some elastic tissue and is important in the maintenance of the normal mucosal pattern. The submucosa and serosa carry the main blood supply and lymphatics of the intestinal wall. The peritoneal covering is a single layer of flat mesothelial cells, supported by a layer of fibrous tissue that includes the well-developed elastic lamina to which the elasticity of the peritoneum is due.

Dissecting microscopy

The dissecting microscope shows the villi of the first part of the jejunum—the part usually sampled when single biopsy specimens are taken—to be predominantly of finger-like and leaf-like configuration. Racial differences in the appearances of the villi have been recognized. In Caucasians the finger-like forms predominate and the villi are five to six times taller than they are thick;[22] in contrast, in many Asians there is a predominance of leaf-like and spade-like forms, which are broader than the finger-like villi but of the same order of height[23] (see also p. 235). Dissecting microscope appearances in duodenal biopsies show more numerous spade forms than are seen in the jejunum. In adults these become more noticeable when, as is not uncommon, there is an associated non-specific duodenitis. We do not now consider that dissecting microscopy has an important part to play in the diagnosis of intestinal disorders, though it continues to be necessary for the correct orientation of biopsy material. It has never been any substitute whatever for careful histological examination.

The mucosa

The mucosa itself is divisible into three zones; a generative crypt zone, the villi which arise from it and the basal layer which also arises from it and lies between it and the muscularis mucosae.

The crypt zone

The crypt zone (Fig. 6.1) contains stem cells in active mitotic division. These give rise to cells which migrate upwards to clothe the villi, mature as they do so and are eventually shed from the surface in 2–4 days. Stem cells also mature into cells which migrate downwards to form the basal layer.[24] The crypt zone increases in extent and activity whenever there is increased cell loss or when the time between maturation and shedding

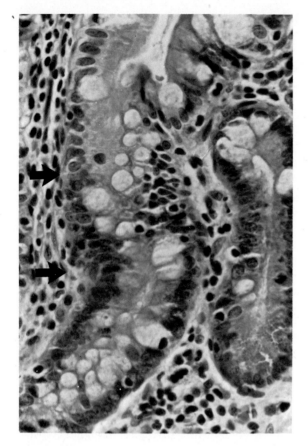

Fig. 6.1 High-power view of jejunal crypt zone showing the stem cell region. The arrows indicate the approximate length of the zone.

Haematoxylin-eosin   × 315

From B.C. Morson & I.M.P. Dawson, Gastrointestinal Pathology, *1979, courtesy of the publishers, Blackwell.*

is shortened, as happens in many forms of intestinal disorders. Minor degrees of increased activity may need careful morphometric techniques for their detection.

Normal villi

Normal villi measure from 320–570 mm in height and from 85–140 mm in width in adults[25] and slightly less in children.[26] The majority of cells covering them are enterocytes concerned with absorption; these are columnar cells which do not contain mucin, contain secretory component, α-1-antitryspin, apo-lipoprotein and lysozyme and have a microvillous brush border in which are histochemically-demonstrable enzymes including disaccharidases and peptidases (Figs 6.2 and 6.3). The remaining cells contain mucin, either as small demonstrable granules or aggregated into globules as goblet cells.

There are three principal types of gastrointestinal mucosubstance: neutral, which are stained red with periodic acid-Schiff techniques; acid non-sulphated, which are stained blue by alcian blue at pH 2.5; and acid sulphated, stained brown by a high iron diamine-alcian blue technique. Intestinal goblet cells may contain all three types, and often there is more than one type in a single cell. Gastric mucus, in contrast, is almost entirely of neutral type.

The basal layer

This contains four different cell types. There are occasional generative cells from the lower zone and

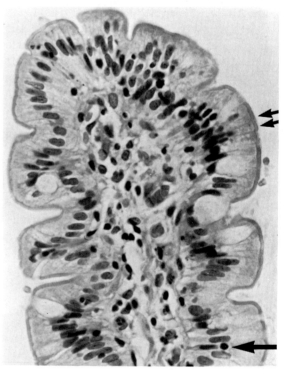

Fig. 6.2 High-power view of the upper part of a jejunal villus. Goblet cells, enterocytes and migrating lymphocytes (single arrow) are all clearly visible and the brush border (double arrow) is well shown.

Haematoxylin-eosin   × 315

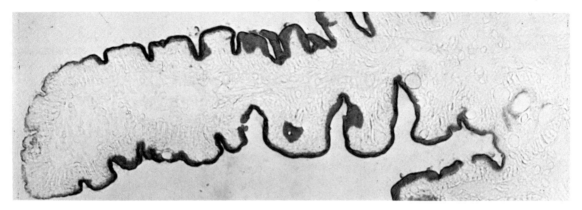

Fig. 6.3 Aminopeptidase in jejunal brush border in a child below the normal height and weight centiles. The enzyme is confined to maturing and mature enterocytes above crypt level and is not seen in the basal layer; in this condition it has also largely disappeared from the villous tips.

Naphthol pararosanilin-fast blue B   × 50

some cells containing variable amounts of mucin. There are also Paneth and endocrine cells.

Paneth cells are normally confined to the small bowel, appendix and proximal colon; they are found in the stomach only in intestinal metaplasia and in the colon as a consequence of inflammatory bowel disease.[27] Individual cells are flask-shaped with large supranuclear intracytoplasmic granules (Fig. 6.4) which stain intensely with eosin or phloxine-tartrazine and contain lysozyme.[28] Their function is unknown.

The endocrine cells of the gut are derived from crypt stem cells and are not, as was previously thought, of neuro-ectodermal origin. They form a part of the so-called diffuse endocrine system,[29–31] and are sometimes designated as APUD cells since some of them are concerned with *a*mine *p*recursor *u*ptake and *d*ecarboxylation. Histologically, they are roughly triangular in shape with a broad base resting on the basement membrane and the apex reaching the lumen; microvilli are present. The cells contain infranuclear cytoplasmic granules which are usually poorly visualized in conventionally fixed and stained material. The granules contain one of a number of polypeptide hormones which include CCK, enteroglucagon, gastrin, GIP, motilin, secretin, somatostatin and VIP.[32] They may also contain a biological amine, usually 5-hydroxytryptamine. Individual cells, and usually, though not invariably, the tumours which arise from them, can be separated from other cells by the use of semi-specific histological techniques

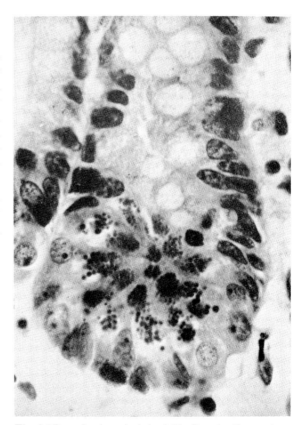

Fig. 6.4 Base of an intestinal gland. The Paneth cells contain large granules: their nucleus is situated at the pole of the cell remote from the lumen of the gland. The endocrine cells are not so easily recognized in the black-and-white photograph: the granules are concentrated in the cytoplasm between the nucleus and the basement membrane of the gland (arrowed).

Silver method for argentaffin granules; phloxin-tartrazine   × 650

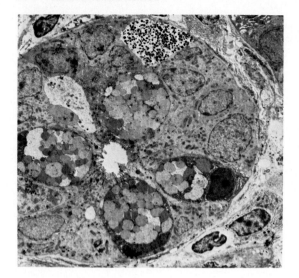

Fig. 6.5 Electron micrograph through the lower end of a crypt to show the relationship of mucus-secreting, absorptive and endocrine cells. Microvilli are visible at the luminal edge

× 1350

of which the most useful are the Grimelius method, Solcia's lead haematoxylin technique[30,33] and possibly the presence of a so-called 'neurone specific' enolase.[34] The granule content can be more specifically investigated for 5-HT using argentaffin techniques or aldehyde-fixed material or by aldehyde-induced fluorescence and for various polypeptide hormones by appropriate immunocytochemical studies with suitable antibodies after appropriate preservation.[32] The electron microscopic appearances of granules may also give some clue as to their hormone and amine content[35] (Figs 6.5 and 6.6).

Brunner's glands

The first and second parts of the duodenum have a number of neutral-mucin-secreting glands (Brunner's) which lie within the submucosa and discharge their secretions through ducts which penetrate the muscularis mucosae and drain into the bases or sides of crypts.[36] They closely resemble, and appear to be an extension of the pyloric antral glands of the stomach, which, at the pylorus, infiltrate and are broken up by the muscularis mucosae (Fig. 6.7).

The lamina propria

The connective tissue, which extends around the crypts and glands of the basal layer and forms the cores of the villi, contains lymphatics and blood

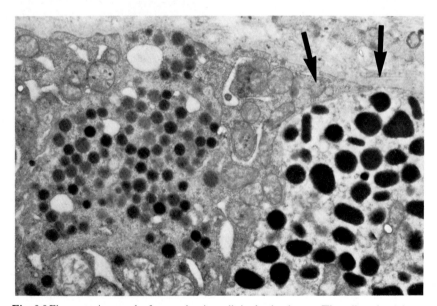

Fig. 6.6 Electron micrograph of two endocrine cells in the duodenum. The cell on the right (arrowed) has the characteristic irregular and cigar-shaped granules of 5-HT. The one on the left is probably a secretin-containing cell.

× 11 000

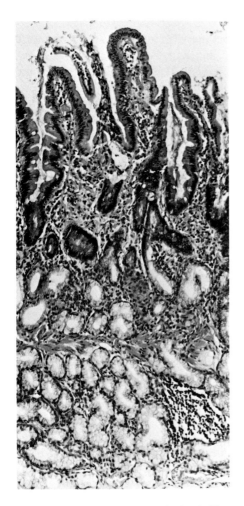

Fig. 6.7 Duodenal mucosa with Brunner's glands. These simple mucus-secreting glands can be seen to lie both above and below the muscularis mucosae.

Haematoxylin-eosin   ×125

vessels, eosinophils, basophils and mast cells and scattered immune competent cells. These include part of the gut-associated lymphoid tissue already described and particularly those thymus-dependent T lymphocytes which emigrate and immigrate between individual enterocytes and are described as inter (or intra-) epithelial.[37] Their numbers vary and they are often counted in relation to the number of enterocytes, the normal then being reckoned as 8–40 per 100 enterocytes. A more accurate and therefore preferable technique is to count their number against a measured length of muscularis mucosae. Minor variations from normal

may be important in detecting early disease or relapse.[38]

ECOLOGY OF THE SMALL BOWEL

The mucosal folds of small intestine already described form niches which are permanently colonized by indigenous organisms. These are strictly or facultatively anaerobic, and most are bacteroides.[39,40] They are more numerous in the ileum then in the jejunum. In the upper small bowel there is, in addition, a more variable, non-indigenous flora of ingested bacteria, mainly aerobes and facultative anaerobes. These cannot normally colonize the bowel permanently, but may do so if the disease conditions allow stagnation of bowel content (see p. 274).

RACIAL AND CLIMATIC DIFFERENCES IN SMALL BOWEL MUCOSA

There is a tendency for healthy people without gastrointestinal symptoms living in developing and/or tropical countries to show some degree of shortening and flattening of villi with an increase in cellularity of the lamina propria and sometimes increased numbers of intra-epithelial lymphocytes.[23,41,42] When these abnormalities are accompanied by asymptomatic evidence of malabsorption the condition is sometimes referred to as a subclinical tropical enteropathy. The histological similarity with the milder changes of tropical sprue has suggested a possible infective condition, endemic and almost to be regarded as 'normal' for the population concerned. These differences may not be as marked as previously believed, and appear to be more related to climate than to race.[43]

SMALL INTESTINE BIOPSY ASSESSMENT

Every laboratory handling small intestinal biopsies should have an agreed and standardized procedure to include proper orientation and processing, informed decision as to whether and when to use paraffin or plastic embedding with conventional or thin section, whether to serialize sections routinely, whether histochemical and immunocytochemical techniques are to be used and when more complex examinations including scanning and transmission electron-microscopy are likely to be of value. This necessitates close co-operation between pathologist and clinician as well as a careful assessment of laboratory facilities and finances.[6,44]

Assessment of the normality or otherwise of a biopsy has, up to now, been largely subjective. Interesting comparisons have beome available between purely subjective assessments, linear measurements, simple stereology using suitable eyepiece graticles and more sophisticated techniques which can generally be classified as 'computer-aided microscopy'.[45] No detailed comment on their relative values can be attempted here but pathologists should be aware of their existence and potential value as well as their cost effectiveness.

CONGENITAL ABNORMALITIES

A recent study of necropsy reports on 8390 children[46] revealed that 1249 (almost 15%) had some form of congenital malformation. Those most commonly found in the gastrointestinal tract included Meckel's diverticulum, anorectal atresia, small bowel atresia, pyloric stenosis and Hirschsprung's disease. In a significant number, more than one anomaly was present.

ATRESIA AND STENOSIS

Atresia (absence of the lumen) or congenital stenosis (narrowing of the lumen) may occur in any part of the small intestine, but most of such abnormalities are found in the duodenum or ileum. The sites of obstruction may be multiple, and abnormalities of other organs are sometimes present. The duodenum and ileum appear particularly subject to vascular insufficiency during the development of the fetus, and this has been invoked in support of the theory that atresia or stenosis are the result of infarction of the bowel during fetal life, with aseptic necrosis and atrophy of the affected segment. There is also experimental evidence that favours fetal vascular insufficiency

as a major factor in their pathogenesis.[47] Atresia is incompatible with survival unless promptly recognized and bypassed surgically. Three patterns are described. There can be a thin membrane stretching across the bowel; a length of bowel can be replaced by a fibromuscular cord with no lumen, or there may be a complete gap between two lengths of bowel with an associated mesenteric defect. Some examples have been associated with segmental absence of muscle coats.[48] Usually only a very short segment of bowel is involved, but the possibility of multiple lesions must be remembered when attempting to deal with the condition. In cases of stenosis—incomplete occlusion—again only a short segment of the bowel is usually involved: the intestine above the level of the obstruction is distended and there is some degree of hypertrophy of its musculature consequent upon the obstruction, while the bowel below the obstructed segment is collapsed.

MALROTATION OF THE INTESTINE

Malrotation is an abnormality in the development of the midgut, which is the part of the intestinal tract between the duodenojejunal flexure and the splenic flexure. Normally at about the fifth week of embryonic development, in the late somite stage, the midgut herniates into the umbilical cord and begins to rotate: it returns to the abdominal cavity at about the 10th week, continuing to rotate through a total of about 270°, so that the caecum reaches the right iliac fossa and the transverse colon lies superficial to the small bowel. This phase is followed by fixation of the bowel.[49] Failure of rotation may result in various anomalies: these include (1) persistence of intestinal eventration at the umbilicus (exomphalos); (2) laevoposition of the caecum, appendix and ascending colon in association with misplacement of the small intestine in the right half of the abdomen; (3) failure of the caecum to descend to its proper position; (4) abnormal mobility of the caecum as a result of persistence of the right mesocolon, and (5) retrocaecal extraperitoneal misplacement of the appendix. All of these are conditions that may be of practical importance by reason of the effects that they may have on the clinical picture, diagnosis and surgical management of acquired diseases affecting the maldeveloped part. Volvulus is a not uncommon complication.

EXOMPHALOS

Rarely, in the course of physiological herniation, the bowel becomes adherent to the hernial sac or fails to return to the abdominal cavity because the neck of the sac is unusually narrow; the hernia then remains until birth and may contain ileum, caecum, ascending colon and sometimes liver. The condition must be distinguished from para-umbilical hernia. Exomphalos is probably related to the condition recently described as peritoneal encapsulation of the bowel.[50]

DUPLICATION, DIVERTICULA AND CYSTS

Duplication

Duplication of the small intestine is extremely rare. In most instances it affects a short length of bowel, usually part of the ileum. The duplicated section may be incorporated within the existing mesentery or, more rarely, possesses a mesentery of its own. It may be blind or communicate at either or both ends with the normal bowel. The mucosa, muscularis mucosae, submucosa and circular muscle coats are usually normal but the longitudinal muscle is often incomplete. The development of carcinoma in later life within the duplicated segment has been described as a complication.[51] Associated volvulus is not uncommon.

Diverticula and cysts

Congenital diverticula (other than Meckel's diverticulum; see below) and cysts of the small intestine are not uncommon. They can lie on the mesenteric or antimesenteric borders, usually the former. The diverticula communicate with the lumen of the bowel; the cysts are closed. Both forms of lesion are surrounded by a more or less imperfect muscle coat, and represent *formes frustes* of duplications. Infarction has been described in them.[52]

Most diverticula of the small intestine are acquired, especially those seen in later life. They can act as stagnant loops (see p. 274).

Meckel's diverticulum and the vitello-intestinal duct

Meckel's diverticulum is the commonest congenital anomaly of the gastrointestinal tract. It can be found in about 2% of all necropsies and is situated on the antimesenteric aspect of the ileum about a metre above the ileocaecal valve. It is commoner in males. It is a true diverticulum, all the layers that normally make up the wall of the intestine being present throughout its whole extent and in their normal relations. Its length in adults is usually from 2–12 cm, and its diameter is about the same as that of the normal bowel into which it opens (Fig. 6.8).

The diverticulum is a remnant of the proximal end of the vitello-intestinal duct. In most cases its blind end is free, but sometimes it remains attached

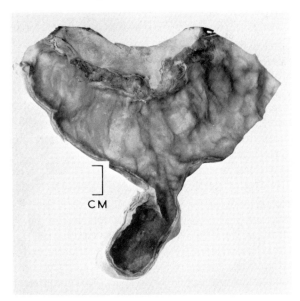

Fig. 6.8 Meckel's diverticulum. The position of the diverticulum on the antimesenteric aspect of the ileum is characteristic. The dark appearance of its lining is due to acute inflammation.

Specimen from the Gordon Museum, Guy's Hospital, London, reproduced by permission of the Curator, Mr J.D. Maynard. Photograph by Miss P.M. Turnbull, Charing Cross Hospital Medical School, London.

by a fibrous cord (the vitelline cord) to the umbilicus. Occasionally, this cord retains a lumen or the diverticulum itself is attached by its tip to the umbilicus, and there can be free leakage of the contents of the ileum.

Meckel's diverticulum is lined by epithelium of small intestinal type. Sometimes islands of gastric mucosa are present, and peptic ulceration may then develop: the ulcer invariably appears in the part of the mucosa that does not contain the acid-secreting glands, and not infrequently it develops in the ileum adjacent to or opposite the opening of the diverticulum. Ectopic pancreatic tissue is also quite commonly found in a Meckel's diverticulum. The other complications of Meckel's diverticulum include perforation and haemorrhage (usually in association with peptic ulceration), acute and chronic inflammation, impaction of foreign bodies, intussusception, mucocele formation (a rare source of pseudomyxoma of the peritoneum; see p. 307), and the development of benign tumours (usually leiomyomas, fibromas or lipomas) or of carcinomas, including adenocarcinomas and carcinoid tumours. In some cases several of these conditions are present together.

Incomplete obliteration of the vitello-intestinal duct may result in other anomalies, any of which may be associated with the presence of Meckel's diverticulum. If only the intestinal end of the duct is obliterated the condition of vitelline sinus results: the sinus opens into the umbilicus and may be the source of a scanty, mucous discharge. In other cases the duct is obliterated at both ends but the intervening part persists and gradually becomes distended by the accumulation of its secretion, forming a vitelline cyst ('enterocystoma'). In exceptional cases adenocarcinoma arises in a vitelline sinus or vitelline cyst, and this accounts for most of the very rare primary carcinomas of the umbilicus, though some may also be of urachal origin. It must be remembered that the commonest malignant tumours of this part are metastatic, often from a primary carcinoma of the ovary.

EPITHELIAL HETEROTOPIA

Heterotopia is defined as the development of a particular tissue—in this case epithelium—in a part where it is not normally expected.[53,54] This contrasts with metaplasia, which is the change of one fully developed adult tissue into another. Heterotopic gastric tissue may be of body or antral type and appropriate specialized cells are also found in it.[55] It is rare in normal small bowel and needs to be carefully distinguished from metaplastic tissue in the duodenum[56,57] (see p. 254) but is not uncommon in congenital duplication, diverticula or cysts and in Meckel's diverticulum. Antral type mucosa is also seen as an acquired metaplastic condition in chronic inflammatory bowel disease.

Heterotopic pancreatic tissue is found in otherwise normal stomachs, in the first and second parts of the duodenum and in Meckel's diverticulum.

MECONIUM PLUG AND MECONIUM ILEUS

A number of cases of intestinal obstruction in the neonatal period are due to the accumulation of viscid mucus and undigested debris of swallowed vernix in the lower part of the ileum. In many, but not all of these cases, the condition is associated with mucoviscidosis (cystic fibrosis of the pancreas). The mass of meconium ('meconium plug') resists the propulsive effort of the peristaltic contractions of the intestinal musculature: the condition known as meconium ileus then results. The dilated bowel proximal to the plug may rupture or undergo torsion. If the meconium gains access to the tissues of the bowel wall, through ulceration or fissuring of the mucosa, a granulomatous reaction develops: subsequent cicatrization leads to organic obstruction that may simulate congenital stenosis.

Histologically, goblet cells are often conspicuous and distended, but there is no diagnostic histological abnormality of the mucus-secreting epithelium.[6,58,59] It remains debatable to what extent an abnormally viscid mucus contributes to the development of meconium ileus; it is now generally agreed that the failure of pancreatic exocrine secretion that accompanies cystic fibrosis of the pancreas plays little part in the pathogenesis of neonatal ileus.

HAMARTOMAS

A hamartoma is a primarily non-neoplastic error of tissue development, in which there is a mixture of tissues indigenous to the organ or tissue from which it arises. It may be apparent at birth or appear later in life. Hamartomas may be predominantly epithelial or predominantly connective tissue in pattern or may containing a mixture of both types of tissue; although originally non-neoplastic, they may later undergo neoplastic change. There is often a familial incidence with a recognizable pattern of inheritance. A number of varieties are seen in the gastrointestinal tract.[60]

Peutz-Jeghers polyposis

The association of gastrointestinal polyposis with excessive melanin pigmentation of parts of the skin and of some mucous membranes has been recognized with increasing frequency in recent years as a distinctive clinicopathological syndrome, often referred to as the Peutz-Jeghers syndrome. It is inherited as an autosomal dominant. The incidence is approximately equal in the two sexes and a considerable proportion of cases are now recognized during childhood. Excessive pigmentation is found principally in the skin round the lips and in the buccal mucosa; it may be present on the fingers and toes, and sometimes elsewhere. The intestinal polyps are found most frequently in the stomach and upper small bowel, particularly the jejunum, and less often in large intestine. Some patients have only a solitary polyp, but this is exceptional, and often there are very large numbers of them throughout the small intestine. *Formes frustes*, in which polyps or pigmentation alone are present, are well described.

The polyps range from sessile nodules a few millimetres across to pedunculated tumours as much as 5 cm in diameter, and there is a tendency for them to appear sequentially in crops. They have a lobulated surface, and do not differ significantly in their gross appearances from adenomatous polyps of the large intestine.

Histologically, there is a branching tree-like core of muscularis mucosae, clothed with epithelium essentially normal for that part of the bowel from which the polyp arises and including any special-

ized cells normally present there, such as simple columnar cells, goblet cells, Paneth cells and endocrine cells of various types. These are present in approximately the same relationship to one another as they are found in normal mucosa (Figs 6.9 and 6.10).

There is usually no evidence of increased mitotic activity, de-differentiation, or structural irregularity, such as is found in the adenomas of the large bowel that are so prone to undergo malignant change.[61-63]

Some reports of malignant change in Peutz-Jeghers polyps are attributable to misinterpretation. This arises because the malformation may involve the deeper tissues of the bowel wall and the appearances that then result can simulate cancerous invasion. However, there have been a few well-documented accounts of undoubted carcinomatous change, with metastasis to regional lymph nodes.[64-65] Recent studies have concentrated on the association of Peutz-Jeghers polyps with breast cancer and ovarian sex cord tumours.[66-68]

The complications of the Peutz-Jeghers syndrome include intestinal haemorrhage, secondary hypochromic anaemia, and intussusception, which tends to be recurrent. The prognosis, however, is in general good.

Juvenile gastrointestinal polyposis

Single or scattered sequential hamartomatous juvenile polyps are common in the large intestine (see p. 363) where they are usually non-familial. Similar polyps occur rarely in the small bowel and slightly more often in the stomach in association with multiple juvenile polyposis syndromes in the large bowel which can but need not be familial.[69-71] Single juvenile hamartomatous polyps confined to the small bowel have not, to our knowledge, been reported. Histologically, the large intestinal polyps of multiple juvenile polyposis resemble single juvenile polyps; there are few reports of the histology of the rare small bowel polyps, but in the examples we have seen there have been dilated spaces filled with mucus, with less surface ulceration than is seen in large intestinal polyps; the glandular elements present have contained endocrine and Paneth cells. There is some evidence that the inherited polyposis syndromes involving the

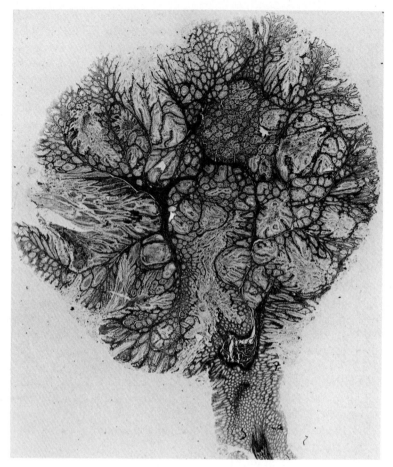

Fig. 6.9 Peutz-Jeghers polyp of small intestine. Note its characteristic branching core, which is composed of smooth muscle.

Haematoxylin-eosin   ×5

whole gastrointestinal tract can be aassociated with other anomalies,[72] and with gastrointestinal carcinoma;[73,74] some of the juvenile polyps in these syndromes have shown concomitant adenomatous epitheliac changes.[71,73,74]

There are also reports of adenomas in the duodenum of patients with familial adenomatous polyposis.[75,76]

Hamartomas of Brunner's glands

These rare hamartomas, which often closely resemble Peutz-Jeghers polyps, arise in the submucosal glands of Brunner in the first and second parts of the duodenum but are not associated with pigmentation or dominant inheritance.[77] They project into the lumen as sessile growths which may become pedunculated and histologically consist of well-formed glands secreting neutral mucin interspersed with smooth muscle (Fig. 6.11).

Cronkhite-Canada syndrome

In this syndrome a polypoid change occurs in the stomach, small intestine and colon. It is associated with protein-losing enteropathy and often also with ectodermal changes which include alopecia, hyperpigmentation and atrophy of the nails.[78] Nutritional defects, including loss of amino acids, may be causative[79] and the lesions may macroscopically resemble those of colitis cystica superficialis.[80] The condition is included here because the poly-

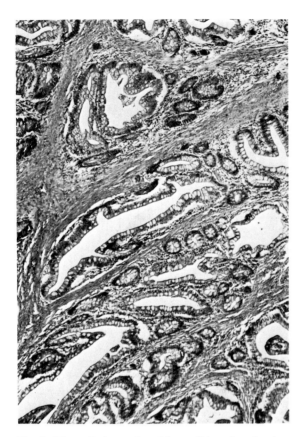

Fig. 6.10 Peutz-Jeghers polyp of the small intestine, showing the bands of smooth muscle in the stroma and the normal appearance of the epithelium lining the tubules.

Haematoxylin-eosin   × 70

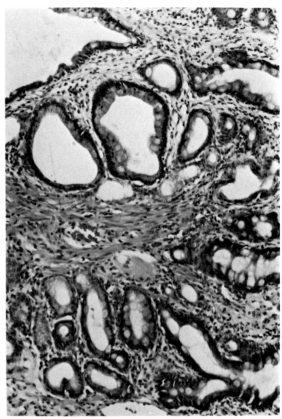

Fig. 6.11 Hamartoma of Brunner's glands. The glands are irregular in shape but are simple mucus-secreting and show no evidence of epithelial hyperplasia. They are interspersed with abundant muscularis mucosae.

Haematoxylin-eosin   × 125

posis, which is often more a diffuse mucosal change than the presence of individual polyps, histologically resembles large bowel juvenile polyposis.

Haemangiomatous malformations

These are rare in the bowel, where the small intestine is the most common site. They may be confined to the bowel, where they can be single or multiple or may be a manifestation of a more generalized angiomatosis.[81] They have, in many reports, been classified as metastases from a primary malignant angiosarcoma because their possible multiple nature has not been appreciated.[82] They usually present with haemorrhage and/or anaemia, the source and cause of which can be difficult to find. Histologically, they can be capillary or cavernous and may project into the lumen with consequent ulceration and bleeding. It is not uncommon to find a haemangiomatous component in other patterns of connective-tissue hamartoma.[83]

Lymphangiomatous malformations

These occur in three forms.

Lymphangiomas

These are probably the counterpart of haemangiomas;[84] they occur almost exclusively in the duodenum and can be distinguished from haemangiomas because some of the cavernous spaces usually contain proteinaceous fluid in which are scattered lymphocytes. They have also been described in the mesentery.[85]

Lymphangiectasia[86]

The lymphatics of the lamina propria and submucosa of a variable length of the small bowel are markedly dilated (Fig. 6.12). Lymphatics in the mesentery and regional lymph nodes may be similarly affected. The dilatation of the vessels is often accompanied by considerable oedema and in consequence there is great distortion of the mucosal villi. Inflammatory changes are usually absent, but focal ulceration may develop. The condition is often accompanied by brown bowel syndrome (see p. 275). Malabsorption and protein loss can also occur.

The cause is unknown. A congenital defect in the lymph drainage of the bowel has been suggested but not convincingly demonstrated. Acquired lymphatic obstruction in the mesentery or elsewhere has also been postulated. Most of the patients are children or young adults. Chylous ascites, hypoproteinaemia, lymphocytopenia and steatorrhoea are clinical findings and there may be associated macroglobulinaemia.[87]

Solitary or multiple lymphatic cysts[88]

These are seldom over 1 cm in diameter and occur in the bowel wall, usually in the submucosa; similar but larger cysts can be found in the mesentery.[89,90] In either situation, they may be accompanied by lymphangiectasia though this is infrequent. They are lined by flattened endothelial cells, often with surrounding fibrosis. The condition is generally harmless and unassociated with functional disturbance—though mesenteric torsion is a rare complication.

Neurofibromatosis

There are occasional examples of neurofibromatosis in the small bowel, with or without a more generalized neurofibromatosis. They are usually complex plexiform lesions involving submucosa and muscle coats.[91,92] Some are associated with somatostatin-secreting tumours (see p. 283).

OBSTRUCTION OF THE SMALL INTESTINE

Causes of obstruction

Any condition that interferes with the onward movement of the intestinal contents may be considered under the heading of intestinal obstruction. The causes may be classified as mechanical, neural and vascular, and they operate in the large as well as in the small intestine: obstruction of the large intestine is usually more gradual in its development.

Mechanical obstruction may be complete or incomplete, and its onset may be sudden or gradual. The lumen of the bowel is narrowed by some condition in the wall of the bowel or within the lumen itself or by external compression. The causes of obstruction include inflammatory strictures (for example, in Crohn's disease), tumours, congenital stenosis or atresia, meconium ileus (see above), ascarids, foreign bodies, gall-stones and food.[93] An

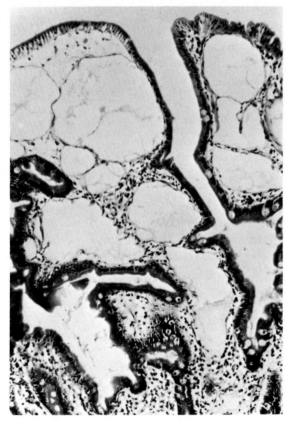

Fig. 6.12 Jejunal lymphangiectasia. The dilated lymphatics have produced marked broadening and distortion at the tips of the villi, but surface enterocytes remain normal.

Haematoxylin-eosin   × 125

annular ulcer of the ileum or lower part of the jejunum that was described as being caused by 'enteric-coated' tablets containing potassium chloride, prescribed to counter hypokalaemia induced by thiazide diuretics, has become increasingly familiar as a benign cause of obstruction of the small bowel: it is considered to be a complication of non-steroidal anti-inflammatory drugs. External compression may result from peritoneal adhesions or bands (the commonest causes of acute intestinal obstruction), incarceration or strangulation of intestine in a hernial sac, intussusception, volvulus, and compression by an intra-abdominal tumour.

The neural type of intestinal obstruction is known as paralytic ileus. The movement of the intestinal contents is halted by paralysis of the intestinal musculature, caused by shock after abdominal operations or by acute peritonitis. The entire small intestine is greatly dilated and filled with gas and fluid faeces.

The vascular causes of obstruction are thrombosis and embolism of the mesenteric blood vessels, commonly the superior mesenteric artery itself. Infarction of the intestinal wall results in paralysis, perforation and peritonitis.

Effects of obstruction

The effects of obstruction vary with the site and the mode of onset. In acute obstruction of the small intestine, the bowel proximal to the obstruction, after a transient initial increase in motor activity, becomes paralysed: it dilates, its wall becomes stretched and very thin, and large amounts of fluid collect within it, providing a rich medium for the growth of intestinal micro-organisms. Antiperistalsis and the accumulation of fluid above the obstruction lead to vomiting, and severe electrolyte disturbances can result from the consequent loss of sodium, potassium and chloride ions.

Chronic obstruction of the small intestine also results in dilatation of the bowel above the site of the obstruction: in contrast to acute obstruction, however, the wall is thickened by compensatory muscular hypertrophy which varies in degree with the duration of the obstruction. Stasis of intestinal contents leads to inflammatory changes in the mucosa, occasionally with the formation of ulcers, which may perforate.

INTUSSUSCEPTION

Intussusception is a variety of intestinal obstruction in which one portion of bowel is invaginated into another (Figs 6.13 and 6.14). Once a portion of the bowel has begun to invaginate in this way into the segment distal to it the latter contracts on the apical part of the entering segment as though it were a bolus of food, and peristalsis then carries it further along the lumen. Because an intussusception is an invagination of part of a continuous tube into the part immediately distal to it, the intruding segment consists of two thicknesses of intestinal wall, the

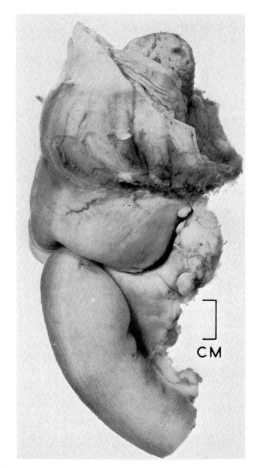

Fig. 6.13 Ileocaecal intussusception. The wall of the caecum has been invaginated by the terminal ileum and its mesentery. The apex of the intruding segment, formed by the ileocaecal valve, is seen at the top of the picture. See also Figure 6.14.

Specimen from the Gordon Museum, Guy's Hospital, London, reproduced by permission of the Curator, Mr J.D. Maynard. Photograph by Miss P.M. Turnbull, Charing Cross Hospital Medical School, London.

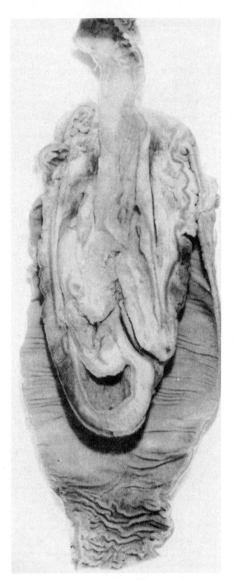

Fig. 6.14 Ileo-ileal intussusception. The bowel has been opened and the intruding segment bisected longitudinally to show the relation of the parts. There is considerable oedema and congestion of the intruding segment, and the apposed serosal surfaces have become adherent over part of their extent.

is continuous at the mouth of the intussusception with the receiving segment, which encloses the intruding segments like a sheath.

Intussusception may occur in the small intestine (jejunojejunal and ileo-ileal intussusception), or at the ileocaecal valve (ileocaecal intussusception, when the valve itself forms the apex of the intruding segment). In ileocolic intussusception the intruding ileum passes through the valve into the ascending colon and the caecum remains in its normal position.

Ileocaecal intussusception is the commonest type.[94,95] It is seen most frequently in children between the ages of 6 and 24 months. Most of them are boys. In contrast to intussusception in adults, there is usually no demonstrable underlying lesion, although it has been suggested that enlargement of the lymphoid tissue in the terminal ileum is one cause.[96] The ileocaecal valve forms the apex of the intussusception, and the caecum is drawn after it into the ascending colon: the apex may even become palpable in the rectum and even appear at the anus!

Occasionally, jejunojejunal and ileo-ileal intussusceptions in children are caused by such lesions as a hamartomatous polyp or Meckel's diverticulum that has become inverted. A more common cause is probably an adenovirus infection[97,98] producing swelling of the gut-associated lymphoid tissue.

In adults there is almost always a predisposing lesion that forms the apex of the intussusception. In the small intestine this is likely to be a foreign body or a benign tumour; in the large intestine it is usually a carcinoma.

Complications of intussusception. These are obstruction of the bowel and gangrene of the intruding segment. Obstruction always results in vascular occlusion, and gangrene, perforation and peritonitis inevitably follow unless the condition is relieved surgically by reduction or resection, or regresses by spontaneous reduction or by sloughing of the intruding segment. Haemorrhagic infarction and gangrene result from constriction of the blood vessels in the mesentery, which is drawn in with the intruding segment. Sloughing of the infarcted length does not necessarily destroy the continuity of the bowel, for adhesions may have formed at the point where the intruding segment is enclosed by

entering and returning parts, which are continuous with each other at the apex of the segment, together with a variable length of the mesentery and the blood vessels within it. The serosal surfaces of the entering and returning parts are opposed and tend to become adherent as fibrinous exudate covers them. The returning part of the intruding segment

the mouth of the intussusception, with the result that union between these parts maintains the integrity of the lumen.

Agonal intussusception

At necropsy, solitary or multifocal intussusceptions may be found in the small intestine of children. There is generally no vascular engorgement of the affected parts of the intestine, and it is clear that the condition has developed in the period immediately before or just after death. The cause, in either case, is irregular peristalsis. Sometimes the direction of the intussusception is the reverse of that ordinarily seen, the intruding segment being drawn into the intestine above it. The condition is of no significance.

STRANGULATION OF THE INTESTINE

The blood vessels in the mesentery of the small intestine may be occluded by torsion in cases of intestinal volvulus, by strangulation in the neck of a hernial sac or by intussusception. The veins, being thin-walled and containing blood under low pressure, become obstructed first and as a consequence the tissue which they drain becomes oedematous: in this way a vicious circle can be built up for the oedema may prevent reduction of the volvulus or hernia, and eventually arterial obstruction follows. Gangrene of the affected part of the bowel results (Fig. 6.15) unless the obstruction is promptly relieved; perforation and peritonitis may occur, either while the intestine is obstructed, or after correction of the obstructing condition if it was not appreciated at the time of the operation that the damaged tissue was no longer viable.

VOLVULUS

Volvulus of the small intestine is less common than volvulus of the colon (see p. 320). A loop of bowel, usually the ileum becomes twisted upon itself, and this results in bowel obstruction and strangulation of the mesenteric blood vessels (see above). The twist may be caused by adhesions, usually to

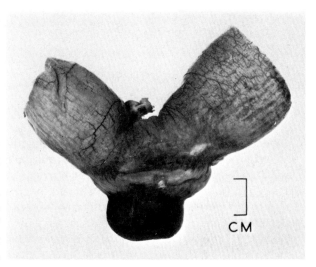

Fig. 6.15 Richter's hernia. In this type of hernia only a part of the wall of the intestine protrudes into the hernial sac. In this case the affected part has undergone strangulation and become gangrenous. The adjoining bowel is hyperaemic, particularly in the immediate vicinity of the line of constriction, which consequently appears as a paler zone between the viable and necrotic tissue.

Specimen from the Gordon Museum, Guy's Hospital, London, reproduced by permission of the Curator, Mr J.D. Maynard. Photograph by Miss P.M. Turnbull, Charing Cross Hospital Medical School, London.

calcified mesenteric lymph nodes; sometimes it is associated with an abnormally short attachment of the mesentery to the posterior abdominal wall or to malrotation or malposition of the bowel.

Other causes of obstruction

Bolus obstruction can follow the ingestion of improperly masticated fruit or vegetables,[99] or high residue diets in hot countries, though this more commonly leads to volvulus.[100]

Stones (often incorrectly called enteroliths) also cause obstruction. Most of those found in the small intestine have been either gall-stones that have ulcerated through from the gall bladder into the upper part of the bowel, fruit stones or true stones that have been swallowed. Very rarely, so-called true enteroliths form as a result of prolonged stasis of the intestinal contents in association with stricture, diverticulum, or the 'stagnant loop syndrome' that results from the formation of a cul-de-sac of bowel in certain surgical procedures, such as partial gastrectomy. These 'true enterol-iths' are mainly composed of bile or calcium salts.[101]

CIRCULATORY DISORDERS[102]

The superior mesenteric artery supplies the whole of the small intestine except for the first part of the duodenum. Occlusion of its main trunk results in infarction of most of the duodenum, the jejunum and all the ileum. Occlusion of a terminal straight artery results in infarction that is confined to the segment of bowel supplied by the affected vessel. Occlusion of one or more of the vessels forming the mesenteric arterial arcades—that is beyond the main trunk of the superior mesenteric artery and before the origin of the straight arteries—usually has little or no effect on the circulation through the bowel.

About 20% of the cardiac output normally flows through the splanchnic circulation. The splanchnic arteries are sensitive to pressor amines; the flow through them is regulated by alteration of their calibre, and a sensitive control of systemic blood pressure is provided by this mechanism. Ischaemia of the small intestine results from organic narrow-ing or obstruction of its arteries or veins, or from reduction of splanchnic blood flow due either to vasoconstriction following severe hypotension or to reduced cardiac output from left ventricular failure; a combination of these factors may be responsible.[103] In this type of hypotension there may be a counter-current exchange mechanism with increased shunting of oxygen across the base of the villi[104] which would explain why the earliest ischaemic lesions occur at the villous tips. There is some evidence that extensive intestinal infarction without obvious arterial disease is occasionally associated with coagulation defects[105] or the intra-vascular deposition of immune complexes.[106,107]

The common cause of arterial narrowing is atheroma, often associated with diabetes, which affects the first 1.0–1.5 cm of the superior mesen-teric artery.[103,108,109] When over 50% of the lumen is occluded symptoms of abdominal angina can occur[110] but infarction is rare unless thrombosis or embolism supervenes. A recent survey covering 20 years indicates that a severe or 'critical' degree of stenosis at autopsy is relatively rare and, when found, does not necessarily relate to symptoms.[111] Local thrombosis undoubtedly occurs in severe atheroma but emboli are probably a more common cause of complete arterial occlusion. Parts of the mural thrombus accompanying myocardial infarc-tion, or intra-atrial thrombi that have formed as a complication of atrial fibrillation, can become detached and may lodge in the main stem or any of the branches of the superior mesenteric artery. When thrombosis does occur it is the main stem of the artery that is occluded, its branches remaining unaffected. A much rarer cause of occlusion of the main mesenteric arteries is polyarteritis.[112] Exten-sion of a dissecting aneurysm of the aorta into the wall of the trunk of a mesenteric artery is another rare cause.

Mesenteric venous occlusion, which is usually the result of external pressure on portal veins, sometimes results from phlebitis in pelvic inflam-mation and occasionally occurs in women taking contraceptive pills. It produces a haemorrhagic pattern of infarction.[103,107]

Something in the order of 20–25% of patients with the symptoms and subsequent operative findings in the bowel of ischaemia have no discoverable arterial lesion. Some have undergone a period of hypotension prior to the onset of symptoms,[113-115] usually as a consequence of my-ocardial infarction, sepsis or major surgery. Low-ering of blood pressure is associated with splanchnic vascular constriction so that the mucosa is deprived of an adequate oxygen supply by two different mechanisms.

ISCHAEMIC BOWEL DISEASE

Interruption or reduction of the small bowel blood supply results in changes which vary in severity from partial or superficial mucosal necrosis, with the possibility of regeneration if the blood supply can be restored, to irreparable full-thickness dam-age with necrosis. There are also marked variations in the extent of involvement and in the degree of healing and repair which take place. In the past a number of terms, including necrotizing and pseu-domembranous enterocolitis have been used de-scriptively; it is now more appropriate to include all degrees of damage from whatever cause under the single term 'ischaemic bowel disease'.

Ischaemic necrosis of the full thickness of the wall of the small bowel is most frequently seen in the middle-aged and elderly. It is commonly associated with shock: this was formerly thought to be secondary to the infarction but is now considered often to be a causative factor. A varying length of bowel is affected: it becomes dark purple and fibrinous exudate develops on the peritoneal surface (Fig. 6.16). The lumen becomes distended and contains blood and fluid faeces. The mucosa is necrotic and there is extensive submucosal hae-morrhage. The muscle coats may be less severely affected. Gas bubbles may be visible in the mesenteric veins. There is haemorrhagic effusion into the peritoneal cavity and fibrinous adhesions form between the loops of infarcted bowel and adjacent structures. Microscopically, the most severe changes are mucosal. In the earliest stages there is patchy necrosis involving villous tips: this later extends to the basal mucosal layer, and necrotic zones coalesce to give total mucosal necrosis, with formation of a surface membrane composed of exudate, red cells, leukocytes and necrotic enterocyte debris. This necrosis tends to

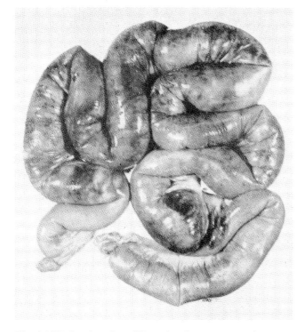

Fig. 6.16 Infarction of small intestine due to mesenteric arterial occlusion. The loops of bowel are distended and dark due to venous congestion.

involve the whole mucosa uniformly and does not have the mushroom-like appearance seen in the large bowel in antibiotic-associated colitis. There is extensive submucosal haemorrhage and oedema, and small fibrin and blood thrombi are often present in vessels.[116] Muscle coats are less severely involved initially and frequently survive; early histologically-recognizable features are poor stain-ing of cytoplasm by eosin, followed by loss of nuclei and finally necrosis with oedema and inflammatory changes (Fig. 6.17).

The lesions of neonatal necrotizing enterocolitis are very similar and it is considered by many to be an ischaemic condition. There is growing evidence that it, and its adult counterpart, result from local ischaemic lesions which are primarily due either to bacterial toxins or to alteration in immune sensitiv-ity.[117,118]

In all patients with extensive infarction, second-ary infection, particularly by anaerobic clostridial organisms, is common and often fatal; it can be difficult on occasions to determine whether the primary cause was ischaemic with subsequent secondary infection or a primary infection by toxin-producing clostridia leading to a secondary ischaemia (see p. 252).

A number of ischaemic lesions produce localized mucosal ulcers but do not involve the full thickness of the bowel wall. Whereas full-thickness necrosis necessitates immediate operation and is often fatal, these ulcers commonly heal. There is a varying degree of mucosal regeneration sometimes associ-ated with pseudo-pyloric metaplasia; more con-spicuous and important is an extensive formation of granulation tissue, often with numerous hae-mosiderin-containing macrophages in the sub-mucosa (Fig. 6.18). This later becomes fibrotic and can lead to severe stenosis and the formation of concentric stricture. The ulcers described in asso-ciation with the taking of non-steroidal anti-inflammatory drugs are of this pattern and are probably due to local vasoconstriction following the lodging of a partly digested tablet in a mucosal fold.[119]

Symptomatology of ischaemia of the small intestine

Full-thickness infarction from sudden complete occlusion of the proximal part of the superior

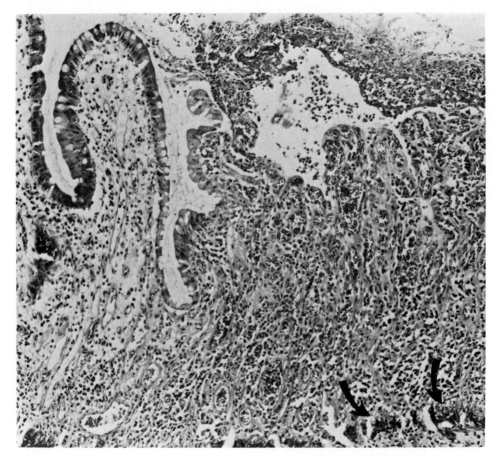

Fig. 6.17 This photomicrograph from the edge of an ischaemic necrotic area of small bowel shows, on the left, an oedematous but relatively intact villus and, on the right, an ulcerated zone. The remains of gland elements can be seen at bottom right (arrowed). There is an exudate consisting of fibrin and debris on the ulcerated surface. The lamina propria contains many inflammatory cells and dilated vessels. Necrosis is not complete and some regeneration with the formation of granulation tissue is beginning.

Haematoxylin-eosin   × 125

mesenteric artery is accompanied by severe continuous abdominal pain, with clinical evidence of intestinal obstruction and peritonitis. Death usually results. When obstruction of the main trunk takes place gradually and is incomplete the patient suffers abdominal pain of anginal type, usually worst after a heavy meal.

Ischaemic necrosis confined to the mucosa and submucosa may present a characteristic 'thumb print' appearance on radiography after an opaque meal: this is attributed to local mucosal distortion by haemorrhage and oedema. When healing results in stricture formation the lesion may or may not be demonstrable radiologically.

It has to be emphasized that among the vascular disorders of the small intestine there is no absolute relation between symptoms and lesions, or between particular forms of lesion and particular causative factors.

Other diseases affecting the vasculature

Polyarteritis,[94] systemic lupus erythematosus and systemic sclerosis may cause necrotizing or occlusive lesions of the small arteries and of the arterioles in the wall of the intestine. These lesions may cause little evidence of ischaemia, or there may be focal necrosis and ulceration, or larger, sometimes confluent, areas of haemorrhagic infarction may result that macroscopically resemble the appear-

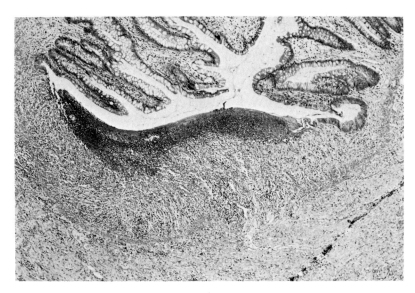

Fig. 6.18 Ischaemic ulcer of jejunum. There is thickening of the lamina propria by oedema and leuocytic infiltration, which extends into the submucosa. The condition presented with acute abdominal colic and melaena. The patient was under treatment for hypertension with reserpine and chlorothiazide. He was given potassium supplements to compensate for hypokalaemia associated with the effects of the thiazide diuretic. The remains of an 'enteric-coated' tablet of potassium chloride were recognizable in the ulcerated area when the surgically excised specimen was examined macroscopically. The relation of local release of potassium salts from tablets and the development of such ulceration is uncertain (see text, opposite). The ulcer in the specimen illustrated almost encircled the bowel.

Haematoxylin-eosin   × 35

Provided by W.St.C. Symmers.

ances associated with embolic occlusion of terminal straight mesenteric arteries. The clinical presentation of these diseases is usually much less abrupt than in cases of the commoner types of mesenteric vascular occlusion in which a major vessel is suddenly closed.

Ischaemic lesions with associated vasculitis have also been described in Schönlein-Henoch purpura, in certain patterns of immune hypersensitivity,[106,117] in diffuse intravascular coagulation in pregnancy,[120] in other vasculitis syndromes including thromboangitis obliterans[121] and following irradiation.

ACUTE INFLAMMATORY CONDITIONS

Typhoid fever

Typhoid or enteric fever (which includes paratyphoid A, B and C) is endemic in the Far and Middle East, Central and South America, Asia and parts of southern, south-western and eastern Europe. In the British Isles and the USA occasional cases and small outbreaks are still seen, mainly in people who have returned from endemic zones, as isolated examples of 'travellers' typhoid'.[122]

The responsible organisms are Gram-negative bacilli. Salmonella fall into two main groups. The first, comprising *Salmonella typhi* and the three types of *Salmonella paratyphi*, A, B and C are ordinarily found only in humans; they are invasive, give rise to generalized infection, have a long (10–14 d) incubation period and do not primarily cause a gastro-enteritis. *S. typhi* and *S. paratyphi A* produce a more severe disease pattern than *S. paratyphi B* which is the one usually seen in Britain. The second group is either adapted to particular animal hosts or unadapted; when they infect human beings they remain confined to the bowel, have a short incubation period and give rise to acute gastro-enteritis. They are discussed under bacterial food poisoning.

Salmonellae are carried in infected food and water or milk and are excreted in the faeces both of those with active disease and of those who, though symptom-free retain viable organisms, usually in the gall-bladder, and are thereby carriers.

The significance of water contamination in the spread of the disease was first recognized in 1856 by William Budd, then a young practitioner in North Devon; his observations provide one of the great milestones in the development of hygiene.[123] The bacilli enter the body through the intestinal mucosa. Patients with hypochlorhydria appear to need a smaller ingested dose of organisms to cause disease than those with normal gastric acidity.[124] The bacilli reach immunologically-competent cells in the solitary lymphoid follicles and Peyer's patches of the ileal mucosa. In the unimmunized individual they stimulate these cells to a primary immunological response. The bacilli invade the bloodstream toward the end of a symptom-free incubation period of 10–14 days: they multiply in the circulation and may be isolated by blood culture during the first week or two after the illness develops. This septicaemia and the accompanying toxaemia are responsible for many of the characteristic clinical features of the disease, such as the eruption of 'rose spots' in the skin, the peculiar type of continued fever and the clouded mental state.

Some of the circulating bacilli are excreted by the liver into the bile and so reach the gall-bladder and return to the lumen of the small intestine. Some are also carried to mesenteric lymph nodes,[125,126] and colonize many organs including bone marrow. In the intestine they come into contact with surface IgA which now contains appropriate antibodies and with lymphoid tissue that now is sensitized: one result may be the characteristic ulceration of Peyer's patches. At this stage, organisms can be cultured from the faeces in an increasing proportion of cases as the disease progresses, the highest incidence of positive stool cultures occurring in the third week of the illness. They are also excreted in the urine, and cultures of urine may be of diagnostic value. Toward the end of the first week of illness specific agglutinating antibodies begin to appear in the patient's blood

and their titre rises to its peak by the end of the third week (Widal reaction).

Macroscopic appearances. The solitary lymphoid follicles and Peyer's patches enlarge as immune competent cells proliferate and they may later become necrotic and ulcerate; there is also submucosal oedema. The ulcerated Peyer's patches are oval lesions with their long axis in the long axis of the bowel (Fig. 6.19) in contrast with those of tuberculosis. Solitary lymphoid follicles do not always ulcerate and when they do, the ulcers are circular and smaller, and are clearly demarcated from the relatively normal surrounding mucosa. Regional lymph nodes are enlarged, soft and hyperaemic.

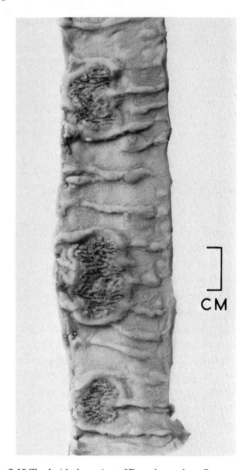

Fig. 6.19 Typhoid ulceration of Peyer's patches. Compare with the picture of tuberculous ulceration in Figure 6.31b.

Specimen from the Pathology Museum, Charing Cross Hospital Medical School, London, reproduced by permission of the Curator, Dr F.J. Paradinas. Photograph by Miss P.M. Turnbull, Charing Cross Hospital Medical School.

THE SMALL INTESTINE 251

Microscopic appearances. The initial lesion is hyperaemia and oedema of lymphoid aggregates and Peyer's patches. Within the lamina propria and submucosa there are large mononuclear cells with deeply-staining nuclei[127] which are modified histiocytes (Fig. 6.20). There are also numerous immune competent cells. It is often said that granulocytes are absent, in keeping with the neutropenia in the blood, but we have seen them in mucosal lesions and in regional lymph nodes in proven cases of typhoid and paratyphoid fever in southern Africa. If the patient recovers mucosal healing occurs by ingrowth from the edge of the ulcer with little granulation tissue formation or subsequent fibrosis. The lesions of paratyphoid fever are similar to those of typhoid, but less extensive and not so severe; they tend to be confined to Peyer's patches in the terminal ileum and complications are rare.

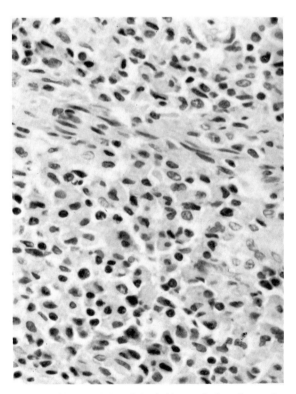

Fig. 6.20 Characteristic cellular infiltrate of affected part of ileum in typhoid fever. Most of the cells are the large, rounded, mononuclear cells with abundant, opaque cytoplasm that are sometimes referred to as 'typhoid cells'.

Haematoxylin-eosin   × 580

Provided by W.St.C. Symmers.

Complications

The two most important in the acute phase are haemorrhage and perforation. In typhoid, the bowel wall becomes soft and friable and single or multiple perforations in association with ulcerated Peyer's patches are common, usually during the fourth week of illness; they may be difficult to diagnose clinically. Surgery, though necessary, can be hazardous because of the general condition of the patient and the friability of the bowel.[128] A minor degree of haemorrhage occurs in most patients whose lesions ulcerate[129] and more serious bleeding is common. Stricture formation after healing is not a complication. Acute cholecystitis is well recognized[130] and probably always precedes the well-known chronic cholecystitis which produces a carrier state. Other rare complications include paralytic ileus, splenomegaly, myocarditis, multifocal necrosis in parenchymatous organs, particularly the liver and kidneys, and in bone marrow, and Zenker's degeneration of the abdominal muscles. Acute bronchitis, meningitis, nephritis, orchitis, arthritis and periosteitis due to the local presence of the typhoid bacillus have all beeen described. Typhoid osteitis may remain in a state of low-grade activity for very long periods; in such cases the organisms may be isolated from the lesion, which are usually solitary, many years after the intestinal infection of which it was originally a complication.

After clinical recovery the organisms may persist in the biliary tract, particularly in the gall-bladder, or in the kidneys. They then continue to be passed, intermittently or more regularly in the faeces or urine, creating the 'carrier state'.[122]

Bacterial food poisoning

'Food poisoning' is caused by three principal groups of organisms: *Staphylococcus pyogenes*, clostridia, principally *Clostridium perfringens*,[131] and salmonellae. Less common causative organisms are *Escherichia coli*,[132] *Bacillus cereus*,[131] *Shigella*,[133] *Clostridium welchii* and *Clostridium botulinum*. Most predominantly affect the large bowel. The term 'food poisoning' has come to be used to describe any acute illness that is attributed to the ingestion of food or drink that has been contaminated by pathogenic bacteria other than those that cause the acute, specific intestinal infections (typhoid, paratyphoid and cholera). The illness may be the result of actual infection of the alimentary tract by these organisms, or of the effect of toxic substances that have been produced by the organisms in the food before ingestion. Bacterial food poisoning usually occurs in outbreaks: these may be confined to a comparatively small number of people who have partaken of the same food, or many hundreds or even thousands may be affected, their illness being traceable to a single source. In almost every instance the outbreak is the result, fundamentally, of a failure to maintain simple standards of hygiene in the preparation and handling of food.

Staphylococcal food poisoning

Staphylococcal food poisoning is so seldom fatal that little is known of the pathological changes that it produces. The symptoms develop within 1–6 hours of ingestion of the food and result from irritation of the mucous membrane of the stomach and, particularly, of the small intestine by the enterotoxin formed by the staphylococci in the food before its ingestion—in other words, the disease is an intoxication and not an infection. It is distinct from pseudomembraneous enterocolitis, which is more properly called antibiotic-associated colitis (see p. 326).

Many outbreaks of staphylococcal food poisoning have been traced to contamination of food that is eaten without further cooking, such as salads, cakes and pastries. The sources of the contamination are food-handlers who are nasal carriers of enterotoxin-producing strains of *Staph. pyogenes*, or who have septic lesions on their hands, or elsewhere on the skin, caused by these organisms.

Clostridial food poisoning[134]

Acute enteritis may follow the consumption of meat contaminated by a strain of *Clostridium perfringens* that is unusually heat-resistant and of relatively low toxigenicity. The attack commonly follows the eating of a meat dish that has been cooked in bulk overnight and allowed to cool slowly over many hours. Food so prepared provides conditions that are notably favourable for the multiplication of an anaerobic spore-bearing organism of this kind and for the formation of its toxin. The resulting infection and accompanying intoxication lead to an acute enteritis that comes on 12 hours later, with sharp colic and diarrhoea, and subsides quickly. The clinical condition has been reproduced in volunteers to whom such strains of *C. perfringens* have been given experimentally by mouth.

Pig-bel enteritis

A more severe form of clostridial food poisoning by *C. perfringens* is the cause of pig-bel, found in the highlands of New Guinea, of which Cooke gave a fascinating description.[135] It is most common in children who have eaten large amounts of imperfectly cooked pig which has been allowed to cool and forms an ideal culture medium for clostridia. Clinically there is abdominal pain with diarrhoea and vomiting followed by distension and constipation. At laparotomy there are multiple distended loops of small bowel often showing full-thickness infarction, and an associated serosal inflammation which can go on to fibrinous peritonitis. The mucosal surface initially shows small greenish spots, resembling the yellow patches of early antibiotic-associated enterocolitis, which soon become confluent. There is submucosal oedema and sometimes gas bubbles form in the bowel wall. Histologically, the green spots represent necrotic villi with little or no inflammatory change; there is a clear dividing line between necrotic villi and viable submucosa, in which intravascular thrombi can be present. Acute secondary inflammatory changes and muscular necrosis often ensue and in those who recover, healing occurs with fibrosis. A somewhat similar condition has been described in sudden over-eating by patients with anorexia nervosa,[136] and forms of enterocolitis sometimes with neutropenia have been attributed to infection with *Clostridium septique*[137] and with various strains of *C. perfringens*.[138]

Botulism

The typically mild and transient illness of the usual form of clostridial food poisoning contrasts strikingly with the far graver condition, with a high case fatality rate, that follows the consumption of food containing the toxins of *C. botulinum*. The disease is caused by the preformed toxin—by weight one of the most poisonous substances known—and there is never any infection of the patients. In Britain, this form of food poisoning is fortunately very rare, in spite of the widespread distribution of toxigenic strains of the organism in farmland soil.

Botulinum toxin has a specific paralysing action on the entire peripheral cholinergic nervous system, both autonomic and somatic.[139] The earliest features are usually diplopia and loss of visual accommodation; death results from failure of the muscles of respiration. It is important to note that several variants of this toxin have been distinguished; they are similar in their toxicological action, but immunologically different. Their neutralization therefore requires specific antitoxins and polyvalent antiserum must be used when the type of intoxication is not known.

'Pseudomembranous' enterocolitis

The term 'pseudomembranous' colitis has been used for a number of conditions, including supposed acute staphylococcal enterocolitis, which are now better understood and categorized.[140,141] Many cases were probably examples of antibiotic-associated colitis which is now known to result from infection by *Clostridium difficile* and is described on page 326. It is rarely seen in the small bowel but when it occurs there it has a close resemblance to the lesions seen in pig-bel. There is a neonatal form,[142] probably also due to clostridial infection, which affects hypoxic stressed infants, in which gas cysts are common. Other patients have had some form of ischaemic bowel disease. In our view the term 'pseudomembranous' is unhelpful and should no longer be used.

Salmonella food poisoning

For many years, *Salmonella typhimurium* (Aertrycke's bacillus) has been far the commonest cause of salmonella food poisoning in Britain. A very large number of other pathogenic organisms of this genus have been isolated from various outbreaks: *Salmonella enteritidis* (Gaertner's bacillus) remains one of the more important of these. Food may become contaminated from two sources: firstly, human carriers and, secondly, infected rats and mice, which are common in most urban communities. The illness is ordinarily an infection and results from the consumption of food that contains the living organisms. It is possible, however, and especially in outbreaks with an incubation period of only a few hours, that the symptoms may sometimes be due to an enterotoxin produced by an organism which has grown in the food, before being killed by cooking. In most cases, the disease runs a short benign course.

Opportunities to study the changes in the alimentary tract are uncommon. The mucous membrane and serosa of the small intestine, particularly the ileum, are hyperaemic and the lymphoid structures in the bowel wall are moderately enlarged. These changes may be accompanied by scattered shallow ulcers in the affected parts of the intestine. When these changes are present in the colon, as is not infrequently the case, they are difficult to distinguish from the appearances of bacillary dysentery. Occasionally the appendix is also involved.

In the severest cases, widespread lesions may develop as a manifestation of salmonella septicaemia. Focal necrosis and focal abscess formation may occur in the liver, and, as in typhoid fever, acute cholecystitis may develop and later become chronic and constitute the source of a carrier state. Salmonella myocarditis, endocarditis and pericarditis have been described, and the organisms may also infect the urinary tract, the meninges, and bones or joints. Unlike typhoid, however, salmonella food poisoning is seldom accompanied by any considerable degree of splenomegaly, even in cases with severe septicaemia.

The microscopic findings in the intestinal and other lesions are often reminiscent of those of typhoid, but with much less striking cellular infiltration, and little or no necrosis. Some of the food poisoning salmonellae cause an inflammatory reaction in which neutrophils are the predominating cell, a response that is seldom found in typhoid or paratyphoid lesions.

Acute bacterial and viral enteritis

Many forms of epidemic diarrhoea, especially in children, are related to infection of the small intestine, particularly the ileum, by viruses, including enteroviruses (particularly echoviruses, rotaviruses, astroviruses and adenoviruses).[143–145] Often in these cases of viral enteritis there is a concomitant infection by an enteropathic strain of *Escherischia coli*. A number of pathogenic strains have now been identified and are subdivided into infantile enteropathogenic, enterotoxin-producing and entero-invasive.[146] Biopsy studies on children with viral, escherichial or mixed infection may show relatively normal mucosa or there can be blunting of villi with some degree of shortening and flattening, crypt zone regeneration and oedema with a mixed cellular infiltration, including some polymorphs, in the lamina propria. Autopsy findings in infants suggest that dehydration plays an important role and it is often difficult to distinguish antemortem from postmortem changes.

Duodenitis

With the increasing use of endoscopic biopsies from the first part of the duodenum for diagnostic purposes, it is important to decide whether minor inflammatory changes and slight degrees of metaplasia are significant. It is now well recognized that in active duodenal ulcer and in its healing phase the adjacent mucosa may show flattening with metaplasia towards a gastric pattern and inflammatory changes in mucosa and submucosa.[147,148] In non-ulcer dyspepsia similar, though often less severe changes are present[149,150] and there is a considerable overlap with the normal in that, as with gastric non-ulcer dyspepsia, some patients with dyspeptic symptoms have normal mucosal histology while others without symptoms show varying degrees of mucosal abnormality. Apart from the difficulties this raises in the confirmation or otherwise of symptomatic duodenitis there is the greater problem of deciding whether, in a biopsy taken from the duodenum to diagnose malabsorption or a suspected specific inflammation

such as an *Esch. coli* infection, positive biopsy changes are to be interpreted as indicative of a specific disorder or merely of an associated but non-specific duodenitis.[151,152] The problem remains not fully resolved; careful morphometric studies will be needed, and many units are now performing these and beginning to publish data from them.

Cholera

Cholera is a form of acute enteritis caused by *Vibrio cholerae* or *Vibrio eltor*.[134] There have been at least six pandemics—those of 1826–37, 1846–62, 1864–75, 1883–96 and 1899–1923, and one that began in 1961. These carried the disease from India to many parts of the world, including Europe and sometimes the Americas, in some instance with a very high mortality. Elimination of cholera from a community depends largely on the prevention of faecal contamination of drinking-water, and the disease remains endemic in many parts of Asia, where periodic outbreaks may cause hundreds of thousands of deaths.

The lesions of cholera are mainly in the lower part of the small intestine, but there is sometimes involvement of the colon also. Biopsy studies[153,154] and electron microscopy[155] have shown that early views on the pathology of cholera, based on histological material obtained at necropsy, were almost totally incorrect. It is now appreciated that the principal lesion is a transient capillary dilatation that allows a marked leakage of fluid with consequent acute dehydration, electrolyte imbalance and circulatory collapse, apparently the result of an enterotoxin which activates adenyl cyclase. There may be comparatively mild, non-specific inflammatory changes in the lamina propria of the mucosa. Ulceration does not occur and erosion is restricted to loss of the surface epithelium from the tips of the villi. The flaky shreds of white matter in the watery, greyish stools are altered mucus and not, as has traditionally been held, pieces of cast-off mucosa. These characteristic 'rice water' stools are a frequent feature of epidemic cholera caused by the classic *V. cholerae*.

The high mortality of cholera is due to the profound shock that accompanies the dehydration and electrolyte imbalance from the severe diarrhoea.

The vibrios are present in enormous numbers in the stools during the illness. If the patient recovers they disappear within a few days in most cases, but occasionally a carrier state results. Most carriers, however, give no history of an attack of the disease.

Yersinia infection

Infection by *Yersinia pseudotuberculosis* or *Yersinia enterocolitica* is increasingly becoming recognized as a cause of enlargement of ileocaecal lymph nodes with symptoms suggesting acute appendicitis or obstruction, particularly in children and adolescents, and often requiring laparotomy; confusion with Crohn's disease is also common.[156-158] At operation the principal finding is enlarged, soft ileocaecal nodes which may show small abscesses on section; there is usually no obvious ileal or appendiceal involvement though mucosal ulceration can be present in the ileum, where the ulcers tend to be longitudinal, or in the colon, where they are small and aphthous.[158] Histologically, lesions are seen in lymph nodes and in submucosa which somewhat resemble those of cat scratch disease. There is initial lymphoid hyperplasia but the architecture remains normal. Histiocytes proliferate and produce a 'starry sky' appearance. This is followed by granuloma formation with central necrosis, polymorph infiltration and the formation of a surrounding zone of epithelioid cells and lymphocytes sometimes with giant cells of Langhans type, and sometimes associated with oedema and the presence of eosinophils (Fig. 6.21). Mucosal ulceration may follow but is by no means constant. Some authors have described the presence of Gram-negative bacilli[158] but these have not been a feature of our own material.

Campylobacter infection

Pathogenic species of campylobacter are curved, Gram-negative, catalase-positive motile rods.[159] They infect both small and large intestines and produce febrile diarrhoea with liquid malodorous stools which usually contain blood. Symptoms and signs suggest a diagnosis of peritonitis and laparotomy has sometimes been performed. In these patients there has been acute inflammation of jejunum and ileum simulating typhoid with associated non-specific inflammatory enlargement of

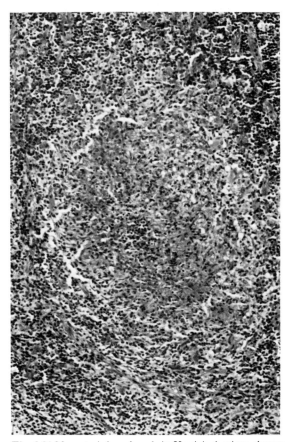

Fig. 6.21 Mesenteric lymph node in *Yersinia.* A micro-abscess with a core of pus cells is beginning to develop.
Haematoxylin-eosin   × 125

mesenteric lymph nodes;[159] colonic appearance can mimic ulcerative colitis.

Whipple's disease

Whipple's disease, first described in 1907, has until lately been of quite uncertain nature. Recent evidence, referred to below, indicates that it may in fact be a bacterial infection. It is usually seen in men of middle age. Clinically, it often presents with migratory polyarthritis, intermittent chronic diarrhoea and steatorrhoea-like malabsorption.[160] The diagnosis can often be made by intubation biopsy of the small intestine. Sometimes lymph node biopsy, either in the course of laparotomy or in the presence of clinical enlargement of superficial nodes, has led to its recognition.

The pathological changes peculiar to the disease are in the small intestine and in mesenteric and, often, pre-aortic lymph nodes. Other parts of the alimentary tract are rarely involved. In some cases lymph nodes outside the abdomen and other organs also show changes. The wall of the small intestine is thickened, especially the mucosa. Minute yellow flecks or streaks mark the position of some of the lymphatics in the serosa of the bowel and there is oedema of the mesentery, often with fibrosis. The regional lymph nodes are enlarged and yellow, and their normal structure may be replaced by thick cheesy material. Microscopically, there is diffuse infiltration of the lamina propria by macrophages. Many of these cells contain granular material that does not react with stains for lipids but gives a positive periodic acid-Schiff reaction and resists digestion with diastase; a proportion of the macrophages also contain lipid material (Fig. 6.22).

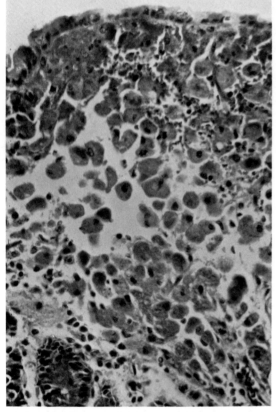

Fig. 6.22 Whipple's disease. The lamina propria is filled with macrophages containing finely granular material, clearly visible in sections stained with H & E, but also readily demonstrable using PAS after diastase digestion. The accumulated macrophages have caused partial mucosal flattening, but the surface enterocytes remain normal.

Haematoxylin-eosin   × 315

Similar cells are present in the lymphatics and in the regional lymph nodes. Multinucleate giant cells are also commonly present, both in the mucosa and in the lymph nodes. In some cases comparable histological changes occur in other organs, particularly the spleen.[161]

In patients treated with antibiotics before biopsy, macrophages containing ingested bacteria may be confined to the submucosa and so be missed in a routine biopsy which includes mucosa only.[162] Rectal biopsy techniques for diagnosis are not always reliable, since muciphages have been wrongly reported as Whipple cells and many macrophages normally present in the rectum contain a lipofuscin pigment akin to the PAS-positive material present in Whipple's disease.[163]

Electron microscopy[164] and immunocyto-chemistry[165] reveal numerous bacilliform bodies 1–2 μm long which are present extracellularly in large numbers immediately beneath the epithelial basement membrane and are ingested by macrophages to form the PAS-positive material described, which is also probably partly lysosomal. Their number diminishes markedly after tetracycline treatment.

Acute non-specific inflammation of the terminal ileum and acute non-specific mesenteric lymphadenitis

Acute non-specific inflammation of the terminal ileum ('acute terminal ileitis') and acute mesenteric lymphadenitis may occur together or the lymphadenitis may be present without obvious disease of the bowel. Most of the patients are children, and the clinical picture is similar to that of acute appendicitis. At operation, however, there is no evidence of any acute lesion of the appendix: instead, the terminal ileum is found to be congested and oedematous, and the lymph nodes in the mesentery of the terminal ileum and in the ileocaecal angle are enlarged. Occasionally, the inflammation of the terminal ileum is sufficiently marked to give rise to local peritonitis and the formation of fibrinous adhesions.[166,167]

The cause of this condition is not clear. It is possible that both the ileitis and the lymphadenitis are manifestations of a non-specific response of the lymphoid tissue to infection, similar in kind to that seen in the tonsillar tissues—in fact, part of the lymphoid hyperplasia that accompanies the development of immunity in children and young adults. Alternatively, such appearances could result from infection by one of the enteric group of organisms or by a virus, and there is now good evidence that a similar clinicopathological picture may result from infection by *Y enterocolitica* (see above). Such observations indicate that ileitis and mesenteric lymphadenitis of the type described here may have a variety of different causes, and should not be considered as an entity.

Phlegmonous enteritis

A small number of patients have recently been described with a condition of the small bowel which resembles phlegmonous gastritis (see p. 159). The mucosa is intact, though there may be focal thromboses and septic inflammation of venules within it, producing local zones of haemorrhage. There is severe submucosal oedema with acute inflammatory changes, and death commonly ensues.[168] Chronic alcoholism[168] and infected venous shunts[169] may be predisposing factors.

Neutropenic enterocolitis

Occasional patients with neutropenia following treatment of haematological conditions with antimitotic drugs develop mucosal and submucosal oedema with transmural inflammation which does not appear to be related to the primary haematological complaint.[170] The pathogenesis is undetermined.

CHRONIC INFLAMMATORY CONDITIONS

Crohn's disease (regional enteritis)

The occurrence of an apparently non-specific chronic granulomatous disease of the terminal ileum has been recognized since the beginning of this century, but the condition attracted little attention until 1932. In that year Crohn and his colleagues described, under the name regional ileitis, a condition that they considered to be a clinical and pathological entity involving the terminal part of the small intestine.[171] Since that

time the same pathological process has been described in other parts of the alimentary tract, and the term regional enteritis was introduced to indicate the more widespread anatomical distribution of the disease. Other expressions such as terminal ileitis, regional jejunitis, ileocolitis and segmental colitis are often used to describe the same disease when it occurs in the corresponding anatomical sites. The names Crohn's disease and regional enteritis are preferred, because they emphasize that the various localized forms of the condition are all manifestations of a single underlying pathological process.

The cause of Crohn's disease is unknown, and attempts to incriminate organisms, such as mycobacteria, dysentery bacilli, protozoa, viruses and fungi, have all failed.[172] The microscopical picture in some cases is that of a sarcoid reaction, but patients with sarcoidosis only very rarely develop involvement of the gastrointestinal tract, while in Crohn's disease the sarcoid-like lesions are not usually seen anywhere but in the bowel and the regional lymph nodes. Interestingly, the Kveim test is not infrequently positive in Crohn's disease:[173] the significance of this observation is not yet evident.

The granulomas of Crohn's disease do not caseate, and there is never any bacteriological evidence of tuberculosis. The Mantoux test is negative in about 80% of patients[174] and this may be used clinically in making the distinction from tuberculosis. In the past, cases of Crohn's disease were regarded as examples of non-caseating hyperplastic ileocaecal tuberculosis, and many pathologists now avoid making the latter diagnosis, in the belief that all such cases are examples of Crohn's disease: however, occasional cases of true fibrocaseous tuberculosis of the ileocaecal region undoubtedly occur and quite closely resemble Crohn's disease clinically and macroscopically (see p. 262).

Other suggested aetiological factors include trauma, and psychosomatic, genetic and racial factors. Sometimes there is a definite familial predisposition to Crohn's disease,[175,176] and some authorities have maintained that its incidence is highest in Jews.[177]

Recent studies have indicated that the lesion of Crohn's disease may result from a disturbance of immunological mechanisms.[178,179] There is certainly pathological evidence that the condition is a disease of lymphoid tissue. It most commonly affects the terminal ileum, which has the largest amount of lymphoid tissue in the gastrointestinal tract, and hyperplasia of lymphoid tissue in the bowel wall is one of the more important histological characteristics of the disease. The regional lymph nodes are always enlarged, and frequently contain the characteristic non-caseating tuberculoid foci. Current opinion is now moving towards the view that there are a number of possible causative factors, all of which act through immune mechanisms. A good recent review of epidemiological factors is available.[180] Crohn's disease occurs at all ages. There are three main peaks of age of onset for both sexes at 20–29, 50–59 and 70–79 years[181] but cases occur in childhood and can lead to growth retardation.[182] Men predominate over women in a proportion of about 5:4. The disease is common in Scandinavia, northern Europe and North America and is becoming more common in southern Europe.[183] It is still rare in tropical and subtropical regions. Large intestinal involvement also appears to be becoming more frequent.

Macroscopic appearances. The pathology of Crohn's disease is fundamentally the same whether it affects the ileum, stomach, duodenum, jejunum, colon or rectum but the early lesions, which are not often seen, form the basis of, but contrast markedly with, the later ones. Characteristically, the terminal ileum and its associated lymph nodes are frequently involved but the primary lesion can be elsewhere in the small[184] or large bowel and multiple discontinuous lesions are not uncommon. In the early stages there is little thickening or rigidity. The mucosal surface may show small discrete superficial ulcers which later become serpiginous while the submucosa and muscle coats are oedematous and gradually become more thickened: there may be an exudate on the serosal surface. The ulcers result from oedema and from enlargement of mucosal and submucosal lymphoid tissue which is the primary lesion in Crohn's disease and which raises the mucosa prior to ulceration and gives rise to fissures which extend upwards to the surface and downwards to the muscularis propria. When this process is extensive the raised islands of mucosa present a cobblestone appearance (Fig. 6.23) but this is not a uniform

finding. Inflammation and fissuring ulceration extend through the muscle coats to involve the serosa and adhesions often bind the gut to adjacent organs and tissues. There is involvement of the peri-intestinal fat and sometimes small granulomas form on the peritoneal surface and are visible as tiny 'tubercles'. Subsequent fibrosis and continuous oedema and inflammation lead to thickening and stricture formation with luminal narrowing and the characteristic 'hose pipe' appearance of the involved segment (Fig. 6.24). The disease is segmental and discontinuous and there are skip areas of normal bowel between involved segments. Regional lymph nodes are often but not always involved.

Microscopic appearances. There are three main features which distinguish Crohn's disease from other chronic inflammatory bowel conditions; though not all are necessarily present in any one patient, all should be carefully looked for. They are lymphoreticular infiltration which is transmural, fissuring ulceration, and the presence of individual granulomas and/or a granulomatous lining to the fissures which are present.[185] There is great thickening of the submucosa, which is oedematous and contains many foci of lymphoid tissue, often with a well-marked follicular structure and the development of germinal centres. Although most numerous in the submucosa, these lymphoid foci often develop throughout the thickness of the bowel wall and particularly in the serosa (Fig. 6.25). Ulceration of mucosa is invariably present, but patchy. It often takes the form of fissures, which may pass right through the bowel wall (Fig. 6.26). These fissures are the basic cause of the intramural abscesses, sinuses and fistulae that are characteristic of the disease; they can be distinguished from artefacts by their lining of granulation tissue. Fibrosis accompanies the other changes in the affected tissues, eventually involving all layers of the bowel wall, with more or less interruption and disruption of muscle coats. In some 50–60% of cases of Crohn's disease, non-caseating tuberculoid foci are found in the bowel wall and in the regional lymph nodes (Figs 6.27–6.29). These foci are sometimes very numerous; in other cases they are found only by examining many lymph nodes using step sections. They consist of a cluster of epithelioid cells, with one or more rather

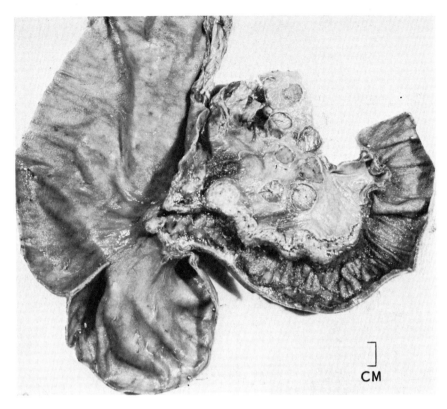

Fig. 6.23 Crohn's disease of the terminal ileum, showing stenosis and the characteristic 'cobblestone' appearance of the mucous membrane. The regional lymph nodes are enlarged (the serosa and subserosal fat have been dissected in places to display them).

small multinucleate giant cells which occasionally contain conchoidal bodies (Fig. 6.28), identical with those that are seen commonly in sarcoidosis (Schaumann bodies) and more rarely in various other tuberculoid granulomatous diseases and in tuberculosis itself.[186] There is no caseation. It is important to examine many lymph nodes when searching for these diagnostically important tuberculoid foci, for they may be found in only one node in a group; also, they may be absent from the more markedly enlarged nodes and yet abundant in small nodes. It has been suggested that the epithelioid cells in the granulomas are reacting to intermittent stimulation by antigens to immune complexes.[187]

The earliest changes in Crohn's disease appear in the lymphoid follicles and in Peyer's patches, which enlarge and become ulcerated. Fresh lymphoid tissue develops throughout the submucosa, pushing up the mucous membrane to give a characteristic cobblestone appearance. Sometimes tuberculoid foci are seen in the lymphoid follicles; more commonly they are to be found along the course of blood vessels and lymphatics. The lymphatics are conspicuously dilated. The granulomatous foci are seen in the serosa also, where they correspond to the tubercle-like structures that are visible macroscopically. They can extend into the mesenteric fat.

Other histological features that have been described in Crohn's disease are less important than those mentioned above, and appear to be secondary effects of the chronic inflammation. They include the presence of metaplastic glands of pseudo-pyloric type in the mucosa, neuromatoid changes in the submucosal nerves, with thickening of the nerve fibres and an increase in vasoactive intestinal polypeptide content,[188,189] marked thickening of the muscularis mucosae, and various changes in the blood vessels.[190] Some transmission and scan-

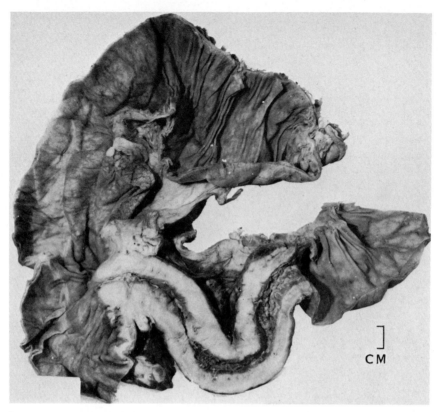

Fig. 6.24 Crohn's disease of the terminal ileum, showing the 'hosepipe' stricture that is typical of the chronic stage.

ning electron microscope studies have been made but are not of great value in laboratory diagnosis.[191]

Complications

The main complications of Crohn's disease are malabsorption and fistula formation. Carcinoma is a less frequent complication, but not so rare as used to be thought (see below).

Malabsorption in Crohn's disease. This is quite common, especially in cases with extensive involvement of the small intestine. The widespread chronic inflammatory changes and ulceration in the mucosa are the anatomical basis for the impairment of absorption of fat, vitamin B_{12}, protein and electrolytes. However, there seems to be no correlation between the extent of the intestinal disease and the severity of the malabsorption. The anatomical site of the lesion may determine the type of deficiency. Impairment of fat absorption is probably the commonest finding, but the resulting steatorrhoea is seldom as severe as that of gluten-induced enteropathy. In general, malabsorption in Crohn's disease is mild: but continued over a long period of time it may lead to severe malnutrition.

Fistulae. Three types of fistula occur in Crohn's disease—internal fistulae between adjacent loops of bowel, enterocutaneous fistulae between loops of bowel and the skin of the abdominal wall, and anal fistulae and fissures. Fistulae of any type may be single or multiple.

Internal fistulae between loops of bowel are found in about 20% of cases of Crohn's disease. The commonest types are ileo-ileal and ileocolic, the latter including the ileorectal fistulae. They are the result of extension of the chronic granulomatous process through the bowel wall, with the formation of intramural fissures or abscesses that reach the serosa and provoke the formation of localized inflammatory exudate on the overlying serosal surface. Another loop of bowel becomes adherent to this area, and eventually the inflam-

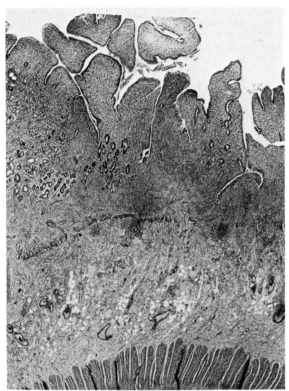

Fig. 6.25 Crohn's disease of the ileum, showing thickening of the submucosa by oedema. There is hyperplasia of lymphoid tissue, particularly in the submucosa and fissuring is present. Haematoxylin-eosin × 25

patient, and are frequently multiple. Actinomycosis has to be considered in the differential diagnosis.

Rectal or anal fistulae and fissures are found in about 30% of patients with Crohn's disease. These fistulae are not continuous with the intestinal lesions. It is of great diagnostic importance that they may precede the development of intestinal disease by a number of years. Alternatively, they may appear at the same time as the clinical manifestations of intestinal disease, or they may not develop until after the latter has become well established. The anal lesions of Crohn's disease may resemble tuberculous lesions clinically, and care is essential that they are not mistaken for tuberculosis on histological examination, for they often contain non-caseating tuberculoid foci similar to those seen in the intestinal lesions.[192,193] However, no tubercle bacilli can be demonstrated in them by histological methods or by culture or guinea-pig inoculation.

Carcinoma. Evidence is steadily accumulating that carcinoma of the small intestine may develop as a late complication of Crohn's disease. There is an increased incidence of both small and large bowel carcinoma which can also occur in a bypass segment; in many patients there is associated epithelial dysplasia.[194–197]

Diagnosis, course and prognosis

Small intestinal Crohn's disease is usually diagnosed only at laparotomy when a resected specimen is available. A careful anal and rectal examination is obligatory and any anal fistula or fissure must be biopsied and searched for a granulomatous reaction which, if present, must be distinguished from tuberculosis or a foreign-body granuloma (see above). Rectal biopsy can also be valuable in clinically suspected cases since small isolated granulomas are sometimes found. Despite claims to the contrary, occasional examples of sarcoidosis are present in the bowel.[198]

The long-term course and prognosis are not good. Surgical resection may be needed for the disease itself (obstruction, fistula formation) but is seldom curative; recurrence is common and the death rate is more than twice that in a matched control group.[199] There is some evidence that a

matory reaction and fissuring extend across from one loop to the other, and then through to the lumen of the second loop, forming the fistula. Sometimes an affected loop of bowel becomes adherent to the parietal peritoneum in the pelvic cavity, with the formation of a chronic pelvic abscess that eventually discharges into the rectum, thus establishing an ileorectal fistula. More rarely, ileovesical or ileovaginal fistulae are formed.

Enterocutaneous fistulae most commonly occur at the site of a surgical scar in patients who have been operated on. Such fistulae sometimes follow appendicectomy and then are the first intimation that the patient may have Crohn's disease. In either case the mechanism of production of the fistula is the same. The diseased bowel becomes adherent to the peritoneal aspect of an abdominal incision or scar, and the granulomatous process spreads through the abdominal wall. Enterocutaneous and internal fistulae may occur together in the same

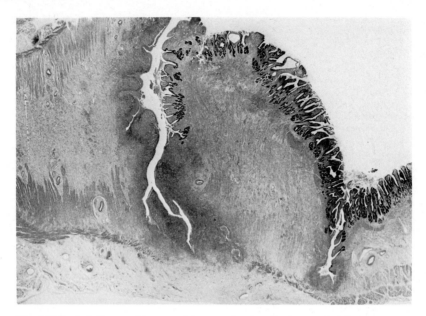

Fig. 6.26 Crohn's disease of the upper jejunum, showing the characteristic fissuring ulceration.

Haematoxylin-eosin   × 10

Provided by Dr R.R. Wilson, Stobhill Hospital, Glasgow.

high granuloma count in a resected specimen indicates a better prognosis in large, but not in small bowel disease.[200]

Tuberculosis

Tuberculosis of the small intestine takes two main forms: (1) primary involvement of the gut-associated lymphoid tissue with spread to the mesenteric lymph nodes, and (2) secondary infection producing intestinal lesions as a result of swallowing infected sputum in cases of open pulmonary tuberculosis.[201-209]

Primary intestinal tuberculosis

Primary intestinal tuberculosis has become an uncommon disease in the indigenous population of the British Isles, although occasional cases are still seen, both in adults and in children. It is still found not uncommonly in recently settled immigrants. Formerly, in Britain and elsewhere, it was usually due to infection by *Mycobacterium bovis*, acquired from cow's milk; the incidence of this type of infection has fallen greatly as a result of the pasteurization of milk supplies in Britain and, more recently, steps to eradicate mycobacteria among cattle. The chances of a child contracting infection by the human type of tubercle bacillus (*Mycobacterium tuberculosis*) from relatives or friends have also been greatly lessened here, as in many other parts of the world, in consequence of the great fall in the number of cases of open respiratory tuberculosis.

It is characteristic of most cases of primary tuberculosis of the intestinal tract, whether of human or bovine origin, that the disease affects predominantly the mesenteric lymph nodes, generally without any recognizable initial intestinal lesion. The nodes are enlarged and matted, and undergo extensive caseation, before eventually healing by fibrosis and calcification. Tuberculosis is the usual cause of the calcification of mesenteric nodes that is seen in abdominal radiographs or during abdominal operation, or at necropsy.

In India, primary tuberculosis involving the small intestine as well as lymph nodes is still quite common; ulcerative and ulcerohypertrophic forms are distinguished.[206] The latter may be difficult to differentiate from Crohn's disease[209] (see p. 257),

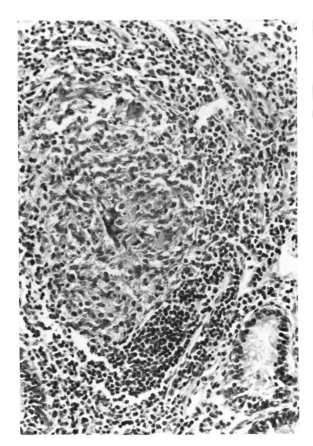

Fig. 6.27 A tuberculoid granuloma without caseation in the ileal mucosa in Crohn's disease.

Haematoxylin-eosin   × 65

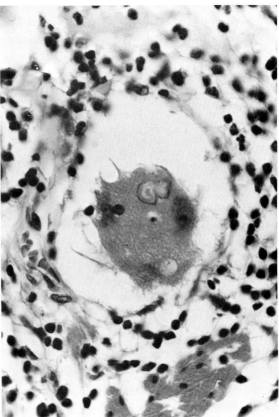

Fig. 6.28 Multinucleate giant cells in Crohn's disease, with included 'conchoidal' bodies, similar to the Schaumann bodies of sarcoidosis.

Haematoxylin-eosin   × 170

and the demonstration of tubercle bacilli by culture or guinea-pig inoculation may be the only certain way of distinguishing between the two, for their gross and microscopic appearances may be very similar (Fig. 6.30). Again there may be no visible lesion at the portal of entry; mucosal lesions form later, presumably either by retrograde spread from involved lymph nodes[201] or, much more probably, as the result of an immune hypersensitivity reaction combined with a continuing exposure to pathogenic mycobacteria.

A number of patients with primary tuberculosis of the small intestine have been reported in Britain[203] and we have seen several in different ethnic groups, including Caucasians. One of the patients was a woman, aged 71. There was an extensive stricture of the terminal ileum, with

dark-grey, ragged ulceration of the mucosa. Histologically, the bowel wall was replaced by a caseating granulomatous mass containing very large numbers of tubercle bacilli. The regional lymph nodes were also involved, and miliary tubercles were present over the peritoneum and in the liver.

Although the incidence of tuberculosis is falling in countries with a high standard of living, it remains important to consider this disease in the differential diagnosis of chronic granulomatous conditions of the small intestine.

Secondary intestinal tuberculosis

Tuberculous ulceration of the small intestine in patients with active pulmonary tuberculosis is also

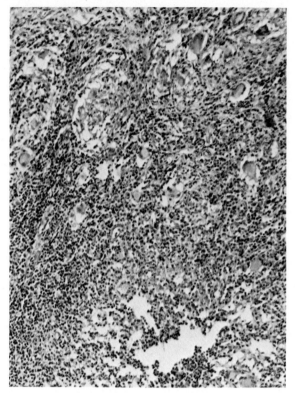

Fig. 6.29 Tuberculoid giant cell reaction in regional lymph node in a case of Crohn's disease of the ileum.

Haematoxylin-eosin   × 120

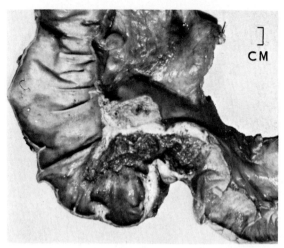

Fig. 6.30 Primary tuberculosis of the terminal ileum, with ulceration. It can be very difficult to distinguish this condition from Crohn's disease unless, as in the case illustrated, the tissues are found to contain many tubercle bacilli.

becoming less common as the incidence of tuberculosis decreases, and in particular with the increasing effectiveness of therapy.

Macroscopic appearances of intestinal tuberculosis

Ulceration involves primarily the lymphoid aggregates and follicles. Ulcers, which are commonly multiple, are therefore most common in the ileocaecal region (Fig. 6.31). When ulcers occur in primary tuberculosis they do not differ in appearance from those in secondary tuberculosis. In both conditions they are oval and lie transversely in the bowel; they have a base of soft white caseous tissue and often give rise to stricture. Small miliary tubercles are commonly present on the serosal surface. As the lesions progress some degree of healing with fibrosis takes place to produce an elongated hard stricture.[202,205]

Microscopic appearances

In the active phase the lesions develop in lymphoid aggregates and Peyer's patches as zones of caseation with a typical tuberculous granulation reaction which spreads round and through the small bowel wall and along the circumvascular and subserosal lymphatics to the regional lymph nodes. Involvement of the peritoneum itself may result in widespread dissemination of the infection throughout the abdominal cavity, with the development of ascites.

The local peritonitis that develops over the sites of tuberculous ulceration may lead to the development of fibrous adhesions between the bowel and neighbouring structures. Because of these adhesions, the eventual penetration of the ulcer through the wall of the ileum is very unlikely to result in generalized peritonitis but contraction of adhesions can lead to kinking and obstruction. Sometimes, when two or more loops of intestine become adherent in this way a fistula ultimately develops, with consequent short-circuiting of the intestinal contents.

In some secondary lesions, healing of the respiratory focus may be accompanied by healing of the ileal ulcers. The contraction of the resulting scar tissue may, in time, lead to the development of strictures and eventual intestinal obstruction.

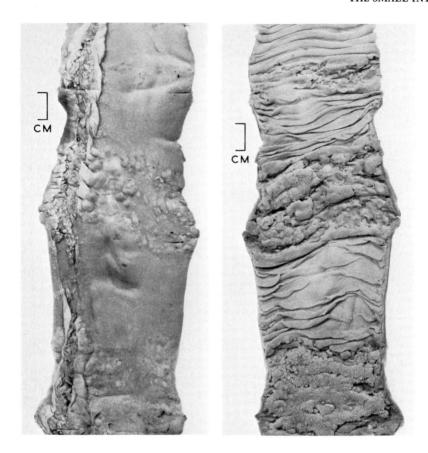

Fig. 6.31a, b (**a**) Secondary tuberculosis of the small intestine, showing the subserosal tubercles overlying the site of the mucosal ulceration (see (**b**)). The lesions are disposed transversely in relation to the long axis of the bowel. (**b**) The mucosal aspect of the specimen illustrated in (**a**). The ulcers encircle the bowel, following the line of distribution of the lymphatic vessels (compare with the longitudinal orientation of the ulcers of typhoid fever, which correspond to the distribution of the intestinal lymphoid tissue; see Figure 6.19).

Specimens from the Pathology Museum, Charing Cross Hospital Medical School, London, reproduced by permission of the Curator, Dr F.J. Paradinas. Photographs by Miss P.M. Turnbull, Charing Cross Hospital Medical School.

Protozoal infections[210]

Giardiasis [210–212]

The commonest protozoon to infect the small intestine is *Giardia lamblia* (*Giardia intestinalis*), a flagellate of worldwide distribution and one of the most frequent parasites of man. Its prevalence is substantially greater in communities with low standards of sanitation and hygiene, and particularly in hot climates, and, along with *Esch. coli*, it is a frequent cause of travellers' diarrhoea.[213] The pear-shaped, binuclear trophozoite, which has four pairs of flagella, is found in the duodenum and jejunum; it is rarely seen in faeces unless there is diarrhoea and a rapid passage of the upper intestinal contents through the bowel. Ordinarily, the giardia has encysted before being passed in the faeces and therefore is found in the latter in the cyst form. The trophozoites may be found in jejunal biopsy specimens; their presence does not necessarily indicate that they have been responsible for whatever symptoms led to the investigation. They are distorted and often difficult to recognize in histological preparation (Figs 6.32 and 6.33),

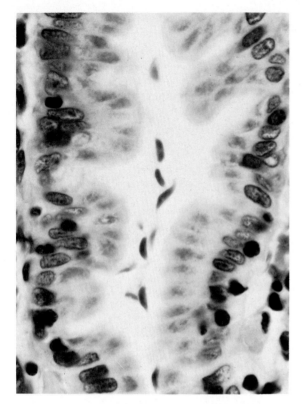

Fig. 6.32 *Giardia lamblia* in the lumen of an intestinal gland. Incidental finding in a jejunal biopsy specimen. The patient had been under treatment for many years for gluten-sensitive enteropathy. No parasites were present in earlier biopsy specimens. Six months before the specimen illustrated was taken in the course of a follow-up examination the patient had spent some days on holiday in a northern European city where giardiasis is reputed to be particularly frequent. There were no symptoms. See also Figure 6.33.

Haematoxylin-eosin   × 750

Provided by W.StC. Symmers.

appearing as slender and generally sickle-shaped structures between the villi. They are rarely seen in the depths of the mucosal glands. Whatever their situation they usually lie free in the mucus covering the epithelial surface; sometimes they are attached to the epithelial cells. The intestinal mucosa is often histologically normal but some degree of villous flattening may be present[214,215] and there may be foci of acute inflammation with small numbers of neutrophils and occasional eosinophils. Some patients have an accompanying nodular lymphoid hyperplasia which may but need not be associated with isolated IgA deficiency or a more generalized hypogammaglobulinaemia.[216,217] There

is also some evidence that careful quantitative histology may reveal a reduction in mucosal surface area in patients who have giardiasis with malabsorption which is less marked in those who are infected but have normal absorption.[218]

Other protozoal infections[210,212]

Amoebiasis (see p. 330) and balantidiasis (see p. 332), which ordinarily affect the large bowel, may

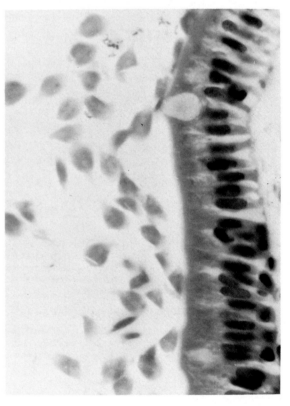

Fig. 6.33 *Giardia lamblia* in a jejunal biopsy specimen. The patient was under investigation for recurrent diarrhoea and symptoms of malabsorption of some 18 months' duration. Recognition of the presence of the parasites and treatment of the infestation led to complete recovery. Note the variation in the appearance of the organisms as illustrated by this specimen and the one shown in Figure 6.32. In this photograph most of the parasites are seen from the dorsal or ventral aspect and in some the paired nuclei can just be made out, separated by the pale line of the axostyles, which run through the body to the pointed posterior end. In Figure 6.32 most of the organisms are seen from the side and appear correspondingly denser.

Haematoxylin-eosin   × 750

Provided by W.StC. Symmers

involve the terminal ileum, particularly in severe cases of chronic infection.

Coccidiosis (isospososis).[210,212,219] Coccidiosis, which is thought to be one of the rarest protozoal infections to occur in man, usually involves the ileum or the caecum. It is caused by *Isospora hominis*, *Isospora belli* and possibly other species. The sporozoites, released from the ingested oocyst in the lumen of the bowel, enter the intestinal epithelial cells. They multiply there in the form of trophozoites, which in turn invade neighbouring epithelial cells. Eventually, a fresh generation of oocysts forms: these pass into the lumen of the bowel, thence to reach other individuals or re-infect the same host through faecal contamination. Occasional cases of intestinal coccidiosis among members of the staff of biological laboratories are possibly due to species of coccidia that ordinarily are confined to animals, particularly *Isospora catti* from cats. Intestinal coccidiosis is usually associated with no more than trivial illness; rarely, severe prostrating diarrhoea has occurred, or there may be recurrent diarrhoea over many years and ultimately the development of malabsorption. It has also been known to cause intractable diarrhoea in infants.[220] We know of a single report of *Cryptosporidiosis* infection with associated cytomegaloviral infection in a male homosexual.[224]

Metazoal infestations

Infestation by cestodes[222]

Taeniasis. The most frequent forms of taeniasis are those caused by *Taenia saginata* and *Taenia solium*. Man is the definitive host of both of these worms, their larval (cysticercal) stage being in cattle and pigs respectively. The adult parasites live in the human small bowel and seldom, if ever, cause any injury to the tissues. This contrasts strikingly with the gravity of the illness that may result when, through ingestion of the ova, the larval state of the infestation (cysticercosis) develops in man. The taeniae are of worldwide distribution.

Diphyllobothriasis. Infestation by *Diphyllobothrium latum* is most frequent in northern Europe, in the Baltic area. The ova of the worm have been found in the intestine of human bodies from peat bogs dating back to the Stone Age. The larval stages develop in freshwater crustacea, particularly species of *Cyclops*, and then in freshwater fish (perch, pike, salmon, trout); the definitive hosts are fish-eating mammals. In man the greatest importance of infestation by diphyllobothrium is the liability to macrocytic anaemia that results from the competition between worm and host for vitamin B_{12}.

Infestation by nematodes

The most frequent nematode infestations of the small intestine are ascariasis,[223] ancylostomiasis[224] and strongyloidiasis.[225]

Ascariasis. Ascaris lumbricoides is the largest and probably the most prevalent roundworm parasite of man.[223,226] The adult ascarids live in the small bowel. In cases of heavy infestation, particularly in children, the worms may become so tangled that they form a mass that obstructs the bowel.[227] Sometimes, in such cases, worms penetrate the bowel wall, reaching the peritoneal cavity: this is almost certainly a consequence of spontaneous perforation in the course of an acute ulcerative inflammation and not due to invasion by the parasite. If the patient survives the accompanying septic peritonitis, the myriads of ascaris ova that may have been shed can cause a sclerosing granulomatous peritonitis that may eventually cause intestinal obstruction. Occasionally, ascarids make their way from the duodenum into the biliary ducts, which they may obstruct.

The ova of *Ascaris lumbricoides* are probably not able to pass through all the states of normal embryonic development unless they spend some time outside the body of the host: in contrast to oxyuriasis (enterobiasis), which can be perpetuated by transfer of freshly-deposited ova from the anal region to the mouth, ascariasis is probably not continually re-established in such a manner. When embryonate ova are swallowed they hatch in the small intestine: the larvae penetrate the mucosa, some then passing to the liver in the portal venous system and then to the lungs in the venous return, while others reach the lungs more directly by way of the lymph flow to the superior vena cava. Many die in transit. The survivors pass from pulmonary alveoli to respiratory passages and thence by way of the oesophagus and stomach to the bowel. The worms reach sexual maturity two to three months after ingestion as ova.

Ancylostomiasis (uncinariasis). Hookworm infestation is one of the most serious of all forms of helminthiasis.[224,228] Two species of these worms are responsible. *Ancylostoma duodenale* is the infesting worm in southern Europe, North Africa, northern India, parts of China and Japan. Fishermen from what is now Japan are thought to have introduced it to the Pacific littoral of South America some 5000 years ago. It has gradually spread to many other parts of the world, including western Australia, south-eastern Asia and West Africa.

Necator americanus is the infesting worm in central and southern Africa, southern Asia, Polynesia and the southern parts of North America, Central America and the northern parts of South America. Its introduction to the Americas is generally believed to have accompanied the slave traffic from Africa.

In Europe, hookworm infestation has largely been eliminated. During the nineteenth century it was prevalent among miners and tunnel workers, often in epidemic form and with a high mortality.[229] Severe anaemia from chronic blood loss, possibly in association with deficiency of iron intake, is the major clinical manifestation. The worms are generally confined to the lower two-thirds of the jejunum. Biopsy studies indicate that histological changes are usually very slight,[230] although severe changes, with flattening and fusion of villi, lymphocytic infiltration and fibrosis of the lamina propria, are seen occasionally.[231] Eosinophils may be numerous throughout the mucosa. Some degree of haemosiderosis is common.

The ova of both types of hookworm are passed in the faeces and then hatch. The third stage larva is formed about a week later and can live in soil for several weeks: it penetrates the skin of man and enters capillaries or is carried in lymph to the regional nodes and, if it survives, to the bloodstream and the lungs. It migrates up the tracheo-bronchial tree and is then swallowed. Further stages in the development of the larvae take place once they have reached the small intestine. Ova are produced within four to eight weeks of penetration of the skin.

Strongyloidiasis.[225,232] Strongyloidiasis occurs throughout the world but is relatively infrequent in temperate climates, particularly Europe. Its cause is *Strongyloides stercoralis*. The adult female worm lives in the duodenum and upper part of the jejunum and deposits her eggs in the mucosa. The rhabditiform larvae usually make their way directly to the intestinal lumen on hatching (Fig. 6.34), but some penetrate the deeper layers of the bowel wall and may even reach the serosa. Auto-infection may result from invasion of the colon or of the skin round the anus by larvae in the faeces. Alternatively, the sexual cycle of the parasite can take place in soil and fresh hosts can be invaded through the exposed skin. The invasive filariform larvae, whether endogenous or exogenous, reach the bloodstream and thence the lungs; they can migrate by way of the trachea and oesophagus to the small bowel. The inflammatory response in the bowel

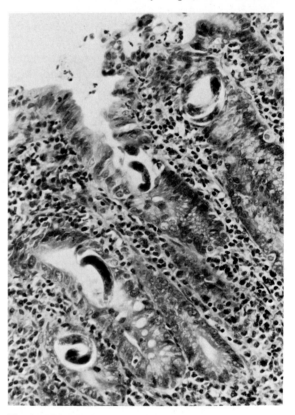

Fig. 6.34 Rhabditiform larvae of *Strongyloides stercoralis* in jejunal glands, freshly hatched from the ovum and making their way to the lumen of the bowel and eventual escape from the host. Compare with Figure 6.35.

Haematoxylin-eosin   × 230

Provided by W.StC. Symmers.

ranges from a mild catarrhal enteritis to oedematous and ulcerative lesions:[233] in the severer form the parasites are not confined to the mucosa but may be found in micro-abscesses or tuberculoid foci (Fig. 6.35) in any part of the wall. Latterly, very widespread and usually fatal dissemination of strongloides larvae through the body has been described as a complication of chemotherapy of lymphomas[234] and comparable diseases, and of the treatment of such diseases as rheumatoid arthritis with corticosteroids or their synthetic analogues. It is notable that such cases may be seen in parts of the world where strongyloidiasis is rare: presumably the patients have become infested while living in endemic areas, and their natural resistance to dissemination of the infestation is somehow significantly lowered by other diseases or their treatment.

Other nematodes known to involve the small bowel on occasion include *Enterobius (oxyuris) vermicularis, Trichuris trichiura*[235] *and species of Toxocara anisakis* and *capillaria.*[236]

Fungal infections

Though these are reasonably common in the stomach and oesophagus of immune compromised patients they are extremely rare in the small bowel. There are reports of candidiasis in the duodenum and jejunum after renal transplant.[237]

MALABSORPTION SYNDROMES

The small intestine absorbs the products of digestion of protein, fat and carbohydrate along with vitamins and other substances.[1-3] Inadequate digestion or absorption leads to deficiency states. These are reflected in nutritional disturbances, including weight loss, anaemia, osteomalacia and dermatoses and in gastrointestinal symptoms which include abdominal discomfort, flatulence and diarrhoea with bulky offensive stools.[238]

Investigation

The first step is to distinguish between malabsorption, malnutrition and maldigestion which may be gastric, pancreatic or hepatic in origin. A full haematological assessment is necessary. The principal causes of primary small bowel malabsorption syndromes are as follows.

1. Damage to or abnormality of enterocytes or their precursors in the crypt zone which interferes with their powers of absorption or prevents them from being replaced rapidly enough to maintain a normal effective absorptive surface. This most commonly results from inherited or acquired enzyme deficiencies, from acquired sensitivity to ingested antigenic food material, from disorders involving the gut-associated lymphoid tissue and from infections.

2. Alterations in small bowel motility which

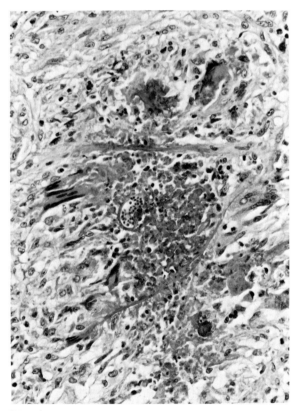

Fig. 6.35 Cross-section of rhabditiform larva of *Strongyloides stercoralis* in a micro-abscess in the subserosa of the jejunum. From a case of local peritoneal irritation complicating a heavy infestation in which great numbers of larvae migrated through the wall of the bowel from the mucosa to the serosa instead of directly entering the lumen (compare with Figure 6.34). The cells in the abscess are eosinophils. There is a tuberculoid reaction in its vicinity.

Haematoxylin-eosin   × 230

Provided by W.StC. Symmers.

produce stagnation of bowel content and consequent alterations to the normal bowel ecology (see p. 274). These usually follow organic disease or defect including resections, anastomoses, strictures, diverticula, and localized areas of disease.

The two patterns are usually readily separable on clinical and radiological grounds. The first, often referred to as primary malabsorption, can be further investigated by absorption studies using xylose and vitamin B_{12} and by estimations of faecal fat, but increasingly clinicians are bypassing these laboratory investigations and proceeding directly to intestinal biopsy. Conventionally this is taken from the jejunum using a single, double or multiple biopsy capsule, but more frequent use is being made of direct endoscopic duodenal biopsy; some of the disadvantages of this are referred to on page 254.

The nature and differential diagnosis of small bowel mucosal damage

In the normal small bowel, cell proliferation occurs in the crypt zone; cells migrate upwards along the sides of the villi, differentiating and maturing as they do so and are shed from the villous tips in 2–4 days.[24,239] They also migrate and differentiate downwards into the basal layer (see p. 231). There are a number of disease processes which damage surface enterocytes so that they are shed more quickly than normal. All of these will produce a basic common pattern of histological change[10] but there will be small but identifiable differences in the uniformity and pattern of the individual lesions in different conditions.[240] To recognize these potentially diagnostic patterns it is often necessary to undertake detailed morphological, morphometric, histochemical and immunocytochemical studies[9,25,241] The basic changes in the mucosa common to all types of visible damage are described below and the variations, with the specialized studies needed to detect them, are described under individual diseases. It must be recognized that some causes of malabsorption, particularly those associated with enzyme defects may not show any recognizable histological abnormality.

When enterocytes are shed more rapidly than normal there is first an increased cell turnover in the crypt zone, which increases in length and contains more numerous mitotic figures. If the enterocyte loss is not severe this may suffice to maintain relatively normal villi. If the shedding remains rapid the enterocytes reach the villous tips before they are fully mature and are smaller than normal, distorted and crowded together. The ratio of enterocytes to goblet cells also changes (Fig. 6.36). The villi themselves become shorter and broader as the enterocytes available to clothe them become fewer. There is often an increase in number of intra-epithelial lymphocytes, though cell counts may be needed to determine this. These changes can progress to a completely flat mucosa covered by a single layer of distorted crowded enterocytes which may appear more than one cell thick (Figs 6.37 and 6.38). At the same time the increased crypt zone proliferation leads to an increase in thickness of the basal layer so that the total

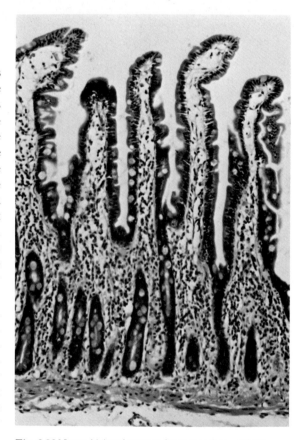

Fig. 6.36 Normal jejunal mucosa for comparison with Figures 6.37–6.39.

Haematoxylin-eosin   × 125

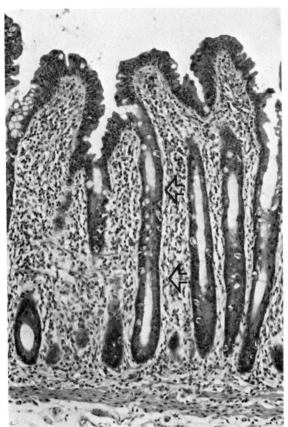

Fig. 6.37 Partial mucosal flattening in gluten-induced enteropathy. The villi are much shorter and wider than normal; the crypt zone (arrowed) is longer and more active than normal; there is piling up and irregularity of surface enterocytes, an increase in migrating interepithelial lymphocytes and a marked increase in cellularity in the lamina propria.

Haematoxylin-eosin ×125

and oriented sections, often with serialization, is necessary; we have not found dissecting microscopic examination of great value apart from the orientation of tissue blocks. Transmission and scanning electron microscopy, though useful for solving individual problems, are not generally of great value either.

Disorders which primarily affect enterocytes

Protein calorie malnutrition (kwashiorkor)

This condition results from dietary protein deficiency and is common in India and in parts of East, West and South Africa. It affects children and adults but in human and experimental animals the changes are more severe in the young and growing

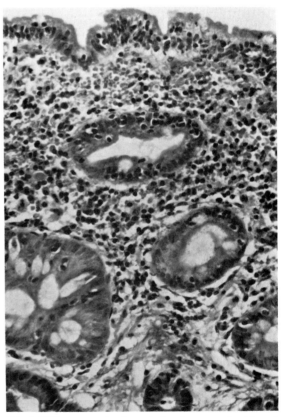

Fig. 6.38 Flat mucosa in gluten-induced enteropathy. There is crowding together of surface enterocytes which are distorted; interepithelial lymphocytes are greatly increased in number and there is an increased cellular infiltrate in the upper part of the lamina propria.

Haematoxylin-eosin ×315

thickness of mucosa may not be greatly altered. Changes in cellularity affecting lymphocytes, plasma cells and histiocytes also occur in the lamina propria, which may need further investigation using immunocytochemical and morphometric methods to allow the delineation of IgA, IgM and IgG in plasma cells, the counting of cell ratios and absolute numbers, and the identification and quantitation of B and T lymphocytes. It may be necessary to demonstrate histochemically or assess biochemically the enzyme content of enterocytes, and to identify and count individual endocrine cells.

To detect and assess these changes, careful microscopic examination of correctly preserved

than in the adult and elderly.[242] The values for volume of lamina propria, villous height, and surface area in jejunal and ileal mucosa are reduced below normal, though individual workers have varied in the degree of crypt hyperplasia which they have described.[243-246] The mucosa tends to return to normal on protein feeding, more slowly in the ileum than in the jejunum. Our own studies and the ultrastructural studies of others[246] suggest that the primary failure may be in normal crypt zone regeneration rather than a too rapid loss of enterocytes.

Defects in enterocyte enzyme systems

Primary autosomal recessive enzyme deficiencies such as inherited disaccharidase deficiency[247] are not usually accompanied by morphological mucosal changes, and histochemical or biochemical techniques are needed to detect the deficiency in a biopsy.[10] Secondary deficiencies and lactose intolerance are usually associated with other diseases including bowel infections, and biopsy may then reflect the secondary disease rather than the induced enzyme defect. The mucosa is often undamaged but electron microscopy may show that microvillous surface area has been reduced.[248]

Food allergies

Hypersensitivity to ingested food, especially protein of cow's milk[249-252] and soy proteins,[253] is becoming increasingly recognized, particularly in babies and young children. The basic lesion is similar to that already described, though mucosal flattening is usually partial rather than complete and much less conspicuous in adults than in children.[251] A notable feature is the increase in intra-epithelial lymphocytes[251,254] which returns to normal when the allergen is removed from the diet. In milk allergy and in other food allergies IgE-containing cells and eosinophils are also often increased in number.[251,252,255]

Gluten-induced enteropathy

This condition has been described under many synonyms, including coeliac disease, adult coeliac syndrome and non-tropical sprue. It commonly begins in childhood (coeliac disease) but sometimes

only becomes evident in adolescence or early adult life. It is characterized by severe steatorrhoea, muscular weakness and failure to grow normally; investigations show poor absorption of xylose but usually normal absorption of vitamin B_{12}.

It affects the proximal small bowel more severely than the distal, and the terminal ileal mucosa can be relatively normal. Within the duodenum and jejunum the severity of change varies so that biopsy findings are not uniform and care is needed in comparing sequential biopsies from the same individual,[256] especially when these are used for assessing the effect of treatment. Histologically, there is partial or more commonly complete villous flattening with distortion and crowding of enterocytes and thickening of the basal layer as already described (Figs 6.36–6.38).

Morphometry and immunocytochemistry play an important role in the differential diagnosis of gluten-induced enteropathy from other causes of mucosal flattening and in the assessment of any improvement on gluten-free diets and of the effects of gluten challenge.

Cytokinetic analysis[257] suggests that convolution of the mucosa is associated with villous shortening and crypt zone hyperplasia, increase in crypt length and mitotic index and an increased cellular infiltration of the lamina propria. This represents a reaction to a moderate surface cell loss; flattening is a reaction to a more serious loss with diminution in the ability of the crypt zone to replace it. It is claimed that the most sensitive parameters for diagnosing gluten-induced enteropathy are the villous/crypt ratio and the length of the surface epithelium as related to a given length of muscularis mucosae.[258]

Intra-epithelial lymphocytes are also of great importance in assessments. Earlier reports claimed that their numbers were increased in gluten-sensitive enteropathy, probably because numbers were counted against 100 surface enterocytes. More careful assessment with counts referred to a given length of muscularis mucosae has indicated that the apparent increase is due to a diminution in number of surface enterocytes,[259,260] and that there may actually be fewer intra-epithelial lymphocytes than normal. Those present may show an accelerated rate of entry into mitosis[261] and a higher proportion are of large lymphocyte or immunoblastic type.[262] This increased activity reverts to normal on a gluten-free diet and is said to be specific for gluten-induced enteropathy.[262]

Paneth cells appear to be decreased in number;[263] it has been claimed that there is an endocrine cell hyperplasia with increased secretion of 5-hydroxy-tryptamine,[264] somatostatin,[265,266] glucagon and other polypeptides[265] and a fall in secretion of secretin.[265] Not all of these studies have commented on the thickening of the basal layer which occurs *pari passu* with the mucosal flattening, and the increase, if it occurs, may be purely secondary.

Within the lamina propria mast cells are increased in number.[267] Plasma cells are also more numerous though opinions vary as to whether there is a significant change in the ratio of IgA/IgM/IgG-containing cells.[268,269] Mast cells, basophils and eosinophils are also increased[270] and there are said to be more nerve fibres in the basal region of the crypts.[271]

When patients are placed on a strict gluten-free diet they improve clinically. The mucosa also shows some reversion to normal, which does not necessarily parallel the clinical improvement and is often not complete;[272] increased numbers of intra-epithelial cells often remain[258] and there may or may not be a reversion to normal of plasma cell numbers and ratios.[273] If gluten is re-introduced, mucosal changes usually occur rapidly[274–276] but clinical deterioration may not be obvious for some time.

The aetiology of gluten-induced enteropathy is still not fully established.[277] Though virtually everyone is exposed to gluten, only certain individuals are affected and these tend to possess certain HLA antigens, particularly HLA B8, HLA DRw3 and HLA DR7.[278,279] Their relatives also have an increased incidence of mucosal abnormalities and of antireticulin antibodies.[280] The actual damage to surface enterocytes may be directly due to the action of gluten products, perhaps associated with the absence of a peptidase,[281,282] but is much more likely to be the result of immunologically-mediated damage in genetically-sensitive individuals.

Dermatitis herpetiformis

It is well recognized that rather over half of all patients with the skin disorder dermatitis herpeti-formis will also suffer from an enteropathy related to gluten and will have a similar distribution of HLA antigens. Both skin and bowel lesions respond to a withdrawal of gluten from the diet.[283,284] Histologically, the mucosal changes present are identical with those of gluten-induced enteropathy, and also improve on gluten withdrawal. There is no correlation between the severity of skin and bowel lesions.[285]

Idiopathic steatorrhoea

There is a small number of patients, almost always adult, who clinically and on biopsy have the symptoms and mucosal changes of gluten enteropathy but who do not respond to a strictly controlled gluten-free diet.[286] There is some evidence that this represents a distinct disorder in which the terminal ileum is also involved, vitamin B_{12} malabsorption is common and plasma cell numbers in the lamina propria are reduced rather than increased. There may be a greater risk of developing malignancy in this group than in gluten-induced enteropathy.

Immunodeficiency syndromes

The majority of recognized immunodeficiency syndromes are not associated with malabsorption or with mucosal abnormality[19] and most patients with malabsorption do not have laboratory evidence of immune defects though some may form antibodies to basement membranes including reticulin.[280] There is, however, a small but significant overlap. A few patients who are sensitive to gluten also have an IgA deficiency, a condition sometimes called hypogammaglobulinaemic sprue.[287] IgA-secreting plasma cells are reduced in number and are replaced by cells secreting IgM. This pattern may also be associated with giardial infestation and improvement often follows treatment of the giardiasis. Immunoproliferative small intestinal disease (alpha-heavy chain disease, Mediterranean lymphoma) is discussed on page 285, nodular hyperplasia on page 284 and acquired immune deficiency syndrome (AIDS) on page 286.

Complications of malabsorption syndromes

Gluten-induced enteropathy has a recognized association with intestinal lymphomas of malignant histiocytic pattern.[288,289] There is some evidence that the development of such lymphomas is linked with the HLA antigen pattern of the patient [290,291] and with hyposplenism and possible abnormal splenic function.[292] There is also a relationship between gluten-induced enteropathy and adeno-carcinomas of small bowel and also squamous carcinomas of the oesophagus.[293] Perhaps the most fascinating problem is the relation between non-specific small bowel ulceration, gluten-induced enteropathy, idiopathic steatorrhoea and lymphoma.[294-5] The ulcers commonly occur in duo-denum or jejunum; they extend into the muscle coats and often perforate. Histological changes are usually described as non-specific, but in a number of patients a lymphoma has subsequently developed[235] and careful retrospective studies may reveal abnormal histiocytes in the ulcer floor or edge which were missed on the initial examination.

Alteration in normal small bowel ecology

Normal small bowel ecology has already been briefly discussed[39,40] (see p. 235). The most common disturbance is for indigenous anaerobes in the upper small intestine to become displaced by non-indigenous organisms, usually pathogenic strains of *Esch. coli*. These may themselves cause direct mucosal damage with partial flattening leading to some degree of malabsorption; they also deconju-gate bile acids which lead to steatorrhoea and they may use up sufficient oxygen to allow the over-growth of strictly anaerobic bacteroides which then bind vitamin B complex.[296,297] Some of the alterations in ecology are associated with gastric conditions which decrease acidity and conse-quently the power to destroy invading organisms. Others are associated with organic and mechanical disorders of the small intestine which lead to stagnation of bowel contents—the so-called stag-nant loop syndromes. Among these are diverticula, fistulae and strictures, and surgical anastomoses with residual blind pouches. Intestinal biopsies from patients with this particular pattern of organic lesion rarely show mucosal abnormality.

Tropical sprue syndromes

These syndromes are now recognized to be of infective origin, usually the result of a persistent *Esch. coli* infection of the upper small bowel.[298,299] They are endemic in the Caribbean, northern South America, Puerto Rico, India, parts of South Asia and in the Philippines and are readily acquired by travellers to these parts.

Histologically, the changes correspond to a moderate degree of the mucosal damage already described. Total mucosal flattening is rare (Fig. 6.39). There is an increase in interepithelial lymphocytes which also involves the crypt zone[300] and the increased cellularity in the lamina propria also includes eosinophils. Lipid may accumulate immediately beneath the epithelial basement mem-brane.[301] Less severe biopsy changes can be difficult to differentiate from the normal mucosal appear-ances in the indigenous symptom-free population.

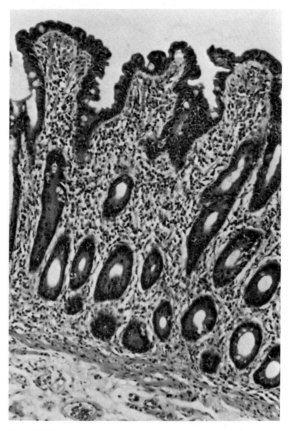

Fig. 6.39 Partial flattening in tropical sprue. Note the resemblance to the partial flattening sometimes seen in gluten-sensitive enteropathy in Figure 6.37. In tropical sprue there is usually a more marked cellular infiltration in the lamina propria.

Haematoxylin-eosin   × 125

Intestinal lipofuscinosis[302,303]

Intestinal lipofuscinosis (the 'brown bowel syndrome') may accompany malabsorption of whatever cause, including pancreatic exocrine deficiency[304] and intestinal lymphangiectasia. A distinctive brown pigmentation of the small intestine and sometimes of part of the stomach is the characteristic feature: it is due to the presence of minute brownish-yellow granules in the cytoplasm of the smooth muscle cells, particularly in the main muscle coats but often also in the muscularis mucosae and even in the muscle cells of the blood vessels in the intestinal wall (Fig. 6.40). Histochemical studies[303] indicate that the pigment consists of lipofuscins and possibly includes ceroid. Its presence has been attributed to malabsorption of vitamin E, associated with deficient fat absorption but is more probably the end-result of a mitochondrial myopathy. Macroscopically, the brown colour is often very noticeable at laparotomy or necropsy, being visible through the serosa.

MISCELLANEOUS CONDITIONS

Protein-losing enteropathies[305]

Excessive loss of protein from the small intestine without a balancing increase in protein synthesis, and leading to hypoproteinaemia, may be a manifestation of a wide range of diseases of the gastrointestinal tract. There is probably no form of the condition that may be regarded as a distinct entity. The diseases that may present with this complication include Crohn's disease, Whipple's disease, malabsorption, eosinophil gastro-enteritis, Ménétrièr's hypertrophic gastritis, ulcerative colitis and intestinal lymphangiectasia. All are conditions in which protein can be lost through the bowel as a consequence of an organic lesion that either permits seepage of protein-rich fluids or limits absorption of the proteins in the diet.

Gas cysts of the intestine

The occurrence of gas cysts in the alimentary tract is a rare condition, sometimes called cystic pneumatosis of the intestine. In most cases the small intestine is predominantly involved, particularly the jejunum, but the stomach and large intestine may be affected. The lesions may be fairly uniformly distributed or confined to a number of isolated segments. The cysts range from a few millimetres to several centimetres in diameter. Most of them are in the submucosa, but some may be found in the subserosa and, occasionally, in the mesenteric tissues close to the bowel wall and in regional lymph nodes. The submucosal cysts, which seldom exceed 1 cm in diameter and usually are very much smaller, bulge into the lumen of the bowel and may resemble polyps. The largest cysts are those in the subserosa or in the mesentery. The cysts do not communicate with one another.

Occasionally, and particularly in infants, the mucosa over submucosal cysts becomes ulcerated

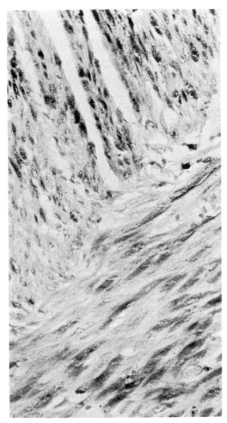

Fig. 6.40. Brown bowel syndrome. Smooth muscle fibres in the circular (top) and longitudinal (bottom right) coats contain granular lipofuscin material which stains positively with PAS after diastase.

Diastase periodic acid-Schiff   × 315

and haemorrhage may then occur and draw attention to the condition. Rarely, rupture of a subserosal or mesenteric gas cyst results in a small spontaneous pneumoperitoneum. In most cases, however, the disease is symptomless and found by chance at laparotomy, on radiological examination or at necropsy.

The cysts are filled with a gas that consists of about 80% nitrogen and small proportions of oxygen, carbon dioxide, methane and hydrogen. Microscopically, the cysts are thin-walled sacs, partly lined by flattened cells, some of which are multinucleate.[306] The histological characteristics are reminiscent of certain types of foreign-body reaction, such, for instance, as that seen in oleogranulomas; the cells concerned are probably histiocytes.

Aetiology and pathogenesis. Gas cysts occur in two age periods: in infancy[307] and, more frequently, in the fourth and fifth decades.[308] Men are affected more often than women. In infants and in some adults the presence of the cysts is associated with mucosal damage, particularly necrotizing enterocolitis. The condition may also occur in adults with severe pulmonary disease, particularly asthma. Two main theories have been suggested to account for the presence of gas. The alimentary theory postulates that gas in the lumen of the stomach or bowel is forced during peristalsis into lymphatics in an area of ulceration. The respiratory theory is based on radiological studies that suggest that the cysts have their origin in decompression of a clinically silent tension pneumomediastinum resulting from rupture of pulmonary alveoli during coughing, for instance. Suction and pulsion in the thorax could then propel air into the sheaths of the pulmonary arteries to reach the fascial sheath of the aorta, thence to track along the lines of the main arterial supply to the intestine. Although the association with chronic pulmonary disease is undeniable, this explanation appears intrinsically unlikely.

Eosinophil enteritis and inflammatory fibroid polyp

These two lesions, which are separate and unrelated, are often confused; both are of undetermined aetiology.

Eosinophil enteritis[309,310] ('eosinophil phlegmon')

This condition, which may be related to similar lesions in the pyloric region of the stomach, and possibly to phlegmonous enteritis (see p. 257), takes the form of diffuse thickening of the wall of one or more segments of the small bowel, with consequent recurrent obstruction which sometimes presents acutely. The affected length of bowel, which may be anything up to 20 cm long, is oedematous and more or less densely infiltrated by eosinophils particularly in the submucosa. Mucosal ulceration is seldom present and never extensive. There is usually an accompanying eosinophilia of the peripheral blood. A 'subgroup' associated with connective-tissue disorders has been described.[311]

The cause of eosinophil enteritis is unknown. Allergy to various foodstuffs, including chocolate, onions and cheese, has been suggested, with little supporting evidence. The role of a herring parasite, *Eustoma rotundatum*, ingested in raw or undercooked fish, originally suggested as a likely factor, now appears improbable. A local sensitivity to foreign protein is possible and the condition can occur as part of a severe allergy.[310]

Inflammatory fibroid polyp[312]

This is a local lesion, rarely larger than 5 cm in longest dimension, and usually solitary, although there is some tendency for it to recur in another part of the bowel following resection. It forms a smooth submucosal mass that becomes ulcerated and causes obstruction. Microscopically, it consists of vascular granulation tissue that contains a variable number of eosinophils and shows more or less tendency to fibrosis. Some of the lesions include areas that are reminiscent of leiomyoma or schwannoma, with palisading of nuclei,[313] and it is possible that some are hamartomatous. Eosinophilia is not present in the blood. A familial relationship affecting three generations has been described.[314]

Endometriosis

Endometriosis of the small intestine can give rise to a tumour-like mass. There is usually evidence of the disease in the pelvic organs or elsewhere in the peritoneal cavity. The endometrial tissue is located mainly in the subserosal and muscle layers of the intestine. Microscopically, endometrial glands and stroma or stroma alone are present, and the presence of haemosiderin pigment should always be looked for.

Backwash (leakback) and stomal ileitis

Ulcerative colitis is normally considered as a disease confined to the large bowel, but in long-standing colitis the ileocaecal valve can become incompetent and the ileal mucosa then becomes reddened and inflamed; it is presumed that this is due to backwash of colonic contents and consequent disturbance of normal ileal bacterial ecology, though this has not been proven.[315,316] Microscopically, there is villous flattening with some destruction and ulceration of the crypt zone with a mixed mononuclear inflammatory reaction and vascular dilatation in the lamina propria. If healing occurs there is some degree of epithelial regeneration but villi are not usually fully reformed; appearances resemble, and may indeed represent, colonic metaplasia.

A somewhat different picture can be seen in the ileum after ileostomy when the stoma becomes inflamed; deep linear ulcers form, with a relatively normal intervening mucosa, and often lead to perforation. They resemble those seen in Crohn's disease but there is no distinctive granulomatous reaction.[317]

The ileum in 'shunt' operations for obesity and after colectomy

After 'shunt' operations, the length and circumference of residual functional small bowel increases. The mucosa becomes thicker and more convoluted and the villi elongate.[318,319] These findings may account for the failure to maintain weight loss which ultimately occurs in many patients.

After total colectomy and permanent ileostomy the lower ileum shows smaller villi and a deeper basal layer than is seen in normal controls. Similar appearances are found in the ileum above an ileorectal anastomosis.[320]

Irradiation damage

This type of damage is less commonly seen than formerly; its appearance and presentation depends on the irradiating dose and on how long after irradiation symptoms appear. It is usually seen as a sequel to radiotherapy for carcinoma of the cervix and the ileum is the common site. In the immediate post-irradiation phase there is interference with crypt zone replication leading to a varying degree of villous flattening; the damage may be severe enough to cause local necrosis and perforation.[321,322] This is followed by slow mucosal regeneration, often associated with submucosal oedema and usually followed by extensive fibrosis and the well-recognized patterns of irradiation vasculitis.

These have been carefully studied both qualitatively and quantitatively in recent well-controlled series.[323,324] In elderly patients who had not received irradiation, there was some atheroma and adventitial fibrosis with patchy medial fibrosis and more extensive intimal fibrosis in extramural arteries, often accompanied by the laying down of longitudinal muscle fibres in the intima. Smaller intramural arteries show moderate or severe fibrosis without medial or adventitial changes. The severity of any lesion present was related to age and diastolic blood pressure.

In those patients, 20 in number, who had received irradiation between 1 and 27 months before bowel symptoms appeared there were numerous fibrin thrombi in capillaries throughout the bowel wall and fibrinoid necrosis with inflammation and infarction was common. Recent thrombus was present in several arteries. More long-term changes, similar to those seen in the control group were also present, but were quantitatively more severe and were not related to age or blood pressure. They did have a relationship with the time between the course of irradiation and the occurrence of symptoms. The final result is often stricture formation which can be difficult to distinguish from ischaemic stricture; points which are helpful are the absence of macrophages containing haemosiderin and the presence of large abnormal nuclei in submucosal fibroblasts.

Behçet's disease

Small bowel ulceration has been described in Behçet's disease.[325] The ulcers are said to have a distinct 'collar stud' appearance with extension into the muscularis propria and consequent risk of perforation. There are no histological features which are distinctive.

Jejunal diverticula

Solitary acquired diverticula occur anywhere in the small bowel but are most common in the duodenum. Multiple acquired diverticula are found, usually in old people along the mesenteric aspect of the jejunum and ileum, and represent herniations of mucosa through the muscularis propria at the points of entry of blood vessels (Fig. 6.41). Often symptomless, they can act as stagnant loops, alter bowel bacterial ecology and lead to steatorrhoea and low levels of vitamin B$_{12}$. Some are apparently related to disorders of smooth muscle or myenteric plexus[326] including systemic sclerosis, but the aetiology of the majority remains undetermined.

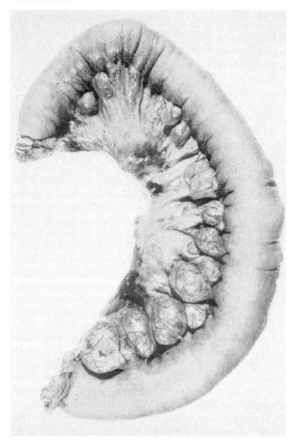

Fig. 6.41 Jejunal diverticulosis. The diverticula are exclusively distributed along the mesenteric attachment.

Small intestinal myopathies

A number of conditions are described under the headings of hollow visceral myopathy or pseudo-obstruction syndromes. Pseudo-obstruction is defined as a clinical syndrome resulting from ineffectual intestinal propulsion in the absence of a lesion which occludes the lumen.[327,328] There are two principal patterns. One, sometimes called secondary, occurs in relation to a recognized underlying disease, usually progressive systemic sclerosis[327,328] or hollow visceral myopathy, which is an inherited (autosomal dominant) condition in which there is a primary degeneration of muscle coats with fibrosis.[329] There is also a primary type of undetermined aetiology and pathogenesis. Many patients also show some degree of mucosal flattening.[330] A good recent review is available.[331]

Other miscellaneous disorders

Among other rare disorders, occasionally described in small bowel biopsies or resected specimens, are duodenal melanosis,[332] malakoplakia,[333] mast cell disease,[334] and hypo-β-lipoproteinaemia.[335,336] There are some experimental studies on the changes in graft-versus-host disease[337,338] and on those which follow the use of cytotoxic drugs,[339] but in general these conditions have been more fully studied in rectal biopsies.

TUMOURS OF THE SMALL INTESTINE

Benign epithelial neoplasms

If the adenomatous lesions arising in the papilla of Vater are excluded, adenomas are rare in the duodenum and ileum and very rare in the jejunum. There is a recognized tendency, as in their large intestinal counterparts, to malignant change (Fig. 6.42) and they can show a predominantly tubular, villous or mixed tubulo-villous structure.[340–344] It is now well recognized that multiple small bowel adenomas occur in Gardner's syndrome[345,346] and in familial colonic polyposis[347] and that there is a less clear distinction than was formerly thought between juvenile and adenomatous polyps (see p. 364). The small bowel carcinomas associated with

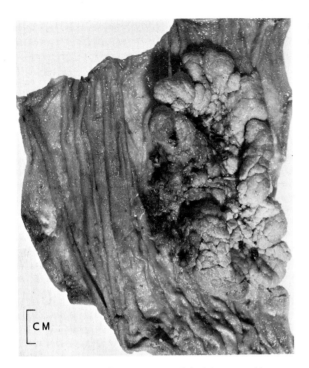

Fig. 6.42 Sessile papillary adenoma of the jejunum, with malignant change.

gluten-induced enteropathy and, as some consider, with Crohn's disease, appear to arise on a basis of dysplasia or *de novo* rather than from pre-existing adenomas. Endocrine cell tumours are described below.

Benign connective tissue tumours

The benign connective tissue tumours include leiomyomas, neurofibromas (sometimes as part of von Recklinghausen's neurofibromatosis) and lipomas. Sometimes they are the starting point of an intussusception.

Haemangiomas and lymphangiomas have been described on page 241.

Malignant tumours

Carcinoma

Carcinomas of small bowel are rare in comparison with carcinomas of stomach or colon; ordinary adenocarcinomas are less common than endocrine cell tumours. Their rarity is probably related to the dilution of potential carcinogens by the succus entericus, the speed of transit of food through the small bowel and perhaps by the efficiency of the gut-associated lymphoid tissue in preventing the access of potential carcinogens to the mucosa.

The ampulla of Vater is the most common site. Carcinomas developing there present as ulcerating or papillary tumours which often obstruct the duct giving rise to painless jaundice and often bleeding (Fig. 6.43). Some at least arise on the basis of a pre-existing adenoma. Microscopically, they are usually well-differentiated tubulo-villous adenocarcinomas, sometimes with considerable mucus secretion, which spread early into the pancreas and to regional lymph nodes.

Duodenal carcinomas in other sites are extremely rare, but carcinomas of jejunum and ileum are well

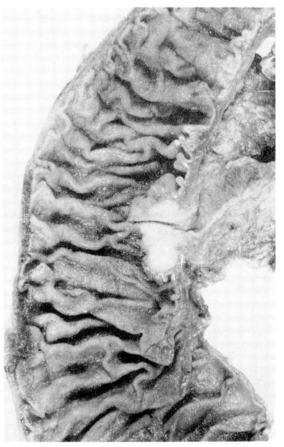

Fig. 6.43 Carcinoma of the hepatopancreatic ampulla. The common bile duct is greatly distended above the tumour. The constriction of the duct as it passes into the tumour has been displayed by cutting a slice from the latter.

described.[348,349] The majority arise on a basis of pre-existing adenoma, as do their large bowel counter-parts; others are associated with gluten-induced enteropathy[350] with or without epithelial dysplasia and there is an association with Crohn's disease[351] which is not accepted by all,[352] and with ileostomy stomas.[353,354] The growths are usually single and annular (Fig. 6.44) but multiple carcinomas have been reported.[355,356] Local and lymph node spread both occur and, since obstructive symptoms are late because of the fluid nature of small bowel contents, metastatic deposits are often present at the time of diagnosis. Histologically, the growths usually have a moderately-differentiated tubulo-villous pattern and invade muscle coats.

Endocrine cell tumours

The endocrine cells normally present in the small bowel have already been described on page 233. They include those which contain the amine 5-hydroxytryptamine (5-HT), the granules of which are argentaffin, diazo positive and show formalde-hyde-induced fluorescence (f.i.f.), and those which

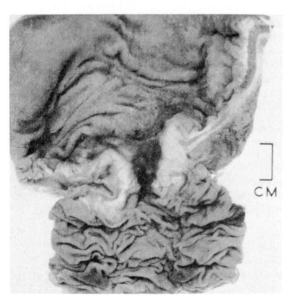

Fig. 6.44 Annular primary carcinoma of the jejunum. The bowel above the obstruction is dilated, and its musculature is hypertrophic.

Specimen from the Gordon Museum, Guy's Hospital, London, reproduced by permission of the Curator, Mr J.D. Maynard. Photograph by Miss P.M. Turnbull, Charing Cross Hospital Medical School, London.

contain polypeptide hormones which include en-teroglucagon, motilin, somatostatin, vasoactive intestinal polypeptide (VIP), gastrointestinal poly-peptide (GIP) and bombesin. The granules of these cells are commonly but not universally argyrophilic and stainable with lead haematoxylin, but are better identified using ultrastructural and immunocytochemical techniques.[29,34] In the fore-gut derivatives of the small intestine (duodenum) gastrin-containing cells are also found and, if pancreatic rests are present, cells containing pan-creatic glucagon and insulin may also be seen.

Tumours of endocrine cells are divided by some workers into two groups; those which secrete 5-HT and are often referred to as 'carcinoids' and those which secrete one or more of the polypeptide hormones and are variously called apudomas or endocrine cell tumours but are best named after their principal secretion, (e.g. glucagonoma) when this can be determined.[357] Some tumours in this group appear to be non-secretory; much depends on the adequacy of the antisera used to identify the secretory product and on proper preservation of tissue.

There are four main histological patterns in this tumour group, the first of which, pattern 'A or 1', usually written A1 is capable of considerable variation,[358,359] and there is some correlation be-tween pattern and function.

So-called 'carcinoid' tumours

Most of the tumours of midgut origin are of histological type A1. They secrete 5-HT and probably also a bradykinin. They arise in the jejunum or ileum, usually in the fifth and sixth decades and are slightly more common in women.[360,361] They grow slowly but invasively, producing gradual narrowing of the bowel lumen with fibrosis and local muscular hyperplasia (Fig. 6.45). After formaldehyde fixation they commonly show a characteristic yellow colour. They are not infrequently multiple and are often associated with a second independent non-endocrine neoplasm in the gastrointestinal tract.[362] They metastasize to liver and mesenteric nodes. Histologically, they have a characteristic 'carcinoid' or A1 pattern[359] of nests and strands of cells with a peripheral border of more solid, deeply-staining smaller cells remi-

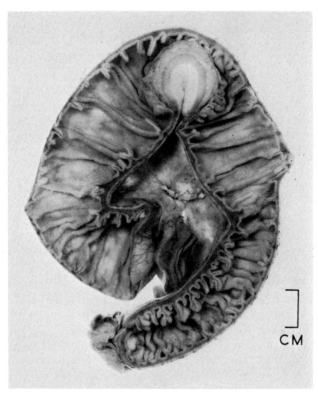

Fig. 6.45 Primary argentaffinoma of the ileum. The original specimen, after fixation in formalin, showed very well the yellow colour that is characteristic of this tumour. Note the hypertrophy of the muscle coat within the tumour and the invasion of the subserosa as well as of the submucosa. The tumour was beginning to undergo intussusception, with the development of some obstruction: the fact that there is little dilatation of the bowel above the growth shows that the latter, in spite of its size, had caused no effective obstruction until shortly before the acute symptoms that necessitated resection.

niscent of basal cell carcinoma of the skin (Fig. 6.46). Individual tumour cells contain argentaffin, diazo-positive granules (Fig. 6.47). Many of the cell nests have a central vascular core. These neoplasms are structurally similar to appendiceal 'carcinoids' but the latter occur in a younger age group and rarely metastasize.

Since all endocrine cell tumours in the gut arise from crypt cells which are capable of maturation into mucus-secreting or enterocyte cells it is not surprising that one sometimes sees a mucus-secreting or glandular component—the so-called A1-A2 pattern—in some 'carcinoid' tumours;[359] there are also examples recorded of pure 'goblet-cell carcinoids' in the ileum, though the usual site for these is the appendix (see p. 309).

The A1 pattern is commonly and the A1A2 sometimes associated with 5-HT and probably bradykinin production. The amine is metabolized to 5-hydroxy indole acetic acid (5-HIAA) by monoamine oxidase in the liver and this compound is excreted in the urine. Once a sufficient volume of functioning metastatic tumour is present in the liver, 5-HT and bradykinins pass via the central veins to the inferior vena cava and reach the right side of the heart where they may give rise to the 'carcinoid syndrome'. This has three components, though not all are necessarily present in any one patient. Episodic diarrhoea may be a paracrine effect from the local tumour in the bowel. Facial

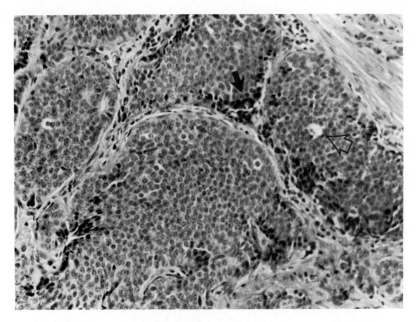

Fig. 6.46 Characteristic pattern of a type A1 'carcinoid' tumour of ileum. There is a band of smaller denser cells (dark arrow) around the edges of many of the cell nests and vascular cores (open arrow) are also visible.

Haematoxylin-eosin   × 200

flushing is more likely to be due to bradykinin than to 5-HT excess. The initial cardiac lesion is a scanty infiltration of subendocardial tissues by mast cells, plasma cells and lymphocytes, associated with an increase in mucopolysaccharide ground substance; subendocardial fibrous and elastic tissue is then laid down in the right atrium, right ventricle and tricuspid and pulmonary valves, and is visible at autopsy as slightly raised plaques of white tissue. A common outcome is pulmonary stenosis with consequent right ventricular hypertrophy not unlike that seen when rheumatic fever affects the pulmonary valve; the tricuspid valve may be stenosed by fibrous tissue or dilated if the pulmonary stenosis has preceded tricuspid involvement. A similar syndrome can be seen when functional 'carcinoid' tumours develop in ovarian teratomas.[363]

Three other histological patterns of endocrine cell tumour exist, all associated with polypeptide hormone rather than 5-HT production. These tumours are most common in the duodenum which is of foregut origin, but are occasionally seen in jejunum and ileum where they are usually readily distinguishable from 'carcinoid' tumours. They tend to affect younger people, sex incidence is usually equal, they grow more quickly and, though fewer of them metastasize than do 5-HT-secreting tumours, they do so earlier. Macroscopically, they may protrude into the lumen or infiltrate the wall but the yellow colour seen in 'carcinoids' after formaldehyde fixation does not occur in them.

Histologically, pattern B, which is more common in the pancreas and hindgut than in the small bowel, where it is usually found only in the duodenum, has a ribbon-like appearance and is often argyrophilic and lead haematoxylin positive. The ribbons form lines or convolutions of single layers of cells lying on a thin connective-tissue stroma (Fig. 6.48). This pattern of tumour is associated with secretion of insulin, somatostatin, gastrin or glucagon but not with 5-HT.

Pattern C is rare; there is a tubulo-acinar appearance with extracellular lakes of PAS-positive

should always be made to determine the polypeptide present either by radioimmunoassay electron microscopy of granules or by tissue immunocytochemistry; recent studies suggest that somatostatinomas may sometimes contain psammoma bodies.[364]

Secondary tumours

Generally speaking, primary tumours of the small intestine are rare and it is always advisable to exclude secondary malignant disease before accepting any tumour as a primary growth. This is particularly relevant when dealing with an adenocarcinoma in the small bowel, which not infrequently results from transcoelomic spread from a primary tumour elsewhere in the abdominal cavity. The commonest secondary tumours of the small intestine are derived from primary growths of the

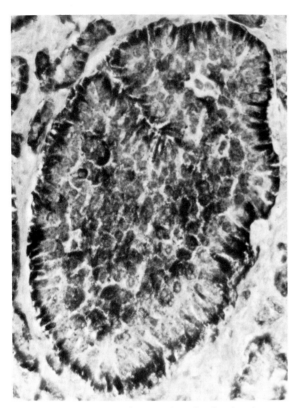

Fig. 6.47 A large cluster of argentaffin cells, showing the typical distribution of the cytoplasmic granules. The peripheral cells have a palisade-like arrangement, and the granules occupy the part of their cytoplasm that is between the nucleus and the outer surface of the cluster. The cells enclosed by the palisade are arranged haphazardly, and their argentaffin granules are distributed more uniformly throughout the cytoplasm.

Masson-Fontana silver method for argentaffin granules × 320

Photomicrograph by Dr J.G. Jackson, Charing Cross Hospital Medical School, London. Preparation by W.StC. Symmers 1938 from a specimen provided by Professor P.T. Crymble, Queen's University and Royal Victoria Hospital, Belfast.

material which is diastase-resistant and does not stain with alcian blue. These tumours are only rarely argyrophilic. Some secrete somatostatin but many have no detectable secretion.

Pattern D is an undifferentiated small cell tumour resembling oat cell tumour of bronchus and can be difficult to classify as of endocrine origin. The granules will not usually stain.

It is not uncommon to find more than one of these four patterns in a tumour and a single tumour can secrete more than one polypeptide. An attempt

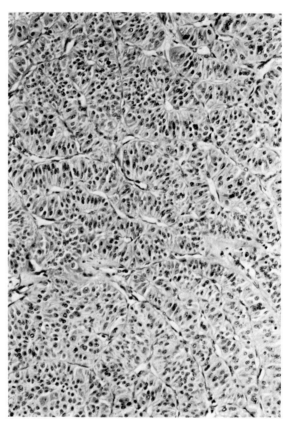

Fig. 6.48 Characteristic ribbon pattern of a type B2 endocrine cell tumour. This example was duodenal in origin and no function could be detected.

Haematoxylin-eosin   × 125

stomach, large intestine and ovary. Squamous carcinoma of the uterine cervix and melanoma of the skin are the commonest extra-abdominal tumours to metastasize to the small intestine.

In very exceptional cases of primary carcinoma of the stomach, a metastatic deposit may grow diffusely in a more or less extensive segment of the small intestine, leading to much thickening of all coats of its wall. Malabsorption may result, but both ulceration and obstruction are infrequent accompaniments. The gastric tumour is of the diffuse scirrhous type (see p. 204): the intestinal involvement follows the same macroscopical and microscopical pattern, and fibrosis may predominate with minimal numbers of malignant epithelial cells present; a PAS stain can be helpful in diagnosis.

Smooth muscle tumours

Smooth muscle tumours are not as common in the small intestine as in the stomach and rectum. They present as bulky, protuberant, spherical or ovoid growths that initially are intramural in position, although they tend to protrude into the lumen and often show some central ulceration. Bleeding with consequent melaena is common.

Microscopically, these tumours typically consist of bundles of recognizable smooth muscle cells. Palisading of the nuclei is common, as in leiomyomas generally, and its presence may sometimes mislead the microscopist into interpreting the tumour as a schwannoma, particularly as the latter may occur in the small bowel. The leiomyomatous tumours are not encapsulated, although condensation of adjoining fibrous connective tissue may form a partial covering; usually, the tissue of the tumour merges gradually with the muscle from which it has arisen.

It is notoriously difficult to forecast the behaviour of leiomyomatous tumours from their histological appearance. Even when there are many bizarre cells with large hyperchromatic or multiple nuclei and abundant eosinophilic cytoplasm, the tumour may prove to be benign. Mitotic counts can be helpful but size is probably the most useful prognostic factor. Tumours less than 30 mm diameter rarely metastasize while those over 50 mm not uncommonly do so.

Lymphomatous lesions

Lymphomatous lesions in the small bowel can be benign, malignant, primary or secondary, diffuse or localized and separate from or associated with other conditions.[365-368] A number of patterns are recognized.

Nodular lymphoid hyperplasia

This is a benign, probably reactive lesion occurring within Peyer's patches and solitary lymphoid follicles of the terminal ileum in infants and young children; it is probably common, but is only recognized clinically when the swelling produces obstruction or intussusception.[166,167] Macroscopically, the follicles enlarge and project into the lumen as polypoid masses but do not usually ulcerate. Germinal centres are conspicuous and there is an increase of lymphocytes in the lamina propria and surrounding submucosa but this does not involve the muscle coats.

A somewhat similar condition occurs in the stomach in adults in association with peptic ulcer or gastritis (sometimes called pseudolymphoma or follicular gastritis) and in the rectum where the swellings are sometimes known as 'anal tonsils'.

A different lesion, often given the same name, occurs in adults rather than in children and is probably initially also non-neoplastic. It has an affinity both with the nodular lymphoid hyperplasia described above and also with the more sinister immunoproliferative small intestinal disease (IPSID) seen in Middle Eastern countries (see below). There is generalized enlargement and hyperplasia of the solitary lymphoid follicles and Peyer's patches in the ileum which cause secondary distortion and flattening of the mucosa though individual enterocytes remain unaffected. In some follicles the normal germinal centres are replaced by aggregates of small lymphoid cells. There is an associated IgA deficiency with a reduction of plasma cell numbers in the lamina propria and this in turn may predispose to giardial infestation. A few patients have been described in whom malignant lymphomatous change has supervened.[369] The condition is not to be confused with multiple lymphamatous polyposis, though it may be related to IPSID.

Multiple lymphomatous polyposis

This rare condition, most commonly seen in the ileocaecal region in late middle age but which also occurs in colon and rectum, consists of numerous submucosal polyps varying in diameter from 5–25 mm;[368-370] in a patient of our own they were present throughout the small and large bowel. Microscopically, the polyps consist of nodules of malignant lymphoid cells, classifiable as of small centrocytic (cleaved cell) type,[370] which surround and compress normal reactive lymphoid follicles, destroying the mantle zone of the germinal centres. There is a distinct tendency to spread outside the confines of the gut, and a generalized lymphoma may supervene.

Immunoproliferative small intestinal disease (IPSID)

This condition, which includes examples of alpha-heavy chain disease and Mediterranean lymphoma, is found mainly in countries on the Mediterranean littoral, in Iran and Iraq and in South Africa.[370-373] It predominates in males in the 10–30-year age group and of low socio-economic status. Clinically there is chronic diarrhoea with weight loss and abdominal pain, all of which improve on tetracycline therapy[374] suggesting an infective origin. Laboratory studies provide evidence of steatorrhoea and malabsorption which are probably related to the presence of abnormal intestinal flora as is seen in the stagnant loop syndrome (see p. 274). In the initial stages small bowel biopsies show variable degrees of mucosal flattening with relatively normal columnar enterocytes; the flattening appears to be predominantly due to a heavy infiltration of the lamina propria by plasma cells and lymphocytes in various stages of maturation, often referred to as a lympho-plasmacytic infiltrate, which tends to obliterate both villi and crypts (Fig. 6.49). A considerable number, but not all, of patients affected also have alpha-heavy chains in the serum. The lamina proprial involvement appears to be diffuse or at least to involve considerable lengths of the intestine.

Although clinical improvement follows tetracycline therapy a lymphoma will ultimately develop in a large number of patients. The first histological

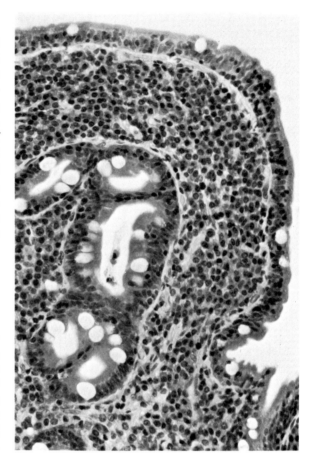

Fig. 6.49 Immunoproliferative small intestinal disease. Plasma cells and lymphocytes pack the lamina propria but are not obviously abnormal, and surface enterocytes appear normal. Haematoxylin-eosin × 315

evidence of this is the appearance in the lamina propria of abnormal immature plasmacytoid cells and immunoblasts in small groups which infiltrate the muscularis mucosae to reach the submucosa. The groups increase in size to form nodules. There is involvement of muscularis propria and serosa and the bowel wall shows patchy thickening with stricture formation and involvement of mesenteric lymph nodes. The growth is probably best classified as an immunoblastic sarcoma.

Lymphomas associated with 'coeliac disease'

The association between 'coeliac disease' and lymphoma is well recognized and it is now appreciated that it holds for gluten-induced enteropathy and dermatitis herpetiformis as well as for idiopathic steatorrhoea.[367,375] The time interval before a lymphoma develops in patients with gluten-induced enteropathy is undetermined since in many patients the duration of the preceding mucosal flattening is also unknown; nor do we know why only certain patients are at risk. The lymphoma itself is described as being of histiocytic origin[376] and is sometimes referred to as malignant histiocytosis of the intestine (MHI): like IPSID (see above) it can be preceded by the presence of small groups of abnormal histiocytes in the lamina propria which need careful search for their detection.[377] Since immunoblasts and malignant histiocytes possess many histological similarities and can be difficult to distinguish apart, one wonders whether similar mechanisms may be involved in the two diseases. The relationship of MHI to the acute 'non-specific' ulcers sometimes seen in the small bowel (see p. 274) is not fully determined but it seems probable that they may be one manifestation of MFI.

Other lymphomas in the small bowel

There remain a number of lymphomas which are not apparently associated with other conditions. The majority are secondary to primary nodal or other lymphomas; for a gut lymphoma to be considered as primary a number of strict criteria must be fulfilled.[368,378] They can be single or multiple and may produce mucosal thickening over a length of bowel or an annular stricture. The most common site is the jejunum. Histologically, they are virtually all non-Hodgkin lymphomas; tumours previously categorized as Hodgkin's disease were probably either secondary or immunoblastic. Immunoblastic or lymphoblastic (large non-cleaved follicular centre cell) patterns are the most common. Lymph node enlargement is not synonymous with secondary involvement; some of the largest nodes in patients with primary lymphoma proved to be reactive on histological examination.

Lesions associated with acquired immune deficiency syndrome (AIDS)

It is now well recognized that AIDS is associated with Kaposi type sarcomas which occur in the skin and are increasingly being identified in the gastrointestinal tract.[379] Gastric and colonic involvement are both more common than small intestinal. There are few reliable reports on any mucosal changes in the small bowel.[380]

REFERENCES

Physiological and anatomical considerations

1. Freeman HJ, Sleisenger MH. Clinics in Gastroenterol 1983; 12: 357.
2. Glickman RM. Clinics in Gastroenterol 1983; 12: 323.
3. Ravich WJ, Bayless TM. Clinics in Gastroenterol 1983; 12: 335.
4. Katz AJ, Grand RJ. Gastroenterol 1979; 76: 375.
5. Hasan M, Sircus W, Ferguson A. Gut 1981; 22: 627.
6. Dawson IMP. In: Stoward PJ, Polak JM, eds. Histochemistry, the widening horizons. Chichester: Wiley, 1981; 127.
7. Mason DY, Piris J. In: Wright R, ed. Recent advances in gastrointestinal pathology. London: Saunders, 1980; 3
8. Carr KE, Toner PG. Cell structure. An introduction to biomedical electron microscopy. 3rd ed. Edinburgh: Churchill Livingstone, 1982.
9. Penna FJ, Hill ID, Kingston D, Robertson K, Slavin G, Shiner M. J Clin Pathol 1981; 34: 386.
10. Dawson IMP. In: Sircus W, Smith AM, eds. Scientific foundations of gastroenterology. London: Heinemann, 1980; 451.
11. Underhill BML. Br Med J 1955; 2: 1243.
12. Hirsch J, Ahrens EH, Blankenhorn DH. Gastroenterol 1956; 31: 274.
13. Morson BC. Proc R Soc Med 1959; 52: 6.
14. Granger DN, Barrowman JA. Gastroenterol 1983; 84: 1035.
15. Gershon MD, Erde SM. Gastroenterol 1981; 80: 1571.
16. Barajas L, Wong P. J Ultrastruct Res 1975; 53: 244.
17. Furness JB, Costa M. Neuroscience 1980; 5: 1.
18. Bienenstock J. In: Asquith P, ed. Immunology of the gastrointestinal tract. Edinburgh: Churchill Livingstone, 1979; 3.
19. Doe WF, Hapel AG. Clinics in Gastroenterol 1983; 12: 415.
20. Greenwood JH, Austin LL, Dobbins WO. Gastroenterology 1984; 52: 501.
21. Kingston D, Pearson JR, Penna FJ. J Clin Pathol 1981; 34: 381.
22. Brackenbury W, Stewart JS. Med Biol Ill 1963; 13: 220.
23. Chacko CJG, Paulson KA, Nathan VL, Baker SJ. J Path 1969; 98: 146.
24. Wright N. In: Anthony PP, MacSween RNM, eds.

Recent advances in histopathology 12. Edinburgh: Churchill Livingstone, 1983; 17.

25. Slavin G, Sowter C, Robertson K, McDermott S, Paton K. J Clin Pathol 1980; 33: 254.

26 de Payer E, France NE, Phillips AD, Walker-Smith JA. Acta Paed Belg 1978; 31: 173.

27. Sandow MJ, Whitehead R. Gut 1979; 20: 420.

28. Peeters T, van Trappen G. Gut 1975; 16: 553.

29. Sidhu GS. Am J Pathol 1979; 96: 5.

30. Dawson IMP. J Clin Pathol 1979; 33 (suppl): 1.

31. Dawson IMP. In: Anthony PP, MacSween RNM, eds. Recent advances in histopathology 12. Edinburgh: Churchill Livingstone, 1983; 111.

32. Polak JM, Bloom SR. In: Wright R, ed. Recent advances in gastrointestinal pathology. London: Saunders, 1980; 23.

33. Dawson IMP. Curr Top Pathol 1976; 63: 221.

34. Bishop AE, Polak JM, Facer P, Ferri G-L, Marangos PJ, Pearse AGE. Gastroenterol 1982; 83: 902.

35. Solcia E et al. In: Bloom SR, ed. Gut hormones. Edinburgh: Churchill Livingstone, 1978; 42.

36. Treasure T. J Anat 1978; 127: 299.

37. Marsh MN. Gastroenterol 1980; 79: 481.

38. Marsh MN. J Clin Pathol 1982; 35: 517.

39. Savage DC. Ann Rev Microbiol 1977; 31: 107.

40. Simon GL, Gorbach SL. Gastroenterology 1984; 86: 174.

41. Baker SJ. Mathan VI. Am J Clin Nutr 1972; 25: 1047.

42. Lindenbaum J. Gastroenterology 1973; 64: 637.

43. Bennett MK, Sachdev GK, Jewell DP, Anand BS. J Clin Pathol 1985; 38: 368.

44. Dawson IMP. Atlas of gastrointestinal pathology as seen on biopsy. Lancaster: MTP Press, 1983.

45. Corazza GR, Frazzoni M, Dixon MF, Gasbarrini G. J Clin Pathol 1985; 38: 735.

Congenital abnoramlities

46. Evans PR, Polani N. Teratology 1980; 22: 207.

47. Louw JH. Ann Roy Coll Surg 1959; 25: 209.

48. Alvarez SP, Greco MA, Geneiser NB. Hum Pathol 1982; 13: 948.

49. Dott NM. Br J Surg 1923–24; 11: 251.

50. Sieck JO, Cawgill R, Larkworthy W. Gastroenterol 1983; 84: 1597.

51. Adair HM, Trowell JE. J Pathol 1981; 133: 25.

52. Fan ST, Lau WY, Pang SW. Am J Gastroenterol 1985; 80: 337.

53. Taylor AL. J Pathol Bact 1927; 30: 415.

54. Willis RA. Br Med J 1968; ii: 267.

55. Dayal Y, Wolfe HJ. Gastroenterol 1978; 75: 655.

56. Spiller RC, Shousha S, Barrison IG. Dig Dis Sci 1982; 27: 880.

57. Kundrotas LW, Camara DS, Meenaghan MA et al. Am J Gastroenterol 1985; 80: 253.

58. Lev R, Spicer SS. Am J Pathol 1965; 46: 23.

59. Park RW, Grand RJ. Gastroenterol 1981; 81: 1143.

60. Dawson I. Gut 1969; 10: 691.

61. Bartholomew LG, Dahlin DC, Waugh JM. Gastroenterol 1957; 32: 434.

62. Rintala A. Acta Chir Scand (Stockholm) 1959; 117: 366.

63. Morson BC. Dis Col Rect 1962; 5: 337.

64. Bussey HJR. Gut 1970; 11: 970.

65. Hsu S-D, Zakaropoulos P, May JT, Costanzi JJ. Cancer 1979; 44: 1527.

66. Trau H, Schewack-Millet M, Fisher BK, Tour H. Cancer 1982; 50: 788.

67. Young RH, Welch WR, Dickersin GR, Scully RE. Cancer 1982; 50: 1384.

68. Burdick D, Prior JJ. Cancer 1982; 50: 2139.

69. Sachatello CR, Pickren JW, Grance JT jr. Gastroenterol 1970; 58: 699.

70. Sachatello CR, Hahn IS, Carrington CB. Surgery 1974; 75: 107.

71. Grigioni WF, Alampi G, Martinelli G, Piccaluga A. Histopathol 1981; 5: 361.

72. Cox KL, Frates RC Jr, Wong A, Gandhi G. Gastroenterol 1980; 78: 1566.

73. Stemper TJ, Kent TH, Summers NW. Ann Int Med 1975; 83: 639.

74. Grotsky HW, Richert RR, Smith WD, Newsome JF. Gastroenterol 1982; 83: 494.

75. Jarvinen H, Nyberg M, Peltokallio P. Gut 1983; 24: 333.

76. Goldman RL. Gastroenterol 1963; 44: 57.

77. Jarnum S, Jensen H. Gastroenterology 1966; 50: 107.

78. Manousos O, Webster CU. Gut 1966; 7: 375.

79. Russell DMcCR, Bhattal PS, St John DJB. Gastroenterology 1983; 85: 180.

80. Melmed RN, Bouchier IAD. Gut 1972; 13: 524.

81. Shepherd JA. Br J Surg 1953; 40: 409.

82. Gentry RW, Dockerty MB, Clagett, OT. Intern Surg 1949; 88: 287 (abstract).

83. Fernando SSE, McGovern VJ. Gut 1982; 23: 1008.

84. Elliott RL, Williams RD, Bayles D, Griffin J. Ann Surg 1966; 163: 86.

85. Dariel S, Lazarevic B, Attia A. Am J Gastroenterol 1983; 36: 30.

86. Mistilis SP, Skyring AP, Stephen DD. Lancet 1965; 1: 77.

87. Harris M, Burton IE, Scarffe JH. J Clin Pathol 1983; 36: 30.

88. Shilkin KB, Zerman BJ, Blackwell JB. J Pathol Bact 1968; 96: 353.

89. Amos JAS. Br J Surg 1958–59; 46: 588.

90. Ford JR. Am J Surg 1960; 99: 878.

91. Christ TD. Arch Int Med 1963; 112: 357.

92. De Schryver-Kecskemeti K, Clouse RE, Goldstein MN. New Eng J Med 1983; 308: 635.

Obstruction

93. Davies GDL, Lewis RH. Br Med J 1959; 2: 545.

94. MacMahon B. Am J Hum Gen 1955; 7: 430.

95. Talwalker VC. Arch Dis Child 1962; 37: 203.

96. Cornes JS, Dawson IMP. Arch Dis Child 1963; 38: 89.

97. Gardner PS, Knox EG, Court SDM, Green CA. Br Med J 1962; ii: 697.

98. Bell TH, Steyn JH. Br Med J 1962; ii: 700.

99. Connelly HJ, del Carmen BV. Am Surg 1969; 35: 820.

100. Saidi F. Gut 1969; 10: 838.

101. Foweather FS. Br Med J 1955; 2: 1010.

Circulatory disturbances

102. Marston A. Clinics in Gastroenterol 1972; 1: 3.

103. Marston A. Gut 1967; 8: 203.

104. Lundgren O. Gut 1974; 15: 1005.
105. Whitehead R. Gut 1971; 12: 912.
106. Grey ES, Lloyd DJ, Miller SS, Davidson AI, Balch NJ, Horne CHW. J Clin Pathol 1981; 34: 759.
107. Meyers S, Dikman S, Schultz N, Janowitz HD. Gut 1981; 22: 61.
108. Johnson CC, Baggenstoss AH. Proc Mayo Clin 1949; 24: 649.
109. Reiner L, Jimenez FA, Rodriguez FL. Am Heart J 1963; 66: 200.
110. Dick AP, Graff R, Gregg DMcC, Peters N, Sarner M. Gut 1967; 8: 206.
111. Marston A, Clarke JFM, Garcia-Garcia JG, Miller AL. Gut 1985; 26: 656.
112. Wold LE, Baggenstoss AH. Proc Mayo Clin 1949; 24: 28.
113. Ming S-C. Circulation 1965; 32: 332.
114. Musa BU. Ann Intern Med 1965; 63: 783.
115. Bounous G. Gastroenterol 1982; 82: 1457.
116. Bircher J, Bartholomew LD, Cain JC, Adson MA. Arch Int Med 1966; 117: 632.
117. Lake AM, Walker WA. Clinics in Gastroenterol 1977; 6: 463.
118. Arseculeratne SN, Panabokke RG, Navaratnam C. Gut 1980; 21: 265.
119. Philpott MG. Br Med J 1971; iii: 251.
120. Rushton DI, Dawson IMP. J Clin Pathol 1982; 35: 909.
121. Herrington JL Jr, Grossman LA. Ann Surg 1968; 168: 1079.

Inflammatory condition

122. Mandal BK. Clinics in Gastroenterol 1979; 8: 715.
123. Budd W. Lancet 1856; 2: 618, 694.
124. Gianella RA, Broitman SA, Zamcheck N. Ann Int Med 1973; 78: 271.
125. Hornick RB, Greiseman S, Woodward TE, DuPont HL, Dawkins AT, Snyder MJ. N Eng J Med 1970; 283: 686.
126. Hornick RB, Greiseman S. Arch Int Med 1978; 138: 357.
127. Chuttani HK, Jain K, Misra RC. Gut 1971; 12: 709.
128. Welch TP, Martin NC. Lancet 1975; i: 1078.
129. Ghosh SK. Public Health 1974; 88: 71.
130. Huckstep RL. Ann Roy Coll Surg Engl 1960; 26: 207.
131. Turnbull PCB. Clinics in Gastroenterol 1979; 8: 663.
132. Rowe B. Clinics in Gastroenterol 1979; 8: 625.
133. Keusch GT. Clinics in Gastroenterol 1979; 8: 645.
134. Wilson GS, Miles A. Topley and Wilson's principles of bacteriology, virology and immunity. 6th ed. vol. 2. London: 1975; 62.
135. Cooke RA. Perspectives in Ped Pathol 1979; 5: 137.
136. Devitt PG, Stamp GHW. Gut 1983; 24: 678.
137. King A, Rampling A, Wight DGD, Warren RE. J Clin Pathol 1984: 37: 335.
138. Severin WJP, de la Fuente AA, Stringer MF. J Clin Pathol 1984; 37: 942.
139. Wright G. Pharmacol Rev 1955; 7: 413.
140. Bartlett JG. Gastroenterol 1981; 80: 863.
141. Price AB, Davies DR. J Clin Pathol 1977; 30: 1.
142. Tait RA, Kealy FW. J Clin Pathol 1979; 32: 1090.
143. Kurtz JB, Lee TW, Pickering D. J Clin Pathol 1977; 30: 948.
144. Ashley CR, Caul EO, Paver WK. J Clin Pathol 1978; 31: 939.
145. Banatvala JE. Clinics in Gastroenterol 1979; 8: 569.
146. Rowe B. Clinics in Gastroenterol 1979; 8: 625.
147. Gregory MA, Moshal MG, Spitaels JM. Scand J Gastroenterol 1982; 17: 441.
148. Morrisay SM, Ward PM, Jayaraj AP, Tovey FI, Clark CG. Gut 1983; 24: 909.
149. Shousha S, Spiller RC, Parkins RA. Histopathol 1983; 7: 23.
150. Hasan M, Hay F, Sircus W, Ferguson A. J Clin Pathol 1983; 36: 280.
151. Holdstock G, Eade OE, Isaacson P, Smith CK. Scand J Gastroenterol 1979; 14: 717.
152. Steer HF. Gut 1984; 25: 1203.
153. Fresh JW, Versage PM, Reyes V. Arch Pathol 1964; 77: 529.
154. Asukura H, Morita A, Morishita T et al. Am J Digest Dis 1973; 18: 271.
155. Asakura H, Tsuchiya M, Watanabe Y et al. Gut 1974; 15: 531.
156. VanTrappen G, Agg HO, Ponette E, Geboes K, Bertrand P. Gastroenterol 1977; 72: 220.
157. El Maraghi NRH, Mair NS. Am J Clin Pathol 1979; 71: 631.
158. Gleason TH, Patterson SD. Am J Clin Pathol 1982; 6: 347.
159. Butzler JP, Skirrow MB. Clinics in Gastroenterol 1979; 8: 737.
160. Comer GM, Brandt LJ, Abissi CJ. Am J Gastroenterol 1983; 78: 107.
161. Haubrich WS, Watson JHL, Sieracki JC. Gastroenterol 1960; 39: 454.
162. Kuhajda FP, Belitsos NJ, Keren DF, Hutchins GM. Gastroenterol 1982; 82: 46.
163. Fisher ER, Hellstrom HR. Am J Clin Pathol 1964; 42: 581.
164. Dobbins WO III, Kawanishi H. Gastroenterol 1981; 80: 1468.
165. DuBoulay CEH. Hum Pathol 1982; 13: 925.
166. Cornes JS, Dawson IMP. Arch Dis Child 1963; 38: 89.
167. Fieber SS, Schaeffer HJ. Gastroenterol 1966; 50: 83.
168. Rosen Y, Won OH. Am J Digest Dis 1978; 23: 248.
169. Blei ED, Abraham C. Gastroenterology 1983; 84: 636.
170. Kies MS, Luedke DW, Boyd JF, McCue MJ. Cancer 1979; 43: 730.
171. Crohn BB, Ginzburg L, Oppenheimer GD. J Am Med Ass 1932; 99: 1323.
172. Golde DW. Lancet 1968; 1: 1114.
173. Mitchell DN, Cannon P, Dyer NH, Hinson KFW, Willoughby JMT. Lancet 1970; 2: 496.
174. Jones-Williams W. Gut 1965; 6: 503.
175. Almy TP, Sherlock P. Gastroenterol 1966; 51: 757.
176. Hislop TG, Kerr Grant A. Gut 1969; 10: 994.
177. Monk M, Mendeloff AI, Siegel CI, Lilienfeld A. Gastroenterol 1969; 56: 847.
178. MacPherson BR, Albertini RJ, Beeken WL. Gut 1976; 17: 100.
179. Fiocchi C, Youngman KR, Farmer RG. Gut 1983; 24: 692.
180. Mayberry JF, Rhodes J. Gut 1984; 25: 886.
181. Garland CF, Lilienfeld AM, Mendeloff AI, Marcowitz JA, Terrell KB, Garland FC. Gastroenterol 1981; 81: 1115.
182. Puntis J, McNeish AS, Allan RN. Gut 1984; 25: 329.
183. Miller DS, Keighley AC, Langman MJS. Lancet 1974; ii: 691.
184. Frandsen PJ, Jarnum S, Malmstrøm J. Scand J Gastroenterol 1980; 15: 683.

185. Morson BC, Dawson IMP. Gastrointestinal pathology. Oxford: Blackwell, 1979: 293–312.
186. Jones-Williams W. J Path Bact 1960; 79: 193.
187. Kraft SC. Gastroenterol 1978; 75: 319.
188. Bishop AE, Polak JM, Bryant MG, Bloom SR, Hamilton S. Gastroenterol 1980; 79: 853.
189. Sjolund K, Schaffalitsky de Muckadell OB, Fahrenkrog J, Hakanson R, Peterson BG, Sundler F. Gut 1983; 24: 724.
190. Antonius JI, Gump FE, Lattes R, Lepore M. Gastroenterol 1960; 38: 889.
191. Marin ML, Geller SA, Greenstein AJ et al. Am J Gastroenterol 1983; 78: 355.
192. Morson BC, Lockhart-Mummery HE. Lancet 1959; 2: 1122.
193. Gray BK, Lockhart-Mummery HE, Morson BC. Gut 1965; 6: 515.
194. Fresko D, Lazarus SS, Dotan J, Reingold M. Gastroenterol 1982; 82: 783.
195. Hawker PC, Gyde SN, Thompson H, Allan RN. Gut 1982; 23: 188.
196. Simpson S, Traube J, Riddell RH. Gastroenterol 1981; 81: 492.
197. Konelitz BI. Am J Gastroenterol 1983; 78: 44.
198. Sprague R, Harper P, McClain S, Trainer T, Beeken W. Gastroenterology 1984; 87: 421.
199. Prior P, Fielding JF, Waterhouse JA, Cooke WT. Lancet 1970; 1: 1135.
200. Chambers TJ, Morson BC. Gut 1979; 20: 269.
201. Crohn BB, Yarnis H. NY State J Med 1950; 40: 158.
202. Anand SS. Ann Roy Coll Surg 1956; 19: 205.
203. Thompson HR, Morson BC. Proc Roy Soc Med 1958; 51: 246.
204. Howells JS, Knapton PJ. Gut 1964; 5: 524.
205. Tandon HD, Prakash A, Rao VB, Prakash O, Nair SK. Indian J Med Res 1966; 54: 129.
206. Tandon HD, Prakash A. Gut 1972; 13: 260.
207. Paustian FF, Monto GL. In: Bockus HL, ed. Gastroenterology 2. 3rd ed. London: Saunders, 1976: 750.
208. Sherman S, Rohwedder JJ, Ravikrishnan KP, Weg JE. Arch Inter Med 1980; 140: 506.
209. Tong-Hua L, Guo-Zone P, Ming-Chang C. J Chir (Paris) 1981; 118: 647.

Protozoal, metazoal and fungal infections

210. Knight R, Wright SG. Gut 1978; 19: 940.
211. Leading article. Br Med J 1977; 3: 538.
212. Knight R. Clinics in Gastroenterol 1978; 7: 31.
213. Nye FJ. Clinics in Gastroenterol 1979; 8: 767.
214. Zamcheck N, Hoskins LC, Winawer J, Broitman SA, Gotleib LS. Gastroenterol 1963; 44: 860.
215. Yardley JH, Takano J, Hendrix TR. Bull Johns Hopkins Hosp 1964; 115: 389.
216. Hartong WA, Gourley WK, Aruanitakis C. Gastroenterol 1979; 79: 61.
217. Ward H, Jalan KN, Maitra TK, Agarwal SK, Makalandakis D. Gut 1983; 24: 120.
218. Wright SG, Tomkins AM. J Clin Pathol 1978; 31: 712.
219. Brandborg LL, Goldberg SB, Breidenbach WC. N Engl J Med 1970; 283: 1306.
220. Liebman WM, Thaler MN, Dehorimen A, Brandborg LL, Goodman J. Gastroenterol 1980; 78: 579.
221. Weinstein L, Edelstein SM, Madara JL, Palchak KR, McManus BN, Trier JS. Gastroenterology 1981; 81: 584.
222. Jones TC. Clinics in Gastroenterol 1978; 7: 105.
223. Pawlowski ZS. Clinics in Gastroenterol 1978; 7: 157.
224. Banwell JG, Schad GA. Clinics in Gastroenterol 1978; 7: 129.
225. Filho EC. Clinics in Gastroenterol 1978; 7: 179.
226. Arean VM, Crandall CA. In: Marcial-Rohas RA, Moreno E, eds. Pathology of protozoal and helminthic diseases with clinical correlation. Baltimore, 1971; 769.
227. Louw JH. Br J Surg 1966; 53: 510.
228. De Leon E, Maldonado JF. In: Marcial-Rojas RA, Moreno E, eds. Pathology of protozoal and helminthic diseases with clinical correlation. Baltimore, 1971; 734.
229. Hunter D. The diseases of occupations. 5th ed. London, 1975; 713.
230. Gilles HM, Watson Williams EJ, Ball PAJ. Quart J Med 1964; NS 33: 1.
231. Sheehy TW, Meroney WH, Cox RS jr, Soler JE. Gastroenterol 1962; 42: 148.
232. Marcial-Rojas RA. In: Marcial-Rojas RA, Moreno E, eds. Pathology of protozoal and helminthic diseases with clinical correlation. Baltimore, 1971; 711.
233. De Paola D. Bol Cent Estud Hosp Serv Estado 1962; 14: 3.
234. Adam M, Morgan O, Persaud C, Gibbs WN. Br Med J 1973; 1: 264.
235. Wolfe MS. Clinics in Gastroenterol 1978; 7: 201.
236. Marsden PB. Clinics in Gastroenterol 1978; 7: 219.
237. Joushi SN, Garvin PJ, Sunwoo YC. Gastroenterol 1981; 80: 829.

Malabsorption syndromes

238. Jeffries GH, Weser E, Sleisenger MH. Gastroenterol 1969; 56: 777.
239. Wright NA, Appleton DR, Marks J, Watson AJ. J Clin Pathol 1979; 32: 462.
240. Manuel PD, Walker-Smith JA, France NE. Gut 1979; 20: 211.
241. Ferguson A, Sutherland A, McDonald TT, Allan F. J Clin Pathol 1977; 30: 1068.
242. Rodrigues MAM, de Camargo JLV, Coelho KIR et al. Gut 1985; 26: 816.
243. Burman D. Arch Dis Child 1965; 40: 526.
244. Brunser O, Reid A, Monckeberg F, Maccioni A, Contreras I. Am J Clin Nutr 1968; 21: 976.
245. Kaschula ROC, Gajjar PD, Mann M et al. Isr J Med Sci 1979; 15: 356.
246. Nassar AM, el Tantawy SA, Khalifa S, Abdel Fattah S, Abdel Hamid J. J Trop Pediatr 1980; 26: 62.
247. Sahi T. Gut 1978; 19: 1074.
248. Phillips AD, Avigad S, Sacks J et al. Gut 1980; 21: 44.
249. Kuitunen P, Visakorpi JK, Savilahti E, Pelkonen P. Arch Dis Child 1975; 50: 351.
250. Iyngkaran N, Robinson MJ, Prathap K, Sumithran E, Yadav M. Arch Dis Child 1978; 53: 20.
251. Rosencrans PMC, Meijer CJLM, Cornelisse CJ, van der Val AM, Lindeman J. J Clin Pathol 1980; 33: 125.
252. Malvenda C, Phillips AD, Briddon A, Walker Smith JA. J Pediatr Gastroenterol Nutr 1984; 3: 349.
253. Haeney MR, Goodwin BJF, Mike N, Asquith P. J Clin Pathol 1982; 35: 319.
254. Phillips AD, Rice SJ, France NE, Walker Smith JA. Gut 1979; 20: 509.

255. Kounai I, Kuitonen P, Savilahti E, Sipponen P. J Pediatr Gastroenterol Nutr 1984; 3: 368.
256. Manuel PD, Walker Smith JA, France NE. Gut 1979; 20: 211.
257. Wright NA, Appleton DR, Marks J, Watson AJ. J Clin Pathol 1979; 32: 462.
258. Rosencrans PMC, Meijer CJLM, Polanco I et al. J Clin Pathol 1981; 34: 138.
259. Guix M, Skinner JM, Whithead R. Gut 1979; 20: 275.
260. Corazza GR, Frazzoni M, Gasbarrini G. Gut 1984; 25: 158.
261. Marsh MN. Gastroenterology 1980; 79: 481.
262. Marsh MN, Haeney MR. J Clin Pathol 1983; 36: 149.
263. Scott H, Brandtzaeg P. Gut 1981; 22: 812.
264. Enerback L, Hallert C, Norrby K. J Clin Pathol1983; 36: 499.
265. Sjolund K, Alumets J, Berg N-O, Hakanson R, Sundler F. Gut 1979; 20: 547.
266. Sjolund K, Hakanson R, Lundqvist G, Sundler F. Scand J Gastroenterology 1982; 17: 969.
267. Strobel S, Busuttil A, Ferguson A. Gut 1983; 24: 222.
268. Scott H, Ek J, Baklien K, Brandtzaeg P. Scand J Gastroenterol 1980; 15: 81.
269. Scott BB, Goodall A, Stephenson P, Jenkins D. Gut 1984; 25: 41.
270. Marsh MN, Hinde J. Gastroenterology 1985; 89: 92.
271. Jones JG, Elmes ME. Diagn Histopathol 1982; 5: 183.
272. Lancaster-Smith M, Kumar PJ, Dawson AM. Gut 1975; 16: 683.
273. Lancaster-Smith M, Packer S, Kumar PJ, Harries JT. J Clin Pathol 1976; 29: 587.
274. Kumar PJ, O'Donoghue DP, Stenson K, Dawson AM. Gut 1979; 20: 743.
275. McNicholl B, Egan-Mitchell B, Fottrell PF. Gut 1979; 20: 126.
276. Bramble MG, Zucoloto S, Wright NA, Record CO. Gut 1985; 26: 169.
277. Kumar PJ. Gastroenterology 1985; 89: 214.
278. Demarchi M, Carbonara A, Ansaldi N et al. Gut 1983; 24: 706.
279. Mearin ML, Biemond I, Pena AS et al. Gut 1983; 24: 532.
280. Pena AS, Mann DL, Hague NE et al. Gastroenterolgy 1978; 75: 230.
281. Cornell HJ, Rolles CJ. Gut 1978; 19: 253.
282. Peters TJ, Bjarnson I. Gut 1984; 25: 913.
283. Fry L, Seah PP, Harper PG, Hoffbrand AV, McMinn RMH. J Clin Pathol 1974: 27: 817.
284. Gawkrodger DJ, Blackwell JN, Gilmour HM et al. Gut 1984; 25: 151.
285. Cooney T, Doyle CT, Buckley D, Whelton MJ. J Clin Pathol 1977; 30: 976.
286. Trier JS, Falchuk ZM, Carey MC, Schreiber DS. Gastroenterology 1978; 75: 307.
287. Eidelman, S. Human Pathol 1976; 7: 427.
288. Isaacson P, Wright DH. Lancet 1978; i: 67.
289. Isaacson P, Wright DH. Hum Pathol 1978; 9: 661.
290. O'Driscoll BRC, Stevens FM, O'Gorman TA. Gut 1982; 23: 662.
291. Swinson CM, Hall AJ, Bedford PA, Booth CC. Gut 1983; 24: 925.
292. Robertson DAF, Swinson CM, Hall R, Losowsky MS. Gut 1982; 23: 666.
293. O'Brien CJ, Saverymuttu S, Hodgson HJF, Evans DJ. J Clin Pathol 1983; 36: 62.
294. Baer AN, Bayless TM, Yardley JH. Gastroenterology 1980; 79: 754.
295. Robertson DAF, Dixon MF, Scott BB, Simpson FG, Losowsky MS. Gut 1983; 24: 565.
296. Banwell JG, Kistler LA, Gianella RA et al. Gastroenterology 1981; 80: 834.
297. Isaacs PET, Kim YS. Clin Gastroenterol 1983; 12: 395.
298. Klipstein FA. Gastroenterolgy 1981; 80: 590.
299. Tomkins AM. Clin Sci 1981; 60: 131.
300. Ross IM, Mathan VI. Q J Med 1981; 50: 435.
301. Schenk EA, Samloff IM, Klipstein FA. Am J Pathol 1965; 47: 765.
302. Fox B. J Clin Pathol 1967; 20: 806.
303. Foster CS. Histopathology 1979; 3: 1.
304. Bauman MB, DiMase JD, Oski F, Senior JR. Gastroenterology 1963; 54: 93.

Miscellaneous conditions

305. Waldmann TA. Gastroenterol 1966; 50: 422.
306. Haboubi NY, Honan RP, Hasleton PS, Ali HH et al. Histopathol 1984; 8: 145.
307. Smith BH, Welter LH. Am J Clin Pathol 1967; 48: 455.
308. Namdaran F, Dutz W, Ovasepian A. Gut 1979; 20: 16.
309. Johnstone JM, Morson BC. Histopathol 1978; 2: 335.
310. Caldwell JH, Sharma HM, Hurtubise PE, Colwell DL. Gastroenterol 1979; 77: 560.
311. De Schryver-Kecksemeti K, Clouse RE. Am J Surg Pathol 1984; 8: 171.
312. Johnstone JM, Morson BC. Histopathol 1978; 2: 349.
313. Navas-Palacios JJ, Colina-Ruizdelgado F, Sanchez-Larrea MD, Cortes-Cansino J. Cancer 1983; 51: 1682.
314. Anthony PP, Morris DS, Vowles KDJ. Gut 1984; 25: 854.
315. Counsell B. Br J Surg 1956; 44: 276.
316. Saltzstein SL, Rosenberg BF. Am J Clin Pathol 1963; 40: 610.
317. Thayer WR, Spiro HM. Gastroenterol 1962; 42: 547.
318. Solhaug JH, Tvete S. Scand J Gastroenterol 1978; 13: 401.
319. Asp N-G, Godmand-Hoyen E, Andersen B, Berg NO. Gut 1979; 20: 553.
320. Bechi P, Romagnoli P, Cortesini C. Histopathol 1981; 5: 667.
321. Wiernik G. Gut 1966; 7: 149.
322. Wiernik G. J Path Bact 1966; 91: 389.
323. Carr ND, Pullen BR, Hasleton PS, Schofield PF. Gut 1984; 25: 448.
324. Hasleton PS, Carr N, Schofield PF. Histopathol 1985; 9: 517.
325. Baba S, Marota M, Ando K, Teramoto T, Endo I. Dis Col Rect 1976; 19: 428.
326. Krishnamurthy S, Kelly MN, Rohrmann CA, Schuffler MD. Gastroenterol 1983; 85: 538.
327. Schuffler MD, Beegle RG. Gastroenterol 1979; 77: 664.
328. Schuffler MD, Rohrmann CA, Chaffee RG et al. Med 1981; 60: 173.
329. Smith JA, Hauser SC, Madara JL. Am J Surg Pathol 1982; 6: 264.
330. Schuffler MD, Kaplan LR, Johnson L. Am J Dig Dis 1978; 23: 821.
331. Mitros FA, Schuffler MD, Teja K, Anuras S. Hum Pathol 1982; 13: 825.

332. Sharp JR, Insalaco SJ, Johnson LF. Gastroenterol 1980; 78: 366.
333. McClure J. Postgrad Med J 1981; 57: 95.
334. Braverman DZ, Dollberg L, Shiner M. Am J Gastroenterol 1985; 80: 30.
335. Glickman RM, Green PHR, Lees RS, Lox SE, Kilgore A. Gastroenterol 1979; 76: 288.
336. Scott BB, Miller JP, Lowsowsky MS. Gut 1979; 20: 163.
337. Mowat AMcI, Ferguson A. Gastroenterol 1982; 83: 417.
338. Weisdorf SA, Salati LM, Longsdorf JA, Ramsay NKC, Sharp HL. Gastroenterol 1983; 85: 1076.
339. Cunningham D, Morgan RJ, Mills PR et al. J Clin Path 1985; 38: 265.

Tumours of the small intestine

340. Perzin KH, Bridge MF. Cancer 1981; 48: 799.
341. Johansen A, Larsen E. Acta Pathol Microbiol Scand 1969; 75: 247.
342. Keeley AF, Gottlieb LS. Gastroenterol 1969; 57: 185.
343. Delvett AF, Cuello R. Gastroenterol 1975; 69: 217.
344. Komorowski RA, Cohen EB. Cancer 1981; 47: 1377.
345. Hamilton SR, Bussey HJR, Mendelsohn G et al. Gastroenterol 1979; 77: 1252.
346. Burt RW, Berenson MM, Lee RG, Tolman KG, Freston JW, Gardner EJ. Gastroenterol 1984; 86: 295.
347. Yao T, Iida M, Ohsato K, Watanabe H, Omae T. Gastroenterol 1977; 73: 1086.
348. Bridge MF, Perzin KH. Cancer 1975; 36: 1876.
349. Barclay TCH, Schapira DV. Cancer 1983; 51: 578.
350. Holmes GTK, Dunn GI, Cockel R, Brookes VS. Gut 1980; 21: 1010.
351. Heathcote J, Knauer CM, Oakes D, Archibald RWR. Gut 1980; 21: 1093.
352. Gyde SN, Prior P, Macartney JC, Thompson H, Waterhouse JA, Allen RN. Gut 1980; 21: 1024.
353. Cuesta MA, Donner R. Cancer 1976; 37: 949.
354. Roth JA, Logio T. Cancer 1982; 49: 2180.
355. Warner TCFS, Peralta J. Cancer 1979; 44: 1142.
356. Wagner KM, Thompson J, Herlinger H. Caroline D. Cancer 1982; 49: 797.
357. Bloom SR, Polak JM. Clinics in Endocrinol and Met 1980; 9: 285.
358. Soga J, Tazawa K. Cancer 1971; 28: 990.
359. Jones RA, Dawson IMP. Histopathol 1977; 1: 137.
360. Zakariah Y, Quan SHQ, Hajdu SI. Cancer 1975; 35: 588.
361. Godwin JD II. Cancer 1975; 36: 560.
362. Peck JJ, Shields AB, Boyden AM, Dworkin LA, Nadel JW. Am J Surg 1983; 146: 124.
363. Sporrong B, Falkmer S, Robboy SJ et al. Cancer 1982; 49: 68.
364. Dayal Y, Doos WG, O'Brien MJ, Nunnemacher G, DeLellis RA, Wolfe HJ. Am J Surg Pathol 1983; 7: 653.
365. Henry K, Farrer-Brown G. Histopathol 1977; 1: 153.
366. Blackledge G, Bush H, Dodge OG, Crowther D. Clin Oncol 1979; 5: 209.
367. Isaacson P, Wright DH. In: Wright R, ed. Recent advances in gastrointestinal pathology. London: Saunders, 1980; 193.
368. Blackshaw AJ. In: Wright R, ed. Recent advances in gastrointestinal pathology. London: Saunders, 1980; 213.
369. Gonzales-Vitale JC, Gomez LG, Goldblum RM, Goldman AS, Patterson M. Cancer 1982; 49: 445.
370. Isaacson PG, Maclenan HA, Subbuswamy SG. Histopathol 1984; 8: 641.
371. Salem PA, Nassar VH, Shahid MJ et al. Cancer 1977; 40: 2941.
372. Haghighi P, Abadi P, Kharazni A et al. Am J Surg Pathol 1978; 2: 147.
373. Al-Saleem T, Zardawi IM. Histopathol 1979; 3: 89.
374. Russell RM, Abadi P, Ismail-Beigi F. Cancer 1977; 39: 2579.
375. Freeman HJ, Weinstein WM, Schnitka TK, Piercey JRA, Wensel RM. Am J Med 1977; 63: 585.
376. Isaacson P, Jones DB, Sworn MJ, Wright DH. J Clin Pathol 1982; 35: 510.
377. Isaacson P. Gut 1980; 21: 381.
378. Dawson IMP, Cornes JS, Morson BC. Br J Surg 1961–62; 49: 80.
379. Salz RK, Kurtz RC, Lightdale CJ et al. Digest Dis Sci 1984; 29: 817.
380. Dobbins WO III, Weinstein WM. Gastroenterol 1985; 88: 738.

The vermiform appendix

THE NORMAL APPENDIX

The appendix is a diverticulum of the caecum, into which it opens some 2–4 cm below the ileocaecal valve. Its length is usually about 7 cm, ranging between 4 and 20 cm, and its anatomical position in the abdomen is variable, usually being situated either behind the caecum or with its distal end in the pelvis, but sometimes lying behind or in front of the ileum.[1] This variability in the relations of the appendix accounts for the diversity of clinical features associated with acute appendicitis. The lumen of the appendix does not usually exceed 2–3 mm in diameter and its normal volume is less than 0.5 ml.[2] In man the appendix serves no evident purpose and its removal is without effect on alimentary function.

The normal appendix is lined by mucosa of colonic type, with crypts lined by absorptive cells, goblet cells producing predominantly sulphated acid mucins, endocrine cells and occasionally a few Paneth cells. This mucosa continually secretes 1–2 ml of mucinous fluid daily.[2]

Most of the endocrine cells of the appendiceal mucosa are situated near the base of the crypts, in between the epithelial cells and the basement membrane. They are of both argentaffin and argyrophil types and immunocytochemistry has shown them to contain a number of peptides including 5-hydroxytryptamine, substance P, somatostatin, enteroglucagon and vasoactive intestinal polypeptide.[3] However, endocrine cells containing 5-hydroxytryptamine are also found in the lamina propria, occurring either singly or in groups, where they form close associations with an intramucosal plexus of fine nerve fibres (Fig. 7.1).[4,5]

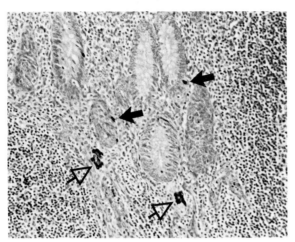

Fig. 7.1 Argyrophilic endocrine cells in the normal appendiceal mucosa occur singly within the crypts (closed arrows) and in clusters in the lamina propria (open arrows).

Grimelius argyrophil reaction   × 170

The lamina propria of the appendix contains relatively more lymphoid tissue than any other part of the intestines. The amount of lymphoid tissue varies with age: there is little in the fetal appendix, but the amount increases after birth to a maximum at the end of the first decade of life and thereafter gradually declines.[6] This atrophy of the lymphoid tissue is often accompanied by an increase in fibrous tissue, first in the submucosa and later replacing the mucosa, especially at the tip. Consequently by late middle life the normal appendix contains little lymphoid tissue and may show fibrous obliteration of the lumen at the tip; such features alone cannot therefore be used as markers of previous inflammation.

The muscularis of the appendix consists of an inner circular coat and an outer longitudinal layer, as in the remainder of the alimentary tract. Granular cells containing PAS-positive material have occasionally been described within the musculature, usually in the inner muscle coat. They are probably degenerate smooth muscle cells.[7] Being developmentally part of the caecum, the appendix has the same pattern of autonomic innervation as that part of the large intestine,[8] although ganglion cells in the submucosal plexus are often inconspicuous. X-ray studies have shown that the normal appendix exhibits irregular peristaltic movements and that its lumen is emptied periodically into the caecum.

CONGENITAL ABNORMALITIES

Duplication of the appendix is a rare anomaly and usually is associated with duplication of the caecum. In the presence of a normal caecum there may be a 'double-barrelled' appendix contained within a single muscle coat, or two well-formed and entirely separate appendices, or a normal appendix accompanied by a rudimentary second appendix arising separately from the caecum.[9] Triple appendix has also been recorded.[10]

Congenital *absence* of the appendix is also rare,[11] but has been described as a possible teratogenic effect of the drug thalidomide.[12] More often, the appendix is *rudimentary*, being no more than 2 cm in length and either of normal width or, more rarely, in the form of a thin muscular cord-like structure lacking a mucosa and having no lumen. In this context it must be remembered that the normal appendix varies greatly in length (see above).

Heterotopias in the appendix are also very uncommon, but heterotopic gastric mucosa, and possibly heterotopic oesophageal tissue, have been described.[13]

Diverticula of the appendix are virtually all acquired (see below) and reports of congenital diverticula, characterized by the absence of inflammation and the presence of all the coats of the appendix in the wall, are exceptional.

INFLAMMATORY CONDITIONS
ACUTE NON-SPECIFIC APPENDICITIS

The term appendicitis was introduced by R. H. Fitz of Boston, whose classic paper in 1886 first drew attention to the significance of acute inflammatory lesions of the appendix as sources of suppurative conditions in the right iliac fossa.[14] The disease is common in western Europe, North America and Australasia, where appendicectomy is the commonest emergency operation, but is rare in tropical Africa and India. In England and Wales appendicitis has its greatest frequency in the second and third decades of life, affecting males and females about equally. It has been suggested that the incidence is falling,[15] but accurate statistics on the frequency of true appendicitis are difficult to obtain and the fall in the frequency in England and Wales may be attributable at least in part to re-classification of patients with abdominal pain in hospital statistics.[16] Deaths from appendicitis are very rare, and usually occur in the elderly, in whom the symptoms are less striking in relation to the severity of the disease, and in whom 'silent' perforation of the appendix with peritonitis is more common. Of 136 deaths from acute appendicitis in England and Wales in 1983, 83 occurred among patients over the age of 70 years.[17] The mortality from acute appendicitis has fallen by about 20 times over the last 50 years, largely because of earlier diagnosis and surgical intervention and the use of antibiotics.

Aetiology and pathogenesis

While some controversy remains over the aetiology and pathogenesis of acute appendicitis it is now generally considered that obstruction of the lumen of the appendix is the most important initiating factor. Experimental studies have shown that the pressure of secretions within an obstructed but otherwise normal human appendix may reach 90 mmHg, well above that normally found in the small blood vessels of the wall, and it is postulated that ischaemic damage to the mucosa allows invasion of the wall of the appendix by faecal organisms and consequent inflammation.[18] Support for this theory comes from the classical work of Wilkie,[19] who showed that if the appendix of a rabbit was ligated while the lumen contained faecal material the animal died within 24 hours from perforated gangrenous appendicitis, but if the luminal contents were sterile then only cystic dilatation of the appendix occurred. Furthermore, bacteriological studies of acute appendicitis have shown that it is usually not a specific infection due to a single bacterial species, but that a wide variety of organisms may be recovered from the inflamed organ, virtually all of them resident flora of the normal large bowel, consistent with the idea of secondary infection.[20]

The best recognized cause of obstruction of the appendiceal lumen in acute appendicitis is a faecolith (Fig. 7.2), a mass of inspissated faecal material which forms around some small foreign

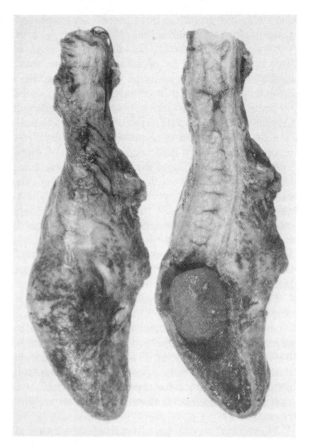

Fig. 7.2 Acute appendicitis. The appendix has been bisected longitudinally. There is a fibrinopurulent exudate on the surface of the hyperaemic serosa (left). A large faecolith is seen obstructing the lumen; the wall of the appendix distal to the obstruction has become gangrenous (right).

Specimen from the Gordon Museum, Guy's Hospital, London, reproduced by permission of the Curator, Mr J. D. Maynard. Photograph by Miss P. M. Turnbull, Charing Cross Hospital Medical School, London.

body in the appendix and grows slowly by the deposition of successive laminae, sometimes with calcification. Estimates of the frequency with which faecoliths are present in acutely inflamed appendices have varied greatly from 9%[21] to 89%[22] but when a faecolith does co-exist with appendicitis the inflammation is almost invariably distal to the obstruction, in keeping with the obstructive theory of pathogenesis. Other proposed causes of luminal obstruction that might lead to acute appendicitis include kinking or constriction of the appendix by peritoneal bands or fibrous adhesions, bezoars, tumours of the appendix or caecum, and lymphoid hyperplasia of the wall. Lymphoid tissue in the appendix is abundant in the pre-pubertal years, when the lumen is at its smallest relative to the thickness of the wall,[6] and hyperplasia of this lymphoid tissue, as may occur during viral and bacterial infections (Fig. 7.3), could lead to obstruction of the appendix and account for the high incidence of appendicitis in childhood.

An obstructive lesion in the lumen of the appendix is not invariably demonstrable in acute appendicitis. Moreover the intraluminal pressure, when measured directly during surgery for appendicitis, is elevated in only about a quarter of cases.[23] The aetiology of so-called non-obstructive appendicitis is controversial. Only in exceptional instances is there proof of a primary infective cause, as in the appendicitis that rarely complicates bacillary dysentery, salmonellosis and intestinal amoebiasis. However, it has been proposed that

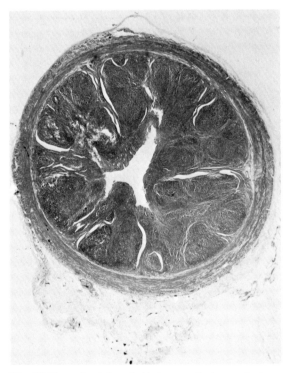

Fig. 7.3 Hyperplastic lymphoid tissue producing marked luminal narrowing of the appendix of a 9-year-old child.

Haematoxylin-eosin   × 6

Histological preparation provided by Dr T. M. Dauncey, East Glamorgan General Hospital, Pontypridd. Photomicrograph by Mr Peter Langham, University of Wales College of Medicine, Cardiff.

primary viral infection of the appendix might damage the mucosal barrier sufficiently to allow secondary invasion by faecal organisms,[24] and serological evidence of recent infection with mumps, adenovirus and influenza B has been described in a minority of patients with acute appendicitis.[25,26] The significance of this is uncertain. An earlier belief that infestation by the threadworm *Oxyuris vermicularis* in children predisposes to acute appendicitis now seems to be unfounded, and a suggestion that *Histoplasma capsulatum* is a frequent cause of appendicitis and mesenteric lymphadenitis was based on misinterpretation of Flemming's 'stainable bodies' in macrophages in the germinal centres of lymphoid follicles as histoplasmas.

Another hypothesis for apparently non-obstructive acute appendicitis proposes that the inflammation is indeed secondary to luminal obstruction but that this is a functional and intermittent obstruction, either due to a sphincter-like mechanism at the base of the appendix where it joins the caecum, or by muscular spasm of the appendix itself. This idea derives mainly from the proposals of Rendle Short,[27] more recently expanded by Burkitt,[28] that the geographical distribution of the disease and other epidemiological data indicate that a low residue diet is the important factor in the aetiology of acute appendicitis. Such a diet results in bowel contents that are firm, tenacious, of low volume and difficult to propel along the lumen, predisposing to faecolith formation. They suggest that even in cases without faecoliths there is exaggerated muscle activity in the wall of the appendix, resulting in an increased intraluminal pressure and a predisposition to muscle spasm. Indeed Burkitt has proposed that the early epigastric colic that is so chacteristic of acute appendicitis is the result of such spasm rather than inflammation.

Macroscopical appearances

The appearance of an acutely inflamed appendix depends on the stage that the inflammatory process has reached when it comes under observation. In the early stages of acute suppurative appendicitis, a part or the whole of the organ is swollen, and its serosal surface may show patches of hyperaemia.

If such an appendix is opened longitudinally, its distended lumen is seen to contain some thin mucopus, and there is often evidence—from alteration in internal diameter—that there has been obstruction, such as might have been brought about by an impacted faecolith (Fig. 7.2) or a fibrous stricture. Often such changes in diameter are best seen when the appendix has been hardened in formalin before being opened.

Later, the swelling increases, especially distal to any obstruction, hyperaemia becomes more extensive, and the peritoneal surface is dulled by pale flecks of fibrin or by purulent exudate. In the absence of surgical intervention, the condition proceeds to the stage known as *gangrenous appendicitis*. The whole organ, or sometimes only its distal part, then becomes softened and friable, and shows areas of haemorrhage and dark greenish-brown patches of necrosis. The interior of the appendix now contains thick mucopus and may be distended to many times its normal capacity; suppurative foci may be found within its wall. These changes may be aggravated by the development of thrombosis in some of the blood vessels, particularly the veins in the appendix itself or in its mesentery.[29]

The speed at which these changes succeed one another is very variable. The clinical and pathological features are not always closely correlated, for occasionally the appendix is found to be already gangrenous within a few hours of the onset of symptoms. As a result of the weakening of its wall by the development of local gangrene, and of the rise in internal pressure due to the accumulation of the infected exudate in the obstructed lumen, perforation is likely to occur, giving rise to the serious complication of peritonitis.

Histological appearances

Acute appendicitis is characterized by oedema and congestion of the wall, a transmural infiltration of neutrophil polymorphs often forming small intramural abscesses, ulceration of the mucosa and a local fibrinopurulent peritonitis (Fig. 7.4). Vascular thrombosis is often present and in the most florid examples the combination of suppurative inflammation and ischaemia leads to gangrenous

appendicitis with necrosis of the wall and perforation.[30]

While the histological diagnosis of established appendicitis is easy, difficulties often arise when an appendix removed from a patient with the clinical features of acute appendicitis shows only mild inflammation confined to the mucosa. It is very tempting to regard this as early appendicitis, but a number of studies have shown that up to 35% of appendices removed electively from asymptomatic patients undergoing abdominal surgery for unrelated reasons show small collections of neutrophil polymorphs in the lumen, focal ulceration of the surface epithelium with pus cells in the adjacent lamina propria, and even a few crypt abscesses.[31] On the other hand, studies of experimental appendicitis give evidence that identical mucosal lesions can progress rapidly to established acute appendicitis with gangrene and perforation.[32] It is obviously impossible to dismiss acute inflammation, even if

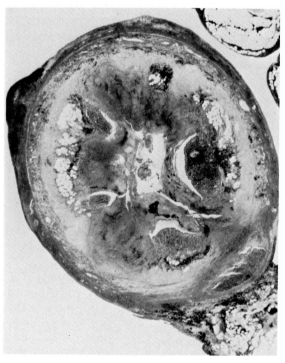

Fig. 7.4 Acute appendicitis. There is haemorrhagic ulceration of the mucosa. All coats of the appendiceal wall are thickened by oedema and an infiltrate of inflammatory cells and there is an overlying peritonitis.

Haematoxylin-eosin   × 10

Photomicrograph by Mr Peter Langham, University of Wales College of Medicine, Cardiff.

confined to the mucosa, in patients with the clinical features of appendicitis but in such cases it must also be prudent to exclude other causes for acute abdominal pain.

Course and complications

Spontaneous healing of acute appendicitis may take place, but the chances that this may occur diminish rapidly as the inflammatory lesions progress. In the absence of complications, such as perforation and peritonitis, the formation of granulation tissue results in healing and fibrosis, leaving the appendix like a thick fibrous cord, its lumen partially or completely obliterated.

Perforation is a particularly grave complication of acute appendicitis. If it occurs suddenly the whole peritoneal cavity may be flooded with bacteria and an acute diffuse peritonitis result. If the inflammatory process has developed more slowly, or if the appendix is retrocaecal in position, the pus that escapes from the lumen will remain localized, being contained by the fibrinous exudate that binds the appendix to adjacent structures. Such developments give rise to the clinically familiar 'appendix abscess' or 'appendix mass'. The infrequent rupture of an appendix abscess back into the caecum gives rise to a so-called 'appendicular granuloma',[33] and similar mechanisms may even more rarely result in *fistulae* between the appendix and adjacent loops of the small or large intestine, the bladder or the abdominal wall.[34] Even in cases of diffuse peritonitis in which appendicectomy is performed, the purulent exudate tends to collect in certain parts of the abdomen, giving rise to pelvic or sub-diaphragmatic abscesses. A pelvic abscess will sometimes perforate spontaneously into the rectum or vagina with consequent resolution, but sub-diaphragmatic abscesses tend to persist and become chronic. These collections of pus, like chronic abscesses at the site of the appendix itself, may become walled off by thick fibrous adhesions: they may then resolve slowly or they may persist for many months.

Infective thrombosis of the veins in the region of the appendix is a common accompaniment of acute appendicitis. Usually it is only a local condition, confined to the small vessels. Occasionally, however, the thrombophlebitis extends into larger vessels, and portions of infected thrombus are then liable to break off and be carried as emboli to the liver, where they lodge in the intrahepatic portions of the portal vein and give rise to multiple liver abscesses. This condition, *suppurative pylephlebitis*,[35] has become considerably rarer since the introduction of antibiotics.

Fibrous adhesions to the greater omentum, small intestine and other abdominal structures may form as a late complication of appendicitis. They predispose to intestinal obstruction and volvulus in the future.

Obliteration of the lumen in the proximal part of the appendix by post-inflammatory scarring can result in distension of the appendix by sterile mucus (Fig. 7.5) and the formation of a *mucocele* (see below).[36] Although usually small and symptomless, this may become infected to give rise to an *empyema* of the appendix. Very rarely rupture of a mucocele causes spilling of mucous material into the surrounding peritoneal cavity to produce a localized *pseudomyxoma peritonei* (see below). Simple mucocele, a lesion caused by luminal obstruction alone, must be distinguished from neoplastic lesions of the appendix with exuberant mucus production, whose macroscopic appearances may be similar (see below).

CHRONIC NON-SPECIFIC APPENDICITIS

There is considerable disagreement about the very existence of chronic appendicitis, mainly because the laboratory examination of appendices removed following a clinical diagnosis of chronic appendicitis does not always reveal pathological changes. Thackray compared 50 appendices from patients who were believed, on clinical grounds, to be suffering from chronic appendicitis with another 50 from a control group of patients whose appendices were removed incidentally during laparotomy for unrelated conditions and who had never had symptoms of gastrointestinal disease.[37] The histological appearances were found to be remarkably similar in the two series and about a quarter of the appendices in both groups were normal.

Fibrosis alone cannot be used as an indication of chronic appendicitis since the amount of appendiceal fibrous tissue increases with age (see above). It is necessary to have such additional evidence of

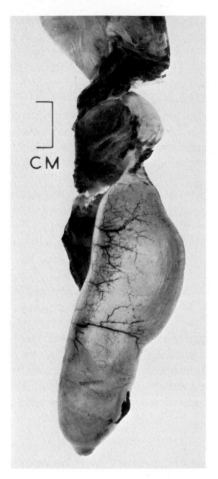

Fig. 7.5 So-called mucocele of the appendix. Retention of mucus in this case has resulted from obstruction, caused by twisting of the base of the appendix, a sequel of fibrosis following appendicitis.

Specimen from the Gordon Museum, Guy's Hospital, London, reproduced by permission of the Curator, Mr J. D. Maynard. Photograph by Miss P. M. Turnbull, Charing Cross Hospital Medical School, London.

active chronic inflammation as infiltration of the muscle layers and subserosa by lymphocytes and plasma cells, or the presence of granulation tissue. The histochemical demonstration of iron may also be a marker of previous haemorrhagic inflammation.[38] Unless histological proof of chronic inflammation is obtained it is wise to consider other causes of chronic or recurrent abdominal pain; nevertheless, some patients are rendered asymptomatic by the removal of what appears histologically to be a normal appendix, suggesting to some clinicians that the symptoms are due to muscular spasm of the appendix ('appendicular colic') but to others that psychological factors are important in the symptoms of chronic appendicitis.

OTHER VARIETIES OF APPENDICITIS

Tuberculosis

Tuberculous appendicitis is most commonly associated with ileocaecal tuberculosis, although secondary spread from pulmonary infection may occur, and apparent primary appendiceal tuberculosis has also been recorded.[39] The macroscopic appearances vary from normal to a thickened, chronically inflamed appendix which is adherent to adjacent structures. A picture identical to acute non-specific appendicitis is another rarer variant. Histologically, the diagnosis is established by the finding of characteristic caseating granulomas, both in the wall of the appendix and in the mesenteric lymph nodes, and the demonstration of tubercle bacilli within the lesions.

Yersiniosis

The appendix may be involved in intestinal yersiniosis, although changes are much commoner and more conspicuous in the terminal ileum and mesenteric lymph nodes.[40] The histological changes in the affected appendix are variable, sometimes being indistinguishable from acute non-specific appendicitis but on other occasions having the characteristic microscopical features of yersiniosis as seen in the ileum (see p. 255), with granulomas, often containing micro-abscesses of polymorphonuclear leukocytes, and lymphoid hyperplasia. The diagnosis is best confirmed serologically.

Actinomycosis

Actinomyces israelii may be a commensal organism in the mouth. From time to time its branching filaments are seen in the lumen of the appendix in histological preparations and sometimes the organism can be cultured from appendicectomy specimens. It is important to appreciate that the presence of *Actinomyces israelii* in the appendiceal lumen does not necessarily indicate pathogenicity, even if the appendix is acutely inflamed. Only if its filaments are seen actually within the inflamed tissues may the diagnosis of actinomycosis be accepted. On the other hand, it is imperative that cases of true acute actinomycotic appendicitis are not overlooked, for failure to treat such cases appropriately is likely to result in progression of the local disease and the risk of spread elsewhere.

In most cases, appendiceal actinomycosis does not produce the clinical picture of acute appendicitis, but takes the form of a more chronic suppurative lesion, with exuberant fibrosis and the formation of sinuses and fistulae between the appendix and adjacent organs, especially other loops of intestine or the anterior abdominal wall. Indeed, the possibility of actinomycosis should be considered in all patients who develop a faecal fistula after appendicectomy. In addition to these local complications, spread of infection into the portal venous system may give rise to metastatic abscesses in the liver.

Schistosomiasis

Appendiceal involvement in schistosomiasis results in similar histological manifestations to schistosomiasis elsewhere in the large intestine, with granulomatous inflammation accompanied by numerous eosinophil leukocytes, related to eggs deposited in the bowel wall.

Oxyuriasis and strongyloidiasis

Infestation of the appendix by *Oxyuris vermicularis* (*Enterobius vermicularis*), sometimes referred to as the threadworm, pinworm or seatworm, is quite common in temperate or cold climates, especially in children. Adult worms in the lumen of the appendix are best recognized by the narrow lateral barb-like alae that protrude from the cuticle (Fig. 7.6). Pinworm infestation produces no symptoms attributable to the appendix and it is now generally considered that it plays no part in the pathogenesis of acute appendicitis.[41] Nevertheless, on rare occasions invasion of the wall of the appendix may occur, resulting in a granulomatous reaction with conspicuous eosinophil leukocytes (Fig. 7.7).

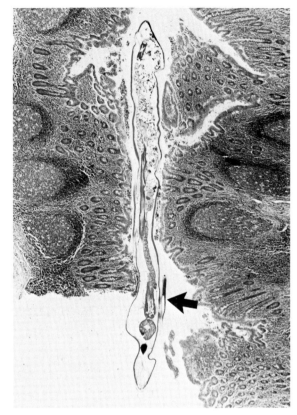

Fig. 7.6 An adult female *Oxyuris vermicularis* worm within the lumen of the appendix. A lateral barb-like ala is present (arrow).

Haematoxylin-eosin   × 30

Photomicrograph by Mr Peter Langham, University of Wales College of Medicine, Cardiff.

Eosinophilic appendicitis has also been described in generalized gastrointestinal strongyloidiasis, with intramural eosinophil-rich granulomas containing the larvae of *Strongyloides stercoralis* (see p. 268).[42]

Miscellaneous causes of appendicitis

Specific *viral* infections of the appendix have been described, usually in childhood. *Measles* infection is the easiest to recognize histologically by its characteristic Warthin-Finkeldey multinucleated giant cells which are usually situated in the margins of briskly reactive lymphoid follicles (Fig. 7.8). *Adenovirus* infection may also produce lymphoid hyperplasia with focal destruction of the surface

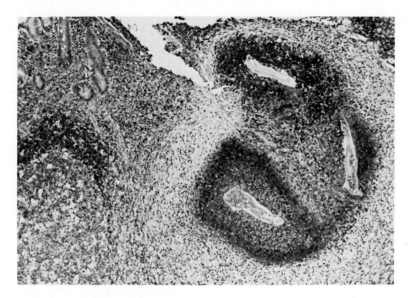

Fig. 7.7 An eosinophil-rich granulomatous reaction to *Oxyuris vermicularis* within the submucosa of the appendix. The overlying mucosa is ulcerated.

Haematoxylin-eosin × 70

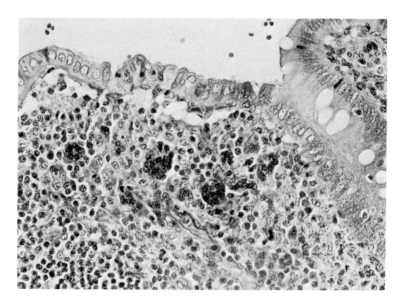

Fig. 7.8 Warthin-Finkeldey giant cells, characteristic of measles infection, in the appendiceal lamina propria adjacent to a lymphoid follicle. The patient developed the typical skin rash 2 days after appendicectomy.

Haematoxylin-eosin × 330

Histological preparation for photography provided by Dr J. Dinnen, County Hospital, Hereford.

epithelium. In some cases intranuclear viral inclusions can be identified on light and electron microscopy.[43] The clinical features of viral appendicitis are usually ill-defined but occasionally the lymphoid hyperplasia may precipitate intussusception of the appendix or, presumably by luminal narrowing, produce features of acute appendicitis.

Acute appendicitis may complicate the course of specific intestinal infections such as *typhoid* and *paratyphoid fever, bacillary dysentery* and *salmonella food poisoning*.[44] The changes in the appendix in such cases reflect those found in the other parts of the intestines. Similarly, appendiceal involvement may also occur in *amoebic dysentery* but there are also recorded cases of apparently localized amoebiasis of the appendix.[45]

Crohn's disease

Involvement of the appendix is said to occur in about 20% of patients with ileocolic Crohn's disease. The pathological features are identical to Crohn's disease elsewhere in the gastrointestinal tract, with transmural focal lymphoid aggregates, fissuring ulceration, granulomatous inflammation and fibrosis (see p. 258).[46,47] Granulomatous appendicitis may be the first manifestation of Crohn's disease—a retrospective review of 11 cases in which appendicectomy had been performed three to nine years before the appearance of specific intestinal lesions revealed appendiceal epithelioid granulomas in five.[48] On the other hand, the risk of recurrent intestinal Crohn's disease following appendicectomy for isolated granulomatous appendicitis seems to be relatively small, probably less than 20%.[46,47]

MISCELLANEOUS CONDITIONS

Diverticula

Diverticula are present in about 1% of appendicectomy specimens; they are often multiple and are usually situated along the mesenteric and antimesenteric aspects of the distal third of the organ (Fig. 7.9). Virtually all are acquired 'false' diverticula resulting from herniation of the mucosa through a defect in the muscular wall, probably as

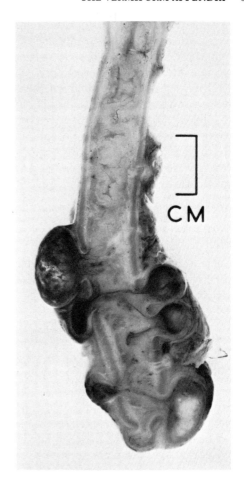

Fig. 7.9 Multiple diverticula of the appendix, which has been bisected longitudinally in order to show the continuity between its lumen and the lumina of the diverticula.

Specimen from the Gordon Museum, Guy's Hospital, London, reproduced by permission of the Curator, Mr J. D. Maynard. Photograph by Miss P. M. Turnbull, Charing Cross Hospital Medical School, London.

a consequence of raised intraluminal pressure: it is pertinent to this view that stenosis of the lumen proximal to the site of the diverticulosis, and hypertrophy of the musculature distal to the obstruction, have been described.[49] Appendiceal diverticula are usually asymptomatic unless secondary infection produces diverticulitis, when the clinical features mimic acute appendicitis.[50]

Intussusception

Intussusception of the appendix is rare.[51] Most cases occur in childhood, especially in boys.

Predisposing factors are said to include a fetal cone-shaped caecum, a thin mesoappendix and increased or irregular peristalsis. It has been associated with intraluminal foreign bodies, faecoliths, worms, lymphoid hyperplasia and tumours of the appendix. Several varieties are described, including intussusception of the tip into the more proximal appendix, intussusception of the proximal appendix into the caecum, either of which may lead to complete inversion of the appendix, or even intussusception of the proximal appendix into the distal appendix.[52]

Torsion

Torsion is also rare. It tends to occur when the appendix is unusually long and has a lax mesentery. It predisposes to acute appendicitis.[53]

Endometriosis

Involvement of the appendix occurs in about 1% of patients with pelvic endometriosis.[54] It is usually an incidental finding at laparotomy, although occasionally symptoms of appendicitis may be present, especially if there has been recent haemorrhage. The deposits may be found in any layer of the appendiceal wall, although they are commonest in the subserosa and the outer muscle coat,[55] often associated with marked localized muscular thickening. Grossly they may be soft and haemorrhagic or pale and fibrotic and on microscopic examination endometrial glands and stroma are found, often with recent or old haemorrhage and fibrosis. Stromal decidualization may occur during pregnancy. The relationship between endometriosis and acute appendicitis is disputed but it has been suggested that haemorrhage into a focus of endometriosis might precipitate acute appendicitis, possibly by causing luminal obstruction.[56]

Vasculitis

Vasculitis in the appendix may occur in collagen diseases, notably polyarteritis nodosa.[57] However, a similar focal necrotizing arteritis of the appendix has been described as an incidental finding, unrelated to appendicitis or any systemic disease, usually in young women.[58] It is manifested by segmental fibrinoid necrosis of arterial walls with destruction of the elastic laminae and an infiltrate of neutrophil and eosinophil leukocytes. Small arteries in the mesoappendix may also be involved. Its significance is unknown.

TUMOURS OF THE APPENDIX

The relative infrequency of tumours of the appendix may be a reflection of the small size of the organ. Nevertheless, any of the tumours and tumour-like lesions that occur in the large intestine, of which the appendix is a derivative, may be found. By far the commonest, however, is the carcinoid tumour which accounts for over 80% of all appendiceal growths.

Metaplastic polyps

Metaplastic polyps are well-demarcated sessile mucosal lesions characterized by elongated crypts with a serrated epithelial lining in which absorptive cells are prominent (see p. 355). Although common in the distal half of the large intestine discrete metaplastic polyps are very rare in the appendix.[59] It is far commoner to find a more diffuse 'metaplastic' change affecting a large area of the appendiceal mucosa (Fig. 7.10). The aetiology of this lesion is unknown. Occasionally it is found in an appendix which is dilated by mucus (a so-called mucocele)[60] but more commonly it is an incidental finding in an otherwise normal organ. The regular differentiation of the epithelium and the lack of cellular or nuclear atypia (Fig. 7.11) allow the lesion to be distinguished from the clinically more important adenoma (see below), with which metaplastic change may co-exist and even merge.[61]

Hamartomatous polyps

Hamartomatous polyps of the Peutz-Jeghers and juvenile types (see pp. 363 and 364) may be found in the appendix. They may even be confined to the appendix, but in the vast majority of cases their presence is part of the Peutz-Jeghers syndrome or of juvenile polyposis, with involvement of other parts of the alimentary tract.[62,63] These lesions,

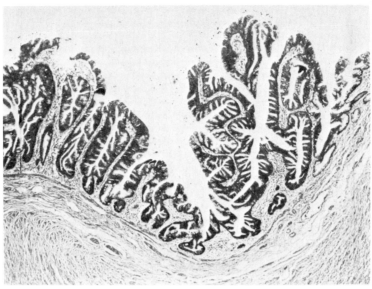

Fig. 7.10 Low-power appearance of the appendiceal mucosa with a diffuse 'metaplastic' change.

Haematoxylin-eosin   × 30

Photomicrograph by Mr Peter Langham, University of Wales College of Medicine, Cardiff.

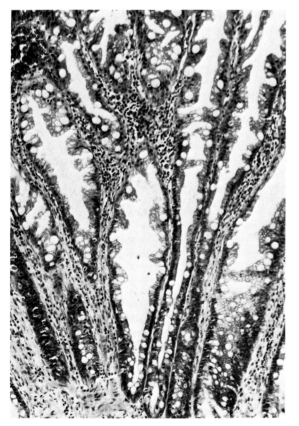

juvenile polyps particularly, should not be confused with adenomas (see below).

Adenomas and cystadenomas

Adenomas of the appendix, like adenomas elsewhere in the large intestine, are neoplastic lesions which may progress to invasive adenocarcinoma. However, unlike adenomas in the remainder of the colorectum, discrete and polypoid lesions with a tubular growth pattern are very uncommon,[64] and most appendiceal adenomas are diffuse villous lesions involving large areas of the appendiceal mucosa (Fig. 7.12).[65] Excessive mucus production commonly causes distension of the appendix to produce a sausage-shaped mass (mucocele) which may reach cystic proportions, in which case the name cystadenoma of the appendix is given.

The hallmark of adenomatous epithelial proliferation throughout the large intestine is dysplasia,

Fig. 7.11 Medium-power appearance of 'metaplastic' change in the appendiceal mucosa. The crypts have a serrated appearance and absorptive cells predominate in the epithelial lining. There is no cytological atypia.

Haematoxylin-eosin.   × 130

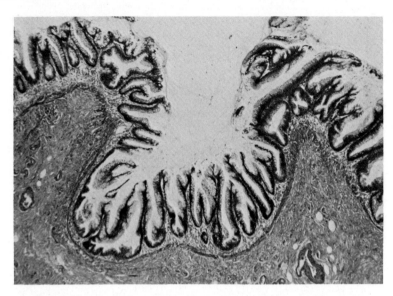

Fig. 7.12 Low-power appearance of a villous adenoma which occupied most of the mucosa of the appendix and which caused luminal distension by mucus.

Haematoxylin-eosin   × 40

Photomicrograph by Mr Peter Langham, University of Wales College of Medicine, Cardiff.

manifested by cytological atypia, cellular crowding, stratification and abnormalities of glandular architecture (see p. 357): the appendix is no exception (Fig. 7.13).[60] However, a number of unusual features often occur in this organ which may cause diagnostic difficulty. Firstly, appendiceal adenomas frequently have a villous configuration with papillary fronds covered by large numbers of mucus-producing cells which often have a deceptively innocuous appearance. In such cases the dysplastic nature of the lesion is best appreciated by examining the epithelial characteristics in the basal half of the mucosa (Fig. 7.13). Secondly, there may be areas with a serrated pattern which can cause confusion with metaplastic polyps, a situation complicated by the occasional co-existence of true metaplastic and adenomatous epithelium within the same appendix.[65] Again, detailed evaluation of the cytology of the basal part of the lesion will allow the regular cells of the metaplastic polyp to be distinguished from the dysplastic cells of an adenoma. Finally, the epithelial lining of a cystadenoma may be particularly difficult to interpret, especially if mucous distension has reduced the mucosa to a single layer of cells. The presence of a few residual villous structures is a helpful pointer to the diagnosis of cystadenoma, but once again cellular characteristics of dysplasia must be identified in the epithelial lining and this may require numerous histological sections (Fig. 7.14).

Appendiceal adenomas rarely produce clinical symptoms and most are discovered incidentally. Nevertheless, a few present with acute appendicitis; more rarely, dystrophic calcification within the abundant mucus may be seen radiologically.[64] Occasionally mucus under pressure may dissect through the wall of the appendix to reach the serosal surface, producing so-called pseudomyxoma peritonei (see below). Histological examination of the appendix in such cases may show the mucus in the wall to be accompanied by epithelial elements, causing confusion with invasive adenocarcinoma. When this 'pseudo-invasion' occurs it is nearly always accompanied by inflammation and abscess formation within the appendiceal wall, unlike true invasion in which the glandular structures are usually surrounded by a desmoplastic reaction.[66]

Adenomas of the appendix are cured by appen-

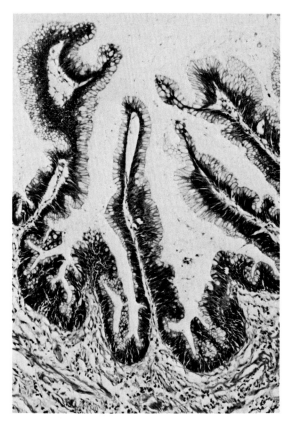

Fig. 7.13 Medium-power appearance of the appendiceal adenoma in Figure 7.12. The epithelium has a villous configuration and shows dysplasia, with crowding and stratification of the cells and nuclear atypia, especially in the basal half.

Haematoxylin-eosin   × 130

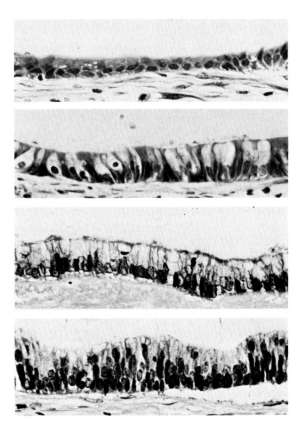

Fig. 7.14 Cystadenoma of the appendix in which the epithelial lining has been reduced to a single layer by mucous distension. Four fields from the same lesion are shown. Dysplasia is easily recognized in the bottom field and nuclear atypia is present in the third field. The diagnosis would not be possible from the two upper fields. Examination of many sections from a so-called mucocele is necessary in order to exclude cystadenoma.

Haematoxylin-eosin   × 340

dicectomy provided the resection line at the base of the appendix is tumour-free. When pseudomyxoma peritonei is the result of an appendiceal adenoma it virtually always resolves after appendicectomy. However, careful scrutiny of the remainder of the large intestine is necessary in patients with appendiceal adenomas because of the strong association with synchronous or metachronous colorectal adenomas and carcinomas.[64]

Adenocarcinoma and cystadenocarcinoma

Adenocarcinoma of the appendix is a rare tumour that presents either as acute appendicitis or as an abdominal mass in a middle-aged or elderly patient.[67] Most, if not all, adenocarcinomas arise in pre-existing adenomas. They may be divided broadly into two growth patterns—mucinous adenocarcinoma (or cystadenocarcinoma), almost invariably arising in a precursor cystadenoma, showing abundant extracellular mucin production, and often having the gross appearance of a mucocele (see below),[60,65] and, less frequently, tubular adenocarcinoma which arises in the more conventional colonic type tubular or tubulo-villous adenoma and, similar to the majority of colorectal carcinomas without exuberant mucus production (Fig. 7.15), produces thickening of the appendiceal wall.[68,69] In both types the diagnosis is established by the identification of true invasion of the wall of the appendix by neoplastic epithelium,[66] and lymph node metastases are present in about a quarter of

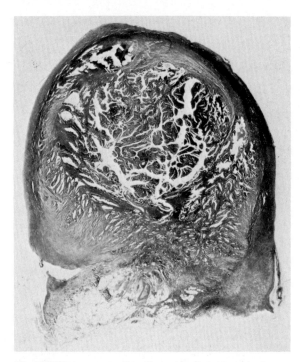

Fig. 7.15 Transverse section of an appendix with a colonic type tubular adenocarcinoma arising in a tubulo-villous adenoma. The tumour has just penetrated the wall and shows early invasion of the mesoappendix (bottom).

Haematoxylin-eosin × 6

Photomicrograph by Mr Peter Langham, University of Wales College of Medicine, Cardiff.

resection specimens. Peritoneal seeding may occur in tumours that have penetrated the wall[60] and these may produce large volumes of mucus and generalized pseudomyxoma peritonei[66] which, because of the persistence of malignant cells in the peritoneum, fails to regress after appendicectomy. Right hemicolectomy is the treatment of choice for carcinoma of the appendix and the prognosis is governed by the degree of differentiation and the Dukes stage (see p. 374);[69] overall the 5-year survival rate is about 60%.

The boundary between adenocarcinomas and endocrine cell tumours of the appendix (see below) is sometimes unclear and colonic type well-differentiated adenocarcinomas may contain conspicuous endocrine cells.[69] The distinction is most blurred, however, in a special group of tumours, discussed in detail below, which often show divergent epithelial differentiation with mucous (and often signet-ring) cells, endocrine cells and

Paneth cells. They have been given many names, including mucinous carcinoid,[70] goblet cell carcinoid,[71] adenocarcinoid,[72] and crypt cell carcinoma.[73] While endocrine cells may be prominent in these tumours they are not invariably present and it is likely that appendiceal tumours reported in the literature as signet-ring carcinoma,[69] microglandular carcinoma[69] and linitis plastica of the appendix[68] are variants of this tumour group.

Finally, it should be stated that metastatic adenocarcinoma in the appendix may mimic primary tumours and that this distinction is obviously important for patient management. The finding of adenomatous changes in the mucosa adjacent to a carcinoma is the best evidence that the latter is primary and in its absence the possibility of another primary abdominal tumour should always be considered, especially if the bulk of the lesion is extramural.

Mucocele of the appendix

There is confusion in the literature over the understanding of this term and it has even been suggested that it should be abandoned.[60] By definition an appendiceal mucocele is simply an appendix that is distended by mucus, and it may be the result of one of two processes. The first, and probably the less common, is dilatation of the appendix consequent upon proximal luminal obstruction (Fig. 7.5), usually from post-inflammatory scarring, and this change has also been called appendiceal ectasia.[60] 'Simple' mucoceles of this sort rarely measure more than 1 cm in diameter and histological examination of the lining usually reveals a flattened, attenuated epithelium which is often partly desquamated to leave a layer of loose connective tissue containing mucin-laden macrophages and giant cells. Very occasionally the mucosal lining of this form of mucocele has a 'metaplastic' appearance (see above).[60,65] The second variety of mucocele is an appendix distended by mucus produced by a neoplasm of the appendix, i.e. by a cystadenoma or a cystadenocarcinoma.[60,65] Mucoceles of this type are commoner and usually much larger than 'obstructive' mucoceles, and are lined by neoplastic epithelium, although, as has been stated above, it may be difficult to recognize this because of flattening of the cells (Fig. 7.14). It behoves the pathologist to take many sections of any mucocele, not only to establish the presence of a neoplastic lining but also, if such a lining is found, to search for an invasive adenocarcinoma.

Pseudomyxoma peritonei

This is another term that has caused confusion in the literature. It is defined as the presence of masses of mucinous material within the peritoneal cavity, and these may be distributed diffusely or localized to one part of the abdomen. Like the term mucocele, pseudomyxoma peritonei is only a description of an appearance, it is not a diagnosis. It is caused by rupture of a mucus-filled viscus, usually an appendix, gall-bladder or a mucinous ovarian cyst, into the peritoneal cavity. Pseudomyxoma peritonei of appendiceal origin results from rupture of a mucocele of the appendix, and the distribution of the extravasated mucus and its clinical effects depend upon the cause of the underlying lesion. If there is rupture of a simple 'obstructive' mucocele or a cystadenoma of the appendix the mucous material is nearly always confined to the right iliac fossa and resolves after appendicectomy. If there is rupture of a cystadenocarcinoma, however, there is a risk of generalized and progressive pseudomyxoma peritonei because of the seeding of mucinous adenocarcinoma over the peritoneal cavity.[65] Such cases may result in a fatal outcome from intestinal obstruction despite therapeutic measures which include omentectomy, radiotherapy and chemotherapy.[74] Although it is claimed by some authors that epithelial cells are present in the mucous masses of pseudomyxoma peritonei only if it is due to malignancy[60] this is disputed by others[69] and consequently the reliability of cytological examination of extravasated mucus is of very limited value for predicting the behaviour in an individual case.

Endocrine cell tumours (carcinoid tumours)

Carcinoid tumours are said to occur in about 0.3% of all appendicectomy specimens.[75] They occur at all ages, including childhood,[76] and are somewhat commoner in females. Most are small tumours measuring less than 1 cm in diameter; about 70%

occur in the tip of the appendix and less than 10% are found in the base of the organ.[75] While carcinoids may co-exist with appendicitis this association is usually coincidental, although tumours at the base of the appendix may cause appendicitis by luminal obstruction. Other clinical manifestations are exceptionally rare, but the carcinoid syndrome[77] and Cushing's syndrome[78] have been described in cases with metastatic spread to the liver. Carcinoid tumours arise from the mucosa of the appendix, and often show an intimate relationship with the basal parts of the crypts. They probably arise from the cells in this zone, although an origin from the endocrine cells that normally populate the lamina propria has also been proposed.[79]

The histological appearances of appendiceal carcinoids are variable but two main patterns are recognized. The first is morphologically identical to the classical ileal or midgut carcinoid tumour, and usually has a yellow colour on gross inspection after formalin fixation. It consists of very uniform endocrine cells arranged in solid masses or packets (Fig. 7.16), sometimes with palisading of the nuclei of the outermost cells. Nuclear pleomorphism is minimal and mitoses are very few. The cells have many similarities with enterochromaffin (EC) cells of the normal intestine and contain cytoplasmic granules which give positive argentaffin and diazo reactions and which are often strongly eosinophilic in routine preparations. Sometimes these granules are scattered throughout the cytoplasm of the cells but more often they are concentrated at the periphery of the tumour masses (Fig. 7.17). Occasionally the cytoplasm has a clear, vacuolated appearance, possibly a degenerative phenomenon.[80] Immunocytochemistry has demonstrated 5-hydroxytryptamine in virtually all of these argentaffin tumours and other peptides may also be present, including neurotensin, somatostatin, motilin and pancreatic polypeptide.[81] While a solid histological pattern is usual in these tumours a small proportion have areas with an acinar arrangement of neoplastic endocrine cells with a small central lumen that may even contain inspissated mucinous material.[80] On rare occasions this acinar pattern, in which virtually all of the cells contain argentaffin granules, dominates the histological picture (Fig. 7.18).

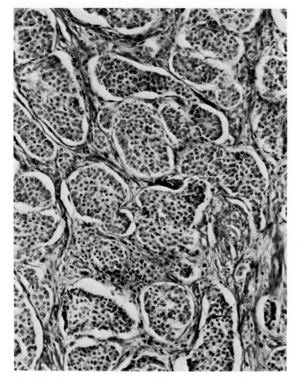

Fig. 7.16 A 'classical' argentaffin carcinoid tumour of the appendix consisting of solid masses of uniform tumour cells. Retraction of the cell masses from the intervening stroma may mimic lymphatic invasion.

Haematoxylin-eosin   × 140

The other main pattern of appendiceal carcinoid, morphologically identical to the usual type of rectal or hindgut carcinoid, is composed of endocrine cells whose granules are non-argentaffin but usually strongly argyrophil.[80] Tumours of this sort are usually small and macroscopically indistinct. Histologically, they consist of small, regular, mitotically inactive endocrine cells arranged in ribbons, trabeculae and, in places, glandular structures (Fig. 7.19). A solid, packeted pattern is not seen. Although small amounts of mucinous material may be found in the glandular lumina intracellular mucus is extremely uncommon and the vast majority of the tumour cells are clearly of endocrine type with argyrophil granules. Once again a variety of peptides may be demonstrable by immunocytochemistry including neurotensin, gastrin, somatostatin, motilin, and glucagon, and some non-

argentaffin tumours may even contain 5-hydroxy-tryptamine.[81]

A common accompaniment of both patterns of appendiceal carcinoid is hypertrophy of the smooth muscle of the wall of the appendix. Another frequent feature, in reality an artefact of fixation, is retraction of the margins of the tumour cell masses from the adjacent stroma (Fig. 7.16) and this may mimic lymphatic invasion. True lymphatic invasion also occurs, as does perineural involvement, but despite this, and the frequent extension of the tumour through the wall of the appendix to reach the subserosa, metastatic spread is exceptionally rare and appendicectomy is almost invariably curative, even when the lesion reaches the serosa or invades the mesoappendix.[75] Indeed a

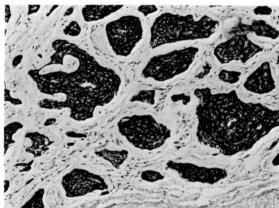

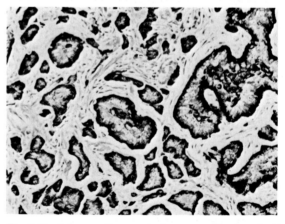

Fig. 7.17a, b Argentaffin granules in an appendiceal carcinoid tumour may be distributed diffusely within the tumour cells (**a**) or concentrated at the periphery of the cell masses (**b**).

Masson-Fontana   × (**a**) × 130; (**b**) × 175

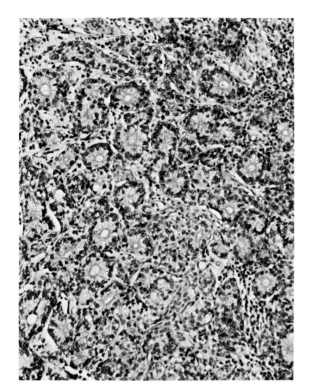

Fig. 7.18 Argentaffin carcinoid of the appendix with a striking acinar pattern, some acini having central lumina. Other areas of this tumour had the 'classical' appearance shown in Figure 7.16.

Haematoxylin-eosin × 140

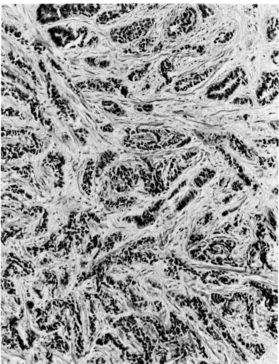

Fig. 7.19 Non-argentaffin carcinoid tumour of the appendix. The cells are arranged in ribbons and trabeculae, with gland-like structures in a few places.

Haematoxylin-eosin × 130

number of studies have found histological features to be of little help in identifying the rare tumours that produce metastases and the best, if not the only, marker of an aggressive clinical behaviour is the size of the primary lesion. Thus it is often recommended that further surgery in the form of right hemicolectomy should be reserved for the very rare primary tumours that measure greater than 2 cm in diameter.[75,82,83]

Mucinous carcinoid

Another tumour which is usually included with appendiceal carcinoids, but which does not fit easily into this category of neoplasms, goes by many names, including mucinous carcinoid,[70] goblet cell carcinoid,[71] adenocarcinoid[72] and crypt cell carcinoma.[73] The tumour seems to hold an intermediate place between carcinoid and adeno-

carcinoma of the appendix, because although the macroscopic features and the pattern of infiltration resemble a conventional carcinoid, endocrine cells often form only a minor component and the overall clinical behaviour suggests a more aggressive neoplasm. The lesion is usually situated in the tip of the appendix and arises in the base of the mucosa to infiltrate the appendiceal wall to a variable degree. It contains a mixture of mucus-producing goblet and signet-ring cells, endocrine cells (usually argyrophil), and sometimes Paneth cells, arranged in strands, nests or small glandular collections (Figs 7.20 and 7.21). In most cases signet-ring cells predominate (Fig. 7.20) but sometimes mucin production is so abundant that pools of extracellular mucus form within the appendiceal wall (Fig. 7.21). Generally speaking, nuclear pleomorphism is absent and mitoses are inconspicuous, although this is not invariably so.

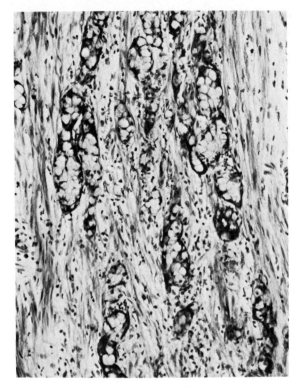

Fig. 7.20 Mucinous carcinoid infiltrating the muscular coat of the appendix. In this example most of the cells are mucus-producing goblet or signet-ring cells arranged in strands and nests but moderate numbers of argyrophil endocrine cells were demonstrable by the Grimelius technique.

Haematoxylin-eosin   × 140

There is little stromal fibrosis and muscular hypertrophy is not a feature. It is possible that the tumour arises from undifferentiated cells in the base of the mucosal crypts, whose progeny subsequently show divergent differentiation towards mucus-producing cells, endocrine cells and Paneth cells. The degree of endocrine cell differentiation varies greatly between tumours. Sometimes it is dominant, in which case endocrine cells are conspicuous, even to the extent that parts of the tumour may have the appearance of a conventional carcinoid.[84] In other cases, there is no recognizable endocrine component and the tumour consists entirely of nests of signet-ring cells[68,69] which may be indistinguishable from metastatic carcinoma.

Although the early reports of mucinous carcinoid and goblet cell carcinoid suggested an excellent prognosis similar to that of conventional carcinoid,

subsequent studies have shown that metastatic spread occurs in up to 20% of cases.[72,85] There seems to be a predilection for ovarian metastasis in the female[85,86] but fatal widespread intra-abdominal dissemination also occurs. Histologically, the metastases may have the appearances of adenocarcinoid, conventional carcinoid or adenocarcinoma.[72] Whether or not right hemicolectomy should be carried out in patients with these tumours is controversial. The behaviour is not related to the presence or absence of an endocrine cell component and, as with conventional carcinoids, perineural and lymphatic invasion are common and poor indicators of future metastasis. Perhaps the best indications for radical surgery are extension beyond

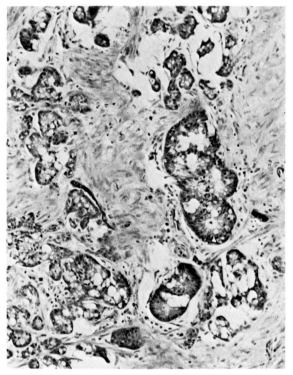

Fig. 7.21 Mucinous carcinoid of the appendix. A glandular pattern is prominent in this example and there is also a little extracellular mucin production in the upper part of this field. Small numbers of argyrophil endocrine cells and Paneth cells were demonstrable. Other areas of this tumour had the pattern shown in Figure 7.20, where endocrine cells were more numerous.

Haematoxylin-eosin   × 130

Histological preparation for photography provided by the late Dr N. Dearnley, Nevill Hall Hospital, Abergavenny.

the appendix and cellular pleomorphism with a high mitotic rate.[72]

Other tumours

Primary appendiceal tumours of non-epithelial origin are rare, but smooth muscle tumours,[87] nerve sheath tumours,[88] ganglioneuromas,[89] granular cell tumours[90] and malignant lymphomas[91] have all been described. Metastatic tumours are rare, but may arise from carcinomas of the breast, stomach and bronchus, among others.[92]

REFERENCES

1. Wakeley CPG. J Anat 1933; 67: 277.
2. Wangensteen OH, Buirge RE, Dennis C, Ritchie WP. Ann Surg 1937; 106: 910.
3. Hofler H, Kasper M, Heitz PhU. Virchows Arch Pathol Anat 1983; 399: 127.
4. Papadaki L, Rode J, Dhillon AP, Dische FE. Gastroenterol 1983; 84: 490.
5. Rode J, Dhillon AP, Papadaki L. Hum Path 1983; 14: 464.
6. Bohrod MG. Am J Clin Path 1946; 16: 752.
7. Sobel HJ, Marquet E, Schwarz R. Arch Path 1971; 92: 427.
8. Emery JL, Underwood J. Gut 1970; 11: 118.
9. Waugh TR. Arch Surg 1941; 42: 311.
10. Tinckler LF. Br J Surg 1968; 55: 79.
11. Collins DC. Am J Surg 1951; 82: 689.
12. Shand JEG, Bremner DN. Br J Surg 1977; 64: 203.
13. Droga BW, Levine S, Baber JJ. Am J Clin Pathol 1963; 40: 190.
14. Fitz RH. Trans Assoc Am Phys 1886; 1: 107.
15. Raguveer-Saran MK, Keddie NC. Br J Surg 1980; 67: 681.
16. Langman MJS. The epidemiology of chronic digestive disease. London: Arnold, 1979: 108.
17. Mortality statistics—cause: review of the Registrar General on deaths by cause, sex and age in England and Wales, 1983 (series DH2, No 11) London, 1984.
18. Wangensteen OH, Dennis C. Ann Surg 1939; 110: 629.
19. Wilkie DPD. Can Med Assoc J 1930; 22: 314.
20. Parker MT In: Wilson GS, Miles AA, Parker MT, eds. Topley & Wilson's principles of bacteriology, virology and immunity. 7th ed. vol 3. London: Arnold, 1984: 170.
21. Horton LWL. Br Med J 1977; 2: 1672.
22. Wangensteen OH, Bowers WF. Arch Surg 1937; 34: 496.
23. Arnbjornsson E, Bengmark S. Am J Surg 1984; 147: 390.
24. Sisson RG, Ahlvin RC, Harlow MC. Am J Surg 1971; 122: 378.
25. Tobe T. Lancet 1965; 1: 1343.
26. Jackson RH, Gardner PS, Kennedy J, McQuillin J. Lancet 1966; 2: 711.
27. Rendle Short A. Br J Surg 1920; 8: 171.
28. Burkitt DP. Br J Surg 1971; 58: 695.
29. Remington JH, McDonald JR. Surg 1948; 24: 787.
30. Butler C. Hum Path 1981; 12: 870.
31. Pieper R, Kager L, Nasman P. Ann Surg 1983; 197: 368.
32. Buirge RE, Dennis C, Varco RL, Wangensteen OH. Arch Path 1940; 30: 481.
33. Le Brun HI. Br J Surg 1958–59; 46: 32.
34. Walker LG, Rhame DW, Smith RB. Arch Surg 1969; 99: 585.
35. Mylliken NK, Stryker HB. N Engl J Med 1951; 244: 52.
36. Carleton CC. Arch Path 1955; 60: 39.
37. Thackray AC. Br J Radiol 1959; 32: 180.
38. Howie JGR. J Path Bact 1966; 91: 85.
39. Bobrow ML, Friedman S. Am J Surg 1956; 91: 389.
40. El-Maraghi NRH, Mair NS. Am J Clin Path 1979; 71: 631.
41. Symmers WStC. Arch Path 1950; 50: 475.
42. Noodleman JS. Arch Pathol Lab Med 1981; 105: 148.
43. Yunis EJ, Hashida Y. Pediatrics 1973; 51: 566.
44. Rubenstein AD, Johnson BB. Am J Med Sci 1945; 210: 517.
45. Peison B. Dis Colon Rectum 1973; 16: 532.
46. Yang SS, Gibson P, McCaughey RS, Arcari FA, Bernstein J. Ann Surg 1979; 189: 334.
47. Allen DC, Biggart JD. J Clin Pathol 1983; 36: 632.
48. Symmers WStC. Unpublished observations, 1974–75.
49. Wilson RR. Br J Surg 1950–51; 38: 65.
50. Deschenes L, Couture J. Garneau R. Am J Surg 1971; 121: 706.
51. Forshall I. Br J Surg 1952–53; 40: 305.
52. Langsam LB, Raj PK, Galang CF. Dis Colon Rectum 1984; 27: 387.
53. De Bruin AJ. Med J Aust 1969; 1: 581.
54. Lane RE. Am J Obstet Gynec 1960; 79: 372.
55. Nielsen M, Lykke J, Thomsen JL. Acta Path Microbiol Immunol Scand A 1983; 91: 253.
56. Mittal VK, Choudhury SP, Cortez JA. Am J Surg 1981; 142: 519.
57. Wold LE, Baggenstoss AH. Proc Staff Meet Mayo Clin 1949; 24: 28.
58. Plaut A. Am J Path 1951; 27: 247.
59. MacGillivray JB. J Clin Path 1972; 25: 809.
60. Higa E, Rosai J, Pizzimbono CA, Wise L. Cancer 1973; 32: 1525.
61. Qizilbash AH. Arch Path 1974; 97: 385.
62. Kitchen AP. Br Med J 1953; 1: 658.
63. Shnitka TK, Sherbaniuk RW. Gastroenterol 1957; 32: 462.
64. Wolff M, Ahmed N. Cancer 1976; 37: 2511.
65. Qizilbash AH. Arch Path 1975; 99: 548.
66. Gibbs NM. J Clin Path 1973; 26: 413.
67. Gilhome RW, Johnston DH, Clark J, Kyle J. Br J Surg 1984; 71: 553.
68. Qizilbash AH. Arch Path 1975; 99: 556.
69. Wolff M, Ahmed N. Cancer 1976; 37: 2493.
70. Klein HZ. Cancer 1974; 33: 770.
71. Subbuswamy SG, Gibbs NM, Ross CF, Morson BC. Cancer 1974; 34: 338.
72. Warkel RL, Cooper PH, Helwig EB. Cancer 1978; 42: 2781.
73. Isaacson P. Am J Surg Path 1981; 5: 213.
74. Fernandez RN, Daly JM. Arch Surg 1980; 115: 409.

75. Moertel CG, Dockerty MB, Judd ES. Cancer 1968; 21: 270.
76. Ryden SE, Drake RM, Franciosi RA. Cancer 1975; 36: 1538.
77. Markgraf WH, Dunn TM. Am J Surg 1964; 107: 730.
78. Johnston WH, Waisman J. Cancer 1971; 27: 681.
79. Aubock L, Hofler H. Virchows Arch Pathol Anat 1983; 401: 17.
80. Dische FE. J Clin Path 1968; 21: 60.
81. Yang K, Ulich T, Cheng L, Lewin KJ. Cancer 1983; 51: 1918.
82. Glasser CM, Bhagavan BS. Arch Pathol Lab Med 1980; 104: 272.
83. Bowman GA, Rosenthal D. Am J Surg 1983; 146: 700.
84. Chen V, Qizilbash AH. Arch Pathol Lab Med 1979; 103: 180.
85. Edmonds P, Merino MJ, LiVolsi VA, Duray PH. Gastroenterol 1984; 86: 302.
86. Heisterberg L, Wahlin A, Nielsen KS. Acta Obstet Gynecol Scand 1982; 61: 153.
87. Jones PA. Dis Colon Rectum 1979; 22: 175.
88. Michalany J, Galindo W. Beitr Path Bd 1973; 150: 213.
89. Zarabi M, LaBach JP. Hum Path 1982; 13: 1143.
90. Johnston J, Helwig EB. Dig Dis Sci 1981; 26: 807.
91. Sin IC, Ling E-T, Prentice RSA. Hum Path 1980; 11: 465.
92. Dieter RA. Dis Col Rect 1970; 13: 336.

8

Jeremy R. Jass

The large intestine

ANATOMICAL CONSIDERATIONS

The large intestine extends from the caecum to the rectum and is divided into six parts—the caecum, ascending colon, transverse colon, descending colon, sigmoid colon, and rectum. The terms colorectum and large intestine are synonymous. The organ is about 1.5 m long, its length being more constant than that of the small intestine.[1] The caecum is the part of the large intestine below the level of the ileocaecal valve. The ascending colon extends from the ileocaecal valve to the hepatic flexure, and the transverse colon from the hepatic flexure to the splenic flexure. The descending colon becomes the sigmoid colon as it crosses the brim of the true pelvis. The rectum cannot be defined precisely, but it begins approximately at the level of the promontory of the sacrum.

The wall of the colorectum consists of a mucous membrane, which includes the muscularis mucosae, separated from the deep muscle layer or muscularis propria by the submucosal layer of loose connective tissue. The large bowel is invested by peritoneum to a variable degree. The caecum and transverse colon are completely invested apart from their mesenteric attachments, whereas the ascending and descending colon are covered anteriorly only. The rectum is covered by peritoneum on the front and sides in the upper third and on the front only in the middle third. The lower third is below the peritoneal reflection. The rectum widens below the peritoneal reflection forming the ampulla, and bends backward to follow the curve of the sacrum. Between the muscularis propria and peritoneum is a variable amount of fat and connective tissue. The serosa includes this layer and the peritoneal membrane. The epiploic appendages are rounded or elongated collections of serosal adipose tissue which cover the colon from caecum to rectosigmoid.

The functions of the colon are complex and not completely understood. They include maintenance of fluid and electrolyte balance, serving as a potential site for the absorption of nutrients, harbouring microorganisms which play an important role in the metabolism of carbohydrates, fatty acids and bile acids and the storage, propulsion and elimination of the luminal contents.[2]

Musculature

The deep muscle coat or muscularis propria has a structure very different from that of the corresponding coat of the small intestine. The inner of the two muscle layers consists of fasciculi of circular fibres forming a continuous sheath. The outer or longitudinal muscle layer also forms a continuous sheath, although in the colon it is mainly concentrated into three narrow bands, the taeniae coli. These are not as long as the intestinal tube to which they belong: they are therefore responsible for the sacculations (haustra) by which the extra length is taken up. The three taeniae fuse in the region of the rectosigmoid junction to form a uniform, complete sheath of longitudinal muscle round the rectum. The muscle is thinnest in the ascending part of the colon and gradually becomes thicker toward the lower part of the sigmoid colon; at the rectosigmoid junction it again becomes thin.

Blood supply

The blood supply to the caecum, ascending colon and most of transverse colon is from the abdominal aorta through the ileocolic and right and middle colic branches of the superior mesenteric artery. The descending colon and rectum are supplied by the inferior mesenteric artery. The junction of these two sources of arterial blood is in the region of the splenic flexure, where the blood supply is rather precarious because of the relatively small size of the communication between the left branch of the middle colic artery (itself a branch of the superior mesenteric artery) and the ascending branch of the left colic artery (which is a branch of

the inferior mesenteric artery). This anatomical fact is fundamental in the pathogenesis of ischaemic disease of the colon (see p. 349). The rectum is supplied by branches of the inferior mesenteric (superior rectal), internal iliac (middle rectal) and internal pudendal arteries (inferior rectal) which anastomose extensively.

The arteries are accompanied, as components of neurovascular bundles, by veins, lymphatics and nerves. These bear the same names as the arteries. The veins form a well-developed submucosal plexus and another, less well-developed, plexus outside the muscularis propria. They are tributaries of the portal system. Portal-systemic anastomoses occur by communication of the superior rectal with the middle and inferior rectal veins.

Lymphatic drainage

The lymph nodes of the large intestine can be divided into those that lie close to the bowel wall (paracolic and pararectal nodes) and those that follow the course of the blood supply. The lymphatic drainage of the lower rectum is through nodes along the superior rectal artery, nodes along the middle rectal artery (to the internal iliac nodes) and to a much lesser extent to the inguinal nodes, probably via presacral lymphatics.

Nerve supply

As in the rest of the gut, the nerve supply is divided into extrinsic and intrinsic components. The extrinsic supply comprises the two arms of the autonomic nervous system: sympathetic and parasympathetic. The parasympathetic supply is via the vagus for the proximal colon and via the sacral spinal nerves for the distal colon and rectum. The preganglionic fibres terminate in the myenteric plexus. The vagus and sacral spinal nerves also contain afferent fibres to complete possible reflex loops. The sympathetic supply is through lower thoracic spinal nerves which mainly end in the superior mesenteric ganglion and lumbar spinal nerves which end in the inferior mesenteric ganglion. These prevertebral ganglia are closer to the spinal cord than the colon. The postganglionic fibres terminate in either the myenteric (Auerbach's) or submucous (Meissner's) plexus. The myenteric plexus is located between the circular and longitudinal muscle coats. The smooth muscle of the internal anal sphincter is supplied by both extrinsic postganglionic sympathetic fibres and by intrinsic postganglionic parasympathetic fibres. The sympathetic nerves also contain afferent fibres whose cell bodies may reside either within the wall of the bowel (e.g. acting as mechanoreceptors) or within the dorsal root ganglia. These will complete short and long reflex arcs respectively.[3]

The denervated colon is capable of co-ordinated peristalsis. This indicates the importance and organizational complexity of the intrinsic component of the nerve supply. The myenteric and submucosal plexuses together comprise a network of intercommunicating ganglia. Within each ganglion are nerve (ganglion) cell bodies, nerve processes and glia. Most of the direct innervation of smooth muscle is through the intrinsic neurons of the two plexuses. The intrinsic neurons acting directly on smooth muscle are either excitatory (mainly cholinergic) or inhibitory (non-adrenergic non-cholinergic—NANC). The former are driven either by intrinsic interneurons or extrinsic parasympathetic fibres. They are inhibited by extrinsic postganglionic sympathetic fibres or indirectly through presynaptic inhibition of excitatory interneurons. The inhibitory NANC fibres supplying smooth muscle are again driven by excitatory interneurons or extrinsic parasympathetic fibres. Some interneurons may also be inhibitory. The NANC neurons probably release vasoactive intestinal polypeptide (VIP). Other important neurotransmitters, apart from acetylcholine and noradrenaline, may include substance P and 5-hydroxytryptamine.[4] The neurons of the myenteric plexus were formerly classified according to whether or not they were argyrophil and cholinesterase positive.[5] These classical light microscopic techniques show no clear correlation with modern functional classifications in which neurotransmitter substances are identified histochemically and ultrastructurally.[6]

Individual smooth muscle cells are not supplied by nerve terminals. Nerve processes with bead-like varicosities surround groups of muscle fibres and neurotransmitters are released into tissue spaces to reach target cells by diffusion. Electrical coupling from cell to cell is achieved through the junctional complexes which are of three types—interdigitations, gap junctions (nexuses) and intermediate junctions.[7]

Mucosal histology

Microscopically, the mucous membrane of the colon and rectum consists of parallel epithelial crypts perpendicular to the mucosal surface, and the lamina propria in which they are situated (Fig. 8.1). There are no villi. The crypts do not branch; this characteristic and the parallel arrangement of the glands are important in distinguishing between normal and abnormal structure. The crypt and surface epithelium are one cell thick. Four main cell types are present. The most numerous are the columnar cells, outnumbering the mucin-distended goblet cells by 5:1.[8] The crypt columnar

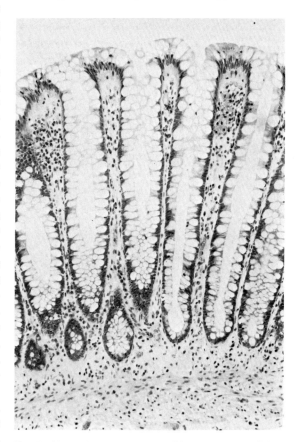

Fig. 8.1 Normal colorectal mucosa. The crypts are parallel to one another and unbranched. The crypt base region is located immediately above the muscularis mucosae.

Haematoxylin-eosin   × 100

cells are compressed inconspicuously between goblet cells and therefore appear less numerous than they are. Paneth cells with large, supranuclear eosinophilic granules are normally limited to the right colon. Endocrine cells with small, subnuclear eosinophilic granules are scattered within the lower crypt (Fig. 8.2). Cell kinetic and morphologic studies indicate that all these cells arise from a single undifferentiated stem cell.[9] Intermediate cells showing features of both Paneth and goblet cells or endocrine and goblet cells point to the common origin of these lines.

Columnar cells function as secretory as well as absorptive units. Secretory functions include IgA translocation,[10] the synthesis of glycocalyceal material and brush border enzymes, and the cellular movement of water and electrolytes. The development of a microvillous brush border accompanies the migration of columnar cells from crypt to the surface. This morphological change signals a switch from the predominantly secretory role to an absorptive function. The goblet cells secrete mainly acid mucins in which sulphate groups and O-acylated sialic acid are well represented. However, the mucin histochemistry varies according to the region of the colorectum, with more neutral mucin in the right colon.[11] This may be related to the fact that blood group substances A, B and H are expressed by the right colon only.[12] Mucins also vary within the different crypt compartments, reflecting the level of cellular maturation.[11] The endocrine cells of the large bowel secrete enteroglucagon, neurotensin, somatostatin, VIP-like peptide and 5-hydroxytryptamine.[13,14] Endocrine cells are more common in the rectum than colon.

The lamina propria forms a connective-tissue framework around the crypts. The pericrypt sheath is probably formed of myofibroblasts. Beneath the basement membrane of the surface epithelium is a collagen plate. Within the lamina propria are small vessels (but few lymphatics), unmyelinated nerve fibres, fibroblasts, plasma cells, lymphocytes, mast cells, histiocytes and eosinophils. Most of the plasma cells are of the IgA type and the lymphocytes are predominantly T cells. The histiocytes may contain mucin (muciphages). Lymphoid follicles with germinal centres are most numerous in the rectum, followed by the caecum.

CONGENITAL ABNORMALITIES[15]

Atresia and congenital stenosis occur more commonly in the anorectal region than in the colon (see p. 398). They are due to complete or partial failure of canalization of the bowel, or perhaps to the effects of local vascular insufficiency during fetal life. Both atresia and stenosis are usually segmental, involving only a few centimetres of bowel.

Duplication of the large intestine is a very rare anomaly. It usually takes the form of a paracolic cyst or tube, with or without an opening into the adjacent normal bowel. Complete duplication of the whole colon has been described.

Anomalies of rotation include mobile caecum, which denotes a failure of fixation and is the commonest type of congenital abnormality of the colon, and transposition of the large intestine.

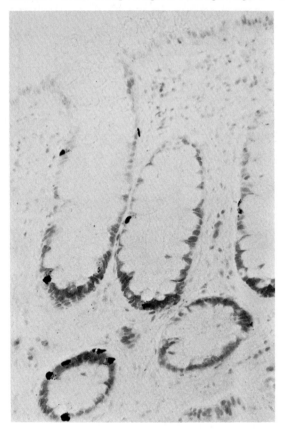

Fig. 8.2 Endocrine cells within normal colorectal epithelium. Grimelius   × 100

Solitary diverticulum

Solitary diverticula of the large bowel are comparatively rare, especially in view of the frequency of diverticulosis (see p. 321). It has not been shown that they are congenital but they may be considered here for convenience. They are found most frequently in the caecum and ascending colon. Diverticula in which all layers of the bowel wall can be demonstrated can certainly be accepted as congenital in origin.

A solitary diverticulum may be an incidental finding at necropsy or in surgical specimens of intestine removed for some other disease. Occasionally, such a diverticulum becomes inflamed, and the patient presents with symptoms suggestive of acute appendicitis. Alternatively, the diverticulitis may be more chronic and present as a mass, usually in the right iliac fossa. There is evidence that some so-called 'solitary ulcers' of the caecum and ascending colon are, in fact, due to inflammation around a congenital diverticulum.[16] Most of the patients with inflammation of a solitary diverticulum of the caecum or ascending colon are in the third decade; this is much below the average age of patients with the common form of colonic diverticulosis and supports the theory of the congenital origin of the solitary lesions. On the other hand, colonic motility studies carried out in Japan suggest that some solitary, right-sided diverticula may be acquired.[17]

Gastric heterotopia

Gastric heterotopia is a rare finding in the large intestine. It occurs most frequently in the rectum, usually presenting as a polyp but occasionally as a flat, plaque-like lesion. It may present with rectal bleeding or as an incidental finding. Some cases have been associated with other congenital anomalies of the gastrointestinal tract. The mucosa is usually of fundic type, but there is no propensity for peptic ulceration.[18]

Hirschsprung's disease

The term megacolon is applied to any form of gross dilatation of the large intestine, whether segmental or involving the whole colon, and whether congenital or acquired.

Congenital megacolon or Hirschsprung's disease has been recognized for many years, but its pathogenesis has only become clear comparatively recently.[19] It is due to a congenital absence of ganglion cells from the intramural plexuses of a segment of the large intestine (usually the rectum): the resulting functional failure of this segment obstructs the passage of faeces from the bowel above, and dilatation of the latter results. Congenital megacolon has to be distinguished from acquired megacolon (see below).

Hirschsprung's disease usually presents with severe constipation. It has been recognized at all ages from 15 days to advanced adult life; nearly all the patients are boys. There is a strong familial tendency to develop the disease, and this suggests that it may be genetically determined.

The large intestine in congenital megacolon usually comprises two segments (Fig. 8.3)—a relatively short, narrow, lower segment, in which there are no ganglion cells either in the myenteric plexus of Auerbach or the submucosal plexus of Meissner, and the dilated upper segment, in which ganglion cells are present in normal numbers. Between these two segments there is a short transitional zone that contains ganglion cells in smaller numbers than in the normal large intestine. There is considerable work hypertrophy of the musculature of the upper segment, which may be

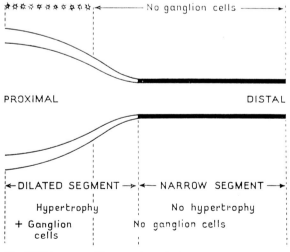

Fig. 8.3 Diagram to illustrate the pathology of Hirschsprung's disease.

Redrawn from Bodian M, Stephens FD, Ward BCH. Lancet 1949; 1: 6 (Fig. 3).

enormously dilated by its contents of faeces, displacing the other abdominal viscera and forcing the diaphragm high into the thorax. The length of the aganglionic or distal segment is variable. In at least 90% of cases the entire rectum down to the anorectal junction is involved, often with part or the whole of the sigmoid colon. Only a very few cases have been reported in which there was a normal segment of bowel below the aganglionic zone as well as the ganglionate segment above it. In some cases the aganglionic segment may be very long, reaching occasionally to the splenic flexure and sometimes involving the entire large intestine and extending even into the terminal ileum: when the aganglionic segment is so extensive the child usually dies in the neonatal period.[20]

Aetiology and neurophysiology

During embryogenesis, ganglion cells derived from the neural crest migrate along a pathway formed by preganglionic parasympathetic fibres which have previously innervated the bowel wall.[21] In Hirschsprung's disease the normal migration fails to occur. There is a marked increase in the number of extrinsic (mainly cholinergic) fibres between the longitudinal and circular muscle coats: these fibres are visible as large, wavy bundles on microscopy (Fig. 8.4). It is now realized that the

disordered function cannot be explained entirely in terms of the adrenergic and cholinergenic nervous systems, but must also implicate the non-adrenergic, non-cholinergic nervous system (see p. 314 for details of the neuroanatomy). A loss of nerves containing vasoactive intestinal peptide and substance P has been described in affected segments.[22]

Rectal biopsy diagnosis

A full-thickness biopsy will provide the most direct evidence of aganglionosis. This should be taken at least 2 cm above the dentate line. The demonstration of large numbers of relatively coarse cholinesterase-positive fibres crossing the muscularis mucosae and entering the lamina propria has been used as a diagnostic finding (Fig. 8.5).[19,23] This method has proved especially successful in the hands of paediatric pathologists and has obviated the need for full-thickness biopsy.[24] The technique has also been employed to document the length of the aganglionic segment. Providing the occasional

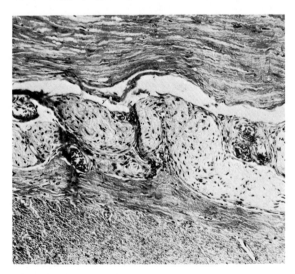

Fig. 8.4 Hirschsprung's disease showing thickened nerves within myenteric plexus.

Haematoxylin-eosin   × 100

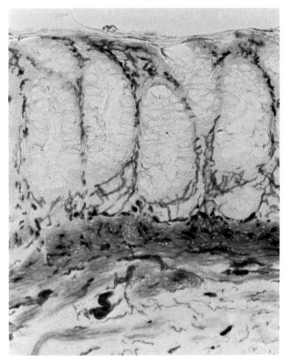

Fig. 8.5 Hirschsprung's disease. Coarse nerve fibres traverse the muscularis mucosae and ramify within lamina propria.

Acetylcholinesterase   × 140

small cholinesterase-positive fibre is ignored, false positives should not occur. However, some authors have described false-negative results.[25]

In cases where a previous colostomy has been performed, the junction between normal dilated and abnormal narrowed aganglionic segments may not be visible to the naked eye. Frozen sections from biopsies taken at the time of operation will help to guide the surgeon. The normal segment is indicated by the presence of normal numbers of ganglion cells and absence of abnormal nerve trunks.

Adynamic bowel syndrome

This term, formerly described as pseudo-Hirschsprung's disease, refers to patients with the clinical and radiological appearances of Hirschsprung's disease, but with apparently normal ganglion cells and nerve trunks. Recent studies have demonstrated that the argyrophil nerve plexus and some cholinergic fibres are absent.[26] A related disorder termed hypogangliosis has been described.[27] Further detailed histochemical studies are needed.

Neuronal intestinal dysplasia[28,29]

This condition gives rise to clinical signs and symptoms resembling Hirschsprung's disease. It is characterized by structural changes affecting the parasympathetic supply, which include hyperplasia of the myenteric plexus, increased acetylcholinesterase activity and the formation of giant ganglia. It may occur in a localized or disseminated form. The former is cured by resection of the affected segment, but the latter is often ultimately fatal. The condition may occur in association with Hirschsprung's disease.

Neuromatosis of the colon may occur in three distinct forms: as a diffuse mucosal lesion (ganglioneuromatosis) in patients with multiple endocrine neoplasia type 2b (associated with phaeochromocytoma and medullary carcinoma of the thyroid); as neurofibromatosis in association with von Recklinghausen's disease; or, more rarely, as a localized, isolated occurrence in any part of the gastrointestinal tract. Megacolon has been described as a complication of neurofibromatosis.[30] Some would regard neurofibromatosis as a form of neuronal

dysplasia, but others see the origin of the former within the sympathetic nervous system as a fundamental distinction between the two disorders.[29]

Idiopathic megacolon[31]

This is a rare condition which usually presents in infancy and affects boys more frequently than girls (2:1). The normal terminal segment of Hirschsprung's disease is not in evidence. The anal canal is short and the rectum is full of faeces. The nature of this disorder is not fully understood.

Rectal biopsy appearances in storage diseases

Inherited metabolic disorders due to the deletion of a single enzyme will result in the abnormal storage of various products of either lipid or carbohydrate metabolism. These products may be detected in macrophages (e.g. glycogen storage disease due to debranching enzyme deficiency, Gaucher's disease, Niemann-Pick disease), in the connective tissue of the lamina propria (e.g. Hurler's disease) or in the neurons of the myenteric plexus (e.g. Fabry's disease, Hurler's disease, metachromatic leukoencephalopathy, Tay-Sachs disease and Niemann-Pick disease). The final diagnosis rests on the demonstration of the enzyme defect (e.g. in cultures of fibroblasts). However, suction rectal biopsy, coupled to electron microscopy, still finds a place in the diagnosis of some storage diseases including neuronal ceroid lipofuscinosis.[32]

ACQUIRED MEGACOLON AND MEGARECTUM

The term megacolon refers to dilatation of the whole of the large bowel; megarectum is dilatation confined to the rectum. The condition may be congenital, as in Hirschsprung's disease, or acquired. The latter group has generally been labelled 'idiopathic'. However, this term will ultimately be abandoned as advances in knowledge of the pathogenesis of the condition under various circumstances are made. The muscle of the affected bowel may be hypertrophic or atrophic, depending on the causative factor.

There are numerous causes of acquired megacolon and megarectum.[33,34] They can be classified as obstructive—usually due to tumours or other forms of stricture; endocrine—as in hypothyroidism; accompanying disorders affecting the central nervous system—these include spina bifida, paraplegia and Parkinson's disease; collagen diseases—such as scleroderma (see p. 386); psychogenic—ranging from faulty bowel habit to severe psychiatric disorders; drugs—particularly those that may have a toxic effect on the nerve supply to the large bowel (chloropromazine, for example, can induce megacolon in rats);[35] and resulting from an acquired loss of ganglia—as in Chagas' disease (South American trypanosomiasis) (see p. 138), in which a gross degree of megacolon is an occasional and striking feature. Endocrine cell hyperplasia has been described in a case of acquired megacolon.[36]

The above disorders may manifest themselves as a condition termed chronic intestinal pseudo-obstruction, though small intestinal involvement usually predominates. So-called familial or hollow visceral myopathy (see p. 387) is probably an important cause of chronic intestinal pseudo-obstruction and may account for some cases of idiopathic megacolon.

MECHANICAL DISORDERS

Obstruction is commoner in the small intestine than in the colon. Moreover, the mechanical and biochemical effects of obstruction of the small intestine are more acute and severe. The commonest cause of obstruction of the large intestine is carcinoma, usually of the sigmoid colon, and this is followed in frequency by volvulus, diverticulitis and incarcerated hernia.[38,39] Less common causes include intussusception, foreign bodies and megacolon.

Volvulus

Volvulus of the large intestine is uncommon in most parts of the world, but there are areas—such as parts of Yugoslavia, Iran, Africa, Scandinavia, Russia and Peru—where it is a frequent disease. In such areas the cause of the volvulus seems to be at least in part related to dietary habits. It usually affects the sigmoid colon or the caecum, although volvulus of the transverse colon[40] and splenic flexure[41] have been described. It is due to torsion of the mesentery and is essentially the result of a large redundant sigmoid loop or a mobile caecum. A mobile caecum is always a developmental anomaly; a redundant loop of sigmoid colon may be acquired, as a manifestation of chronic constipation or, possibly, due to long-standing subsistence on a high-fibre diet. Sigmoid volvulus can also be the result of extrinsic factors, such as adhesions.

Intussusception

Intussusception of the large intestine is uncommon. It is usually due to a tumour, which may be benign or malignant.[42] The main cause is carcinoma of the sigmoid colon. In children it is often not possible to detect a cause. In West Africa, caecocolic intussusception is the commonest variety.[43] Intussusception of the rectum (internal procidentia) is related to the solitary ulcer syndrome (see p. 352).

Foreign bodies

Foreign bodies are seldom a fundamental cause of large bowel obstruction, although they may be contributory. For example, impaction of a fruit stone in a constricting carcinoma of the colon may precipitate acute obstruction, and chicken bones, buttons and other foreign articles have been found impacted in bowel affected by diverticulitis and may then partly or completely occlude the lumen. Unless symptoms draw attention to the condition, the pressure of such foreign bodies on the tissues may result in perforation of the bowel wall, causing local abscess formation or peritonitis. Foreign bodies inserted through the anus for purposes of concealment or sexual gratification may cause obstruction, laceration, pressure necrosis and perforation, sometimes with fatal results.[44]

Barium granulomas

These are rare, but may present as polypoid masses mimicking a tumour. They may be discovered many years after the causative barium enema. The rectum is most often affected and macroscopically the raised lesions vary from white to grey-pink in colour. The histological appearances vary with the age of the lesion, but the crystals of barium sulphate are always present (Fig. 8.6). They range in size and shape from small granular crystals to large rhomboidal forms. These are anisotrophic in polarized light, may be identified histochemically by the Rhodinozata method and characterized further by energy dispersive X-ray analysis.[45] Early lesions show acute inflammation, with barium crystals surrounded by granulation tissue. Later, foreign-body type granulomas develop, in which macrophages and multinucleate giant cells containing phagocytosed barium are identified.

Trauma

Traumatic perforation of the rectum can be caused by sigmoidoscopy and during administration of enemas, including barium enemas, as well as by impalement and other accidents and assaults. An especially dangerous practice is a form of horseplay in which the nozzle of a compressed air hose is pointed at the buttocks: when the tap is opened, even though the nozzle is still some distance from the victim's clothing, the jet of air forcing its way through the anus causes pneumatic rupture of the lower part of the colon.[46]

Spontaneous rupture of the colon

'Spontaneous' rupture of the colon, particularly the sigmoid, has been reported in adults as a complication of constipation and undue straining during attempted defaecation.[47] In babies, mucoviscidosis accompanying cystic fibrosis of the pancreas may be complicated by rupture of the colon,[48] again in association with obstruction by intestinal contents (meconium plug).

DIVERTICULAR DISEASE

Diverticula of the colon are pouches of mucosa that protrude through the wall of the gut. Inflammation (diverticulitis) is a frequent complication.

Diverticulosis

Diverticulosis of the colon is a common condition, being found in about 5% of all necropsies. There is no special liability of either sex to the disease. It is uncommon under 35 years of age, and its incidence then gradually increases. About two-thirds of all who are in their eighth and ninth decades have diverticula.[49] The age incidence leaves little doubt that the condition is acquired. Congenital diverticula occur, but are usually solitary (see p. 317).

From an anatomical point of view, acquired colonic diverticula are typical pulsion diverticula, their wall consisting of mucous membrane (including muscularis mucosae). They penetrate the bowel wall and appear on the outside of the intestine, covered by serosa or fat according to their location. Their appearance is globular and they communicate with the lumen of the bowel by a narrow neck (Fig. 8.7). The sigmoid colon is the site of the

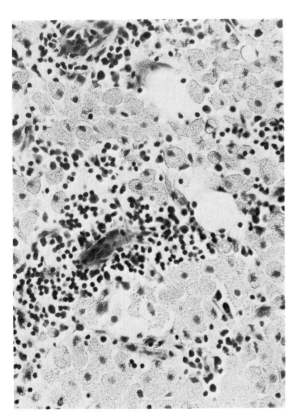

Fig. 8.6 Barium granuloma. Histiocytes contain phagocytosed barium sulphate crystals.

Haematoxylin-eosin × 400

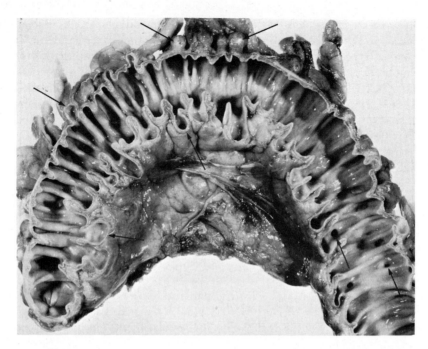

Fig. 8.7 Diverticular disease of the sigmoid colon with arrows indicating either the orifices or the submucosal protrusions of the diverticula. The bowel wall shows characteristic thickening and corrugation.

disease in about 80% of cases. The descending colon is the next commonest site, followed by the transverse colon, ascending colon and caecum, in decreasing order of frequency. Rarely, the entire colon is affected. The diverticula are generally situated between the mesenteric taenia coli and the antimesenteric taeniae, and only very rarely between the two antimesenteric taeniae. In fact, it is usually only in cases of very advanced and long-standing diverticulosis that multiple diverticula—often only 2–3 mm in diameter—are found between the antimesenteric taeniae. They appear to form at the weakest parts of the bowel, such as the gaps in the circular muscle coat through which the blood vessels pass that supply the wall.[50] On opening a surgical specimen of diverticulosis the orifices of the diverticula are seen in two parallel rows between the mesenteric and antimesenteric taeniae. Each diverticulum has a narrow neck, and although semifluid or fluid faeces can easily pass in, they tend to stagnate and become inspissated within the diverticulum, forming a spheroidal faecolith.

The most striking abnormality in diverticular disease of the sigmoid colon is a pronounced thickening and corrugation of the smooth muscle layers.[51] This anomaly of the muscle contributes much more to the intestinal mass that is felt clinically and at laparotomy than do any changes due to inflammation, fibrosis or excess of pericolic fat. The taeniae coli in the affected part of the gut appear thick, assuming an almost cartilaginous consistency. The circular muscle is also thick and has a corrugated, concertina-like appearance (Fig. 8.7). Between these muscular corrugations the bowel wall is sacculate, and it is at the apex of the sacs or pouches that the diverticula are found as they penetrate the bowel wall to lie in the pericolic fat. The corrugations are interdigitating processes of the circular muscle. They are not continuous round the circumference of the bowel, being only arcs of muscle confined to the two zones between the mesenteric and the antimesenteric taeniae. Each arc consists of a double layer of circular muscle and the thin investing layer of longitudinal muscle. This muscle abnormality is present whether there is inflammation or not. It accounts for the characteristic saw-tooth appearance seen on X-ray examination of the colon.[52]

It is probable that these changes are the accompaniment of a gross exaggeration of the normal physiological action of the muscle of the sigmoid colon.[53] The thickening is due to shortening and not to true hypertrophy or to hyperplasia of muscle cells. Other evidence that incriminates shortening as the cause of the muscle thickening is the distinctive redundancy of the mucous membrane. Also, the excessive amount of fat round the sigmoid colon is explained by bunching of the pericolic tissues consequent upon shortening of the bowel by musculature contraction. It has recently been shown that increased amounts of elastin are laid down between the smooth muscle cells of the taeniae coli as compared to age-matched controls. This may be the cause of shortening.[54]

There is uncertainty about the actual mechanism of formation of diverticula.[55] The simple distension theory is still influential despite evidence to the contrary. It is probable that muscle activity converts the colon into a series of pouches or bladders, the outflow from which is obstructed so that high pressures develop locally.[56] In some surgical specimens of diverticular disease it is possible to see separation of the circular muscle fasciculi where the bowel is sacculate, giving a curious ribbed appearance reminiscent of the change in the appearance of the vesical musculature in cases of chronic obstruction of the outflow from the urinary bladder. The separation of the circular muscle fibres causes widening of the gaps through which the blood vessels of the colon pass, and it is through these that the pouches of mucosa are pushed.

Diverticulitis

The most important complication of diverticulosis is inflammation, or diverticulitis. This may be acute or chronic, but in either case the pathogenesis is the same. As the faeces in a diverticulum becomes inspissated and hard the mucosal lining becomes eroded and a mild inflammatory reaction follows. This extends through the wall of the diverticulum, which consists only of mucous membrane, and eventually involves the pericolic fat, with abscess formation and eventual fibrosis (Fig. 8.8). If the affected diverticulum is in direct contact with peritoneum rather than buried in mesenteric fat, a

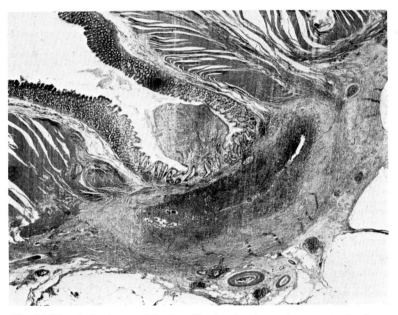

Fig. 8.8 Diverticular disease of the sigmoid colon showing an abscess at the tip of a diverticulum. An inflammatory polyp composed of granulation tissue and covered by an outgrowth of columnar surface epithelium projects into the lumen. The apex of the diverticulum lies in the serosal plane, having penetrated the bowel wall.

Haematoxylin-eosin   × 8

local peritonitis is set up, with the formation of fibrinous exudate and local adhesions.

Diverticulitis occurs most commonly in the descending and sigmoid parts of the colon, particularly the latter. The faeces are normally more fluid in the upper parts of the colon, and therefore less likely to stagnate in a diverticulum. Once an inflammatory reaction is set up in relation to diverticula, the course of the disease tends to alternate between remissions of the inflammatory process and reactivation by the passage of more infected material from the bowel lumen into the diverticulum. The clinical picture is therefore characterized by repeated attacks of fever. In addition to the local peritonitis the affected part of the bowel is surrounded by oedematous fibrofatty tissue. When there is very extensive pericolic inflammation the accompanying fibrosis has a restrictive effect on the normal freedom of movement of the affected segment of colon, which may acquire the most bizarre and irregular shapes and form a tumour-like mass of fibromuscular tissue.

From a surgical point of view, diverticulitis presents as a hard mass that may not be distinguishable from carcinoma until the bowel is opened. The mass is mainly due to muscle thickening and only partly to an excess of surrounding fibrofatty tissue. Foreign bodies such as fruit stones tend to become stuck in areas of diverticulitis, and may on occasions precipitate obstruction of the bowel. It must also be remembered that diverticulitis and carcinoma of the colon are both common diseases, have a similar age distribution, and may be present together in the same segment of intestine. Moreover, the obstructive effects of a carcinoma can lead to the development or aggravation of diverticulosis and diverticulitis of the bowel above the growth.

When examining a surgical specimen of diverticulosis it is necessary to make a careful inspection of every diverticulum for evidence of inflammation. The juxtacolic abscesses are often very small, and difficult to find in the mass of fat and fibrous tissue. The openings of the diverticula should also be inspected, for vascular granulation tissue may be found there that has been the source of haemorrhage into the bowel lumen (Fig. 8.8).

Histological appearances. Microscopically, the diverticular abscesses often include foci of a foreign-body reaction to vegetable material from the faeces. Occasionally, barium granulomas are seen. Otherwise, the inflammatory response in diverticulitis is quite non-specific.

It must be emphasized that inflammation begins at the apex of a diverticulum and then spreads directly into the soft pericolic or mesenteric fat. Diverticula are mainly external to the bowel wall, and so the inflammation in diverticulitis is extramural and only rarely involves mucosa other than that within a diverticulum. A diverticulum becomes inflamed because of the failure of faecal matter to be discharged through its narrow neck as it passes through the circular muscle layer. No doubt contraction of circular fibres helps to keep the neck narrow. The trapped faeces become inspissated and hard, causing low-grade chronic inflammation in the adjacent mucosa. The mucosal lymphoid tissue undergoes hyperplasia and the earliest signs of abscess formation can often be demonstrated within such lymphoid masses at the apex of the diverticulum. Often only one diverticulum is inflamed, and it is unusual for more than three or four to be affected.

Sometimes the inflammation spreads from the apex of a diverticulum along the outer aspect of the deep muscle layers, forming a dissecting abscess. In other cases it extends deeply into the mesenteric fat.

Complications of diverticulosis and diverticulitis

The complications of diverticulosis and diverticulitis include perforation, haemorrhage, intestinal obstruction and vesicocolic fistula. Perforation is rare. Occasionally it is due to a sharp foreign body, such as a chicken bone, penetrating a diverticulum. Haemorrhage is also uncommon.[57] It usually stems from granulation tissue at or near the orifice of a diverticulum. Sometimes it follows erosion of the wall of the diverticulum by hard faeces. Diverticulitis is second to carcinoma among the causes of obstruction of the large intestine. In obstructive cases the muscular thickening of the bowel is very marked, and contributes significantly to the stenosis. Vesicocolic fistula is another uncommon complication.[58] It occurs in cases of sigmoid diverticulitis and results from the formation of adhesions between the urinary bladder and a focus of peritonitis overlying a pericocolic abscess. The abscess, continuing to enlarge, erodes the wall of the bladder until eventually a fistula is established through which gas and faeces may enter the bladder. Pneumaturia and cystitis result.

Diverticulosis of the ascending colon

Diverticulosis confined to the ascending colon seems to be a condition distinct from diverticulosis of the sigmoid colon. It is also distinct from the common solitary diverticulum of the caecum or ascending colon (see p. 317). There is a curiously high incidence in Asia.[59] The contrast between the right-sided diverticulosis seen in eastern countries and the predominantly sigmoid disease of the Western world may well reflect differing dietary habits; the full explanation is not apparent.

The pathological findings and complications are essentially the same in right-sided and sigmoid diverticulosis.

INFLAMMATORY DISORDERS
BACTERIAL COLITIS AND PROCTITIS

The diagnosis of an infective colitis or proctitis requires either the isolation of the organism or the demonstration of a rising antibody titre. Improved bacteriological methods have contributed to the identification of 'new' pathogens including *Clostridium difficile*,[60] *Campylobacter fetus* subsp. *jejuni*,[61] *Yersinia* species[62] and *Edwardsiella tarda*.[63] Campylobacter is now realized to be a relatively common cause of enterocolitis and is isolated more frequently than either *Salmonella* or *Shigella* species. Rectal biopsies from patients with infectious diarrhoea can usually be distinguished from idiopathic inflammatory bowel disease, especially when taken at an early stage.[61,64] However, it is rarely possible to identify the bacterial cause from biopsy appearances; these are non-specific. Immunohistochemical methods have been employed to identify micoorganisms in rectal biopsies.[65]

The mechanism by which bacteria cause disease include the elaboration of a preformed toxin, production of toxins following gut colonization and invasion with consequent damage to mucosal epithelium.[66] Disease caused by the elaboration of a toxin (Salmonella, Yersinia) causes less tissue damage than mechanisms involving tissue invasion (Shigella, Campylobacter). The former present clinically with diarrhoea whereas agents causing more tissue damage are associated with the dysenteric symptoms of fever, abdominal pain and the passage of numerous small-volume stools containing blood, pus and mucus. The latter group will present the greatest diagnostic difficulty with respect to the differentiation from idiopathic inflammatory bowel disease.

Campylobacter colitis

Bacteria of this genus were recognized as a cause of human disease in 1946,[67] but their importance was not appreciated until the development of simple methods of isolation in 1977.[68] The enterocolitis affects young adults, who present with fever, abdominal pain, diarrhoea and the passage of blood after a few days. The disease was assumed to affect only the small bowel, but involvement of colon, rectum and appendix is now well documented. The sigmoidoscopic appearances include oedema, hyperaemia, granularity and contact bleeding. Rectal biopsy shows oedema with a patchy inflammatory infiltrate composed mainly of neutrophils (Fig. 8.9). These are present in both the lamina propria and crypt epithelium, producing incipient crypt abscesses.[61] Microgranulomas are not uncommon but distinct epithelioid (sarcoid) granulomas are absent. Unlike ulcerative colitis, distorted crypts, mucus depletion and chronic inflammation are inconspicuous. However, patients with inflammatory bowel disease show an increased susceptibility to all forms of infective colitis. This should always be borne in mind, as exacerbations of inflammatory bowel disease may be due to a bacterial pathogen and therefore amenable to treatment with appropriate antibiotics. Campylobacter has been identified in rectal biopsies with the aid of immunohistochemistry.[65]

Salmonella colitis

The organisms *Salmonella typhi* and *Salmonella paratyphi* cause septicaemic illnesses whereas salmonella infection of food-poisoning type is gener-

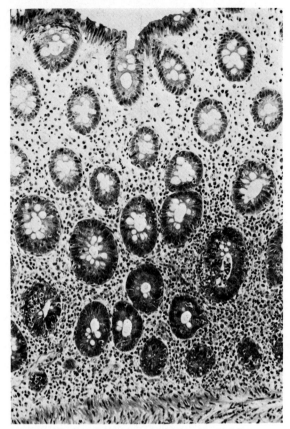

Fig. 8.9 Infective colitis (Campylobacter) showing characteristic patchy inflammation and oedema. The crypts are infiltrated by neutrophils (incipient crypt abscesses).

Haematoxylin-eosin   × 100

ally confined to the gastrointestinal tract. In some patients this results in vomiting, profuse watery diarrhoea and colicky peri-umbilical abdominal pain suggesting predominantly gastric and small intestinal involvement. In others, dysenteric features such as frequent small-volume bloody motions, tenesmus and tenderness over the sigmoid colon are present. The appreciation of colonic involvement in salmonellosis has only recently gained widespread acceptance. The rectal biopsy appearances are similar to those of campylobacter colitis.[64]

Shigellosis and bacillary dysentery

Shigella sonnei is the commonest cause of bacillary dysentery in the Western world. Epidemics of severe disease are usually due to *Shigella flexneri*. The inflammation involves the large intestine and occasionally the terminal ileum. There is discrete serpiginous ulceration and the intervening mucosa is granular and haemorrhagic. The inflammation remains superficial, accounting for the rarity of perforation. It is most severe in the rectum and sigmoid colon. However, deep ulceration of the colon has been demonstrated radiologically in one case of infection with *Sh. flexneri*.[69] The regional lymph nodes are enlarged. The earliest inflammation is seen in the lymphoid follicles of the mucosa which break down to form ulcers. Inflammatory changes include the formation of crypt abscesses, indistinguishable from those of ulcerative colitis. The rectal biopsy appearances are those of other forms of bacterial colitis. The complications of acute bacterial dysentery include myocarditis, splenitis, liver abscess and joint effusions, but these are only found in severe infections, usually with *Shigella shigae*, which produces a powerful exotoxin.[70]

Acute bacillary dysentery can be followed by a chronic state in which organisms remain in the bowel and ulceration of the intestine persists. Alternatively, the initial inflammation may have been so severe that, despite healing, permanent structural changes are found. These include the appearance known as colitis cystica profunda in which mucus retention cysts are found in the submucosa.[71]

Clostridium difficile and pseudomembranous colitis

It is now well established that antibiotic-associated diarrhoea may be due to colonization of the colorectum by toxin-producing *C. difficile*.[60,72] Most cases have been associated with the oral administration of lincomicin, clindamycin and ampicillin. The endoscopic and biopsy appearances of antibiotic-associated diarrhoea range from normal through non-specific inflammation to the definitive changes of pseudomembranous colitis. The latter represents the severest manifestation of antibiotic-associated diarrhoea. The rectum is frequently involved and the sigmoidoscopic appearances are those of pale plaques of mucus, fibrin and pus adhering to a hyperaemic mucosa (Fig. 8.10). Early

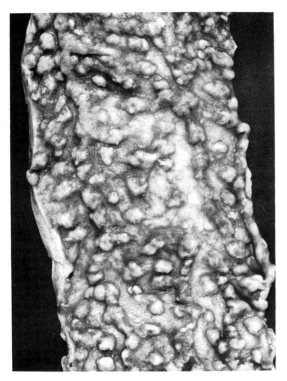

Fig. 8.10 Pseudomembranous colitis due to infection with *C. difficile*. Pale plaques of inflammatory exudate are surrounded by a reddened mucosa.

lesions appear microscopically as disruption of the surface epithelium with tufts of inflammatory exudate (Fig. 8.11).[73] As the disease progresses, the tufts become plaques and the underlying mucosa is disrupted. Ultimately the changes become indistinguishable from acute ischaemic colitis. Acute toxic dilatation may ensue. Membranous inflammation due to *Staphylococcus* species is uncommon.

Yersinia colitis

Yersinia enterocolitica and *pseudotuberculosis* are Gram-negative rods belonging to the family Enterobacteriaceae. Infection affects infants or older children and adults. The former present with an acute gastro-enteritis whilst the disease in older children may simulate appendicitis. Laparotomy in the last reveals terminal ileitis and mesenteric adenitis with variable involvement of colon and appendix. Most descriptions of the microscopic changes in the colon are based upon surgical resections or autopsy studies.[74] *Y. enterocolitica* infection leads to a necrotizing process with microabscesses involving the lymphoid tissues of the bowel wall and mesenteric lymph nodes. Histiocytes are conspicuous, especially around the edges of the micro-abscesses. Discrete granulomas are

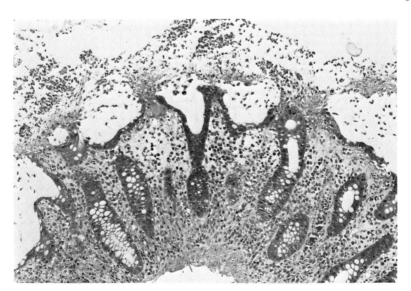

Fig. 8.11 Pseudomembranous colitis due to infection by *C. difficile*. Summit lesions composed of plumes of fibrin and pus occur at sites of superficial ulceration.
Haematoxylin-eosin   × 100

more likely to be associated with *Y. pseudotuberculosis*. Involvement of lymphoid follicles may result in aphthous ulceration as seen in Crohn's disease.[62]

Tuberculosis

Both primary and secondary forms usually involve the terminal ileum, caecum and appendix.[75] Involvement of the rest of the colon and rectum is unusual,[76] but has been documented in countries where the disease is frequently encountered.[77] The macroscopic appearance includes the formation of a few sharply-defined ulcers with thickening and induration of the surrounding bowel. Miliary tubercles may be seen on both serosal and mucosal surfaces. In contrast, Crohn's disease usually involves a greater length of bowel, shows more superficial ulceration and a cobblestone pattern of mucosal ulceration. The diagnosis of tuberculosis should not be accepted without the demonstration of caseating granulomas or tubercle bacilli in the histological sections or alternatively by culture or guinea-pig inoculation with fresh tissue. Pulmonary tuberculosis should always be excluded.

Infection with *Mycobacterium avium-intracellulare* is seen in immunosuppressed patients, including male homosexuals with the acquired immune deficiency syndrome (see p. 348).

Actinomycosis

The appendix is the commonest site of actinomycosis within the abdominal cavity. The disease is rare in the colon, but rather more common in the rectum where it is usually associated with anal fistulas.[78] There are two varieties of rectal involvement. In one the disease is primary in the rectum and in the other it is due to spread from the ileocaecal region. Actinomycosis should be considered in the differential diagnosis of strictures of the rectum. It is likely that actinomycosis is invasive only when the intestinal wall has been breached by some other condition such as diverticulitis[79] or trauma.

Gonorrhoea

Rectal gonorrhoea presents with an acute superficial inflammatory lesion of the lower rectal mucosa and should always be considered in the differential diagnosis of proctitis in the male. The gonococcus is detected by direct smear and Gram stain of pus from the mucosal surface of the rectum. In female patients gonococci can be found in the rectum in association with a urogenital tract infection in 30% of all cases. This is due to spread of the disease from the vagina and not necessarily to sexual practices. In males, however, gonococcal proctitis is invariably due to homosexual activities. The diagnosis can be aided by examination of rectal biopsies in which the appearances resemble other bacterial infections (see p. 325).

Syphilis

The primary lesion of anorectal syphilis is usually a chancre in the anal canal or at the anal margin, and much less commonly in the rectum.[80] Gumma of the rectum is extremely rare, but may be mistaken clinically for carcinoma.

Spirochaetosis

Intestinal spirochaetosis represents the infection of colorectal epithelium by spirochaetes belonging to the genus Borrelia. In histological preparations this is evidenced by a basophilic fringe along the apical border of surface epithelial cells (Fig. 8.12). It is not clear whether this infection produces symptoms. However, recent clinical studies have sug-

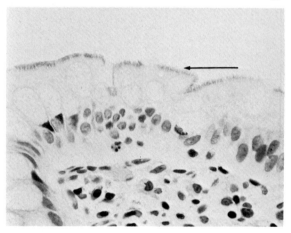

Fig. 8.12 Spirochaetosis. The basophilic border (arrow) at the apical margin of the surface columnar cells is formed by a row of spirochaetes.

Haematoxylin-eosin   × 400

gested that intestinal spirochaetosis may be a cause of diarrhoea[81] and it is of interest that an ultrastructural investigation demonstrated spirochaetes within the cytoplasm of epithelial cells and within macrophages in the lamina propria.[82] An association between spirochaetosis and homosexual activity has been suggested.[83]

Chlamydial proctitis and lymphogranuloma venereum

The microorganisms of the genus Chlamydia were formerly classed as viruses, but are now known to occupy a position intermediate between viruses and bacteria. The species *Chlamydia trachomatis* includes the agents responsible for lymphogranuloma venereum (LGV), a disease found in tropical and subtropical countries. The primary infection is transmitted by sexual contact. Males develop a lesion on the genitalia, followed by involvement of the inguinal lymph nodes. Rectal involvement may occur through anal intercourse in males. In females the disease spreads to the rectum from the primary site (vagina) presumably via lymphatics. Subgroups of *Chlamydia trachomatis* which do not cause LGV are additional causes of proctitis in homosexual males, but the lesions of the LGV subgroup are more severe.[84]

Chlamydial proctitis presents with anal pain, tenesmus and an anal discharge of blood and pus. On sigmoidoscopy the mucosa is granular, friable and ulcerated. The histological appearances are non-specific and resemble active ulcerative colitis.[85] There may be associated peri-anal abscesses and fistulae. Granulomas have been described in the rectal mucosa and inguinal lymph nodes.

A chronic stage of the disease is characterized by the formation of tubular strictures in which the wall of the rectum is thick, rigid and severely ulcerated.[86] The perirectal tissues show fibrosis and there is extensive anal scarring with bridging of the peri-anal skin. 'Burnt-out' strictures in which the mucous membrane is smooth and intact are not uncommon. Microscopically, there is non-specific chronic inflammation and fibrosis. Carcinomas, both adenocarcinoma and squamous carcinoma, have been described in lymphogranulomatous strictures.[87]

VIRAL INFECTIONS

Herpes simplex virus colitis and proctitis have been described in immunosuppressed patients[88] and homosexual males.[89] The biopsy appearances include mucosal erosions and inflammatory changes simulating ulcerative colitis. The diagnosis is established by the demonstration of multinucleated giant cells and intranuclear inclusions. The herpes virus antigen may be demonstrated immunohistochemically.

Cytomegalovirus (CMV) infection also occurs in immunosuppressed individuals, especially following renal transplantation.[90] It has been suggested that colonic involvement, typically manifested by multiple ulceration, is due to an underlying vasculitis.[90] Cytomegalic inclusions are found in endothelial cells, fibroblasts and macrophages, but rarely in epithelial cells (Fig. 8.13). CMV infection may complicate ulcerative colitis and precipitate toxic megacolon.[91]

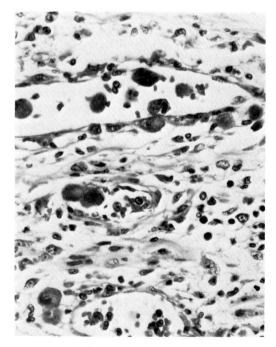

Fig. 8.13 Cytomegalic inclusions which appear to be mainly within endothelial cells. The rectal biopsy was from a patient with the acquired immunodeficiency syndrome.

Haematoxylin-eosin   × 400

FUNGAL INFECTIONS

Fungal infections may be of two types. Firstly are those in which bowel involvement is the principal if not primary manifestation of the disease and the picture may simulate granulomatous bowel disease.[92] Causative organisms include *Paracoccidioides brasiliensis* which is seen in the Americas, particularly South America, *Histoplasma capsulatum*, particularly prevalent in North America and, in West Africa, *H. duboisii*. Secondly, and more common, are the fungal infections associated with disseminated disease in immunosuppressed patients. These cases are not associated with a granulomatous reaction. Such opportunistic fungal infections include candidosis, mucormycosis and histoplasmosis.

PROTOZOAL INFECTIONS

Amoebic dysentery

This is a disease of the large intestine due to infection with *Entamoeba histolytica*. It is worldwide in its distribution, though more prevalent in the tropics than in temperate climates. Active vegetative forms are present in the large bowel in patients with dysentery. These are passed in the stools, encyst into a more resistant form and are re-ingested. The cysts are unharmed by gastric juice and pass into the intestine where their wall is dissolved liberating the active forms of amoebae. These secrete an enzyme which enables them to pass through the intestinal epithelium, disrupting the tissue and liberating red blood cells which they ingest.

Amoebic dysentery may occur in individuals who have never left Britain, and such cases may be readily confused with other inflammatory conditions of the colon such as diverticulitis and ulcerative colitis.[93] Amoebiasis is being described with increasing frequency in homosexual males. Infections may be both sporadic and epidemic.

The earliest lesions are small, yellow elevations of the mucosal surface containing semifluid necrotic material infected with the parasite (Fig. 8.14). When these lesions rupture into the lumen, the amoebae continue to proliferate, undermining the adjacent intact mucous membrane to leave a

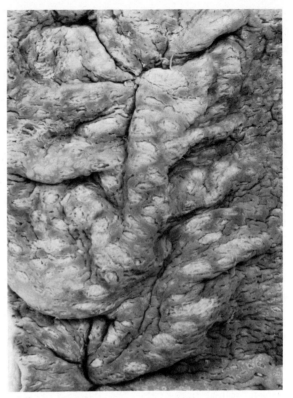

Fig. 8.14 Amoebic colitis showing characteristic ulcerated elevations and oedema of the intervening mucosa.
Specimen from the Gordon Museum, Guy's Hospital, London, reproduced by permission of the Curator, Mr J.D. Maynard. Photograph by Miss P.M. Turnbull, Charing Cross Hospital Medical School, London.

discrete oval ulcer with overhanging edges and extending into the submucosa.

Amoebic ulcers are most frequent in the caecum and rectum, but may be scattered throughout the large intestine and are especially numerous in the region of the flexures. Diffuse amoebic colitis involving the entire large bowel is the most dangerous form of the disease. In surgical specimens the ulcers are oval in shape and lie with their long axis transversely across the bowel. They are flat, without induration of the underlying bowel wall and have a characteristic hyperaemic edge. The floor of the ulcer, especially in severe cases, is covered by a ragged, yellowish-white membrane. In severe cases the ulceration becomes confluent leaving isolated patches of intact, hyperaemic mucosa among extensive areas of necrosis. Extensive inflammatory polyposis has been demonstrated as a complication of amoebic colitis and this may be a source of confusion with idiopathic inflammatory bowel disease.[94]

The inflammatory reaction of amoebic dysentery is found around the ulcers, and in severe cases passes right through the bowel wall. There is oedema, vascular congestion and infiltration with leukocytes, especially eosinophils. Amoebae are found on or just beneath the surface of the ulcers particularly beneath the overhanging margin, but in severe cases they accompany the inflammatory reaction into the bowel wall and may be seen within blood vessels. They are readily recognized in haematoxylin and eosin preparations by their round contour and large size relative to other cells. Diastase PAS can be a useful method for demonstrating them in histological preparations.

The diagnosis of amoebic dysentery may be made by finding cysts or active forms of *E. histolytica* in the stools, in scrapings from the surface of rectal ulcers or in rectal biopsies. The biopsy should be taken from the edge of an ulcer. Amoebae are easily recognized as large, round cells with small, dark nuclei. The proportion of cytoplasm to nucleus is greater than in other cells and the cytoplasm often contains ingested red blood corpuscles which differentiate *E. histolytica* from *Entamoeba coli* and other ordinarily non-pathogenic intestinal amoebae (Fig. 8.15).

Complications either result from the migration of amoebae through the bowel wall or following amoebic invasion of veins. Local complications are partly caused by secondary bacterial infection.

Perforation of the colon is rare and usually fatal.[95] Massive necrosis has been reported and is probably the result of superimposed bacterial infection.[96] In these severe cases the clinical, radiological and pathological appearances may simulate the toxic megacolon of ulcerative colitis.[97] Invasion of the skin of the peri-anal region causes ulcerative lesions which can be very extensive. Likewise, amoebic ulceration of the abdominal wall will sometimes occur around colostomy openings and following the drainage of pericolic and appendicular abscesses. In cutaneous amoebiasis the amoebae can be recovered from the surface of the lesions. Other complications include polyarthritis[98] and postdysenteric colitis.[99] The latter may be difficult to distinguish from idiopathic inflammatory bowel disease.

A common complication of amoebic dysentery is the appearance of an amoeboma, which can develop months or many years after the original infection. It is a chronic form of the disease in which localized secondary infection and fibrosis have led to the formation of a tumour which may be mistaken for carcinoma or diverticulitis. Amoebomas are usually single and involve a short segment of colon. They are commonest in the caecum and rectum.[100] Both cysts and active forms of *E. histolytica* can usually be found in the affected tissues although in very chronic cases these may be few or absent. Immunohistochemistry may facilitate the identification of organisms in chronic amoeboma.

The most serious complication of amoebic colitis is invasion of veins in the bowel wall and subsequent metastasis of amoebae to the liver in the portal bloodstream with the development of amoebic hepatitis or amoebic liver abscess. In amoebic hepatitis there is a non-specific inflammatory reaction in the portal tracts without necrosis or abscess formation. Amoebae are not found and the disease may be due to hypersensitivity to the organism. In amoebic liver abscess small zones of necrosis of the parenchyma enlarge and coalesce to form cavities filled with bacteriologically sterile pus. A zone of hyperaemia surrounds the lesions which are often in the right lobe. Bleeding occurs into the abscess, the contents of which become a

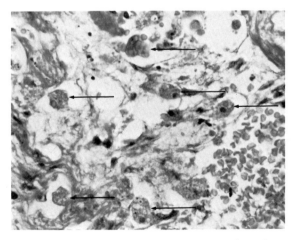

Fig. 8.15 Amoebic colitis. The field includes several amoebae showing engulfment of red blood cells (arrows). The lack of an inflammatory reaction is characteristic.

Haematoxylin-eosin   × 300

dark reddish-brown colour and have been likened
to anchovy sauce. Microscopically, the 'abscess' is
an area of necrosis of liver parenchyma in which
amoebae may be found except in very chronic
cases. Such an abscess may progress to a chronic
state, become encapsulated with fibrous tissue and
undergo calcification. It can rupture into the
peritoneal cavity, through the diaphragm into the
pleural cavity causing amoebic empyema or into
the substance of the lung. Metastatic lesions in the
brain, kidneys and spleen may result from invasion
of the blood stream.

Balantidium coli

Infestation by this large ciliated protozoon produces changes similar to those seen in amoebic
dysentery.

Cryptosporidiosis

The small intestine is the usual site of involvement
but examples of colonic involvement resembling
Crohn's disease have been described (Fig. 8.16).[101]
Cryptosporidiosis usually occurs in immunodeficient individuals[102] including male homosexuals
with the acquired immune deficiency syndrome.[103]

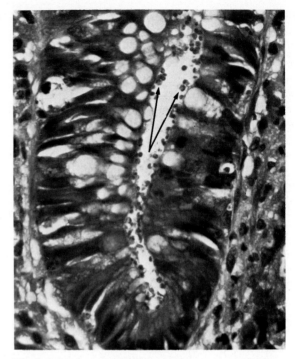

Fig. 8.16 Cryptosporidiosis. Numerous round organisms line
the luminal border of the crypt (arrows). From a case of
acquired immunodeficiency syndrome.

Haematoxylin-eosin   × 400

TREMATODE INFESTATIONS

Schistosomiasis (bilharziasis)

Infestation of the large intestine is caused most
commonly by *Schistosoma mansoni* and *Schistosoma
japonicum*, but may also be caused by *Schistosoma
haematobium*.[104] The first is endemic in African and
Central and South American countries, including
the Caribbean Islands. *S. japonicum* is found in
Japan, China, the Philippine Islands and the
countries of South-East Asia. *S. haematobium* is
found in Africa, particularly Egypt, and in countries of the Near and Middle East.

Infection occurs in man while wading or bathing
in water contaminated with the larval stage of the
worm, or cercaria. This penetrates the skin and
enters venules to be carried through the heart and
systemic circulation to the liver where the cercariae
mature to form the mature worms (Fig. 8.17).

These migrate to the mesenteric veins, and particularly to the submucosal vessels of the gut, where
they lay their eggs (Fig. 8.18). The latter pass
through the intestinal wall into the faeces. The
cycle is completed in water contaminated with
faeces containing eggs. The latter hatch out,
liberating the larvae, which are ingested by the
intermediate host, a snail, within which the second
larval stage of cercariae develops and eventually
emerges in a free-swimming form.

The pathological changes in schistosomiasis are
essentially the result of an inflammatory reaction
to the eggs in the tissues of the intestinal wall.
Lesions are commonest in the rectum and left
colon where they are usually due to *S. mansoni*. If
the lesions are in the right side of the colon and the
appendix, *S. haematobium* may be responsible.[105]

In the early stages there is an acute proctitis and
colitis accompanied by oedema, haemorrhage and
discharge of eggs into the bowel lumen. Chronic
infection leads to a great variety of morphological
appearances. Ulceration, localized or diffuse, stric-

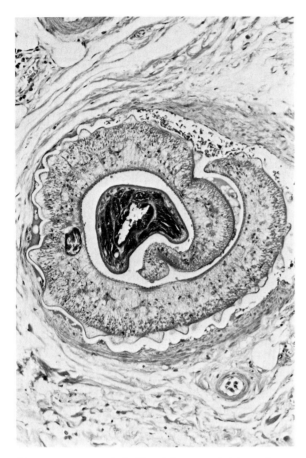

Fig. 8.17 Schistosomiasis. The adult trematode is located within a submucosal vein and was discovered in a bilharzial polyp.

Haematoxylin-eosin   × 40

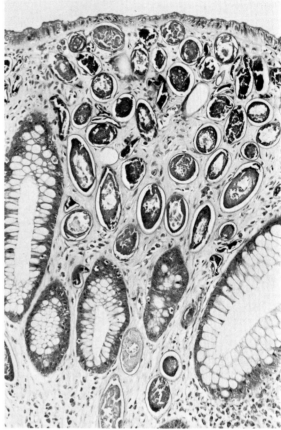

Fig. 8.18 Schistosomiasis. This section through a bilharzial polyp shows numerous eggs within the lamina propria. Many are calcified and there is a lack of surrounding inflammation.

Haematoxylin-eosin   × 100

tures due to extensive granulomatous inflammation, pericolic masses and polyps are the main types. Schistosomal polyposis may be confused with other types, including familial polyposis. Lesions may also be distributed throughout the abdominal cavity, particularly in the omentum. Involvement of the terminal ileum is described in *S. haematobium* infestation.

Histological examination shows eggs surrounded by epithelioid cell histocytes and giant cells together with infiltration by eosinophils and proliferation of fibroblasts. In chronic cases a characteristic concentric fibrosis develops around the granuloma. Not infrequently, eggs may be embedded in tissue without any surrounding inflammatory reaction

(Fig. 8.18). The eggs of *S. mansoni* are oval and possess a lateral spine. In *S. haematobium* the egg is much the same size and shape but has a terminal spine. The lateral spine of *S. japonicum* is smaller than that of *S. mansoni* and the egg is more spherical. The diagnosis of schistosomiasis can be made by finding the bilharzial granulomas in rectal biopsies.

Long-standing chronic infestation may be complicated by the development of carcinoma. In *S. japonicum* infection the pathogenesis of carcinoma has been described and compared with the pathology of malignant change in ulcerative colitis, including the development of precancerous dysplasia.[106]

Anisakiasis

This infestation is caused by species of the larval ascarid *Anisakis* and results from the consumption of raw fish. Most reports stem from Japan and Scandinavia.[107,108] The stomach and small intestine are involved more commonly than the colon. In the last, macroscopic changes resembling Crohn's disease have been described.[109] Acute lesions contain an inflammatory infiltrate which includes neutrophils and eosinophils. Granulomas are found in more advanced lesions.

Strongyloidiasis

The clinical manifestations of this condition usually relate to the lung and upper small intestine (see p. 268). Colonic involvement occurs rarely and is associated with diarrhoea, abdominal pain and melaena.[110] Fatal, widely-disseminated disease may occur in immonosuppressed individuals (Fig. 8.19).

ULCERATIVE COLITIS

Ulcerative colitis is an inflammatory condition of the mucous membrane which begins in the rectum and may spread proximally to involve the entire colon. Involvement of the appendix is seen in about half of all cases. The terminal ileum can be affected in cases of total colitis, but this is of little importance in relation to pathology and treatment. Idiopathic or granular proctitis represents a distal form of ulcerative colitis.

Aetiology and pathogenesis

A large number of experimental models for ulcerative colitis now exist. Most of these have a disorder of immunity as their basis. It is not possible to review these mechanisms in detail, but an attempt will be made to link current evidence concerning the pathogenesis of ulcerative colitis to the characteristic histopathological changes observed in this condition.

The earliest changes in ulcerative colitis are vascular congestion and the passage of an inflammatory exudate including neutrophils into the lamina propria. This acute inflammation could be mediated on an anaphylactic basis (type I hyper-

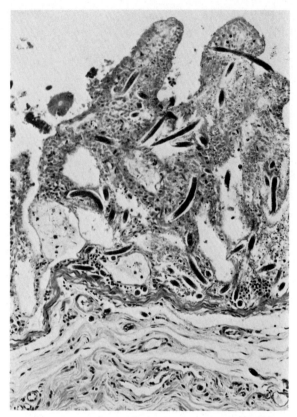

Fig. 8.19 Strongyloidiasis. This massive intestinal infestation occurred in an immune-deficient patient with disseminated lymphoma.

Haematoxylin-eosin   × 100

sensitivity), through cytotoxic antibodies (type II hypersensitivity) or through immune complex formation (type III hypersensitivity). Degranulation of mast cells and release of histamine or other mediators of acute inflammation would depend on the local production of IgE. Increased numbers of IgE-containing plasma cells within the lamina propria have been reported in rectal biopsies from patients with inflammatory bowel disease.[111] However, it has been suggested that patients with an allergic basis to their disease may represent a distinct and separate subgroup who respond to therapy with sodium cromoglycate (cromolyn sodium).[112,113]

Cytotoxic antibodies directed against surface epithelial cells could inflict damage that would initiate the activation of complement and/or release chemical agents to bring about an acute inflammatory response. Anticolon antibodies have been described in patients with inflammatory bowel disease.[114] Alternatively, antibodies against entero-bacteria may cross-react with gut epithelium.[115] These antibodies could also be linked to antibody-dependent cell-mediated cytotoxicity in which neutrophils, lymphocytes and monocytes have been implicated.[116]

Immune complexes may be derived either from the circulation or be formed locally within the vessels of gut mucosa, giving rise to an Arthus reaction. In attempting to engulf the large insoluble immune complexes associated with the Arthus reaction, neutrophils would discharge lysosomal enzymes and thereby amplify the inflammatory damage. The concept of circulating immune complexes could be linked to the extra-intestinal manifestation of ulcerative colitis. Circulating immune complexes have been identified in patients with inflammatory bowel disease[117] and experimental models lend support to their involvement in its pathogenesis.[118] However, others have reported conflicting findings or were unable to relate disease severity with the numbers of circulating immune complexes.[119] However, the possibility of a local production of immune complexes remains an attractive hypothesis.

Most workers agree that increased numbers of plasma cells are found in the lamina propria of patients with ulcerative colitis. When active disease exists there is a significant increase in plasma cells secreting IgA, IgM and IgG.[120] This increase could be secondary to local antigenic stimulation following epithelial damage. Alternatively, the plasma cells could be producing antibodies that are contributing to the tissue damage.

Delayed or cell-mediated hypersensitivity is presumably more likely to operate in Crohn's disease, which is characterized by lympho-histio-cytic infiltration and granuloma formation.

Most of the other mucosal changes associated with ulcerative colitis, such as mucus depletion and crypt distortion, are likely to be secondary to inflammation, regeneration and repair. The muscle thickening in chronic ulcerative colitis is probably due to sustained muscle spasm. This may be related to the release of peptides by the intrinsic neurons of the myenteric plexus or histamine by mast cells. Contraction of smooth muscle could also influence disease progression by causing mucosal hypoxia.

Incidence

The peak age incidence for either sex on first attendance at hospital is in the third decade. The disease has been described in a child of 3 weeks[121] and there are reports of the condition developing in childhood and at puberty. It can also occur for the first time in patients over the age of 50 but, in many of these, mild but suggestive symptoms have been present for some time previously.[121]

In most adult series the disease is more common in women than men (ratio 3:2). In children below the age of 14 the sex incidence appears about equal. The condition is stated to be more common in Jews[122] than in other races and seems to be less common in Blacks than in Whites.

Macroscopic appearances in surgical specimens

The serosa is intact and retains its normal shiny surface. The only exception to this is in acute fulminating disease, when involvement of the full thickness of the bowel wall, with or without perforation, causes acute inflammatory serosal changes. The regional lymph nodes are sometimes enlarged. The length of the colon and rectum is always reduced. This is most obvious in the distal colon and rectum. Fibrosis makes little contribution and is largely lacking. Shortening is sometimes reversible. The contraction is accompanied by a reduction in the transverse calibre. The mucous membrane has a granular or velvety surface appearance and is extremely friable (Fig. 8.20). Vascular congestion may be marked. In its earliest form, the ulceration is little more than a superficial erosion. Full-thickness ulceration of the mucous membrane is usually patchy, but any intact intervening mucosa is always diseased. The ulceration may have a linear distribution, especially in the colon, where it is related to the line of attachment of the taeniae coli. It must be emphasized that the inflammatory changes in ulcerative colitis are continuous, although severely affected areas may sometimes be separated by patches of less obviously involved mucosa.

The mucosal changes of ulcerative colitis involve the rectum and rectosigmoid in the first place and spread proximally in continuity until the entire

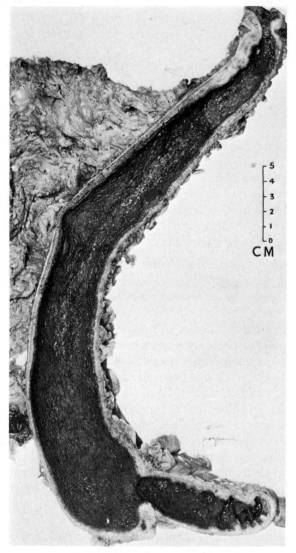

CM

5
4
3
2
1
0

Fig. 8.20 Chronic ulcerative colitis involving the whole of the colon. The gut is shortened with muscular thickening of the wall and loss of the haustral pattern. The usual pattern of mucosal folding is lost and there is diffuse, superficial ulceration with the surface covered by haemorrhagic slough.

large bowel may be involved. True ulcerative colitis with a sigmoidoscopically and histologically normal rectum could only occur in very mild cases in which the disease regressed completely. Such cases are rare. Occasionally the rectal mucosa may look sigmoidoscopically normal, but will show signs of disease when examined microscopically. The severity of the mucosal changes in surgical specimens is usually greatest in the distal large bowel and tends to diminish proximally. Even in total colitis

the disease is usually more severe in the left colon and rectum. In occasional specimens the proximal limit of the disease shows an abrupt transition from diseased to normal mucosa but a gradual change is more usual.

Polypoid change in ulcerative colitis is extremely common. The term 'pseudo-polyp' is used but inflammatory polyp is a better expression as it indicates the way in which polyps are formed. They are the result of full-thickness ulceration of the mucous membrane with undermining of adjacent mucosa which is relatively raised up so that it projects into the lumen. These inflammatory polyps or mucosal tags may be present in large numbers and adopt bizarre shapes. They may stick to one another forming mucosal bridges. If healing takes place the polyps remain as evidence of past disease, so-called *colitis polyposa*. The polyposis of ulcerative colitis is more prominent in the colon than the rectum (Fig. 8.21).

When the terminal ileum is involved the mucosal changes are similar to those seen in the colon. They are always in continuity with disease in the large bowel and are associated with a rigid, dilated and incompetent ileocaecal valve (Fig. 8.20). The expression 'backwash' ileitis is widely used, but there is, as yet, no evidence that ileal disease is the result of such a mechanism. Ileitis is found in about 10% of colectomy specimens for ulcerative colitis. The extent of involvement varies from 5–25 cm but is only very rarely longer. It is extremely rare for ascending enteritis to occur following colectomy and ileostomy and this is usually a fatal complication. It is probable that it is not due to the ulcerative colitis but is a complication of the ileostomy operation, so-called prestomal or stomal ileitis. Ulcers are scattered throughout the ileum and jejunum. The intervening mucosa is normal or oedematous. The ulcers readily perforate, giving rise to peritonitis and the formation of faecal fistulas.

Segmental fibrous strictures of the colon do not occur in ulcerative colitis. If true fibrous strictures are present in the colon showing diffuse inflammation, the diagnosis of Crohn's disease rather than ulcerative colitis should be considered. Alternatively, stricture formation can be the result of localized muscular thickening or malignant change.

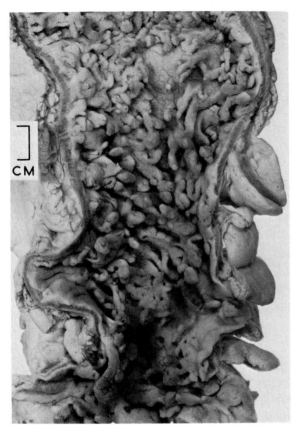

Fig. 8.21 Healed ulcerative colitis showing the formation of inflammatory pseudo-polyps. These are characterized by their bizarre shapes.

Specimen from the Gordon Museum, Guy's Hospital, London, reproduced by permission of the Curator, Mr J.D. Maynard. Photograph by Miss P.M. Turnbull, Charing Cross Hospital Medical School.

Fulminating colitis

Some 5–10% of all patients with ulcerative colitis have a fulminating episode either as a first attack or in an acute relapse, and in these cases the colon may be resected as an emergency measure. A segment of large bowel, most commonly the transverse colon, becomes acutely dilated (so-called *toxic megacolon*), and all coats including the muscle are thinned (Fig. 8.22). The wall has the consistency of wet blotting-paper. There is extensive mucosal ulceration with surviving islands of mucous membrane showing intense congestion. Perforation, either spontaneous or surgical, is common.

Microscopic appearances in surgical and biopsy specimens

The fact that ulcerative colitis is essentially a mucosal disease is readily appreciated in surgical specimens. The muscularis propria and serosa are only inflamed in cases of acute fulminating colitis.

In active disease, one of the most striking features is congestion and dilatation of thin-walled vessels in the mucosa and submucosa, accompanied by oedema (Fig. 8.23). Inflammatory cell infiltration of the lamina propria includes plasma cells, eosinophils and smaller numbers of neutrophils. Lymphocytes are less conspicuous in routine sections, but hyperplasia of mucosal lymphoid follicles is seen in the rectum in chronic cases (*follicular proctitis*). Histiocytes occur in the vicinity of disrupted crypt abscesses but do not form the typical non-caseating granulomas of Crohn's disease. Giant cells of foreign-body type are seen occasionally.

An important feature of active ulcerative colitis is infiltration of the crypt epithelium by neutrophils and the formation of crypt abscesses (Fig. 8.23). However, crypt abscesses are a non-specific finding, occurring also in appendicitis, infective colitis and Crohn's colitis. Crypt abscesses either discharge their pus into the lumen or spread in the loose tissues of the submucosa giving rise eventually to undermining ulcers. Inflammation does not extend beyond the submucosa, except in acute fulminating disease.

Submucosal inflammation usually involves the upper submucosal compartment only and is always in proportion to the overlying mucosal inflammation. Fibrosis is not a prominent feature, even in chronic ulcerative colitis. Involvement of the appendix does not lead to purulent appendicitis because inflammation is mucosal.

In the acute fulminating disease, there is transmural inflammation and extensive loss of mucosa. Surviving mucosa shows intense vascular congestion and oedema with a relatively mild inflammatory cell response. The submucosal tissues may disappear leaving bare muscle covered by only a very thin layer of granulation tissue. The fibres of the muscularis propria become stretched and separated by oedematous exudate. This may lead to perforation. The dilatation associated with acute

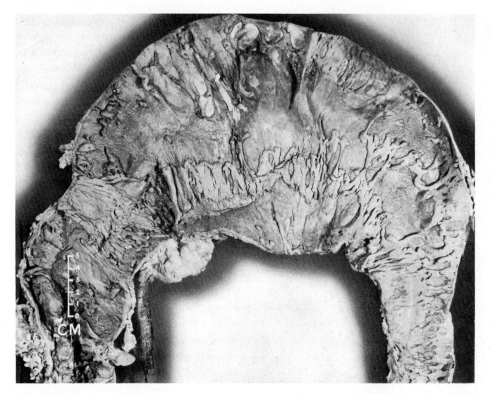

Fig. 8.22 Fulminating ulcerative colitis with marked dilatation of the transverse colon ('toxic megacolon').

fulminating disease may be due to a primary toxic atrophy of the smooth muscle. Acute fulminating disease may lead to the condition known as *acute toxic dilatation*, which is associated with a high mortality. Acute dilatation complicates other forms of colitis, including Crohn's disease, amoebic colitis, ischaemic colitis, pseudomembranous colitis and bacillary dysentery.

Sequential rectal and colonoscopic biopsies provide one with an opportunity to monitor the natural history of the disease. This may be divided into an active phase (Fig. 8.23) of varying severity, a resolving phase (Fig. 8.24) and a phase of remission (Fig. 8.25). Not all biopsies can be thus classified, however. Some patients show a continuous, albeit low-grade colitis (quiescent). Partial treatment may lead to the appearances of resolution though inflammation is still active and the patient is extremely unwell.

In the active phase of ulcerative colitis there is mucosal inflammation of variable severity with an increase in the plasma cell content of the lamina propria and polymorphonuclear infiltration which is usually focal and often in the form of crypt abscesses. The mucosal surface is irregular and covered with pus. Vascular congestion and haemorrhage are prominent. The epithelium shows a variable degree of destruction, especially of the superficial part of the crypts. This is accompanied by mucin depletion of the goblet cells and reactive hyperplasia of surviving epithelium. Mucin depletion is a very important sign of active disease (Fig. 8.23).

Ulcerative colitis in an active phase can be graded subjectively into mild, moderate, or severe. In mild cases the epithelial membrane can show mucin depletion but otherwise remains almost intact. At the other extreme, the entire mucous membrane consists only of a zone of inflammatory cells with a few surviving tubules and the muscularis mucosae is identifiable only as a line across which cells infiltrate into the submucosal layer. In biopsies from very severe active ulcerative colitis it is even possible for the mucous membrane to be completely

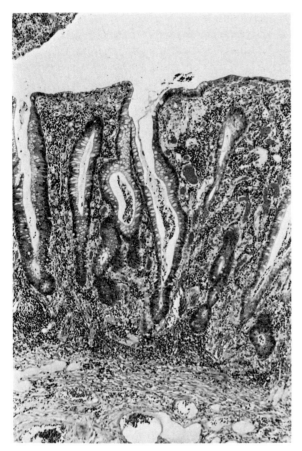

Fig. 8.23 Active phase of chronic ulcerative colitis showing diffuse mucosal inflammation with marked vascular dilatation. The crypts show partial mucus depletion and a collection of neutrophils within a gland results in the formation of a crypt abscess.

Haematoxylin-eosin   × 80

denuded of the epithelium. In such patients the severity of the disease can be underestimated at sigmoidoscopy.

The resolving phase is characterized by a reduction in vascularity and gradual disappearance of polymorphs and crypt abscesses; the increased content of plasma cells and lymphocytes is the last to decline. The restoration of the goblet cell population is among the earliest signs of resolution and is accompanied by reactive hyperplasia of the epithelium, especially at the base of the crypts, and restoration of epithelial continuity (Fig. 8.24). Attempts to restore the normal architecture of the mucosa are accompanied by branching and irregularity of the epithelial tubules. In cases where

there has been very severe mucosal loss, a single layer of columnar cells will cover an ulcerated area and form tubules which grow in the direction of the muscularis mucosae, but usually fail to reach it. This leaves a permanent gap between the base of the crypts and the luminal side of the muscularis mucosae. This gap is an important sign of mucosal atrophy.

During the phase of resolution of an attack of colitis the inflammation, especially the presence of lymphocytes and plasma cells, may become patchy or focal, and this can give rise to difficulties in the differential diagnosis of Crohn's disease.

In patients with ulcerative colitis in remission, the sigmoidoscopic appearances can be quite normal. It does not follow that the rectal mucosa will be normal histologically (Fig. 8.25). The

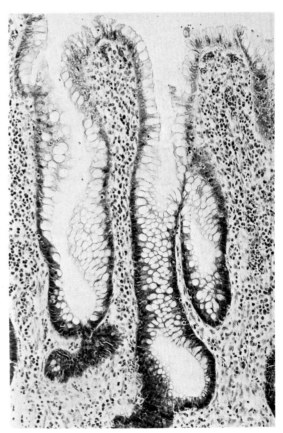

Fig. 8.24 Resolving phase of chronic ulcerative colitis. There is crypt hyperplasia and replenishment of the goblet cell population. Some residual active inflammation is evident.

Haematoxylin-eosin   × 100

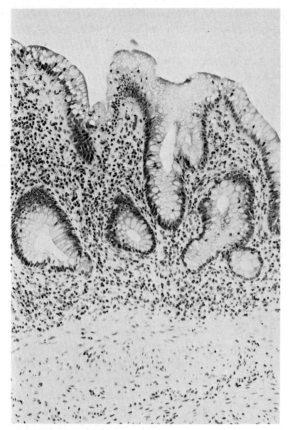

Fig. 8.25 Chronic quiescent ulcerative colitis. The crypts show branching and atrophy and the muscularis mucosae is thickened. The patient was clinically in remission but there is some residual active inflammation.

Haematoxylin-eosin   × 100

inflammatory content of the rectal mucosal is within normal limits, epithelial continuity is restored and the goblet cell population has returned to normal. However, there are nearly always some signs of mucosal atrophy. They may be minor, such as slight loss of parallelism, separation of the tubules, or branching of the crypts. In patients with a long history of severe disease there is shortening of the crypts, which fail to reach the muscularis mucosae, leaving a characteristic gap. The muscularis mucosae itself is usually thickened with a tendency to splaying of its fibres. Paneth cell metaplasia, endocrine cell hyperplasia and fat in the lamina propria are all features of long-standing disease. The salient features on rectal biopsy of the various phases of ulcerative colitis are summarized below.

1. Active phase
   a. Irregular mucosal surface with luminal pus
   b. Loss of epithelium with ulceration
   c. Increased chronic inflammatory cell content of lamina propria
   d. Focal polymorph infiltration with crypt abscesses and oedema
   e. Vascular congestion
   f. Mucin depletion of goblet cells
2. Resolving phase
   a. Reduction in vascular congestion
   b. Gradual disappearance of polymorphs and crypt abscesses
   c. Restoration of goblet cell population
   d. Reactive epithelial hyperplasia and restoration of epithelial continuity
   e. Declining population of lymphocytes and plasma cells
3. Colitis in remission
   a. Loss of parallelism, unequal separation and branching of crypts
   b. Short tubules of varying length, separated from one another (mucosal atrophy)
   c. Thickening of muscularis mucosae
   d. Paneth cell metaplasia
   e. Endocrine cell hyperplasia
   f. Fat in lamina propria.

Dysplasia in ulcerative colitis

Recognition of precancerous changes in biopsies from patients with ulcerative colitis is not straightforward. Inflammatory and reparative changes may mimic dysplasia (Fig. 8.26). However, the term dysplasia should only be used when there is unequivocal evidence of a neoplastic alteration. A new classification[123] for precancerous change in ulcerative colitis has been proposed, and encourages the use of an indefinite category (Table 8.1). Biopsies indefinite for dysplasia fall into two

Table 8.1 Classification of dysplasia in ulcerative colitis

Negative	
Indefinite	probably negative
	unknown
	probably positive
Positive	low grade
	high grade

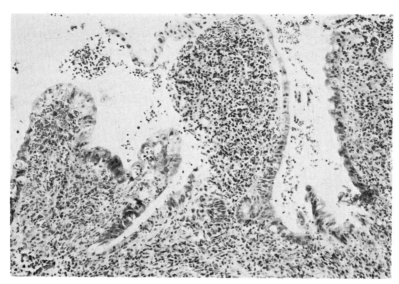

Fig. 8.26 Inflammatory and regenerative changes in ulcerative colitis. There is considerable distortion of architecture and the cytological appearances mimic dysplasia. However, there is intense acute inflammation and the changes can be expected to regress.

Haematoxylin-eosin × 100

groups. The epithelial changes may be accompanied by active inflammation which precludes the confident recognition of a neoplastic process. Alternatively, the various histological features that constitute dysplasia may be represented only in part or to a mild degree. Villous change without cytological atypia, basal cell hyperplasia and other patterns of incomplete maturation fall into the latter category. There are two main types of dysplasia. The easiest to recognize is *adenomatous dysplasia* which often shows a villous configuration (Fig. 8.27). Macroscopically, this presents as a nodular or velvety mucosa. Dysplasia arising in flat mucosa may lack the usual architectural features associated with adenomatous dysplasia and reliance is placed on cytological atypia and disordered differentiation (Fig. 8.28).

In *villous dysplasia* cytological atypia may be very mild or limited to the intervillous (crypt) epithelium. Nevertheless, apparently low-grade villous dysplasia may give rise directly to carcinoma, which is often mucinous in type. Poorly-differentiated, diffusely infiltrating carcinoma is more frequently associated with dysplasia arising in flat mucosa.[124] Some changes are peculiar to dysplasia in ulcerative colitis, including Paneth cell metaplasia and goblet cell inversion or dislocation. However, these alterations are sometimes seen in nondysplastic colitic mucosa. The principal cytological features of dysplasia are an increase in the nucleo-cytoplasmic ratio, nuclear hyperchromatism, variation in nuclear size and shape, loss of nuclear polarity and increased mitotic activity. Elongation and pseudostratification of nuclei are typical of adenomatous dysplasia, but not dysplasia in flat mucosa.

Cancer in ulcerative colitis

The incidence of cancer in ulcerative colitis lies between 3 and 5% of all cases.[125] The risk is highest in patients with long-standing and extensive disease. In patients who have had the disease for 10–20 years the risk is 23 times that expected in the general population.[126] However, since patients who have had the disease for 10–20 years will still be relatively young, it may be misleading to compare them with an age-matched population. Thus patients who develop carcinoma may be predisposed to such a complication, the effect of ulcerative colitis being merely to bring about its earlier development. Not only has the risk of cancer been exaggerated by attempts to estimate the cumulative probability of malignant change from retrospective

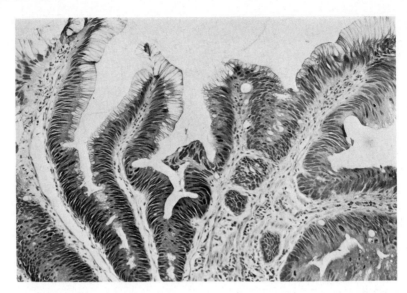

Fig. 8.27 Dysplasia in ulcerative colitis. The mucosa shows a villous configuration and is lined by mucin-secreting columnar cells. The nuclei are enlarged, hyperchromatic and pseudostratified but there is little pleomorphism. The changes amount to low-grade dysplasia.

Haematoxylin-eosin   × 100

data, but the prognosis of this complication may be less grave than was first thought, particularly when patients are kept under close supervision and information is gathered prospectively.[127]

Cancers arise anywhere in the colorectum. They are often multiple, flat and diffusely infiltrative, like gastric carcinoma (Fig. 8.29). Mucinous and poorly-differentiated carcinomas occur frequently. It is important to distinguish between well-differentiated carcinomas and the misplaced epithelium of colitis cystica profunda.[123]

It is now becoming clear that cancer is more likely to arise in patients who show precancerous changes or dysplasia.[123] However, it is not always possible to demonstrate dysplasia in patients who develop carcinoma, though intra-epithelial neoplasia must have been present if only for a relatively short duration and within a very limited area. Thus the detection of dyplasia will be successful when the change is widespread and diffuse and less successful when it is patchy or focal yet unstable.

Liver disease in ulcerative colitis

The liver is not infrequently affected in ulcerative colitis and liver function tests may be abnormal, the most common single abnormality being a raised serum alkaline phosphatase. A wide range of changes has been described in biopsy material,[128] with diffuse fatty change and non-specific reactive hepatitis being common. Less commonly, but more seriously, there may be acute hepatitis, chronic active hepatitis and cirrhosis.[129] Large duct obstruction can result from primary sclerosing cholangitis,[130] bile duct carcinoma[131] or cholelithiasis. Pericholangitis may occur alone or in association with primary sclerosing cholangitis.

Miscellaneous complications

Skin lesions, arthritis, iridocyclitis, amyloidosis, lymphoma, endocrine cell tumours and squamous cell carcinoma have all been described as complicating factors. However, one review suggests that the reported cases of ulcerative colitis complicated by amyloidosis were examples of colonic Crohn's disease.[132]

CROHN'S DISEASE OF THE LARGE INTESTINE

The pathology of Crohn's disease is discussed in detail in Chapter 7 (p. 257). Consideration will

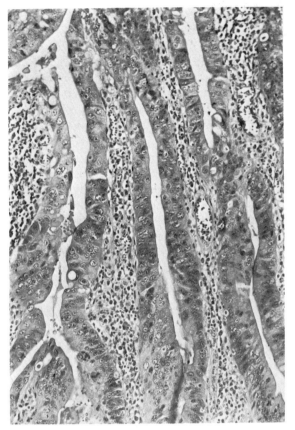

Fig. 8.28 High-grade dysplasia within flat mucosa in ulcerative colitis. The nuclei are enlarged, pleomorphic and show loss of polarity.

Haematoxylin-eosin   × 100

ment of the terminal ileum is much commoner in Crohn's disease than ulcerative colitis. Also anal lesions are more frequent and severe in Crohn's disease. These include ulceration, fistulae and extensive lymphocytic inflammation.

Crohn's disease shows a characteristic pattern of mucosal changes ranging from early aphthoid ulceration, to serpiginous and deep fissuring ulceration, associated with a cobblestone appearance (Fig. 8.30). In severely affected segments, the wall is thickened and the bowel lumen is narrowed. Serosal involvement with or without granuloma formation is a regular feature of Crohn's colitis. Deep fissuring may lead to the formation of fistulae (internal or enterocutaneous). These are never found in ulcerative colitis. Inflammatory polyps may occur in Crohn's disease, but are not as prominent or as extensive as those of ulcerative colitis.

The regional lymph nodes are often enlarged and fleshy and may contain sarcoid-like granulomas.

Microscopic features

The contrasting microscopic features in ulcerative colitis and Crohn's disease of the large intestine

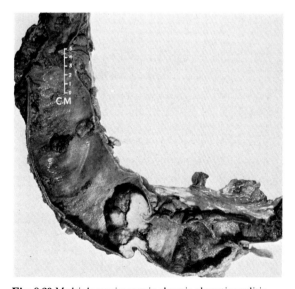

Fig. 8.29 Multiple carcinomas in chronic ulcerative colitis. Five primary carcinomas are included in the length of bowel illustrated and there were three further carcinomas in the rest of the colon. The surrounding mucosa shows villous change which was dysplastic on histological examination.

now be given to the macroscopic and microscopic features which distinguish Crohn's disease of the large intestine from ulcerative colitis.

Macroscopic features

Crohn's disease is often a discontinuous process in which diseased areas are separated by entirely normal tissue. Even when involvement is extensive, there are usually small patches of uninvolved bowel. The rectum may be uninvolved in Crohn's disease, whereas it is always affected in ulcerative colitis. Thus a normal rectal biopsy in a patient with inflammatory bowel disease is highly suggestive of Crohn's disease. However, it is possible to find near-normal rectal biopsies in some patients with mild ulcerative colitis in remission. Involve-

are summarized in Table 8.2. Transmural inflammation is never found in ulcerative colitis, except in acute fulminating disease. Rectal biopsies may sometimes include submucosa; disproportionate inflammation of the submocosa is a feature of Crohn's disease. Not only may the width of the submucosa be increased, but this may be accompanied by marked fibrosis in Crohn's colitis.

The character of the mucosal inflammation often differs in Crohn's disease and ulcerative colitis. In Crohn's disease inflammation is patchy and the inflammatory cell population frequently includes a greater proportion of lymphocytes and histiocytes. Patchy inflammation may also be seen in ulcerative colitis, especially in the resolving phase.

Sarcoid-like granulomas are virtually diagnostic of Crohn's disease but multiple sections may be needed to identify them (Fig. 8.31). Focal collections of histiocytes or microgranulomas may often be observed. Aggregates of lymphocytes in relation to the base of the crypts are also a feature of Crohn's colitis. The crypt architecture is typically well preserved in Crohn's disease. The crypts are parallel and unbranched and there is little atrophy. Indeed the crypts may be taller than normal. The

goblet cell population is well maintained even in the presence of active inflammation. Crypt abscesses may occur but are not numerous and often are distensive rather than disruptive. Paneth cell metaplasia may be found in Crohn's disease, but not to the same extent as in ulcerative colitis. Reactive epithelial changes occur focally in Crohn's disease but are generally more widespread in ulcerative colitis.

Fissuring ulcers are an important hallmark of Crohn's disease, but are rarely present in biopsies of the colon or rectum. A true fissure is lined by granulation tissue. Aphthoid ulcers are superficial ulcers, usually in relation to an underlying lymphoid aggregate.

The most important microscopic features in rectal biopsies that help to distinguish between ulcerative colitis, infective colitis and Crohn's disease are summarized in Table 8.3.

Cancer in Crohn's disease

The frequency of colorectal cancer is slightly increased in patients with Crohn's colitis. How-

Table 8.2 Microscopic differences in the pathology of ulcerative colitis and Crohn's disease of the large intestine

Ulcerative colitis	Crohn's disease
1. Mucosal and submucosal inflammation (except in acute fulminating colitis)	1. Transmural inflammation
2. Width of submucosa normal or reduced	2. Width of submucosa normal or increased
3. Very intense vascularity Little oedema	3. Vascularity seldom prominent Oedema marked
4. Focal lymphoid hyperplasia restricted to the mucosa and superficial submucosa	4. Focal lymphoid hyperplasia in mucosa, submucosa, serosa and pericolic tissues
5. 'Crypt abscesses' very common	5. 'Crypt abscesses' fewer in number
6. Mucus secretion grossly impaired	6. Mucus secretion slightly impaired
7. Paneth cell metaplasia common	7. Paneth cell metaplasia rare
8. Sarcoid type granulomas absent from bowel and lymph nodes	8. Sarcoid-type granulomas in 60–70% of cases in bowel and lymph nodes
9. 'Fissuring' absent	9. 'Fissuring' very common
10. Dysplasia occurs	10. Dysplasia very rare
11. Anal lesions—non-specific inflammation	11. Anal lesions; sarcoid foci often present
12. Neuronal hyperplasia not marked	12. Neuronal hyperplasia marked
13. No lymphangiectasia	13. Lymphangiectasia

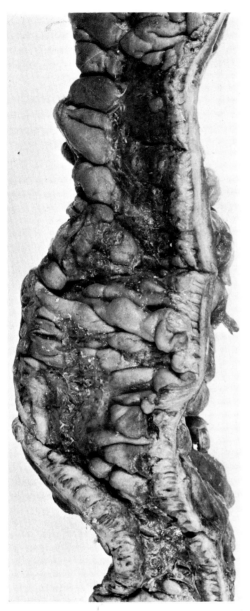

Fig. 8.30 Crohn's disease of the colon with stricture formation, ulceration and marked submucosal oedema giving the characteristic 'cobblestone' appearance.

ever, precancerous dysplasia is rarely observed.[133,134]

Indeterminate colitis

This term has been used to describe the 5–10% of surgical specimens which do not conform to the standard macroscopic and microscopic features of ulcerative colitis and Crohn's disease.[135] These cases are usually examples of extensive, acute and severe colitis, with some degree of dilatation of the colon. In this state, maximal overlap of the pathology of Crohn's disease and ulcerative colitis can be demonstrated and the usual differences may be lacking. A misleading appearance is the discontinuous ulceration. However, minor histological changes in intact mucosa between ulcerated areas may suggest previous inflammation which has resolved. Fissuring ulceration is an accepted parameter of Crohn's disease, but is occasionally seen in very acute ulcerative colitis, except that the quality of fissuring is different. The fissures in

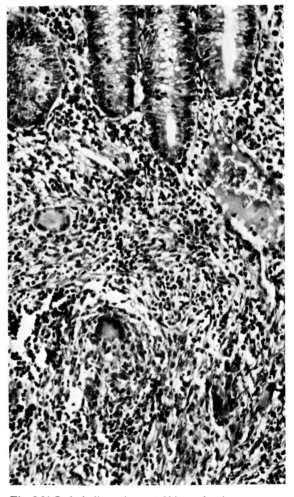

Fig. 8.31 Crohn's disease in a rectal biopsy showing non-caseating granulomas within the submucosa.

Haematoxylin-eosin × 210

Table 8.3 Differential diagnosis of infective colitis, ulcerative colitis and Crohn's disease in rectal biopsies

Histological features	Infective colitis	Active ulcerative colitis	Crohn's disease
Mucosal oedema	+ +	+	+ +
Vascularity	+	+ + +	+
Mucosal inflammation			
(a) polymorphs	+ + +	+ +	+
(b) mononuclear cells	±	+ + +	+ + +
Distortion of crypt architecture	–	+ + +	+
Mucus depletion	±	+ + +	±

acute colitis are clefts sparsely lined by inflammatory cells whereas in Crohn's disease they are lined by granulation tissue. Transmural inflammation with myocytolysis of the muscularis propria can occur in both types of idiopathic inflammatory bowel disease and are common to acute toxic dilatation of any cause. The clues to the correct diagnosis are found in the study of pre-operative or postoperative rectal and colonic biopsies and, of course, in the subsequent progress of the disease, which may, in later surgical material, reveal diagnostic criteria.

Bizarre polyposis in inflammatory bowel disease

Bizarre or giant inflammatory polyposis of the colon occurs in both Crohn's disease and ulcerative colitis. In such cases the mucous membrane is replaced by a thick layer of polypoid tissue composed of a dense mass of mucosal fronds. This 'seaweed' type of polyposis is often segmental or patchy and may completely fill the lumen of the colon, producing obstructive symptoms. Ulceration is conspicuous by its absence on macroscopic inspection and the adjacent flat mucosa can appear quite normal. The histological diagnosis is achieved by searching for the ordinary discriminating criteria of Crohn's disease and ulcerative colitis.

Idiopathic inflammatory bowel disease and diverticular disease

Crohn's disease is more likely than ulcerative colitis to co-exist with diverticular disease of the sigmoid colon.[137] Patients with documented diverticular disease may present with diverticulitis, which is subsequently shown to be Crohn's disease. The pathological demonstration of co-existing Crohn's disease and diverticular disease may not be straightforward. Crohn's disease is suggested by the presence of non-caseating granulomas (to be distinguished from foreign-body granulomas), involvement of mucosa between diverticula, and deep, fissure-like ulceration. The latter may be simulated in diverticulitis, but the ulcers are usually broader than those of Crohn's disease. Fistulous tracts occur in both conditions.

Eosinophilic colitis

Recently a number of patients with eosinophilic gastro-enteritis (see pp. 170 and 276) have been shown to have colonic involvement.[138] However, increased numbers of mucosal eosinophils may be observed in a number of conditions, including Crohn's disease and ulcerative colitis. Eosinophilic colitis should therefore not be diagnosed unless the clinical context is appropriate.

Radiation colitis

Most patients with radiation colitis are women who have had radiotherapy for carcinoma of the uterine cervix. The injuries may begin during the course of radiotherapy or they can appear months, years or even several decades later.[139]

Patients with acute radiation injury present with diarrhoea, including the passage of mucus, abdominal distension, tenesmus and colicky abdominal pain. On sigmoidoscopy the rectal mucosa appears oedematous with a loss of the vascular pattern. The earliest histological changes include nuclear pyknosis, flattening of the cells, loss of nuclear polarity, enlargement of nuclei, reduced mitotic activity and mucin depletion (Fig. 8.32). The surface epithelium is lost and the lamina propria and crypt epithelium are infiltrated by eosinophils.

Delayed radiation effects may be manifested clinically by diarrhoea, colicky abdominal pain, nausea and vomiting. Macroscopically, the mucous membrane is granular and haemorrhagic, with loss of mucosal folds. Ulcers are covered by slough. The bowel wall shows a fusiform type of stenosis

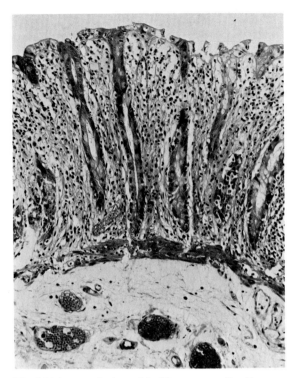

Fig. 8.32 Acute radiation colitis. The crypts are lined by an attenuated epithelium showing mucin depletion and there is submucosal telangiectasia.

Haematoxylin-eosin × 100

and there is serosal fibrosis with adhesions. The formation of internal fistulae has been described.[140] The most characteristic changes are seen within connective tissue and include oedema, fibrosis, telangiectasia and fibroblasts with bizarre nuclei. It is not clear to what extent these changes reflect direct radiation injury or secondary ischaemic damage. Vascular lesions are prominent and include swelling of endothelial cells, the subendothelial accumulations of foam cells, thrombosis and arteriosclerotic changes. The mucosa is atrophic and may show distorted crypt architecture and cytological atypia.

Drug-induced colitis

The effects of laxative abuse are described on page 388. Antibiotic-associated diarrhoea and pseudomembranous colitis are considered on page 326. An acute haemorrhagic right-sided colitis has been described in patients taking penicillin[141] and ampicillin.[142] Gold[143] and methyldopa[144] have been documented as causes of a non-specific colitis. Treatment of leukaemia or other forms of cancer with chemotherapeutic agents such as 5-fluorouracil may cause changes similar to radiation colitis.[145] The administration of enemas to prepare the colon for endoscopy may cause changes simulating mild inflammatory bowel disease.[146]

Colitis in defunctioned bowel

Defunctioning of the whole or part of the large intestine by ileostomy or colostomy may result in pathological changes which are peculiar to this state. The severity of these changes depends on the length of time that the intestine has been defunctioned. Before the development of colectomy and ileostomy for extensive inflammation it was customary to perform caecostomy alone, and such patients were sometimes left with a defunctioned bowel for many years.

With increasing time the bowel contracts until its lumen is as small as 1 cm in diameter. The mucosa is granular in appearance and shows diffuse non-specific inflammation of a relatively mild character. The submucosa and serosa contain an excess of adipose tissue and the muscularis propria is thickened. The inflammation is almost certainly due to stasis of intestinal contents with bacterial invasion of the mucous membrane. These changes, unless very extreme, are reversible if bowel continuity is restored.

Collagenous colitis

The first case was reported in 1976 by Lindstrom.[147] Most patients have been middle-aged women with watery diarrhoea. The main microscopic change is the formation of a dense eosinophilic band of collagen beneath the basement membrane of the surface epithelium (Fig. 8.33).[148,149] The mucosa is otherwise normal, though some authors have described an increased lymphocytic infiltrate in the lamina propria.[150] The change may be patchy and is most marked in the left colon and rectum, though involvement of the right colon has been described.[151] The collagenous band ranges from 10–100 μm in thickness. Stains for amyloid and immunoglobulin are negative. Ultrastructural

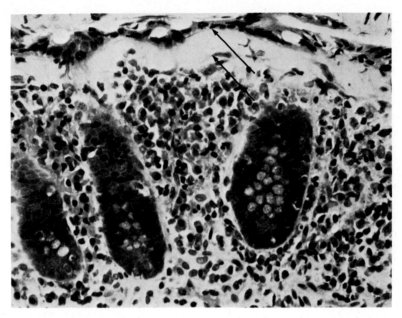

Fig. 8.33 Collagenous colitis. A thickened collagenous plate (located between arrows) underlies the surface epithelium.

Haematoxylin-eosin   × 400

studies have confirmed that the band consists of collagen and have shown changes in the basement membrane and endothelial cells of superficial capillaries.[152] The collagenous plate has been observed to regress following treatment.[150,151] It is not clear whether the diarrhoea is due to an absorptive or a secretory defect.[153] The underlying pathogenesis is unknown but suggestions include infection,[150] hypoxia and a disturbance of the pericryptal sheath.[153]

Colitis in graft-versus-host disease (GVHD)

Colitis in the recipients of bone marrow transplants may be due to the underlying condition, the effects of chemotherapeutic agents, radiation and opportunistic infection as well as GVHD itself. The earliest changes of GVHD are seen in the immature crypt base cells, which show vacuolar degeneration. However, the endocrine cell population is preserved. Crypt abscess formation ensues, proceeding ultimately to crypt destruction and ulceration.[154,155] Some of the conditions which are treated by bone marrow transplantation may be accompanied by

gastrointestinal abnormalities, including colitis. These include chronic granulomatous disease of childhood[156] and immunodeficiency syndromes.[157]

Proctitis in homosexuals and the acquired immune deficiency syndrome (AIDS)

Non-specific inflammation of the rectal mucosa is a common finding in male homosexuals.[158] Aetiological factors include mechanical trauma, the insertion of various materials, including drugs, per anum, and infection. Sideroplages are a useful sign of traumatic haemorrhage. Certain infections are being described with increasing frequency in male homosexuals, though not limited to this population. They include gonorrhoea (see p. 328), spirochaetosis[158,159] (see p. 328), lymphogranuloma venereum[160] (see p. 329) and amoebiasis[161,162] (see p. 330). There may be co-existing anal and perianal lesions (see p. 403).

The acquired immune deficiency syndrome (AIDS) may be accompanied by severe enterocolitis due to a number of opportunistic pathogens (Fig. 8.34). These include *Mycobacterium avium-intracellulare*, (Fig. 8.34).[163] cytomegalovirus (see

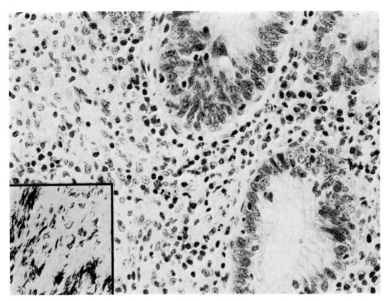

Fig. 8.34 *Mycobacterium avium-intracellulare* colitis from a patient with acquired immunodeficiency syndrome. The lamina propria contains a diffuse infiltrate of pale histiocytes. These are filled with acid-fast bacilli (inset).
Haematoxylin-eosin   × 250; Ziehl-Neelsen (inset)   × 250

p. 329), herpes simplex virus (see p. 329), cryptosporidium[164] (see p. 332) and candida (see p. 330). Two or more of these infections may co-exist in the same patient. Kaposi's sarcoma commonly involves the gut, including the colon, when this complication develops during the course of the disease. Gastrointestinal lymphoma is a rarer complicating malignancy.

VASCULAR DISORDERS

ISCHAEMIC BOWEL DISEASE

This term refers to the alterations to the bowel wall which follow an hypoxic episode. The spectrum of change ranges from complete recovery in mild cases, through partial resolution with fibrosis, to transmural infarction.[165] The extent and pattern of disease depend on the state of the vessels, anatomy of the blood supply, blood pressure, duration of the hypoxic episode and the bacterial population within the bowel lumen. Immune mechanisms may play a role and intravascular coagulation due to a 'single organ' Shwartzman reaction may

represent one of the underlying mechanisms.[166] Complete occlusion of the arteries supplying the affected bowel wall is rarely demonstrated. Ischaemia plays an important role in the pathogenesis of a variety of conditions. These include classical ischaemic colitis, necrotizing enterocolitis of infancy, necrotizing enterocolitis associated with neutropenia, certain forms of infective colitis, radiation colitis, uraemic colitis, colitis associated with intestinal obstruction, stercoral ulceration, simple ulcer, solitary ulcer syndrome and haemolytic uraemic syndrome. Various terms have been used to describe the spectrum of changes associated with ischaemic colitis. Membranous or acute ischaemic colitis refers to mild disease with involvement limited to the mucosa. Haemorrhagic or acute colonic necrosis has been applied to severe and extensive disease involving the full thickness of the bowel. When infarction is accompanied by gangrene due to secondary invasion by organisms from the faeces, the term necrotizing colitis has been used.

Ischaemic colitis is probably underdiagnosed and it is now realized that even young patients are not exempt. Oestrogen therapy[167] (leading to thrombotic occlusion of small vessels) and sickle cell disease[168] are causes of ischaemic bowel disease in the young. Vasculitis is discussed on p. 353.

Acute ischaemia

The reaction of the colon to ischaemia can be divided into three phases: (1) acute, with haemorrhage and necrosis; (2) reparative, with granulation tissue formation and fibrosis, and (3) later forms of residual pathology with ischaemic stricture and chronic complications.

The colon has a relatively poor blood supply, particularly the left side.[169] The splenic flexure and the descending colon are the areas of maximum susceptibility, but disease may involve any segment and even the whole colon. Rectal involvement is being recognized with increasing frequency.[170] Combined involvement of small and large intestine is not infrequent.

In the early stages the bowel is dilated and darkly congested, with a red, oedematous mucosa. The wall is friable and is usually thinner than normal. Mucosal ulceration may be superficial only; it may also be deep and linear in distribution, with extensive denudation of mucous membrane, sometimes with perforation. The lumen is filled with altered blood and there is an inflammatory peritoneal reaction. Inflammatory polyposis due to undermining ulceration of mucosa with the formation of mucosal tags is not uncommon. The whole appearance can mimic that seen in fulminating ulcerative colitis with toxic megacolon (see p. 337). When infarction of the colon is partial thickness only, mucosal necrosis may give rise to a grey membrane loosely adherent to the surface. In some cases there are patches of gangrene present due to complete necrosis of the tissues of the bowel wall. If a patient has survived an episode of infarction for some days or longer, then signs of resolution will appear. The bowel wall becomes thicker, contracted and indurated and the very dark appearance is replaced by signs of revascularization. These changes fade imperceptibly into the stage of ischaemic stricture.

The histological changes are often confined to the mucosa and submucosa. The muscularis is relatively resistant to the effects of hypoxia. The mucosal involvement is usually patchy with intact and normal intervening mucosa which is raised up by submucosal oedema or haemorrhage. This gives a cobblestone appearance and accounts for the diagnostic 'thumb-printing' radiological sign.

The microscopic pathology of ischaemic colitis is distinctive and readily distinguished from other inflammatory bowel disease. There is haemorrhage into the mucosa, and sometimes the submucosa, accompanied by oedema and necrosis. Epithelial tubules often appear to be 'bursting' and are covered with a layer of fibrin and necrotic tissue (Fig. 8.35). In severe cases with coagulative necrosis, only a shadowy outline of the normal structure remains. There is only a moderate leukocyte infiltration during the early stage, but this increases later and is accompanied by sloughing with mucosal ulceration. Fibrin thrombi within mucosal and submucosal capillaries are particularly characteristic. Gram stains will often reveal colo-

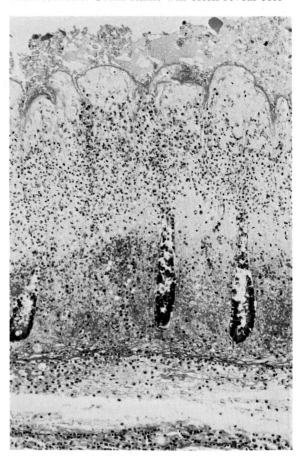

Fig. 8.35 Ischaemic colitis. The infarcted mucosa shows disrupted crypts and haemorrhage within the lamina propria. Haematoxylin-eosin   × 100

nies of bacteria in the mucosa and submucosa. The muscularis propria is destroyed in severe cases, but often relatively spared. However, as in early stages of intestinal ischaemia, the muscle fibres can show poor staining and loss of nuclei when the more obvious pathology is in the mucosa and submucosa.

Reparative phase

The effects of acute ischaemia are followed by subacute and chronic inflammation with the formation of granulation tissue. Microscopic fissures may lead down to or into the muscularis propria at points of deeper hypoxic damage. The granulation tissue reaction is exuberant and, in conjunction with the residual islands of inflamed and sometimes hyperplastic mucosa, presents a pattern mimicking Crohn's disease or chronic active ulcerative colitis. Eosinophils and iron-pigment-laden histiocytes are a variable feature. The latter are evidence of prior haemorrhage in the submucosa and mucosa. This is important in differentiating ischaemic from inflammatory bowel disease. Epithelial cell regeneration is visible at the margin of the mucosal ulcers in the form of young cells growing in a thin sheet over the bed of inflamed granulation tissue.

Ischaemic stricture

Most cases of severe and extensive infarction of the colon never reach the stage of stricture, because the small intestine is often involved and the patient dies of shock. Ischaemic strictures treated by surgical excision are relatively short and usually are situated at the splenic flexure.[165] The strictures may be tubular or fusiform and at the site of some there is sacculation of the gut wall. In all cases there is obvious fibrosis and this may extend deeply into the pericolic tissues. The submucosa is characteristically widened and filled with granulation tissue. Mucosal ulceration is patchy (Fig. 8.36). The differential diagnosis from segmental Crohn's disease of the colon may be difficult prior to microscopic examination.

The principal histological feature of ischaemic stricture is full-thickness loss of mucosa in the ulcerated areas, the surface of which is covered by

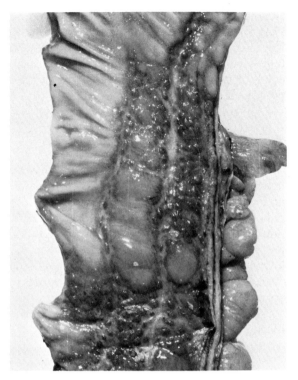

Fig. 8.36 Ischaemic stricture of colon. The mucosal ulceration is patchy with a serpiginous outline and a longitudinal orientation.

granulation tissue. At the edge of the ulcerated areas, epithelial regeneration is present with columnar epithelium beginning to grow over the surface. Neighbouring intact mucosa may show patchy atrophy. The adjacent muscularis mucosae shows splaying of its fibres and fibrosis. The submucosa is widened and filled with a characteristic granulomatous reaction with a marked proliferation of fibroblasts. Macrophages, full of haemosiderin pigment, are a feature of the cellular infiltrate. The muscularis propria is relatively spared but may show patchy fibrosis with replacement and separation of its fibres by granulation tissue identical and continuous with that seen in the submucosal layer.

Neonatal necrotizing enterocolitis[171]

This is a rare and often fatal form of ischaemic bowel disease which affects premature infants, especially when there has been a period of stress.

Infants present with abdominal distension, vomiting and bloody diarrhoea. The disease may be restricted to the colon, which shows extensive mucosal ulceration, vascular congestion and thickening of the bowel wall. Submucosal cysts are a prominent feature (pneumatosis coli).

Transient ischaemic colitis[165,172]

There is a transient or reversible form of ischaemia in which the patient presents with crampy abdominal pain, diarrhoea and rectal bleeding. The radiological features of ischaemia quickly revert to normal. Although the diagnosis is usually clinical the pathologist may obtain material when the disease involves the rectum or sigmoid colon or at colonoscopy. Sequential biopsies show features of acute haemorrhagic necrosis of the mucosa with subsequent return to normal or to a regenerative mucosal pattern.

Neutropenic enterocolitis[173]

This is a haemorrhagic necrotizing enterocolitis which mainly affects the right colon. Patients usually have an underlying leukaemia or lymphoma.

Obstructive colitis[174]

Colitis may occur in association with obstruction of the large bowel, particularly carcinoma. Ten per cent of cases are due to other obstructing lesions such as diverticulitis, volvulus, Hirschsprung's disease and faecal impaction. The colitis takes the form of ulcers which are often linear, run longitudinally and are covered by fibrinopurulent material. Intervening mucosa is congested and raised up by submucosal oedema and haemorrhage. In nearly all cases described, the colitis has been proximal to the obstruction and separated from it by a short zone of relatively normal mucosa. The histology is essentially the same as for the earlier stages of ischaemic bowel disease. It has been suggested that a rise in intraluminal pressure related to the obstruction results in a fall in intramural blood flow with resulting ischaemic necrosis.

Stercoral ulceration

This is not infrequently seen at autopsy in elderly patients with a history of intractable constipation. The appearances resemble ischaemic injury and are probably brought about by the pressure of impacted faecal material in the presence of circulatory deficiency. The ulcers are sharply demarcated and histology shows mucosal loss and transmural inflammation.

Non-specific ulcer of the colon

This may present acutely with perforation, mimicking acute appendicitis, or in a chronic form in which the patient complains of abdominal pain and diarrhoea and is found to have a tender mass in the right iliac fossa.[175] The right colon is the most usual site of involvement. Multiple ulcers occur in a minority of patients. Left-sided disease may resemble diverticulitis. The aetiology is not understood, but ischaemia probably plays an important role. Predisposing factors include steroid and other anti-inflammatory drug therapy, oral contraceptives, renal transplantation and non-specific stress. Cytomegalovirus has been identified in a series of seven out of nine cases but its presence could be secondary.[176]

The ulcers are usually found on the antimesenteric border of the colon. They are sharply punched out and, if chronic, show a bed of granulation and fibrous tissue. Small vessels may contain fibrin thrombi.

Solitary ulcer/mucosal prolapse syndrome

The term solitary ulcer syndrome is a misnomer in as much as ulceration is a late feature of the disease and may be multiple. The characteristic mucosal changes are probably the result of ischaemia due to stretching of vessels within prolapsed mucosa. Trauma may also play a role. The mucosal prolapse is internal and may result from faulty motility of the puborectalis muscle. This causes the patient to strain at defaecation. The commonest symptoms are rectal bleeding, passage of mucus, perineal pain and tenesmus. The lesions are usually located on the anterior or anterolateral walls of the rectum and vary in shape and size.[177]

The earliest microscopic changes are fibrosis of the lamina propria and upwards extension of smooth muscle fibres from the thickened muscularis mucosae (Fig. 8.37). The crypts may appear hyperplastic and sometimes a villous configuration is seen. These changes may lead to a mistaken diagnosis of adenoma. The misplacement of cystic glands into the submucosa may mimic invasive carcinoma. This appearance has been referred to as 'localized colitis cystica profunda'.[178] Ulceration is usually superficial, if present, and never extends beyond the submucosa. Identical mucosal changes are seen in the apex of a complete rectal prolapse, the apex of a prolapsing haemorrhoid and the tip of a colostomy. Ischaemia may be the common pathogenetic mechanism in all these conditions.

Vasculitis

The gastrointestinal tract is involved in up to 50% of patients with polyarteritis nodosa, but colonic manifestations are rarely the cause of the initial presentation (Fig. 8.38). Colonic involvement may present with the signs of ischaemic bowel disease, perforation or an apple-core lesion on examination by barium enema simulating carcinoma.[179] Vasculitis associated with systemic lupus erythematosus may also present as diffuse ischaemic bowel disease.[180] Behçet's disease[181] may involve the colon with the formation of discrete, symmetrical, punched-out ulcers (Fig. 8.39). It is not clear whether these are due to an underlying vasculitis.

Buerger's disease

Involvement of sigmoid colon (among other intestinal lesions) has been recorded in Buerger's disease (thromboangeitis obliterans).[182]

Polycythaemia rubra vera

Thrombosis of the middle colic artery causing gangrene and perforation of the transverse colon has been described.[183]

Vascular anomalies

A spectrum of vascular anomalies occurs in the colon and rectum. Attempts to classify this group have met with only partial success. One detailed classification is based upon the type and size of vessels involved as well as any associated systemic or cutaneous lesions.[184] The defects of such classifications are twofold. Firstly, the pathogenesis of

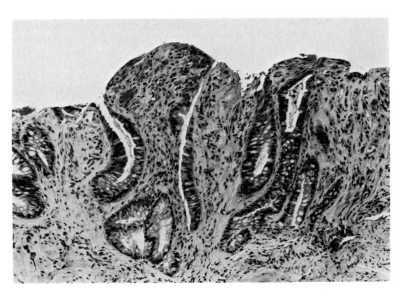

Fig. 8.37 Solitary ulcer syndrome. Bundles of smooth muscle extend up into the lamina propria and the crypts appear hyperplastic and show mucin depletion.
Haematoxylin-eosin   × 100

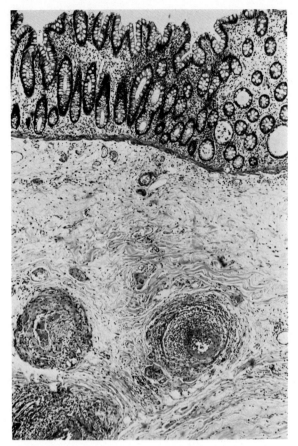

Fig. 8.38 Polyarteritis nodosa. Medium-sized arteries with the submucosa are infiltrated and cuffed by an acute inflammatory infiltrate.

Haematoxylin-eosin   × 100

many anomalies is unknown. Secondly, it is difficult to be certain whether a dilated, thin-walled vessel is a capillary vessel or an arteriole.

Cavernous haemangioma

This is a hamartoma or congenital malformation which increases in size *pari passu* with the viscus. Rectal bleeding is the usual presenting sign; intussusception is rare.[185] The rectum and sigmoid colon are the sites of predilection.[186] The abnormality involves the entire blood supply, including the perirectal or pericolic tissues and sometimes surrounding viscera. Macroscopically, the mucous membrane is plum-coloured, but otherwise normal. Large, tortuous vascular channels can be seen in the bowel wall and adjacent tissues. These are lined by endothelium, which may appear hyperplastic. Thrombosis leads to hyalinization and calcification (phleboliths). More localized types of cavernous haemangioma may project from the mucosal surface to form a polypoid lesion.

Angioectasia

A bewildering profusion of names has now been linked to one of the commonest vascular anomalies and an important cause of gastrointestinal bleeding—angiodysplasia, vascular ectasia, phlebectasia, arteriovenous malformation, haemangioma and telangiectasia. Our preferred term is angioec-

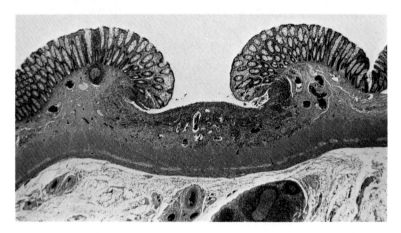

Fig. 8.39 Behçet's disease involving colon. A characteristically symmetrical ulcer is bordered by normal colonic mucosa.

Haematoxylin-eosin   × 16

tasia, which is purely descriptive. The pathogenesis of this lesion is unknown. Some workers regard the anomaly as an age-associated phenomenon,[187] but the condition has been reported in an adolescent.[188] Nonetheless, most patients are elderly and present either with acute colonic haemorrhage, or more commonly with chronic blood loss leading to iron-deficiency anaemia.[189] The lesion comprises clusters of dilated, thin-walled vessels in the mucosa and submucosa. The right colon opposite the ileo-caecal valve is the site of predilection, but jejunal and gastric involvement has been described. Angiography has been the traditional method of diagnosis, but colonoscopy coupled with electrocoagulation therapy has become popular as a method for combining diagnosis with treatment.

Angioectasias of various types have been described in association with von Willebrand's disease, Rendu-Osler-Weber syndrome (hereditary haemorrhagic telangiectasia), Turner's syndrome, calcinosis-Raynaud's-sclerodactyly-telangiectasia (CRST) syndrome, systemic sclerosis, Peutz-Jeghers syndrome, blue rubber-bleb naevus syndrome (Bean's syndrome) and Klippel-Trenaunay-Weber syndrome.[184]

Lymphangioma

These are very uncommon and are usually incidental findings. They typically involve mesenteric tissues rather than the wall of the bowel itself. They may occasionally present as polypoid lesions, but are more usually diffuse and ill-defined. The pathogenesis is unknown. Some cases of diffuse colonic lymphangiectasia have presented with malabsorption, protein loss and potassium depletion.[190] This probably represents a hamartomatous abnormality, similar to lymphangiectasia of the small intestine (see p. 242).

EPITHELIAL POLYPS

A polyp is a circumscribed tumour projecting above an epithelial surface and may be either sessile or pedunculated. Many lesions may assume such a form, but non-epithelial causes of polyp formation will be considered separately. A histological classification of benign epithelial polyps is given in Table 8.4.

Hyperplastic (metaplastic) polyp

This is a frequently encountered, non-neoplastic epithelial lesion, whose aetiology is unknown. It occurs less commonly in Japan, but increased numbers are found in Japanese who have migrated to Hawaii.[191] This suggests that environmental factors, possibly dietary, are involved in their causation. The underlying defect is a form of dyskinesis in which the proliferative compartment of the crypt becomes elongated or hyperplastic. Migration of cells above the proliferative zone is slowed because surface cells are retained longer than their normal counterparts.[192] These cells become hypermature[192,193] and their metabolic

Table 8.4 Histological classification of epithelial polyps of the large intestine based on underlying pathogenesis

Type	Single or small numbers	Multiple
Dysmature	Hyperplastic (metaplastic) polyp	Hyperplastic (metaplastic) polyposis

Neoplastic	Adenoma—tubular
	            tubulo-villous
	            villous
		Adenomatosis (familial polyposis)

Hamartomatous	Juvenile polyp Peutz-Jeghers polyp	Juvenile polyposis Peutz-Jeghers syndrome Cowden's syndrome ?Cronkhite-Canada syndrome
Inflammatory	Inflammatory polyp (pseudo-polyp)	Inflammatory polyposis (pseudo-polyposis)

exhaustion is evidenced by the synthesis of incomplete mucins,[194,195] cytoplasmic accumulation of carcinoembryonic antigen,[194] failure to translocate IgA[196] and several enzymatic deficiencies.[197,198] Columnar cells of normal colorectal epithelium are compressed inconspicuously between adjacent goblet cells. However, the volume of columnar cell cytoplasm in hyperplastic polyps is much greater than normal. This is in part due to an accumulation of intracytoplasmic mucin. The slowed migration increases the number of these filled-out cells per crypt and the resulting excess of cytoplasm is accommodated by crypt infolding or serration (Fig. 8.40).

Hyperplastic polyps were once considered to represent a form of senile degeneration.[199] Their age dependence is not well demonstrated in recent population studies[200] and cases of large, multiple polyps have been recorded in young individuals.[201]

Hyperplastic polyps appear as pale, sessile nodules arising on the mucosal folds (Fig. 8.41). They are usually less than 5 mm in diameter. Larger varieties may become pedunculated and be mistaken for adenomas. They occur throughout the colon (including the appendix) but are more common in the rectum and sigmoid colon. They are frequently discovered in very large numbers clustering around a carcinoma of the sigmoid colon or rectum. Although there is little evidence that

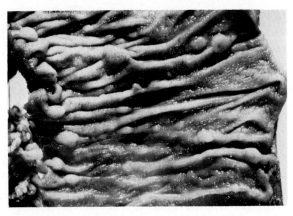

Fig. 8.41 Hyperplastic (metaplastic) polyposis. Characteristic pale nodules are situated mainly on the mucosal folds.

hyperplastic epithelium is more prone to neoplastic change than normal epithelium, it has been suggested that hyperplastic polyps might signal the presence of an environmental factor implicated in colorectal carcinogenesis.[202] Convincing reports of dysplastic or carcinomatous change are few, and limited to cases of large multiple polyps (*hyperplastic polyposis*).[203–205] Hyperplastic polyposis has been described in young individuals and may mimic familial adenomatosis coli.[201]

Histological examination reveals a slightly thickened mucosa. The cells lining the proliferative compartment show enlarged vesicular nuclei with prominent nucleoli. The nuclear membrane is delicate and there is no hyperchromatism. Mitotic figures may be numerous. There may be pseudo-invasion with disruption of the muscularis mucosae, mimicking malignant infiltration. Above the level of the proliferative zone, the crypts become serrated and are lined by goblet cells and columnar cells (Fig. 8.42). The latter show a distinct brush border and contain apical mucin droplets which are more PAS positive than normal colonic mucus. The columnar cell cytoplasm is typically pale and eosinophilic. Hyperplastic change of this type may occasionally be observed in adenomas[201] and juvenile polyps and not uncommonly in chronic ulcerative colitis.[206]

Adenoma

This is a benign neoplasm with the potential for malignant change. It may be described as a

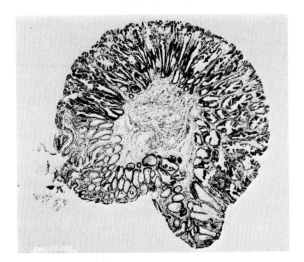

Fig. 8.40 Hyperplastic (metaplastic) polyp of the large intestine. The characteristic serrated contour of the hyperplastic crypts contrasts with the normal crypts (below). Haematoxylin-eosin ×20

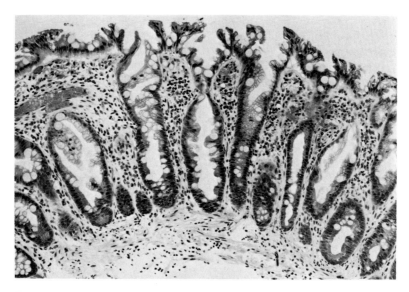

Fig. 8.42 Hyperplastic polyp showing characteristic serrated crypt contour.
Haematoxylin-eosin   × 100

circumscribed focus of dysplastic epithelium.[207] Most cases present either as a sessile or pedunculated polyp, but a small percentage may be entirely flat. The transition into the adjacent normal mucosa is always abrupt. The configuration may be either tubular, tubulo-villous or villous and it is upon this basis that adenomas are classified.[208] This replaces the earlier terminology of adenomatous polyp, papillary adenoma and villous papilloma respectively. Adenoma may present as a solitary lesion, but some patients produce several adenomas, with new crops being demonstrated on successive examinations of the colon and rectum.

Adenomas are larger and occur with greater frequency in populations at a higher risk of developing colorectal cancer.[209] They occur with greater frequency in males. It is thought that genetic factors determine the susceptibility to adenoma formation whereas environmental factors may cause the adenoma to grow, show increasing dysplasia and ultimately transform into a malignant neoplasm.[210] Population studies have shown adenomas to be evenly distributed throughout the colon and rectum.[211] However, the largest adenomas are found in the left colon and rectum, which are the sites of predilection for carcinomas.[212,213]

Microreconstruction and cell kinetic methods employing tritiated thymidine have suggested that neoplastic transformation first takes place in the proliferative zone at the crypt base. This extends to replace the compartment of maturing cells so that dividing cells in various states of maturity are found in the upper crypt and surface epithelium.[214–216] Uncontrolled crypt division, budding and surface folding may then occur to produce a polypoid growth with its particular architectural characteristics. The above view of the morphogenesis of adenoma is not universally accepted. A recent detailed microreconstruction study in specimens of adenomatosis coli suggests that the buds of single-gland adenomas originate in the proliferative zone but then sprout into the lamina propria whilst migrating upwards to form a single-gland adenoma in the upper part of the mucosa.[217]

All adenomas are dysplastic, but not all dysplastic epithelium is polypoid. Not only may the occasional flat adenoma be encountered, but dysplasia may occur in flat mucosa in such conditions as ulcerative colitis.[206] For this reason the concept of the adenoma-carcinoma sequence has been superseded by the dysplasia-carcinoma sequence.[213] Dysplasia is regarded as synonymous with intra-epithelial neoplastic change and is recognized by a combination of cytological atypia, architectural disorder and aberrant differentiation. A series of adenomas will show all grades of dysplasia ranging from mild or low grade, which deviates minimally from normal, through to severe or high-grade dysplasia, which amounts to carcinoma-in-situ.[213] It is wise to avoid the term carcinoma-in-situ when reporting one's observations, as misinterpretation may lead to overzealous treatment. Furthermore, mucin[218] and enzyme[197,198] histochemistry as well as DNA flow cytometric,[219] cytogenetic, cell culture and animal transplantation studies[220] have indicated fundamental differences between adenomatous (dysplastic) and carcinomatous cells. The suggestion that all adenomas represent carcinoma-in-situ should be resisted from the experimental as well as the clinical standpoint.

Tubular adenoma

This is the commonest of the three types of adenoma. The size varies from less than 0.1 cm to several centimetres in diameter, but most are a little less than 1 cm. Small adenomas are sessile but lesions approaching 1 cm in diameter are usually pedunculated (Fig. 8.43). Tubular adenomas resemble miniature cauliflowers with an irregular surface which is darker than the surrounding mucosa.

Microscopic examination reveals closely-packed epithelial tubules with little papillary infolding (Fig. 8.44). In mild dysplasia both goblet cells and columnar cells are recognized (Fig. 8.45). With loss of differentiation these cell types are replaced by a single population of immature columnar cells secreting little or no mucus. These usually show a dark, amphophilic cytoplasm. Nuclei in mild dysplasia are a little enlarged and crowded and mitoses are numerous (Fig. 8.45). With increasing dysplasia the nuclei enlarge further and become hyperchromatic, elongated and pseudostratified (Fig. 8.46). In severe or high-grade dysplasia they may assume a more rounded configuration with a prominent nucleolus (Fig. 8.47). There are also notable architectural changes, with excessive budding and branching producing—in severe dysplasia—a gland-within-gland pattern. Paneth cells and endocrine cells may be scattered haphazardly throughout adenomatous epithelium.

Villous adenoma

These are often large sessile tumours, but may also be pedunculated. The surface is shaggy or velvety and the neoplastic tissues are soft and fragment easily (Fig. 8.48). Occasionally, villous adenomas may be initially flat, making their endoscopic diagnosis difficult. Multiple villous adenomas are rare, but villous adenomas often co-exist with tubular adenomas. Most are said to occur in the sigmoid colon and rectum, but a colonoscopic survey from St Mark's Hospital indicates a wider distribution throughout the colon.[213]

Low-power microscopy shows slender villi with the intervillous epithelium lying directly above the muscularis mucosae (Fig. 8.49). Dysplastic change as described under tubular adenoma is seen in the lining epithelium. Not uncommonly, the dysplasia is very mild and the epithelium comprises tall mucous cells. Excess secretion of mucus may lead to the clinical presentation of dehydration and electrolyte depletion. The propensity for malignant change is high.[221] Mucinous carcinomas show a significant association with villous adenomas;[221] this is not surprising in view of their similar cytology.

Tubulo-villous adenoma

These may be regarded as intermediate between the tubular and villous adenomas in terms of their architectural configuration, size and malignant potential (Fig. 8.50).[221] Although the majority are pedunculated like tubular adenomas, sessile forms are sometimes seen (Fig. 8.51).

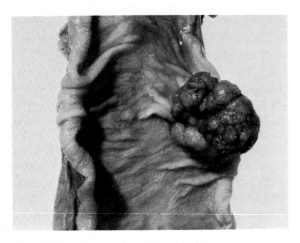

Fig. 8.43 Tubular adenoma of sigmoid colon.

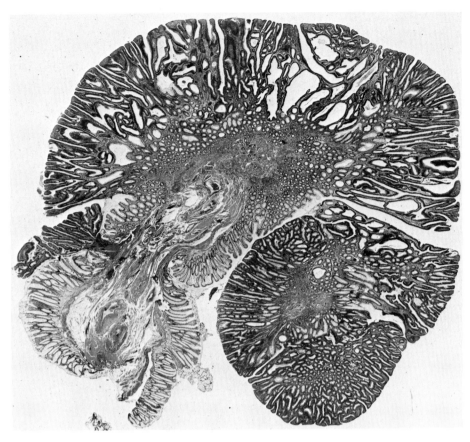

Fig. 8.44 Tubular adenoma.
Haematoxylin-eosin   × 9

Malignant adenoma

The great majority of adenomas do not undergo malignant change. In a series of adenomas, only 1% of those under 1 cm (74% of adenomas) contained invasive cancer.[221] On the other hand, 35% of adenomas over 2 cm showed malignant change (Fig. 8.52). The risk of malignant change is also increased in patients with multiple adenomas, in villous lesions and, perhaps most importantly of all, in adenomas showing high-grade or severe dysplasia.[213,221] Carcinoma is only diagnosed when neoplastic epithelium has penetrated the muscularis mucosae. The mucosa contains few lymphatics.[223] Neoplastic tissues confined to the mucosa are unable to metastasize and the term intramucosal carcinoma is inappropriate and potentially misleading. It is important to distinguish between malignant infiltration and pseudo-invasion (Fig. 8.53). The latter is due to traumatic implantation of adenomatous epithelium into the stalk of an adenoma. This will be accompanied by evidence of haemorrhage such as macrophages containing haemosiderin. On the other hand, the cytological and architectural features of malignancy and an associated desmoplastic response will be lacking.[224]

Malignant infiltration within the stalk of an adenoma is not an indication for further surgery provided that the carcinomatous glands have been completely excised. The completeness of excision is demonstrated by the careful examination of well-orientated step sections through the core of the polyp. Further treatment is advised for poorly-differentiated carcinoma. This form of management requires endoscopic removal of the polyp as

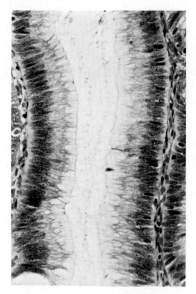

Fig. 8.45 Adenoma showing mild dysplasia. The nuclei are slightly enlarged and show crowding and elongation. Mucin secretion is reduced but still evident and polarity is retained.

Haematoxylin-eosin   × 150

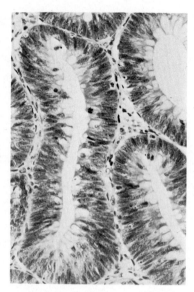

Fig. 8.46 Adenoma showing moderate dysplasia. There is focal loss of nuclear polarity, an increase in the nucleocytoplasmic ratio and further loss of mucin production. The nuclei are still slender with finely stippled chromatin; the cytological appearances fall short of malignancy.

Haematoxylin-eosin   × 150

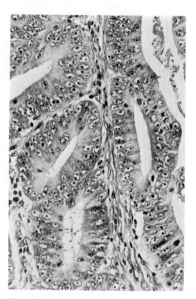

Fig. 8.47 Adenoma showing severe dysplasia. The nuclei are ovoid and vesicular and contain prominent nuclei; the cytological appearances resemble those of malignant epithelium (carcinoma-in-situ). There is no mucin secretion.

Haematoxylin-eosin   × 60

a 'total excisional biopsy'. Although this practice has been successful at St Mark's Hospital,[225] some authors regard endoscopic polypectomy as inadequate treatment for invasive carcinoma.[226] In a detailed review of this subject it is suggested that lymphatic permeation should be added to the above criteria for further surgery.[227]

Adenomatosis coli (familial polyposis coli)

In this condition, many hundreds and often thousands of adenomas are present throughout the colon. This is associated with the inevitable development of colorectal cancer in untreated cases. It is inherited as an autosomal dominant condition and affects both sexes equally. The child of an affected parent therefore has a 50% chance of inheriting the disease. The adenomas begin to appear in the second or third decades of life, though later development can occur. The figure of 100 adenomas has been suggested as a convenient distinction between adenomatosis coli and multiple adenomas.[228]

The usual symptoms are increasing bowel motions which later become associated with the passage of mucus and blood. The average age at diagnosis in propositus cases is 35 years and two-thirds will have developed a carcinoma by this time. The average age of propositus cases with carcinoma is 39 years and without carcinoma 27 years. This suggests that adenomas exist for an average of 12 years before malignancy appears, and even then only one or two out of several thousand will have become malignant.

Inspection of a colectomy specimen will show numerous polyps, most of which are tubular adenomas (Fig. 8.54). Small polyps are less pedunculated and the smallest are sessile nodules on the mucosal surface. Histological examination often shows the presence of micro-adenomas consisting of a few (sometimes single) dysplastic tubules; these would not have been visible on gross inspection of the mucosal surface.

Cancer prevention is dependent upon early diagnosis and colectomy before the adenomas have undergone malignant change. This is achieved by

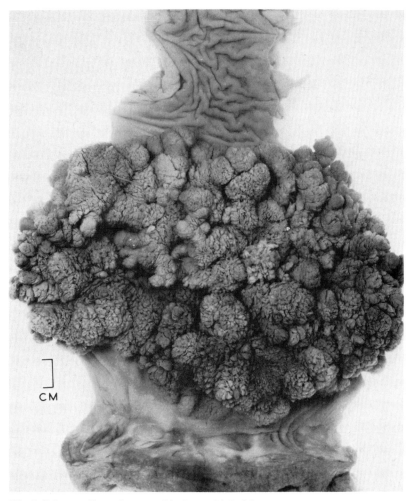

Fig. 8.48 Large villous adenoma of the lower third of the rectum.
Specimen from the Pathology Museum, Charing Cross Hospital Medical School, London, reproduced by permission of the Curator, Dr F.J. Paradinas. Photograph by Miss P.M. Turnbull, Charing Cross Hospital Medical School.

preparing a family pedigree and examining the siblings of the propositus straight away and all children from the age of about 14.

Ornithine decarboxylase has been proposed as a marker of clinically normal family members who carry the polyposis genotype.[229]

Gardner's syndrome

Adenomatosis coli may be associated with various extracolonic lesions.[230] Gardner and co-workers reported a syndrome consisting of adenomatosis coli, multiple osteomas of the skull and mandible, multiple cysts and soft tissue tumours of the skin.[231] The syndrome has been modified by Gardner and others as an increasing range of extracolonic manifestations has been recorded. These include osteomas of the entire skeleton,[232] abdominal and intra-abdominal desmoid tumours,[233] diffuse fibrosis of the mesentery and retroperitoneum,[234] dental abnormalities,[235] adenomas of the small intestine, periampullary region of the duodenum and stomach,[236-238] carcinoma of the periampullary region, fundic gland cyst polyps in the stomach,[239] papillary carcinoma of the thyroid,[240] tumours of the central nervous system,[241] hepatoblastoma[242] and multiple

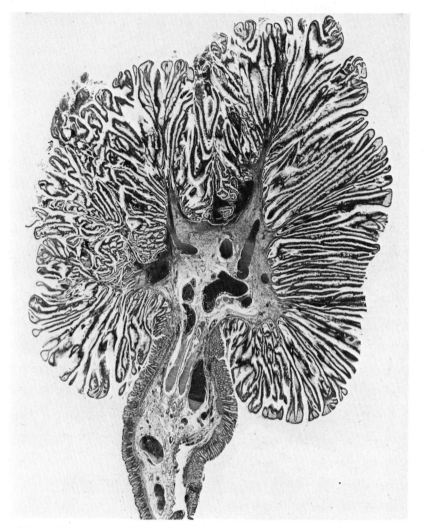

Fig. 8.49 Pedunculated villous adenoma. Serial reconstruction has shown that the villi are in fact epithelial folia or leaves.

Haematoxylin-eosin   × 6

endocrine adenomatosis type IIb.[243] The multiple combinations and permutations of extracolonic lesions make it virtually impossible to define Gardner's syndrome. Not only are the colorectal adenomas of adenomatosis coli and Gardner's syndrome indistinguishable, but subclinical osteomas of the mandible have been described in patients with otherwise typical adenomatosis coli.[244]

It is probably reasonable to regard adenomatosis coli as a single disease, in which varied extracolonic manifestations occur with a frequency yet to be determined.

Turcot's syndrome

The association between adenomatosis of the colon and malignant tumours of the central nervous system has been termed Turcot's syndrome.[241] The syndrome is apparently inherited on an autosomal recessive basis, although this remains controversial.[245] It appears to be distinct from familial adenomatosis not only in the mode of inheritance, but also because the adenomas are relatively few in number and cancer arises at an earlier age.

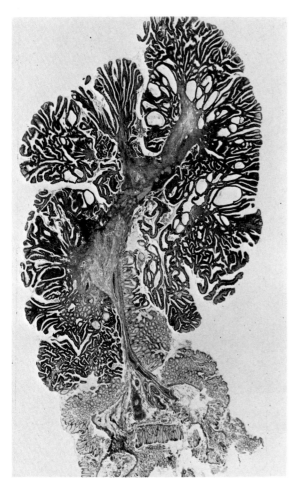

Fig. 8.50 Tubulo-villous adenoma.
Haematoxylin-eosin   × 8

Juvenile polyp

This is a non-neoplastic epithelial polyp composed of tissues indigenous to the site of origin, but arranged in a haphazard manner. Most are found in young children and they may occur as multiple familial lesions in association with various congenital defects.[246] These findings suggest that the juvenile polyp is a hamartoma rather than an acquired inflammatory lesion. However, inflammatory polyps may have a similar if not identical appearance.[247] It is possible that the lamina propria in affected individuals is especially prone to overgrowth at a particular developmental stage, but that this overgrowth is caused by a relatively trivial inflammatory stimulus. Colectomy for ju-venile polyposis (see below) affords an opportunity to examine juvenile polyps at the earliest stages of their development. They appear as a focus of oedematous and hyperaemic lamina propria with overlying epithelial ulceration.

The usual childhood lesion is solitary, but several may be present. Most occur in the rectum and present between the ages of 1–10 (peak at ages 4–5). Males and females are affected equally. Bleeding is the commonest symptom, but some may undergo amputation or prolapse through the anus. Macroscopically, the typical lesion has a smooth, spherical, red head and a narrow stalk. The cut surface shows cysts filled with mucin. The thin stalk lacks muscularis mucosae and the polyp is liable to torsion, venous congestion, haemorrhage and infarction.

Microscopically, the polyp consists of epithelial tubules, which may be dilated or cystic, embedded in an excess of lamina propria (Fig. 8.55). The tubules are lined by an essentially normal epithelium (Fig. 8.56). The surface is frequently ulcerated and there may be purulent inflammation of the lamina propria. There may occasionally be stromal metaplasia to cartilage or even bone. Muscularis mucosae is not included within the stroma. Solitary lesions are not thought to have any malignant potential, but one case with malignant change has been described[248] and dysplasia has also been observed in a solitary polyp.[249]

Juvenile polyposis

In this condition numerous polyps of juvenile type are found in the large bowel (Fig. 8.57) and sometimes in the small bowel and stomach.[250] One rare form occurs in infancy and is associated with diarrhoea, haemorrhage, malnutrition, intussusception and death at an early age.[251] No family history is found. The remaining cases vary in their age of onset and may either be familial or sporadic. Sporadic cases may be associated with various congenital defects including abnormalities of the cranium and heart, cleft palate, polydactyly and malrotations. Familial cases have been reported in three generations, suggesting an autosomal dominant inheritance.[252] There is often a significant excess of colorectal cancer in these families and the number of reports of patients with both juvenile

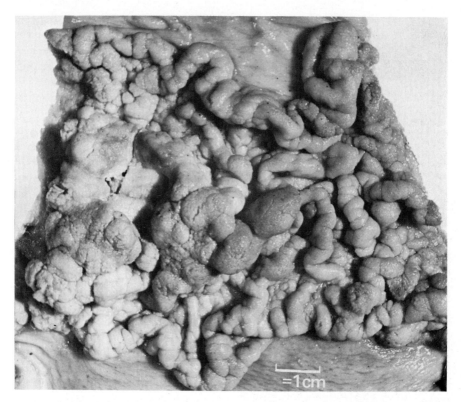

Fig. 8.51 Large sessile tubulo-villous adenoma of the upper third of the rectum. Malignant change has developed at the left of the mass, resulting in ulceration.

polyposis and cancer of the colon or rectum has risen in recent years.[253] It has been suggested that the risk of colorectal cancer may be 10%, which is at least three times the expected figure. The polyps in juvenile polyposis may adopt an atypical appearance, with papillary infolding, a relative reduction in the amount of lamina propria and absence of surface ulceration.[254] Polyps of this type are more prone to the development of dysplasia and this probably accounts for the increased propensity for malignant change.[255]

Juvenile polyposis has recently been described in association with ganglioneuromatous polyposis (see p. 385).[256]

Peutz-Jeghers polyps

Peutz-Jeghers syndrome has been discussed on page 239. In about half of all cases one or more small polyps are found in the colon or rectum, but these are rarely of clinical significance. However,

there are recent reports on colorectal cancer arising in association with the Peutz-Jeghers syndrome.[257–259] Occasionally one or more polyps of the Peutz-Jeghers type are found in the colon or rectum without any evidence of polyps in the stomach or small intestine. Such tumours show the typical tree-like branching of smooth muscle derived from the muscularis mucosae and are covered by an entirely normal colorectal epithelium. Grossly, such lesions mimic adenomas and the correct diagnosis depends upon microscopic examination.

Cronkhite-Canada syndrome

This rare form of non-neoplastic gastrointestinal polyposis does not show any familial tendency. The disease presents with alopecia, pigmentation of the skin, dystrophy of the nails, diarrhoea, protein-losing enteropathy and severe electrolyte disturbances.[260] The symptoms may suggest a diagnosis of

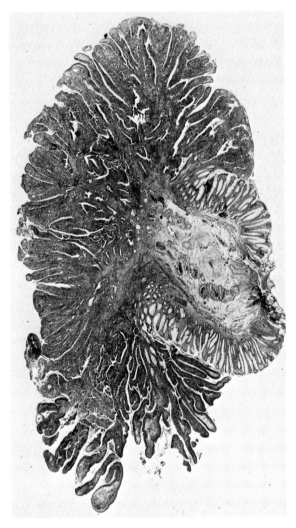

Fig. 8.52 Early malignant change within a pedunculated villous adenoma. The relatively small amount of residual adenomatous epithelium occupies the lower portion of the polyp.

Haematoxylin-eosin   × 15

ulcerative colitis.[261] There is often a fatal outcome. The mean age at presentation is 60 and there is a slight male predominance.

The gross appearances range from diffuse nodularity of the mucosa to the formation of large polyps which may appear gelatinous. Ulceration is not seen. Microscopically, the epithelial cysts show cystic dilatation with flattening of the lining epithelium. The lamina propria is oedematous with focal chronic inflammation and hyaline change.

The appearance resembles 'colitis cystica superficialis', a complication of pellagra.

Cowden's syndrome[262, 263]

This rare condition, named after the family in which it occurred, is characterized by the presence of gastrointestinal and cutaneous hamartomas and proliferative lesions of the breast and thyroid. Inheritance is probably autosomal dominant. The gastrointestinal lesions resemble juvenile polyposis and it is possible that Cowden's syndrome is a variant of juvenile polyposis. However, our knowledge of this syndrome is far from complete.

Inflammatory polyps

Non-neoplastic proliferations of either mucosa or granulation tissue may be due to various injuries of the colorectal epithelium. The most frequent cause is ulcerative colitis, but others include Crohn's disease and ischaemic bowel disease. Pseudo-polyposis is an alternative but less satisfactory term. The polyps range in their gross appearance from finger-like projections to rounded masses. Finger-like polyps are often fused or bifid, giving rise to bizarre shapes (see Fig. 8.21). Bridges, beneath which a probe can be passed, may be formed. Inflammatory polyps are usually multiple. Histologically, inflammatory and granulation tissue are present to a variable degree. Cystic dilatation of glands may produce an appearance resembling the juvenile polyp. This is especially true for inflammatory polyps arising at the site of ureterosigmoidostomy. However, juvenile and inflammatory polyps are distinguished by the appearance of the surrounding mucosa and the clinical history. Bizarre or giant pseudo-polyposis is discussed on page 346.

MALIGNANT EPITHELIAL TUMOURS
ADENOCARCINOMA

Adenocarcinoma is the commonest malignant tumour of the colon and rectum. Other much less frequently encountered neoplasms include undifferentiated, adenosquamous, squamous and endocrine cell carcinomas. In England and Wales there

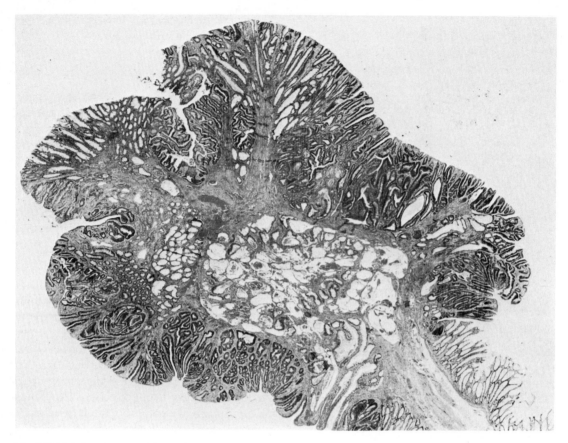

Fig. 8.53 Tubular adenoma with pseudo-invasion of the stalk.
Haematoxylin-eosin   × 10

are 6000 deaths per annum from rectal cancer and 10 000 from cancer of the colon. The actual incidence is higher, because approximately one third of all cases are cured by surgery. The incidence is rising and in the USA this is now the second most common malignant tumour (excluding skin cancer).

There are certain pathological and epidemiological differences between cancer of the colon and cancer of the rectum. However, it is convenient to consider the two regions together as the anatomical junction is arbitrarily defined (opposite the sacral promontory) and many carcinomas arise at the rectosigmoid junction itself.

Epidemiology

There are marked variations in the incidence of colorectal cancer throughout the world. Whilst the disease is common in North America, northern Europe, Australia and New Zealand it is seen much less frequently in South America and is rare in Africa and most parts of Asia. There is a good correlation between the consumption of meat and the incidence of colorectal cancer in various populations. Seventh Day Adventists, who consume little or no meat, show a relatively low rate of colorectal cancer as compared to their fellow Americans.[264] However, there may be two epidemiological subtypes of colorectal cancer: one related to diet and socio-economic status and the other not. One survey has shown that the incidence of cancer of the lower third of the rectum in countries with a low risk of colorectal cancer in general is similar to the incidence of cancer in the lower third of the rectum in countries with a high risk of colorectal cancer.[265] In Japanese who have adopted a Western-style diet the incidence of

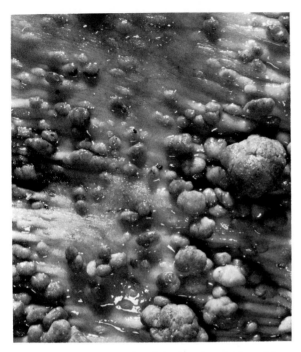

Fig. 8.54 Adenomatosis or familial polyposis coli. Most of the tubular adenomas show a lobulated and fissured surface.

colonic cancer is increased whereas the figure for rectal cancers is unaltered.[266,267] Colonic carcinoma may therefore represent a variable disease in which dietary factors are important, whereas rectal cancer appears to be an aetiologically more stable disease.[267] Nonetheless, there is evidence that the incidence of rectal cancer is falling in high-risk countries.[268] This supports the epidemiological distinction between rectal and colonic cancer, but indicates that environmental factors may in fact influence the development of rectal cancer.

Age and sex incidence

Colorectal cancer becomes more frequent with increasing age. The average age at the time of diagnosis is 60. In low-risk populations the average age at diagnosis is lower and the tumours typically arise in the right colon and include a high proportion of poorly differentiated mucinous or signet-ring cell subtypes. Rectal cancers are more common in males than females. Moving proximally to the right colon the ratio alters, becoming greater for females. The sex incidence is influenced by age with younger patients including more females. In later life the disease is more common in males.[254,269,270]

Aetiology

Epidemiological studies indicate the importance of environmental factors in the causation of colorectal cancer. The increased consumption of meat by high-risk populations will lead to a higher intake of animal fat and in turn to increased bile acid synthesis. Bile acids may promote tumour growth or may be converted into carcinogens by the intestinal microflora, which is itself modified by diet.[271,272] Cholesterol from the diet may also promote tumour growth directly.[273] Endogenous cell products, including sex hormones,[274] growth factors and locally-produced hormones, may also act as promoters. Western diets are low in 'fibre' or cellulose derived from plant cell walls.[275] This factor is probably not so much of importance in altering intestinal transit time[277] but may dilute the concentration of potential carcinogens by increasing the bulk of the stool or binding bile acids. 'Fibre' also acts as a substrate for fermenting microorganisms.[277] The products of fermentation are short-chain fatty acids including butyric acid. Acidification of the colon may prevent the degradation of bile acids into carcinogens.[278] In addition, n-butyrate acts as a differentiating agent and could play a role in the morphogenesis of colorectal cancer.[279] Other dietary factors may include calcium[280] and selenium[281] deficiency.

Family studies suggest that genetic factors may be implicated in the aetiology of colorectal cancer. Adenomatosis (familial polyposis coli) is inherited on an autosomal dominant basis. Veale suggested that all adenomas have a genetic aetiology, small numbers of adenomas being inherited in an autosomal recessive fashion.[282] However, in one very large family pedigree, multiple adenomas were shown to be inherited on an autosomal dominant basis.[283] Even if this interesting observation is confirmed, it is important to distinguish multiple adenomas from familial adenomatosis coli. In the last, hundreds and often thousands of adenomas appear at an early age, the development of cancer is inevitable and extracolonic manifestations are described (see p. 360).

Genetic factors may also be of importance in a

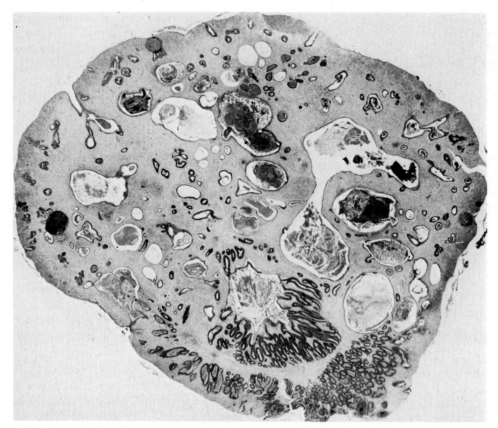

Fig. 8.55 Juvenile polyp of the large intestine showing tubular and cystic structures within an abundant cellular stroma. The darkly-staining areas contain mucus.

Mucicarmine and haemalum   × 5

particular subgroup of patients with colorectal cancer. Such patients are typically young with tumours of the right colon and multiple carcinomas, both of the colon and other organs.[284,285] The underlying mechanism may be a reduced capacity for DNA repair.[286]

The time-scale of the multistep theory of carcinogenesis (which involves firstly initiation and then promotion) precludes all but fixed stem cells as potential targets for carcinogens. Precancerous lesions may be regarded as signals of an underlying population of initiated stem cells which are not yet committed to the formation of an infiltrating neoplasm.

Precancerous lesions and conditions

Most colorectal carcinomas arise from pre-existing benign adenomas. The evidence for this is summarized as follows.

1. Similar site predilection for large adenomas and carcinomas (left colon and rectum)[287]
2. Similar site predilection for severe dysplasia and carcinoma (left colon and rectum)[287]
3. Fewer and smaller adenomas in countries with a low incidence of colorectal cancer[288]
4. Residual adenoma in specimens of colorectal cancer. This is more probable in cases where the growth is at an early stage and has therefore not had sufficient time to destroy the adenoma.[289,290]
5. A series of adenomas exhibits all grades of dysplasia up to carcinoma-in-situ and early malignant change[287,289]
6. Adenomas are more frequently detected in surgical specimens in cases of colorectal cancer than in other diseases[291]
7. Removal of adenomas reduces the incidence of colorectal cancer[292]

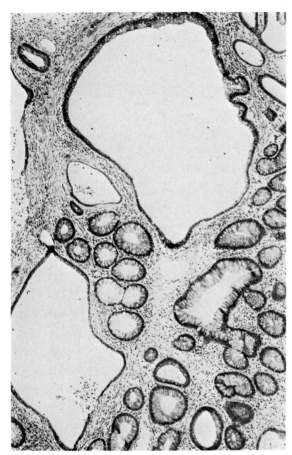

Fig. 8.56 Juvenile polyp. At higher magnification the crypts are seen to be lined by normal colorectal epithelium.

Haematoxylin-eosin   × 25

8. Rarity of reports of 'de novo' carcinoma
9. Increased risk of metachronous carcinoma in patients with adenomas[293]
10. Average age of patients presenting with adenomas approximately five years less than average age of patients with carcinoma.[294]

Adenomatosis coli or familial polyposis coli leads to the inevitable development of colorectal cancer if left untreated. The cancer risk in patients with juvenile polyposis is now considered to be at least as high as 10% (see p. 363). A slight risk is also observed in the Peutz-Jeghers syndrome (see p. 364). Occasional examples of malignant change have been described in hyperplastic (metaplastic) polyps (see p. 356), but the risk of this occurrence has not been shown to be higher than that for normal colorectal mucosa.

Inflammatory bowel disease (ulcerative colitis (see p. 341), Crohn's disease[295] and schistosomiasis japonica[296]) predisposes to colorectal cancer. Surgical procedures including ureterosigmoidostomy,[297] cholecystectomy[298] and gastrectomy[299] have been associated with an increased incidence of colorectal cancer, possibly by altering the colonic micro-environment. Carcinomas often arise in anastomoses in both humans and experimental animals.[300] The anastomotic site may be responsible for promoting tumour development. It is still not clear whether the mucosa adjacent to colorectal cancer 'transitional mucosa', which differs histologically and histochemically from normal,[301] represents a carcinogen-induced field effect or a non-specific alteration due, for example, to growth-promoting tumour products.

Dysplasia is the histological change common to the majority of precancerous lesions and conditions described above. The magnitude of the risk of

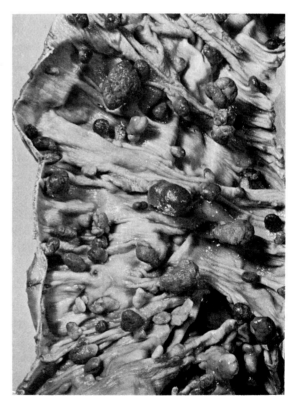

Fig. 8.57 Juvenile polyposis. This may be mistaken for familial polyposis but the polyps show a characteristically smooth and glistening surface in this example.

malignant change appears to be closely related to the grade of dysplasia. It is therefore advantageous to unify the precancer-cancer hypothesis by employing the term dysplasia-carcinoma sequence.[302]

Early colorectal cancer

This may be defined as cancer involving but limited to the submucosa. Eighty per cent show evidence of arising in a benign adenoma. The management of early colorectal cancer (malignant adenoma) is discussed on page 359.

Pathology

About one half of all large bowel cancers occur in the rectum and rectosigmoid area. The sigmoid colon accounts for a further 25% and the remaining one quarter of all cases is roughly equally distributed between the caecum, ascending, transverse and descending parts of the large intestine. As noted above, the distribution varies in different populations and has changed with time.[303]

Macroscopic appearances

Most cancers of the colon and rectum are ulcerating tumours with raised, everted edges (Figs 8.58 and 8.59). The 'string-carcinoma' is of this type, but surrounds the lumen, producing the effect of a string tied tightly around the bowel (Fig. 8.60). These small, annular growths cause stenosis and proximal dilatation. Symptoms of obstruction are usually late in onset because 'string-carcinomas' are commonest in the proximal colon where the faeces are normally fluid and pass easily through a constriction which would soon obstruct the passage of solid stool. Protuberant types of intestinal cancer are less frequent and are often of a relatively low grade of malignancy. Some of them have a villous or papillary surface configuration, a type which accounts for about 7% of all carcinomas of the colon.[304] About 10% of intestinal cancers show a colloid appearance on the cut surface of the tumour due to abundant secretion of mucin by tumour cells.

Most cancers of the colon and rectum remain relatively small and circumscribed compared with gastric carcinoma. Moreover, they rarely show much submucous or intramural spread beyond

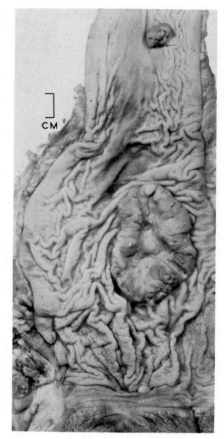

Fig. 8.58 Ulcerated protuberant carcinoma of the rectum. There is a second primary carcinoma about 6 cm above the main tumour.
Specimen from the Gordon Museum, Guy's Hospital, London, reproduced by permission of the Curator, Mr J.D. Maynard. Photograph by Miss P.M. Turnbull, Charing Cross Hospital Medical School.

their macroscopic borders. This characteristic is important in the consideration of surgical treatment. The diffusely infiltrating scirrhous type of carcinoma which is typically seen in the stomach as 'linitis plastica' is very rarely seen in the large bowel.[305] When it does occur it is more likely to be a secondary manifestation of an occult carcinoma of the stomach than a true primary of the colon or rectum.

Microscopic appearances

About 85% of adenocarcinomas of the colorectum are composed of relatively well-differentiated tubules secreting small quantities of mucin. About 20% are well differentiated, 60% moderately

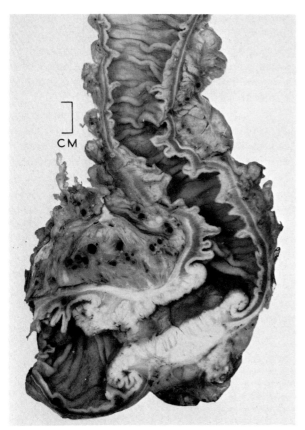

Fig. 8.59 Large ulcerated annular carcinoma of the colon.
Specimen from the Gordon Museum, Guy's Hospital, London, reproduced by permission of the Curator, Mr J.D. Maynard. Photograph by Miss P.M. Turnbull, Charing Cross Hospital Medical School.

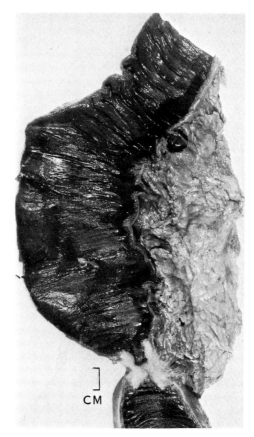

Fig. 8.60 Melanosis coli accompanied by an annular or string carcinoma of the transverse colon. The mucosal surface of the tumour was not pigmented.

differentiated and 20% poorly differentiated. Scattered Paneth cells and cells containing argentaffin or agyrophil granules are not an unusual feature, but are few in number. The criteria for grading differentiation are discussed below.

Between 10 and 15% of colorectal cancers are mucinous, implying that substantial quantities of mucin are retained within the tumour. This is usually visible macroscopically to give the well-known appearance of a 'colloid' (mucoid) cancer. Two main growth patterns of mucinous adenocarcinoma may be encountered: (1) glands filled with mucin, together with interstitial mucin (Fig. 8.61), and (2) chains or clumps of cells surrounded by mucin. Often a tumour may show both growth patterns. In some tumours the cells are so obscured by masses of mucin that assessment of the degree of differentiation is made difficult. Tumours com-

posed only of signet-ring cells are rare in those countries with a high incidence of colorectal cancer, but are more frequent in low-risk areas.

The term 'undifferentiated' carcinoma is used to describe a type which shows no attempt at tubular differentiation. Such tumours differ from anaplastic carcinoma in the lack of pleomorphism and bizarre mitotic figures. They do not secrete mucin but do contain scanty argyrophil cells. These tumours are rare, but have a good prognosis.[306] Older terms such as carcinoma simplex, medullary carcinoma and trabecular carcinoma are discouraged. The histology of undifferentiated carcinoma has to be distinguished from malignant carcinoid (see p. 378). It is good practice to examine sections from different parts of a tumour when considering this differential diagnosis.

The so-called 'nephrogenic' adenocarcinoma of

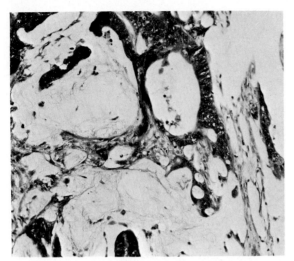

Fig. 8.61 Mucinous adenocarcinoma. The tubules are disrupted by pools of mucus.

Haematoxylin-eosin   × 100

the colon and rectum is extremely rare. In such cases the glands are lined by clear cells, giving some resemblance to adenocarcinoma of the kidney.

Calcification and ossification (Fig. 8.62) of carcinomas in the large intestine are very rare.[307] They can occur in metastatic deposits as well as in the primary growth. Psammomatous calcification may occur in papillary tumours. Ossification is seen within adenocarcinomatous tubules as well as among areas of necrosis and lakes of mucin. There is no evidence that the presence of ossification or calcification affects prognosis, although it seems to be more commonly seen among the younger age groups with colorectal cancer.

The diagnosis of carcinoma in a rectal biopsy should never be made unless there is unequivocal evidence of invasion by malignant cells. Tumour that has crossed the line of the muscularis mucosae is clearly invasive and radical surgical treatment is usually indicated except for selected early colorectal cancers. Invasive adenocarcinoma is recognizable by its accompanying desmoplastic reaction. A cautious approach to the histological diagnosis of carcinoma is important because superficial biopsies of benign adenomas can closely mimic the appearances seen at the surface of a carcinoma.

Histochemistry

Enzyme studies, mucin and lectin histochemistry and immunohistochemistry have helped to probe the functional characteristics of colorectal cancer.

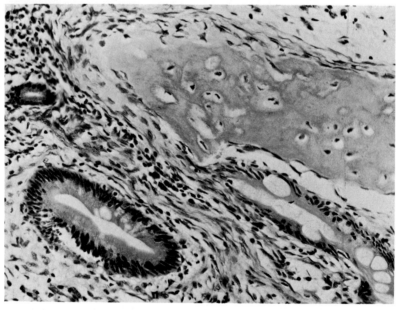

Fig. 8.62 Osseous metaplasia in the stroma of a well-differentiated primary adenocarcinoma of the rectum.

Haematoxylin-eosin   × 225

Photograph provided by W. StC. Symmers.

Enzyme studies reveal the abandonment of respiratory or aerobic metabolism and the adoption of the anaerobic glycolytic and pentose shunt pathways.[308-310] Similar changes are seen in villous adenomas and areas of high-grade dysplasia. Changes in secretory or cell surface glycoconjugates (glycoproteins and glycolipids) may be demonstrated by mucin or lectin histochemistry or immunohistochemistry. For example, mucin histochemistry demonstrates the loss of O-acetyl sialomucins: this accompanies neoplastic transformation.[311] Changes in glycoconjugate structure are brought about either by their defective or incomplete synthesis, the induction of inappropriate glycosyl transferases to give new sugar sequences or a combination of both. Important cell surface glycoconjugates include HLA and blood group antigens, tissue-specific antigens and tumour-associated antigens. None of the tumour-associated antigens so far described is both tumour and tissue specific. The growing list includes T blood group antigen[312] (cross-reacts with the peanut lectin receptor), 19–9 antigen[313] (sialylated Lewis[a] blood group), Lewis[x][314] (stage-specific embryonic antigen 1), sialylated Lewis[x][315] and Lewis[y].[316] These changes may in time be shown to be important in relation to invasiveness, metastatic potential and tumour immunity. Other cell products which have been shown to be associated with tumour grade, stage and prognosis are described below (see p. 374).

Genetic studies

Direct chromosome analysis requires the isolation of cells in mitosis and is therefore time-consuming. Automated flow cytometry is less sensitive, but more applicable to the routine study of colorectal cancer. Colorectal cancers are arbitrarily divided into either near diploid or aneuploid by the degree of deviation of DNA content from a standard. Relationships have been demonstrated between ploidy and tumour grade and stage.[317]

The mutational theory of carcinogenesis has been bolstered by the discovery of oncogenes in various human tumours. It has been suggested that the normally-occurring proto (cellular) oncogenes (which probably regulate cell growth) are converted into transforming oncogenes. Several mechanisms may underly oncogene activation including point mutations,[318] translocation of genetic material and gene amplification.[319] Oncogenes implicated in human colorectal carcinogenesis include c-myb,[319] c-myc[320] and members of the ras family.[320] It is now understood that the c-myc gene plays an important role in cell cycle regulation.[320]

Relationship of type and grade of tumour to prognosis

A number of histological parameters are linked to prognosis, though it is not possible to predict the outcome for individual patients. Tumour size is irrelevant.[322] Adenocarcinomas showing a papillary configuration are uncommon, but confer a more favourable prognosis than the normal tubular adenocarcinoma.[323] In one study, the 5-year survival figures for non-mucinous and mucinous carcinomas were 53 and 34% respectively. When individual sites in the colon and rectum were compared, 5-year survival figures for non-mucinous and mucinous tumours were similar, except in the rectum (49 and 18% respectively).[324] However, this study included signet ring cell carcinomas with mucinous carcinomas. Signet-ring cell carcinomas represent the most ominous subtype.[305] Tumours showing an expanding pattern of spread with a 'pushing' growth margin have a better prognosis than diffusely infiltrating carcinomas.[323] A dense band of lymphocytes at the growing margin is also a marker of a good prognosis[323,325] as is a prominent infiltration by eosinophils.[326]

Division into three histological grades of malignancy should be attempted for adenocarcinoma.[327,328] *Well-differentiated adenocarcinoma* shows well-formed tubules and nuclei that are of uniform size and shape. The nuclei may or may not show crowding and stratification, but polarity is well maintained. Thus the apex and base of the cell are easily discerned. The overall appearance is often reminiscent of adenomatous epithelium (Fig. 8.63). Twenty per cent of adenocarcinomas are well differentiated and the survival rate is 80% at five years. In *moderately-differentiated adenocarcinoma*, glandular structures are still present, though they may adopt an irregular outline. Nuclei have become larger and more pleomorphic and polarity is discerned with difficulty, if at all (Fig. 8.64).

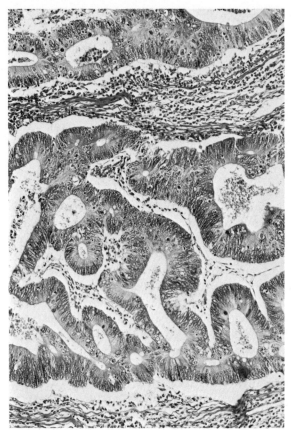

Fig. 8.63 Well-differentiated adenocarcinoma. Tubules are well formed, nucler polarity is retained and the nuclei are uniform in size and shape.

Haematoxylin-eosin   × 60

Sixty per cent of tumours are moderately differentiated and show a 60% 5-year survival. In *poorly-differentiated adenocarcinoma*, tubular structures are highly irregular or not formed at all. Instead, the tumour cells are grouped into cords, clumps or sheets (Fig. 8.65). Twenty per cent of adenocarcinomas are poorly differentiated and only 25% of cases survive five years.[329] Architecture and, to a lesser extent, cytology are the best guides to tumour differentiation. Functional differentiation shows little relationship to prognosis. Loss of staining for secretory component and epithelial IgA has been shown to correlate with loss of differentiation, but offers no advantage over conventional grading and staging.[330,331] Carcinoembryonic antigen expression is related to differentiation in as much as loss of polarity and diffuse cytoplasmic staining are features of poorly-differentiated carcinomas.[332]

The Dukes classification (Fig. 8.66) of rectal cancer was introduced at St Mark's Hospital, London, in 1928 and is now accepted all over the world as a valuable guide to prognosis.[333] The Dukes 'A' case (15% of all operable cancers) is one in which the cancer has spread into the tissues of the bowel wall, but not beyond the muscularis propria and there are no lymph node metastases. A patient with cancer of the colon or rectum at the Dukes 'A' stage can be almost invariably cured of his disease by appropriate surgical treatment. A Dukes 'B' case (35% of all operable cancers) is one in which the growth has spread beyond the muscularis propria into the pericolic or perirectal tissues in continuity but there are no regional lymph node metastases. Such patients have a 70% chance of cure. Once the lymph nodes are involved (Dukes 'C' case) the prognosis becomes very much

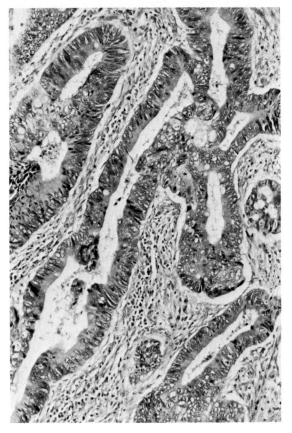

Fig. 8.64 Moderately-differentiated adenocarcinoma. Tubules are discernible but irregular in their configuration. There is loss of nuclear polarity and variation in nuclear size and shape.

Haematoxylin-eosin   × 60

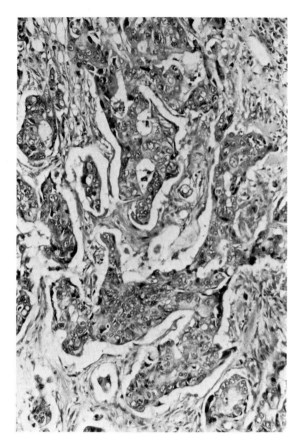

Fig. 8.65 Poorly-differentiated adenocarcinoma. There is little attempt at tubule formation.

Haematoxylin-eosin ×60

poorer with only about one in three patients surviving five years. About 50% of all surgically treated cancers are in this stage. 'C' cases that have not penetrated the bowel wall are associated with fewer positive lymph nodes than those which have,[322] and are therefore likely to have a more favourable prognosis.[334]

Local spread

Direct spread of the primary tumour in continuity occurs along those tissue planes which provide the least resistance. The submucosa is composed of loose connective tissue which is readily involved, but the muscularis propria offers considerable resistance to infiltration by malignant cells because of its dense structure. As a result, adenocarcinoma spreads through gaps in the muscle through which the blood supply to the mucous membrane travels. It is also quite common to see infiltration along the myenteric plexus between the circular and longitudinal layers. Beyond the muscularis propria the soft adipose and connective tissues of the serosa or mesenteric border offer little resistance, but the peritoneal membrane is a tough structure which often remains intact despite being stretched over the carcinomatous mass. It is unusual to find much direct upwards or downwards spread in continuity in the submucosal layer beyond the visible borders of the tumour (in contrast to what is usually seen in gastric or oesophageal carcinoma). However, extensive downward intramural spread of rectal cancer can occur with tumours of a high grade of malignancy, which is the main reason why low anterior resection for high-grade rectal cancer should be avoided. This illustrates the practical importance of grading biopsied tumours. The relationship between local spread in continuity and prognosis after surgical treatment has been described: in 'B' cases without lymph node metastases the corrected 5-year survival rate is 90% with slight spread, 80% with moderate spread in continuity, and 57% with deeply invasive tumours. There is a much higher incidence of high-grade tumours in operation specimens showing extensive local spread than slight or moderate extension. The depth of tumour penetration beyond the muscularis propria may be measured, as well as the deep or lateral margin of surgical clearance for rectal tumours below the peritoneal reflection. This would make the assessment of the extent of local spread more objective and reproducible.

Lymphatic spread

Carcinoma can be seen permeating lymphatic channels, particularly in the submucosal and extramural tissues. The distinction between lymphatics and capillaries is often made with difficulty, if at all.

Lymph node metastasis appears to be a progressive process in which carcinoma spreads from node to node. It is rare to find involved nodes at a distance from the primary tumour and unaffected nodes intervening. In the great majority of cases of carcinomas of the colon and rectum, lymphatic spread follows the most direct route to the regional

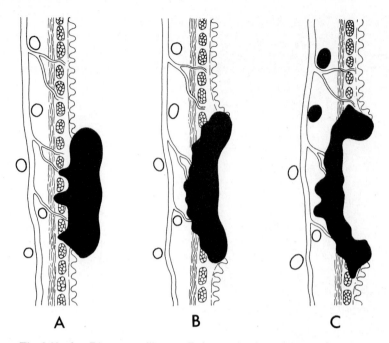

Fig. 8.66a, b, c Diagrams to illustrate Dukes staging for rectal carcinoma. A. Growth limited to the bowel wall with no lymph node involvement. B. Spread beyond muscularis propria with no lymph node involvement. C. Lymph node involvement present.

lymph nodes (Fig. 8.67). If these become involved, lymph flow can be blocked, and so-called retrograde lymphatic metastasis may then arise.[335] This is only apparent in advanced cancer and is associated with a very poor prognosis.

The presence of lymph node metastases in an operation specimen of colonic or rectal cancer (Dukes 'C' cases) greatly worsens prognosis. The prognosis also varies with the number of involved lymph nodes. Thus, the 5-year survival rate is about 60% with only one node affected, 35% with two to five involved and only 20% when six or more nodes are affected. Involvement of the lymph node lying nearest to the surgical suture placed near the origin of the superior haemorrhoidal artery (Dukes 'C2') in cases of rectal adenocarcinoma is associated with about a 15% 5-year survival.[329] The influence of lymph node metastasis on prognosis is also closely related to the grade of malignancy of the primary tumour and the extent of local spread. There is a progressive increase in the percentage of cases with lymphatic metastases when passing from well- through moderate- to poorly-differentiated adenocarcinoma.

Spread to the inguinal lymph nodes may occur in rectal cancer. In the St Mark's Hospital series of operation specimens, only 2% of all rectal cancers showed involvement of inguinal nodes, but if cancers of the lower third of the rectum are taken alone the figure rises to 7%. Inguinal node involvement mostly occurs when the haemorrhoidal lymph nodes are already affected.

Sinus histiocytosis of regional lymph nodes occurs in about one third of operation specimens for cancer of the colorectum. It has been suggested that this could be an indication of host resistance.[336]

Peritoneal involvement

Once malignant cells have penetrated through the peritoneum they can be disseminated through the peritoneal cavity. Fortunately the peritoneum forms a relatively sound barrier to such spread and is often intact, though tightly stretched over the underlying growth. Poorly-differentiated tumours cause multiple deposits throughout the abdominal cavity, whereas well-differentiated carcinomas produce relatively few metastases by transcoelomic

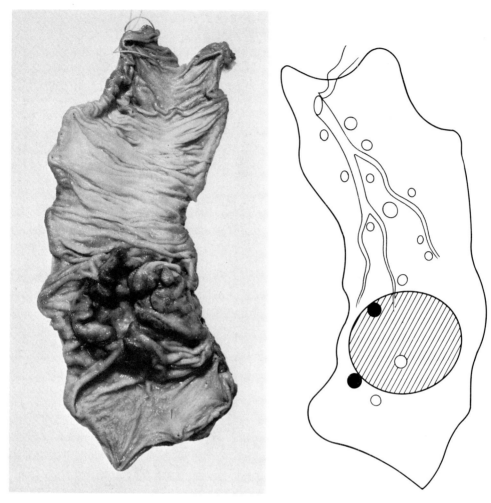

Fig. 8.67a, b (**a**) Ulcerating carcinoma of sigmoid colon. (**b**) Chart of the lymphatic spread of the carcinoma shown in (**a**), as viewed from behind. The affected nodes are indicated by the solid black areas. The tumour is a Dukes 'C' type (see Fig. 8.66).

spread. The ovary is a site of predilection for tumours spreading transcoelomically (Krukenberg tumour). Peritoneal penetration may be obvious macroscopically or only detected on histological examination.

Venous spread[337]

Permeation of large extramural veins by tumour reduces the overall 5-year survival rate from 55 to 30% (Fig. 8.68). Submucosal venous involvement has little effect on prognosis. Intravenous growth is often covered by organizing granulation tissue and thrombus, especially when well differentiated.

This host response may effectively seal the tumour within the vein and so prevent malignant embolism. This may explain why the involvement of extramural veins is not inevitably associated with the development of metastatic spread. It may be relevant that the production of plasminogen activator by tumours is associated with an enhanced metastatic potential.[338]

Implantation

Metastasis may arise by the implantation of malignant cells into any raw or traumatized surface. This includes fistulas or other wounds at the anus

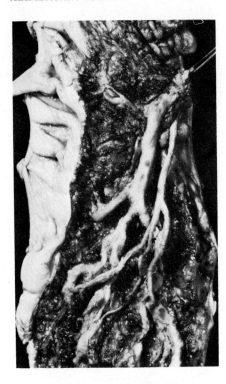

Fig. 8.68 Specimen dissected to show spread of carcinoma with the lumen of veins draining the rectum.

such as those which follow haemorrhoidectomy. Recurrence in abdominal incisions, around colostomies and in the perineum following rectal excision are probably due to implantation. Many recurrences at the anastomotic line will be due to implantation, but other causes include regrowth of residual tumour and possibly the development of a metachronous (new primary) anastomotic tumour.[339]

Pelvic recurrence

The incidence of regrowth of carcinoma in the pelvis after excision of the rectum is 10%.[340] This mostly occurs with carcinomas of the lower (extraperitoneal) rectum, because this is encased by the narrowing pelvic funnel which makes adequate surgical removal of the primary tumour difficult. Pelvic recurrence is commonest in rectal cancers at the Dukes 'C' stage, in those which have extensive local spread in continuity and in tumours that are poorly differentiated.

Complications

Intestinal obstruction is the commonest complication of carcinoma of the large bowel. It seems to have an unfavourable effect upon prognosis after surgical treatment, which is probably due to the fact that obstruction is often associated with relatively advanced disease. Free perforation is uncommon and also indicates an unfavourable prognosis, due to peritonitis and the escape of malignant cells into the abdominal cavity. Penetration of the wall of the colon by carcinoma is sometimes associated with the development of a pericolic abscess. Internal fistula is very rare. Intussusception of the colon in adults is more often caused by carcinoma than by benign tumours or other causes.[341]

Acute appendicitis can be precipitated by proximal large bowel growths causing back pressure on the caecum with obstruction of the lumen of the appendix.[342] Colonic ulceration proximal to obstructing carcinomas is due to associated ischaemic colitis (see p. 352). It must be distinguished from cancer arising in ulcerative colitis.

Non-metastatic cutaneous manifestations (such as dermatomyositis and acanthosis nigricans) of cancer of the colon and rectum are infrequent.

A frequent complication of carcinoma in the lower rectum is the presence of secondary haemorrhoids. These are important because they may be the presenting sign and a cursory examination may not reveal the carcinoma above them, with consequent delay in the diagnosis.

ENDOCRINE ('CARCINOID') TUMOURS

These are relatively uncommon, the sites of predilection being caecum and rectum. Caecal and colonic neoplasms are often large on first presentation and approximately 50% have metastasized at the time of diagnosis.[343] The caecum, like the appendix and small bowel is a midgut derivative. Most midgut endocrine tumours, including those of the caecum, show the characteristic 'carcinoid' pattern (type A1 pattern).[344,345] This comprises solid clumps or islands of uniform, pale cells with peripheral cords or trabeculae. Cells at the periphery of the nest may show hyperchromatic nuclei and a bright, eosinophilic granular cytoplasm. It is not uncommon for tumours to show tubular differentiation with luminal periodic acid-Schiff positive material (A2). Mixed solid and tubular (A1–A2) patterns are uncommon. Some caecal endocrine tumours complete their likeness to the typical carcinoid by a positive, argentaffin reaction indicating the secretion of 5-HT. This is especially seen in the peripheral cells with an eosinophilic cytoplasm. However, an associated carcinoid syndrome is uncommon, even in the presence of metastases.

Rectal endocrine tumours. These present in two macroscopic forms.[346,347] The usual finding is that of a small, firm submucosal nodule less than 1 cm in diameter and discovered fortuitously. The cut surface is pink or tan. These can be treated by local excision only, provided that removal is complete. Less commonly the tumour presents as a large growth which may be ulcerated or polypoid and is often associated with metastases.

Microscopically, three patterns are encountered of which the ribbon type (B) is the commonest. The ribbons consist of two or more layers of cells arranged along a delicate core of vascular connective tissue and may be straight, convoluted or interlacing (Fig. 8.69). The next commonest pattern is a mixed A1–A2, often with a conspicuous tubular component (Fig. 8.70). Rectal or hindgut endocrine tumours are rarely argentaffin, but the majority are argyrophil by the Grimelius technique.[348] Immunocytochemical studies have documented the secretion of a variety of polypeptide hormones including pancreatic polypeptide, glucagon, somatostatin, substance P, insulin, beta-endorphin and enkephalin.[348] One tumour may secrete several different hormones.

The distinction between benign and malignant rectal endocrine tumours may be difficult, but guidelines can be offered. Apart from the size of the tumour, there are a number of histological features associated with malignant endocrine tumours. These include spread beyond the muscularis propria, nuclear pleomorphism, high mitotic activity, a diffusely infiltrating pattern of growth and tumour necrosis. The majority of malignant

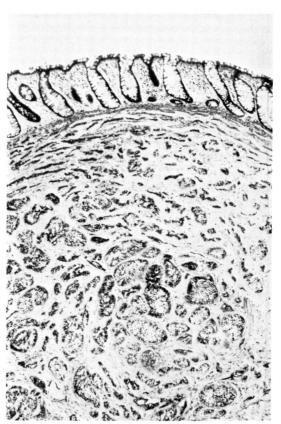

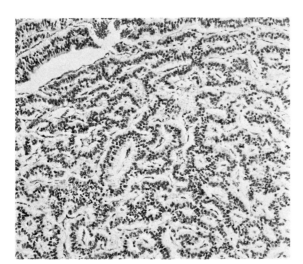

Fig. 8.69 Rectal carcinoid showing pattern of interlacing ribbons (type B) supported by a delicate stromal network. This was a malignant tumour extending through the bowel wall and involving local lymph nodes.

Haematoxylin-eosin   × 100

Fig. 8.70 Rectal carcinoid showing a mixed pattern comprising tubule formation and peripheral cords (A_1–A_2). The tumour was small and confined to the submucosa.

Haematoxylin-eosin   × 25

rectal endocrine tumours show a ribbon (B) pattern.[349] Some tumours are more appropriately classified as adenocarcinomas that include a population of endocrine cells. This is certainly true of one variant of the so-called goblet cell carcinoid which has been described in the colon[350] as well as the appendix (see p. 309). The rare small cell undifferentiated carcinoma (oat cell carcinoma) is similar to its lung counterpart in terms of its histogenesis, histology and behaviour. These tumours must be distinguished from metastatic carcinoma, lymphoma and melanoma and from the cloacogenic squamous carcinoma of the anal canal transitional zone (see p. 410).

Squamous carcinoma

Primary squamous carcinoma of the colon and rectum occurs only very rarely.[351] The possibility of metastatic carcinoma should always be excluded and the cervix is the most likely primary site. Squamous carcinoma may complicate chronic ulcerative colitis[352] and squamous metaplasia within adenocarcinoma is not an uncommon finding. Some squamous carcinomas may represent upward extension of a carcinoma of the anal canal. Others could arise in squamous epithelium representing either congenital heterotopia or an acquired metaplasia due to an unknown stimulus. This is supported by the finding of normal and dysplastic squamous epithelium in the vicinity of a primary squamous carcinoma. Minor degrees of upgrowth of squamous epithelium from the anal canal into the lower rectum are quite common in prolapsing haemorrhoids. Extensive upgrowth producing 'leukoplakia' has been described accompanying a squamous carcinoma.[353] Finally, it is possible that neoplastic transformation and metaplastic change could arise concomitantly.[354]

Adenosquamous carcinoma

Both adenocarcinomatous and squamous carcinomatous tissues are present as separate but contiguous elements. This distinguishes this rare tumour from the more common squamous metaplasia within an adenocarcinoma. Intercellular bridges and keratin should be demonstrated in the squamous part.

Secondary carcinoma

The stomach is one of the commonest sources of both solitary and multiple secondary deposits in the large intestine. These may present as single or multiple strictures mimicking primary colorectal cancer or Crohn's disease. Widespread diffuse spread may give rise to a shortened tubular colon mimicking ulcerative colitis. Often the primary gastric lesion is difficult to demonstrate, even at laparotomy. Histological findings suggesting the correct diagnosis are the presence of diffuse infiltration, poor differentiation and signet-ring cells, all of which are unusual features in primary colorectal carcinoma. Other primary sites to be considered are breast,[355] skin (malignant melanoma), ovary, bladder, kidney,[356] cervix[357] and lung. Involvement of the rectum by carcinoma of the prostate is unusual.[358]

NON-EPITHELIAL TUMOURS

TUMOURS OF LYMPHOID TISSUE

Benign lymphoid polyps

These present as smooth, round, submucous tumours in the lower third of the rectum.[359] Whilst the majority are sessile lesions, pedunculated lymphoid polyps may occur. They are usually single, but can number up to four or five. They are slightly more common in men than in women and present in the third or fourth decades of life. They are found incidentally during examination for other complaints and vary in size from a few millimetres to 3 cm in diameter. Ulceration is very rare.

Microscopically, they are composed of normal lymphoid tissue including lymphoid follicles with germinal centres (Fig. 8.71). Sarcoid-like foci are sometimes present. They lie mainly in the submucosa and are covered by attenuated mucosa. Involvement of the deep muscle layer of the bowel wall is exceptional. Their small size, follicular pattern, lack of mucosal ulceration and non-involvement of muscle coats usually allows them to be easily differentiated from malignant lymphoma.

Benign lymphoid polyps are harmless lesions

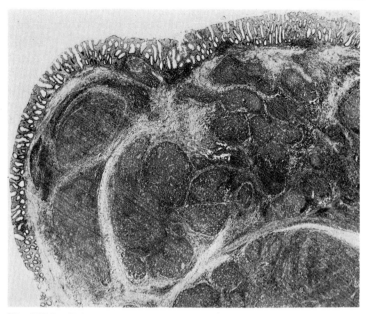

Fig. 8.71 Sessile benign 'lymphoid polyp' of the rectum showing well-formed follicles with germinal centres.

Haematoxylin-eosin   × 12

Photograph provided by W. StC. Symmers.

and are probably a response to local inflammation. They frequently regress if left untreated.

Benign lymphoid polyposis

This is a rare condition, usually occurring in childhood, in which there is overgrowth of the lymphoid follicles normally present in the colon and rectum.[360] Many cases represent an exaggerated hyperplasia of the lymphoid tissue of the gut occurring in young children with viral infections (echovirus, adenovirus),[361] but the condition may be familial[360] and may be found in patients with immune deficiency syndromes.[362] The condition may present as a rectal prolapse.[361] Macroscopically, the mucosa bulges with many grey sessile nodules measuring 0.3–0.6 cm in diameter. The condition has to be distinguished from multiple lymphomatous polyposis (see below) when the same criteria as those described above for benign lymphoid polyps are used, and also from familial adenomatous polyposis.

MALIGNANT LYMPHOID TUMOURS

There are three types. The commonest form is found in association with generalized malignant lymphoma. Second, malignant lymphoma can be a primary growth in the colon or rectum. Third, it may present as lymphomatous polyposis. Lymphoid tumours are more frequently found in the small intestine than the large intestine but sometimes both segments of the intestinal tract are involved together.[363]

Bowel involvement in generalized disease

The bowel can be involved directly or as the result of invasion from without.[364] The latter is less common than the former, and the usual clinical presentation is as a presacral mass. The histological diagnosis is made by deep rectal biopsy. Direct secondary involvement of the colon and rectum presents as a circumscribed mass, which is more often polypoid than ulcerative, or as diffuse nodular or plaque-like lesions. The latter can involve long segments of bowel and multiple tumours are common. The mucosal surface may have a rugose or brain-like appearance, but this may also be seen in multiple lymphomatous polyposis. Microscopically, all histological varieties of malignant lymphoma can be seen. The submucosa, in particular, is widely infiltrated.

Primary malignant lymphoma

The criteria for making a diagnosis of a primary malignant lymphoma tumour are: (1) no lymphadenopathy at presentation; (2) a normal chest X-ray; (3) a normal white cell count; (4) bowel lesion predominates at laparotomy, and (5) liver and spleen are free of tumour.[365] Three macroscopic types are seen. Annular or plaque-like thickenings are the most common, followed by bulky protuberant growths and, rarely, thickening and dilatation of the bowel. The cut surface of the aneurysmal unfixed tumour has a characteristically uniform, fleshy appearance. The surface of tumours is sometimes covered by an exuberant slough of necrotic tumour.

Sixty per cent of primary malignant lymphomas of the large bowel occur in the caecum, 20% occur in the rectum, and the remainder are distributed throughout the colon. This reflects the normal distribution of lymphoid tissue in the large intestine. The high proportion of caecal tumours includes some that have spread locally from the terminal ileum, which is particularly rich in lymphoid tissue. Multiple primary foci are quite common. Primary malignant lymphoma can be associated with ulcerative colitis,[366] with small intestinal malabsorption, adenocarcinoma in a different part of the large bowel, as well as with malignant disease in other organs. There is a report of colonic malignant lymphoma developing during immunosuppressive therapy following renal transplantation.[367]

The histological appearances will depend upon the grade of lymphoma which is in turn dependent on the cell type.[368,369] High-grade tumours, such as the immunoblastic (undifferentiated large cell) lymphoma, are well represented in the colon. They show fissuring ulceration and for this reason are prone to perforation. The tumour shows an expanding pattern of growth leading to effacement of normal structures. Another high-grade lymphoma is the lymphoblastic (poorly-differentiated lymphocytic) which occurs mainly in children and in the ileocaecal region. The tumour cells characteristically replace fat and dissect between the fibres of the muscularis propria, which is left largely intact. Lymphomas of centrocytic type (small follicle centre cells) usually present as multiple lymphomatous polyposis (see below). Lymphoplasmacytoid lymphoma is less common and there are rare reports of plasma cell lymphoma.[370] True histiocytic lymphoma is probably very uncommon and primary Hodgkin's disease must be regarded as an extreme rarity. A collection of 71 primary lymphomas of the colorectum from St Mark's and St Bartholomew's hospitals, London, includes 30 cases of multiple lymphomatous polyposis (centrocytic), 14 immunoblastic, 6 lymphoplasmacytoid, 5 lymphoblastic, 2 centroblastic/centrocytic, 1 centroblastic, 1 plasmacytoma and 12 unclassified.

Primary lymphoma and carcinoma of the colon spread in similar fashion and should be staged by similar systems.[368] However, no universally accepted method of staging yet exists.

The distinction between lymphoma and poorly-differentiated carcinoma has been greatly facilitated by the development of immunological markers for lymphoid and epithelial cells. The subsequent typing of lymphomas is dependent upon good morphological preparations and the application of immunocytochemical techniques.[368,369,371]

Multiple lymphomatous polyposis

This condition appears to occur exclusively in adults. The large bowel and other segments of the gastrointestinal tract are diffusely involved by malignant centrocytic lymphoma, causing widespread areas of polypoid thickening of the mucosa (Fig. 8.72). The polyps may be pedunculated but the gross appearances merge with those of brain-like convolutions and diffuse mucosal nodularity. The latter patterns are particularly seen in the stomach and rectum. The clinical presentation is of diarrhoea and even steatorrhoea. Histologically, there is diffuse infiltration by centrocytic lymphoid cells (Figs 8.73 and 8.74).[368,371] In many cases a leukaemic blood picture develops, even when the disease is apparently localized to the gut at its onset. Splenomegaly, generalized lymphadenopathy and bone marrow involvement all commonly occur preterminally, and there are many similarities with chronic lymphocytic leukaemia. Unlike other gastrointestinal lymphomas, perforation of the bowel

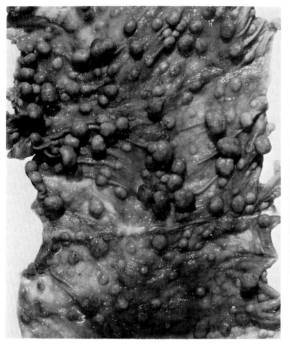

Fig. 8.72 Multiple lymphomatous polyposis.

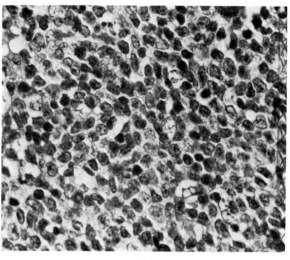

Fig. 8.74 Multiple lymphomatous polyposis. A high-power view shows a uniform cell population comprising cells whose nuclei show irregular outlines (cleaved cells) and inconspicuous nucleoli. Cytoplasm is scant. The cells are centrocytes (small follicle centre cells).

Haematoxylin-eosin   × 400

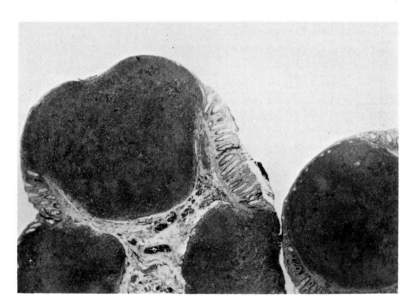

Fig. 8.73 Multiple lymphomatous polyposis. Four neoplastic nodules are illustrated showing absence of germinal centres, which are a feature of normal lymphoid follicles.

Haematoxylin-eosin   × 6.5

rarely occurs, but there may be intestinal obstruction from large tumour masses. Despite the widespread distribution of the disease it is rarely rapidly fatal having a slow but relentlessly progressive course in most instances.

Large intestinal manifestations of leukaemia

Plaque-like thickening, nodular lesions, diffuse infiltrations, a convoluted brain-like appearance and leukaemic polyposis are all seen in the colon and rectum. Such involvement is most frequent in poorly-differentiated leukaemias. These changes are usually multiple. Most leukaemic lesions are symptomless and are found at autopsy. On rare occasions, abdominal or rectal symptoms are the presenting feature of the disease. Microscopically, the lesions seem to represent enlargement and leukaemic replacement of the lymphoid follicles normally present in the large intestine. The proximal colon is affected more frequently than the distal colon and rectum.

The macroscopic and microscopic features may closely resemble lymphoma, but myeloblastic leukaemia is distinguished by the demonstration of chloroacetate esterase activity.[372]

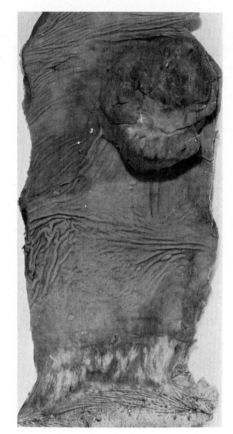

Fig. 8.75 Malignant smooth muscle tumour of rectum (leiomyosarcoma) presenting as a protuberant mass with central ulceration.

TUMOURS OF SMOOTH MUSCLE

Tumours of smooth muscle arise occasionally from the muscularis mucosae but more often from the muscularis propria. They are rare in both colon and rectum but slightly more numerous in the latter. A predilection for males (M:F = 1.8:1) was observed in a series of anorectal smooth muscle tumours from St Mark's Hospital, London.[373] They may occur at any age. Smooth muscle tumours which arise from the muscularis mucosae present as small, hard nodules or polyps. They are seldom more than 1 cm in diameter and are discovered as incidental findings. Tumours arising from the muscularis propria may be intraluminal, intramural, extramural or dumb-bell (intra- and extramural) in position. They vary greatly in size, from 1–20 cm in diameter, and tend to ulcerate the overlying mucosa (Fig. 8.75). The larger ones commonly undergo cystic change and haemorrhage. On section they are hard and lobulated. Microscopically, there is a more or less orderly arrangement of branching and interlacing bands of smooth muscle cells.

Most malignant tumours, as judged by metastasis, tend to be larger and cystic degeneration is frequent. Lymph node metastases are rare, and occur only with very anaplastic tumours. Extensive local spread in continuity with the main tumour can make adequate local removal difficult and lead to a high local recurrence rate. A high local recurrence rate for smooth muscle tumours arising in the muscularis propria of the anorectal region (including internal sphincter) is not related to grade of differentiation.[373] The presence of bizarre cells is not a reliable indication of malignancy since these may be the result of degeneration. The bizarre or epithelioid variety of smooth muscle tumour not uncommonly seen in the stomach is rare in the large intestine. The best criteria of malignancy are anaplasia[373,374] and the numbers of mitotic figures. Tumour necrosis and a high cellularity are also suggestive of an aggressive behaviour. It is important that each tumour is adequately sampled for histological examination since marked variability in appearance can occur in different areas of the same tumour. The survival rate after surgery is variable,[375] and in some patients local recurrence and hepatic or pulmonary metastases may appear as long as 10 years after the initial treatment.

A unique case has been reported in which an apparently benign but infiltrating multicentric smooth muscle tumour involved the proximal colon along its entire circumference with nodules in the mesocolon; this has been termed leiomyomatosis of the colon.[376]

NEUROGENIC TUMOURS

Solitary benign neurofibroma of the rectum and colon is rare, only a few cases having been reported.[377] They occur in the submucosal layer and within the myenteric plexus. There is one case report of a solitary tumour of the rectum presenting in a patient with von Recklinghausen's disease.[378]

Multiple neurofibromas of the gastrointestinal tract are quite common in von Recklinghausen's disease, though the colon seems to be involved less frequently than the small intestine.[379] Plexiform neurofibromatosis of the colon has been reported.[380] Diffuse intestinal ganglioneuromatosis, medullary carcinoma of the thyroid, phaeochromocytoma and multiple mucosal neuromas may co-exist in an inherited syndrome.[381] There are cases of polypoid ganglioneurofibromatosis of the large bowel mixed with multiple polyps of the juvenile type.[382-384] This seems to be an example of how one hamartomatous disorder may be accompanied by other tissue malformations. Localized ganglioneuromatosis in the absence of systemic disease is rare, but has been described throughout the gastrointestinal tract. Most cases seen at St Mark's Hospital, London, have presented as ulcerating strictures of the small bowel simulating Crohn's disease.

TUMOURS OF FAT

Simple lipomas

Lipomas of the colon and rectum are uncommon.[385] They usually arise in the submucosa, although subserosal tumours occur occasionally. Most examples are single, but multiple lipomas have been recorded. Small submucosal lipomas are sometimes found incidentally in operation specimens removed for other conditions. Lipomas less than 2 cm in diameter are probably always symptomless. Presenting symptoms for larger lipomas include pain (due to acute or chronic intussusception) and bleeding per rectum (from ulceration of overlying mucosa). It seems that lipomas are found rather more often in the right colon than in the left colon or rectum. Macroscopically, a lipoma is characteristically round and very soft, with a short pedicle. Microscopically, the appearances are those of simple adipose tissue. Necrosis and haemorrhage may be such prominent features in tumours which have presented because of intussusception, that all microscopic evidence of adipose tissue has been obliterated with replacement by vascular granulation tissue. In such cases the macroscopic appearance of the tumour might suggest the correct diagnosis.

Lipomatous polyposis

There are several case reports of lipomatous polyposis of the colon.[386,387] In one of these, the small intestine was also extensively affected.[387] The lipomas are submucous in position and project into the lumen as large polypoid tumours. Enlargement of the appendices epiploicae without any submucous tumours is probably hamartomatous rather than neoplastic.[388]

Lipohyperplasia of the ileocaecal valve

In this condition there is an excess of adipose tissue in the submucosa at the ileocaecal valve producing thickening and pouting of the valve, which protrudes into the caecum.[389] There may be some narrowing of the lumen. The appearance has been likened to a boggy, reddened cervix and to prolapsed haemorrhoids. Mild degrees of lipohyperplasia of the ileocaecal valve are quite commonly found in operation specimens removed for other conditions. It is usually a localized manifestation of generalized obesity and only occasionally gives rise to symptoms when it is one cause of the 'ileocaecal valve syndrome'.[390] It may be mistaken radiologically for a carcinoma or some other type of tumour.

Microscopically, the adipose tissue in the submucosa is in excess of normal, but is not encapsulated and fades away in both sides of the valve. Occasionally, there is congestion of the thickened valve with erosion of the overlying mucosa which leads to bleeding. The condition should not be confused with lipoma or with true intestinal lipomatosis which is hamartomatous.

MISCELLANEOUS TUMOURS

Isolated case reports of soft tissue tumours involving the large bowel include granular cell myoblastoma of the rectum[391] and caecum,[392] and fibrosarcoma of the rectum.[393] These tumours are uncommon. Involvement of the large bowel by rhabdomyosarcoma[394] and haemangiopericytoma[395] has been described, but these tumours probably arose outside the bowel wall.

Vascular tumours and tumour-like lesions are discussed on p. 353.

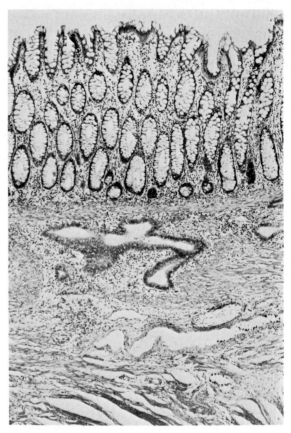

Fig. 8.76 Endometriosis. Endometrial tissue, including characteristic stroma, occupies the submucosa.
Haematoxylin-eosin   × 100

MISCELLANEOUS CONDITIONS

Endometriosis

The large intestine is involved by endometriosis in as many as 20% of women with this condition.[396] However, most cases are not associated with symptoms referable to the bowel. For this reason endometriosis is often discovered in surgical specimens removed for other conditions. When symptoms do arise, the commonest are abdominal pain, constipation and intestinal obstruction. Rectal bleeding is uncommon. The sigmoid colon and rectum are the sites of predilection.

Endometriomas are ill-defined firm tumours up to 5 cm in diameter. They are found in the subserous and muscular coats of the bowel, but may involve the submucosa (Fig. 8.76). The cut surface is a glistening grey colour with haemorrhagic foci. The lesion may project into the lumen as a non-ulcerated polypoid mass. Biopsy may cause ulceration and subsequent biopsy of endometrial tissue sprouting through the defect may produce a histological appearance that could be mistaken for adenocarcinoma.

The peritoneal surface of the bowel, particularly within the pouch of Douglas, may become studded by endometrial tissue resembling secondary deposits of carcinoma.

Systemic sclerosis (scleroderma)

Involvement of the large intestine is commonly seen in systemic sclerosis. Alternating thickening and thinning of the bowel wall results from patchy replacement of the muscularis propria by collagen and elastic tissue. Multiple sacculations develop in the weakened bowel wall. The taeniae coli are relatively spared, even in advanced cases. Submucosal changes are not pronounced and the mucous membrane may be atrophic or show non-specific inflammatory changes with patchy ulceration. Some of these changes may be the result of ischaemia due to arterial involvement.[397]

Patients may present with the syndrome of 'chronic intestinal pseudo-obstruction' in which there is intractable constipation or alternating constipation and diarrhoea. This syndrome is secondary to a variety of causes (see p. 320) but the most important differential diagnosis is 'hollow visceral myopathy'[398] (see below).

Hollow visceral myopathy[398]

This familial condition has been described comparatively recently; its pathogenesis is poorly understood. Any segment of the gastrointestinal tract may be involved, but the duodenum is the site of predilection. The affected bowel is dilated and thin-walled. The smooth muscle of the muscularis propria, particularly the longitudinal coat, shows vacuolation, degeneration and fibrosis. Deposition of lipofuscin may be prominent but this is probably a non-specific feature of malabsorption; severe cases involving the small intestine have been referred to as the 'brown bowel syndrome' (see p. 275).[399] Distinctive abnormalities of the colonic myenteric plexus have been demonstrated by silver impregnation techniques in a series of women with hollow visceral myopathy.[400]

Pseudo-melanosis coli

The occurrence of melanin-like pigmentation in the mucosa of the colon and rectum has been related to chronic constipation and to the consumption of purgatives of the anthracene group. It is relatively uncommon today, but still occasionally seen in surgical specimens removed for a variety of large bowel disorders including megacolon, volvulus and carcinoma (see Fig. 8.60). In most cases the presence of pigment is only apparent on microscopic examination, although in severe cases it may be obvious to the naked eye, when the large bowel mucosa assumes a colour varying from black

to brown. Although the right side of the colon, including the appendix, is more markedly affected than the left, the terminal ileum and other parts of the small intestine are never involved. The lymphoid follicles in the colonic mucosa do not contain pigment and stand out against the dark background as tiny white spots. Occasionally the regional lymph nodes may contain pigment. Adenocarcinomas and carcinomas arising within the affected colon are also free of pigment.

Microscopic examination shows that the pigment is present in macrophages within the lamina propria. It is a golden-brown colour in haematoxylin and eosin preparations (Fig. 8.77).

Histochemical stains show that the pigment is not a true melanin, but that it has staining properties of lipofuscin.[401] Both the pigment-containing macrophages and the epithelial cells

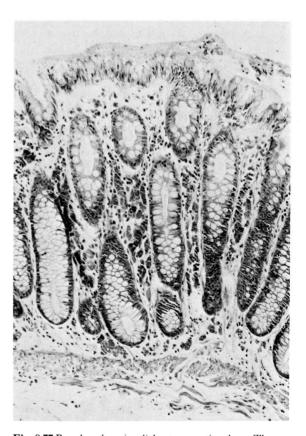

Fig. 8.77 Pseudomelanosis coli due to purgative abuse. The lamina propria contains large numbers of pigment-laden macrophages.

Haematoxylin-eosin   × 100

have been shown to contain numerous cytolysosomes.[402,403] These are membrane-bound cytoplasmic structures formed by the accumulation of damaged cellular organelles within lysosomes. Hydrolysis of these damaged organelles by lysosomal enzymes leads to the production of lipofuscin. The initial damage may be brought about by a variety of noxious agents including anthracene purgatives.

Cathartic colon

The ingestion of excessive quantities of any purgative can lead to a diarrhoeal state with potassium deficiency, excessive loss of water, steatorrhoea or protein-losing gastroenteropathy.[404] This condition is clinically and radiologically distinctive. Such patients always have melanosis coli but in addition they have a curious macroscopic appearance of the mucosal surface, particularly in the proximal colon, which has been variously compared to the skin of a toad's back, snake skin or alligator skin. Sacculation of the bowel wall may be present. There can also be mucosal atrophy and thickening of the muscularis propria.

The pathogenesis of cathartic colon has become clearer as a result of neuropathological studies on the myenteric plexus of the colon, and with the realization that anthraquinones (taken as a remedy for constipaton) are potent cell poisons, even in minute doses.[405,406] These are concentrated in the colon, particularly on the right side. They probably stimulate the nervous tissue to produce a purgative action. In surgical specimens of early cases of cathartic colon the only abnormality of the myenteric plexus is gross swelling and pallor of the neurons, suggesting overstimulation. Later there is loss of myenteric neurons, with Schwann cell proliferation. Finally there is toxic damage to the smooth muscle cells resulting in muscular atrophy, so that there is failure of gut motility. The colon is converted into a dilated, thin-walled tube.

Gas cysts of the colon and rectum (pneumatosis coli)

Cystic pneumatosis is a rare condition in which gas cysts appear in the submucosal and serosal layers of the gastrointestinal tract, most commonly in the small intestine but also in the colon.[407] The pathology is the same whatever the level involved. The entire colon and rectum can be affected or only a part. The diagnosis is made by sigmoidoscopy and rectal biopsy and the radiological appearances are also characteristic.[408] The disease is often symptomless but can present with diarrhoea, rectal bleeding due to erosion of mucous membrane covering the cysts, or rarely pneumoperitoneum from rupture of a gas cyst into the abdominal cavity.[409] It can also simulate polyposis coli. The condition can apparently resolve spontaneously.

The aetiology of pneumatosis coli is unknown. It can affect both children (especially neonates; see p. 351) and adults and has been associated with a variety of intestinal disorders of inflammatory, neoplastic, vascular or mechanical aetiology, and (in adults) with pulmonary emphysema and chronic lung disease.[410] Among the theories of pathogenesis are the entry of gas-forming bacteria after damage to the bowel wall.[411] Mechanical theories have suggested that intestinal gas may enter the bowel wall from the lumen after mucosal damage, or that air from ruptured pulmonary alveoli may dissect through the mediastinum and retroperitoneum and along the mesenteric vessels into the bowel wall,[412] or that the gas cysts represent dilated lymphatics.[413] Biochemical theories refer to variations in acid–base balance in the intestinal wall and excessive carbohydrate fermentation within the bowel lumen.[414]

The mucosal surface has a coarse, cobblestone appearance due to large numbers of submucosal cysts, the apices of which may show intramucosal haemorrhage. Cysts also project from the serosal surface. The gas appears to be under pressure, as rupture of cysts through the sigmoidoscope or in fresh surgical specimens causes a popping sound.

The rectal biopsy appearances are distinctive. Cystic spaces lying in the submucosa immediately beneath the muscularis mucosae are lined by large macrophages. These may be multinucleate with eosinophilic cytoplasm, which may contain fatty droplets.[413] The connective tissue between the cysts, which are often multilocular, shows little or no evidence of inflammation. The covering mucous membrane is attenuated and sometimes contains small haemorrhages. The appearances are most likely to be confused with lymphangioma and oleogranuloma. In the former there are no macrophages and the lymphatic spaces are lined by a flattened endothelium without any interstitial inflammation. In oleogranuloma there is a macrophage response but also much inflammation and fibrosis around fat-filled spaces (see p. 404).

Malakoplakia

Although this condition is most frequently found in the urinary tract there are increasing reports of its occurrence in the large intestine[415] where it may present with abdominal pain, diarrhoea and rectal bleeding. It usually appears either as a single tumour or as multiple polypoid lesions, but there is one report of diffuse thickening affecting the majority of the colon.[416] Histologically, the lesion is composed of an infiltrate of large macrophages with an eosinophilic granular cytoplasm in which characteristic PAS-positive iron-containing calculospherules (Michaelis-Gutmann bodies) are found (Fig. 8.78). The lesion often occurs in patients with co-existing debilitating illnesses or malignancy. There is increasing evidence that the condition represents an abnormal macrophage response to bacterial infection.[417]

Epiploic appendages

The importance of these structures is their occasional liability to torsion, with thrombosis and infarction, giving rise to symptoms which mimic acute appendicitis.[418] Aseptic necrosis with separation, hyalinization and calcification is quite common.[419] Probably most loose bodies in the peritoneal cavity (so-called peritoneal 'mice') are due to torsion and separation of appendices epiploicae (see p. 314). They can cause intestinal obstruction by becoming adherent to the abdominal wall with the formation of a fibrous band or

adhesion through which a loop of bowel becomes incarcerated. There are reports of torsion of appendages occurring within hernia sacs causing pain which may resolve spontaneously or require surgical intervention. It is not uncommon to find minor degrees of inflammation and fibrosis in and around epiploic appendages in surgical specimens of colon removed for a variety of unrelated conditions.

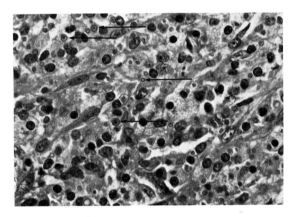

Fig. 8.78 Malakoplakia complicating a rectal adenocarcinoma (not shown). The large histiocytes have a granular cytoplasm and many contain Michaelis-Gutmann bodies (arrows).
Haematoxylin-eosin   × 300

Muciphages

Macrophages distended by granular material which on staining can be shown to contain mucosubstances[420] are a common finding in rectal biopsies. Such cells have been mistaken for manifestations of Whipple's disease[421] or carbohydrate and other storage disorders. They are in fact 'muciphages'—normal phagocytic cells which have taken up mucus liberated into the lamina propria following damage to the mucosa. They are probably a non-specific manifestation of mucosal damage.

REFERENCES

Anatomical considerations

1. Underhill BML. Br Med J 1955; 2: 1243.
2. Phillips SF. In: Polak JM, Bloom SR, Wright NA, Butler AG, eds. Basic science in gastroenterology. Physiology of the gut. Glaxo Group Research, 1984: 283.
3. Baumgarten HG. In: Bertaccini G, ed. Mediators and drugs in gastrointestinal motility. I. Morphological basis and neurophysiological control. Berlin: Springer, 1982: 7.
4. Furness JB, Costa M. In: Bertaccini G, ed. Mediators

and drugs in gastrointestinal motility. I. Morphological basis and neurophysiological control. Berlin: Springer, 1982.
5. Smith B. Gut 1970; 11 : 271.
6. Burnstock G. Scand J Gastroenterol 1981; 16 (suppl 70) : 1.
7. Gabella G. Br Med Bull 1979; 35/3: 213.
8. Cheng H, Bjerknes M. Am J Gastroenterol 1984; 86: 76.
9. Cheng H, Leblond CP. Am J Anat 1974; 141 : 537.
10. Brandtzaeg P. Clin Exp Immunol 1981; 44: 221.
11. Filipe MI. Invest Cell Pathol 1979; 2 : 195.
12. Wiley EL, Mendelsohn G, Eggleston JC. Lab Invest 1981; 44: 507.
13. Bloom SR, Polak JM. In: Gut hormones. Edinburgh: Churchill Livingstone, 1981.
14. Sjolund K, Sanden G, Hakanson R, Sundler F. Gastroenterol 1983: 85 : 1120.

Congenital abnormalities

15. Gross RE. In: The surgery of infancy and childhood. Philadelphia, 1953; chs 11, 12, 14, 17.
16. Williams KL. Br J Surg 1960; 47: 351.
17. Sugihara K, Muto T, Morioka Y, Asano A, Yamamoto T. Dis Col Rect 1984; 27: 531.
18. Wolff M. Am J Clin Pathol 1971; 55 : 604.
19. Meier-Ruge W. Curr Topics in Pathol 1974; 59 : 131.
20. Careskey JM, Weber TR, Grosfeld JL. Am J Surg 1982; 131 : 160.
21. Smith B. In: The neuropathology of the alimentary tract. London: Arnold, 1972.
22. Bishop AE, Polak JM, Lake BD, Bryent MG, Bloom SR. Histopathol 1981; 5 : 679.
23. Trigg PH, Belin R, Haberkorn S et al. J Clin Pathol 1974; 27: 207.
24. Lake BD. In: Filipe MI, Lake BD, eds. Histochemistry in pathology. Edinburgh: Churchill Livingstone, 1983.
25. Hamoudi AB, Reiner CB, Boles ET, McClung HJ, Kerzner B. Arch Pathol Lab Med 1982; 106: 670.
26. Puri P, Lake BD, Nixon HH. Gut 1977; 18: 754.
27. Howard ER, Garrett JR, Kidd A. Scand J Gastroenterol 1982; 71 (suppl): 151.
28. Puri P, Lake BD, Nixon HH, Mishalany H, Claireaux AE. J Ped Surg 1977; 12: 681.
29. Scharli AF, Meier-Ruge W. J Ped Surg 1981; 16: 164.
30. Feinstat T, Tesluk H, Schuffler MD et al. Gastroenterol 1984; 86: 1573.
31. Bodian M, Stephens FD, Ward BCH. Lancet 1949; i: 6.
32. Rapola J, Santavuori P, Savilahti E. Hum Pathol 1984; 15: 352.

Acquired megacolon and megarectum

33. Todd IP. Proc Roy Soc Med 1961; 54: 1035.
34. Ehrenpreis T, Bentley JFR, Nixon HH et al. Arch Dis Child 1966; 41: 143.
35. Zimmerman GR. Arch Pathol 1962; 74: 59.
36. Lindop GBM. Gut 1983; 24: 575.
37. Faulk DL, Anuras S, Christensen J. Gastroenterol 1979; 74: 922.

Mechanical disorders

38. Byane JJ. Am J Surg 1960; 99: 168.
39. Becker WF. Surg Gyn Obstet 1953; 96: 677
40. Eisenstat TE, Raneri AJ, Mason GR. Am J Surg 1977; 134: 396.
41. Sachidananthan CK, Soehner B. Dis Col Rect 1972; 15: 466.
42. Bond MR, Roberts JBM. Br J Surg 1964; 51: 818.
43. Cole GJ. Br J Surg 1966; 53: 415.
44. Israel GI. Dis Col Rect 1961; 4: 139.
45. Levison DA, Crocker PR, Smith A, Blackshaw AJ, Bartram CI. J Clin Pathol 1984; 37: 481.
46. Comline SC. Br Med J 1952; ii: 745.
47. Dickinson PH, Gilmour J. Br J Surg 1961; 49: 157.
48. Thomas CS, Brockman SK. Ann Surg 1966: 164: 853.

Diverticular disease

49. Welch CE, Allen AW, Donaldson GA. Ann Surg 1953; 138: 332.
50. Slack WW. Gastroenterol 1961; 39: 708.
51. Morson BC. Br J Radiol 1963; 36: 385.
52. Williams IP. Br J Radiol 1963; 36: 393.
53. Morson BC. Proc Roy Soc Med 1963; 56: 798.
54. Whiteway JE, Morson BC. Gut 1985; 26: 258.
55. Eastwood MA, Watters DAK, Smith AN. In: Connell AM, ed. Clinics in gastroenterology 11/3. London: Saunders, 1982.
56. Painter NS. In: Diverticular disease of the colon. London: Heinemann, 1975.
57. Mobley JE, Dockerty MB, Waugh JM. Am J Surg 1957; 94: 44.
58. Lockhart-Mummery HE. Proc Roy Soc Med 1958; 51: 1032.
59. Sugihara K, Muto T, Morioka Y. Gut 1983; 24: 1130.

Inflammatory disorders

60. Bartlett JG, Moon N, Chang TW et al. Gastroenterol 1978; 75: 778.
61. Price AB, Jewkes J, Sanderson PJ. J Clin Pathol 1979; 32: 990.
62. Vantrappen G, Agg HO, Ponette E et al. Gastroenterol 1977; 72: 220.
63. Marsh PK, Gorbach SL. Gastroenterol 1982; 82: 336.
64. Day DW, Mandal BK, Morson BC. Histopathol 1978; 2: 117.
65. Price AB, Dolby JM, Dunscombe PR, Stirling J. J Clin Pathol 1984; 31: 1007.
66. Evans N. Clinics in Gastroenterol 1979; 8: 599.
67. Karmali MA, Fleming PC. Can Med Assoc J 1979; 120: 1525.
68. Skirrow MB. Br Med J 1977; ii: 9.
69. McElfatrick RA, Wurtzebach LR. Gastroenterol 1973; 65: 303.
70. Van Heynnigen WE, Gladstone GP. Br J Exp Pathol 1953; 34: 202.
71. Goodall HB, Sinclair ISR. J Path Bact 1957; 73: 33.
72. Burdon DW, George RH, Mogg GAG et al. J Clin Pathol 1981; 54: 548.
73. Price AB, Davies DR. J Clin Pathol 1977; 30: 1.
74. El-Maraghi NRH, Mair NS. Am J Clin Pathol 1979; 71: 631.

75. Anscombe AR, Keddie NC, Schofield PF. Gut 1967; 8 : 337.
76. Hawley PR, Wolfe HRI, Fullerton JM. Gut 1968; 9 : 461.
77. Tandon HD, Prakash A, Rao VB, Prakash O, Nair SK. Ind J Med Res 1966; 54 : 129.
78. Morson BC. Proc Roy Soc Med 1961; 4 : 723.
79. Powers PW, Kramer SG, Drake WL. Am J Surg 1961; 102 : 713.
80. Smith D. Dis Col Rect 1965; 8 : 57.
81. Douglas TG, Crucioli V. Br Med J 1981; ii : 1362.
82. Antonakopoulous G, Newman J, Wilkinson M. Histopathol 1982; 6 : 477.
83. Tompkins DS, Waugh MA, Cooke EM. J Clin Pathol 1981; 34 : 1385.
84. Quinn TC, Goodell SE, Mkrtichian E et al. N Engl J Med 1981; 35 : 195.
85. Levine JS, Smith PD, Brugge WR. Gastroenterol 1980; 79 : 563.
86. Miles RPM. Br J Surg 1957; 45 : 180.
87. Levin I, Romano S, Steinberg M, Welsh RA. Dis Col Rect 1964; 7 : 129.
88. Boulton AJM, Slater DN, Hancock BW. Gut 1982; 23 : 247.
89. Goodell SE, Quinn TC, Mkrtichian EE et al. Gastroenterol 1981; 80 : 1159.
90. Foucar E, Kiyoshi M, Foucar K et al. Am J Clin Pathol 1981; 76 : 788.
91. Cooper HS, Ruffensperger ED, Jones L et al. Gastroenterol 1977; 72 : 1253.
92. Smith JMB. Gut 1969; 10 : 1035.
93. Morton TC, Neal RA, Sage M. Lancet 1951; i : 766.
94. Berkowitz D, Bernstein LH. Gastroenterol 1975; 68 : 786.
95. Turner GR, Millikan M, Carter R, Thompson RJ, Hinshaw DB. Am Surg 1965; 31 : 759.
96. Essenhigh DM, Carter RL. Gut 1966; 7 : 444.
97. Faegenburg D, Cheal H, Mandel PR, Ross ST. Am J. Roent 1967; 99 : 74.
98. Rappaport EM, Rossien AX, Rosenblum LA. Ann Intern Med 1951; 34 : 1224.
99. Powell SJ, Wilmot AJ. Gut 1966; 7 : 438.
100. Ruiz-Moreno F. Dis Col Rect 1963; 6 : 201.
101. Nime FA, Burek JD, Page DL et al. Gastroenterol 1976; 70 : 592.
102. Weinstein L, Edelstein SM, Madara JL et al. Gastroenterol 1981; 81 : 584.
103. Chiampi FP, Sundberg RD, Klompus JP, Wilson AJ. Hum Pathol 1983; 14 : 734.
104. Azar JE, Schraibman IG, Pitchford RJ. Trans Roy Soc Trop Med Hyg 1958; 52 : 562.
105. Gelfand M, Hammar B. Trans Roy Soc Trop Med Hyg 1966; 60 : 231.
106. Ming-Chai C, Chi-Yuan C, Pei-Yu C, Jen-Chun H. Cancer 1980; 46 : 1661.
107. Yokogawa M, Yoshimura H. Am J Trop Med Hyg 1967; 16 : 723.
108. Ashby BS, Appleton PJ, Dawson IMP. Br Med J 1964; i : 1141.
109. Pinkus GS, Coolidge C, Little MD. Am J Med 1975; 59 : 114.
110. Stemmermann GN. Gastroenterol 1967; 53 : 59.
111. O'Donoghue DP, Kumar P. Gut 1979; 20 : 149.
112. Heatley RV, Calcraft BJ, Rhodes J, Owen E, Evans BK. Gut 1975; 16 : 559.
113. Rosekrans PCM, Meyer CJLM, Van der Wal AM, Lindeman J. Gut 1980; 21 : 1017.
114. Carlsson HE, Lagercrantz R, Perlman P. Scand J Gastroenterol 1977; 12 : 707.
115. Bull DM, Ignaczak TF. Gastroenterol 1973; 64 : 43.
116. Shen L, Fanger MW. Cell Immunol 1981; 59 : 75.
117. Jewell DP, MacLennan ICM. Clin Exp Immunol 1977; 14 : 219.
118. Mee AS, McClaughlin JE, Hodgson HJF, Jewell DP. Gut 1979; 20 : 1.
119. Soltis RD, Hasz D, Morris MJ, Wilson ID. Gastroenterol 1976; 76 : 1380.
120. Keren DF. In: Norris HT, ed. Pathology of the colon, small intestine and anus. Edinburgh: Churchill Livingstone, 1983.
121. Law DH, Steinberg H, Sleisenger MH. Gastroenterol 1961; 41 : 457.
122. Acheson ED. Gut 1960; 1 : 291.
123. Riddell RH, Goldman H, Ransohoff DF et al. Hum Pathol 1983; 14 : 931.
124. Riddell RH. In: Morson BC, ed. Current topics in pathology, vol 63. Berlin, 1976.
125. Edwards FC, Truelove SC. Gut 1964; 5 : 15.
126. Lennard-Jones JE, Morson BC, Ritchie JK, Shove DC, Williams CB. Gastroenterol 1977; 73 : 12.
127. Lennard-Jones JL, Morson BC, Ritchie JK, Williams C. Lancet 1983; ii : 149.
128. Perrett AD, Higgins G, Johnston HH, Massarella GR, Truelove SC, Wright R. Quart J Med 1971; 40 : 211.
129. Holdsworth CD, Hall EW, Dawson AM, Sherlock S. Quart J Med 1965; 34 : 211.
130. Thorpe MEC, Scheuer PJ, Sherlock S. Gut 1967; 8 : 435.
131. Ritchie JK, Macartney AJ, Thompson H, Hawley PR, Cooke WT. Quart J Med 1974; 43 : 263.
132. Shorvon PD. Am J Dig Dis 1977; 22 : 209.
133. Warren R, Barwick W. Am J Surg Pathol 1983; 7 : 151.
134. Cooper JD, Weinstein MA, Korelitz BI. J Clin Gastroenterol 1984; 6 : 217.
135. Price AB. J Clin Pathol 1978; 31 : 567.
136. Joffe N. Clin Radiol 1977; 28 : 609.
137. Schmidt GT, Lennard-Jones JE, Morson BC, Young AC. Gut 1968; 9 : 7.
138. Lee FI, Costello FT, Cowley DJ, Murray SM, Srimankar J. Am J Gastroenterol 1983; 79 : 164.
139. Berthrong M, Fajardo LF. Am J Surg Pathol 1981; 5 : 153.
140. DeCosse JJ, Rhodes RS, Wentz WB et al. Ann Surg 1969; 170 : 369.
141. Toffler RB, Pingoud EG, Burrell MI. Lancet 1978; ii : 707.
142. Sakurai Y, Tsuchiya N, Ikegami F et al. Dig Dis Sci 1979; 24 : 910.
143. Martin DM, Goldman JA, Gilliam J et al. Gastroenterol 1981; 80 : 1567.
144. Ingle JN. N Engl J Med 1981; 304 : 1044.
145. Floch MH, Hellman L. Gastroenterol 1965; 48 : 430.
146. Leriche M, Devroede G, Sanchez G et al. Dis Col Rect 1978; 21 : 227.
147. Lindstrom CG. Pathol Eur 1976; 11 : 87.
148. Bogomoletz WV, Adnet JJ, Birembaut P, Feydy P, Dupont P. Gut 1980; 21 : 164.
149. Nielsen VT, Vetner M. Histopathol 1980; 4 : 83.
150. Pieterse AS, Hecker R, Rowland R. J Clin Pathol 1982; 35 : 338.
151. Eaves ER, Wallis PL, McIntyre RLE, Korman MG. Aus NZ J Med 1983; 13 : 630.

152. Teglbjaerg PS, Thaysen EH. Gastroenterol 1982; 82: 561.
153. Grouls V, Vogal J, Sorger M. Endoscopy 1982; 14: 31.
154. Epstein RJ, McDonald GB, Sale GE et al. Gastroenterol 1980; 78: 764.
155. Sale GE, McDonald GB, Shulman HM et al, Am J Surg Pathol 1979; 3: 291.
156. Werlis SL, Chusid MJ, Caya J et al. Gastroenterol 1982; 82: 328.
157. Strauss RG, Ghishan F, Mitros F et al. Dig Dis Sci 1980; 25: 798.
158. McMillan A, Lee FD. Gut 1981; 22: 1035.
159. Tompkins DS, Waugh MA, Cooke EM. J Clin Pathol 1981; 34: 1385.
160. Levine JS, Smith PDF, Brugge WR. Gastroenterol 1980; 79: 563.
161. Burnham WR, Reeve RS, Finch RG. Gut 1980; 21: 1097.
162. McMillan A, Gilmour HM, McNeillage G, Scott GR. Gut 1984; 25: 356.
163. Gillin JS, Uramacher CM, West R, Shike M. Gastroenterol 1983; 85: 1187.
164. Chiampi P, Sundberg RD, Klompus JP, Wilson AJ. Hum Pathol 1983; 14: 734.

Vascular disorders

165. Marston A, Murray TP, Lea Thomas M, Morson BC. Gut 1966; 7: 1.
166. Mori W. Histopathol 1981; 5: 113.
167. Barcewicz PA, Welch JP. Dis Col Rect 1980; 23: 109.
168. Gage TP, Cagnier JM. Gastroenterol 1983; 84: 171.
169. Marston A, Kieny R, Szilayi E, Taylor GW. Arch Surg 1976; 111: 107.
170. Marston A. Clin Gastroenterol 1972; 1: 539.
171. Tait RA, Kealy WF. J Clin Pathol 1979; 32: 1090.
172. Dawson AMP, Schaeffer JW. Gastroenterol 1971; 60: 577.
173. Kies MS, Luedke DW, Boyd JF et al. Cancer 1979; 43: 730.
174. Feldman PS. Dis Col Rect 1975; 18: 601.
175. Blundell CR, Earnest DL. Dig Dis Sci 1980; 25: 494.
176. Sutherland DER, Chan FY, Foucar E et al. Surg 1979; 86: 386.
177. Rutter KRP, Riddell RH. Clin Gastroenterol 1975; 4: 505.
178. Rosengren J-E, Hildell J, Lindstrom CG, Leandoer L. Gastrointest Radiol 1982; 7: 79.
179. Lee EL, Smith HJ, Miller GL, Burns DK, Weiner H. Am J Gastroenterol 1984; 79: 35.
180. Kistin MG, Kaplan MM, Harrington JT. Gastroenterol 1978; 75: 1147.
181. Baba S, Maruta M, Ando K et al. Dis Col Rect 1976; 19: 428.
182. Herrington JL, Grossman LA. Ann Surg 1968; 168: 1079.
183. Deprophetis N, Khubchandani IT. Dis Col Rect 1969; 12: 142.
184. Camilleri M, Chadwick VS, Hodgson HJF. Hepato-gastroenterol 1984; 31: 149.
185. Weinstein EC, Moertel CG, Waugh JM. Ann Surg 1963; 157: 265.
186. Parker GW, Murney JA, Kenoyer WL. Dis Col Rect 1960; 3: 358.
187. Boley SJ, Sammartano R, Adams A, DiBiase A, Kleinhaus S, Sprayregen S. Gastroenterol 1977; 72: 650.
188. Allison DJ, Hemingway AP. Lancet 1981; ii: 979.
189. Richter JM, Hedberg SE, Athanasoulis CA, Schapiro RH. Dig Dis Sci 1984; 29: 481.
190. Ivey K, Denbesten L, Kent TH, Clifton JA. Gastroenterol 1969; 57: 709.

Epithelial polyps

191. Stemmermann GN, Yatani R. Cancer 1972; 31: 1260.
192. Hayashi T, Yatani R, Apostol J, Stemmermann GN. Gastroenterol 1974; 66: 347.
193. Kaye GI, Fenoglio CM, Pascal RR, Lane N. Gastroenterol 1973; 64: 926.
194. Jass JR, Filipe MI, Abbas S et al. Cancer 1984; 53: 510.
195. Boland CR, Montgomery CK, Kim YS. Gastroenterol 1982; 2: 664.
196. Jass JR, Faludy J. Histochem J 1985; 17: 373.
197. Wattenberg LW. Am J Pathol 1959; 21: 165.
198. Czernobilsky B, Tsou K-C. Cancer 1968; 35: 113.
199. Arthur JF. J Clin Pathol 1968; 21: 735.
200. Vatn MH, Stalsberg H. Cancer 1982; 49: 819.
201. Williams GT, Arthur JK, Bussey HJR, Morson BC. Histopathol 1980; 4: 15.
202. Jass JR. Lancet 1983; i: 28.
203. Sumner HW, Wasserman NF, McClain CJ. Dig Dis Sci 1981; 26: 85.
204. Estrada RG, Spjut HJ. Am J Surg Pathol 1980; 4: 127.
205. Cooper HS, Patchefsky AS, Marks G. Dis Col Rect 1979; 22: 152.
206. Riddell RH, Goldman H, Ransohoff DF et al. Hum Pathol 1983; 14: 931.
207. Morson BC, Jass JR. In: Precancerous lesions of the gastrointestinal tract. London: Bailliere Tindall, 1985.
208. Morson BC, Sobin LH. In: The typing of intestinal tumours, vol 15. World Health Organization: Geneva, 1976.
209. Muto T, Ishikawa K, Kino I et al. Dis Col Rect 1977; 20: 11.
210. Hill MJ, Morson BC, Bussey HJR. Lancet 1978; i: 245.
211. Williams AR, Balasooriya BAW, Day DW. Gut 1982; 23: 835.
212. Sato E, Gann 1974; 65: 295.
213. Konishi F, Morson BC. J Clin Pathol 1982; 35: 830.
214. Deschner EE, Lipkin M. Cancer 1975; 35: 413.
215. Lane N, Lev R. Cancer 1963; 16: 751.
216. Maskens AP Gastroenterol 1979; 77: 1245.
217. Nakamura S, Kino I. J Nat Cancer Inst 1984; 77: 41.
218. Greaves P, Filipe MI, Abbas S, Ormerod MG. Histopathol 1984; 8: 825.
219. Goh HS, Jass JR. J Clin Pathol 1986; 39: 387.
220. Paraskeva C, Buckle BG, Sheer D, Wigley CB. Int J Cancer 1984; 34: 49.
221. Muto T, Bussey HJR, Morson BC. Cancer 1975; 36: 2251.
222. Sundblad AS, Paz RA. Cancer 1982; 50: 2504.
223. Fenoglio CM, Kaye GI, Lane N. Gastroenterol 1973; 64: 51.
224. Muto T, Bussey HJR, Morson BC. J Clin Pathol 1973; 26: 25.
225. Morson BC, Whiteway JE, Jones EA, Macrae FA, Williams CB. Gut 1984; 25: 437.
226. Colacchio TA, Forde KA, Scantlebury VP. Ann Surg 1981; 194: 704.

227. Cooper HS. In: Norris HT, ed. Pathology of the colon, small intestine and anus. Edinburgh: Churchill Livingstone, 1983: 201.
228. Bussey HJR. In: Anthony PP, MacSween NM, eds. Recent advances in histopathology, vol. 12. Edinburgh: Churchill Livingstone, 1984.
229. Luk GD, Baylin SB. NEJM 1984; 311: 80.
230. Cohen SB. J Med Gen 1982; 19: 193.
231. Gardner EJ. Am J Hum Gen 1953; 5: 139.
232. Gardner EJ. Am J Hum Gen 1962: 14: 376.
233. McAdam WAF, Goligher JC. Br J Surg 1970; 57: 618.
234. Simpson RD, Harrison EG, Mayo CW. Cancer 1964; 17: 526.
235. Gardner EJ. Proc Utah Acad 1969; 46: 1.
236. Bussey HJR. Proc Roy Soc Med 1972; 65: 294.
237. Utsunomiya J, Maki T, Iwama T et al. Cancer 1974; 34: 745.
238. Yao T, Iida M, Ohsato K, Watanabe H, Omae T. Gastroenterol 1977; 73: 1036.
239. Watanabe H, Enjoji M, Yao T, Ohsato K. Hum Pathol 1978; 9: 270.
240. Thompson JS, Harned RK, Anderson JC, Hodgson PE. Dis Col Rect 1983; 26: 583.
241. Turcot J, Despres JP, St Pierre F. Dis Col Rect 1959; 2: 465.
242. Kingston JE, Herbert A, Draper GJ, Mann JR. Arch Dis Child 1983; 58: 959.
243. Perkins JT, Blackstone MO, Riddell RH. Cancer 1985; 55: 375.
244. Utsunomiya J, Nakamura T. Br J Surg 1975; 62: 45.
245. Lewis JH, Ginsberg AL, Toomey KE. Cancer 1983; 51: 524.
246. Bussey HJR. Gut 1970; 11: 970.
247. Franzin G, Zamboni G, Dina R, Scarpa A, Fratton A. Histopathol 1983; 7: 719.
248. Tung-hua L, Ming-chang C, Hsien-chiu T. Chin Med J 1978; 4: 434.
249. Friedmann CJ, Fechner RE. Dig Dis Sci 1982; 27: 946.
250. Veale AMO, McColl I, Bussey HJR, Morson BC. J Med Gen 1966; 3: 5.
251. Sachatello CR, Carrington CG. Surg 1974; 75: 107.
252. Smilow PC, Pryor CA, Swinton NW. Dis Col Rect 1966; 9: 248.
253. Jarvinen H, Franssila KO. Gut 1984; 25: 792.
254. Lipper S, Kahn LB, Sandler RS, Varma V. Hum Pathol 1981; 12: 804.
255. Ramaswamy G, Elhasseiny AA, Tchertkoff V. Dis Col Rect 1984; 27: 393.
256. Mendelsohn G, Diamond MP. Am J Surg Pathol 1984; 8: 515.
257. Monga G, Mozzucco G, Castello R, Mollo F. Ital J Gastroenterol 1983; 15: 119.
258. Tweedie JH, McCann BG. Gut 1984; 25: 1118.
259. Stockdale AD, Ashford RFU, Leader M. Clin Oncol 1984; 10: 229.
260. Cronkhite LW, Canada WJ. NEJM 1955; 252: 1011.
261. Ryall RJ. Proc Roy Soc Med 1966; 59: 614.
262. Lloyd KM, Dennis M. Ann Intern Med 1963; 58: 136.
263. Carlson GJ, Nivatvongs S, Snover DC. Am J Surg Pathol 1984; 8: 763.

Malignant epithelial tumours

264. Wynder EL. Cancer Res 1975; 35: 3388.
265. Correa P. Cancer Res 1975; 35: 3395.
266. Wynder EL, Kajitani, Ishikawa S, Dodo H, Takano A. Cancer 1969; 23: 1210.
267. Sugano H, Kato Y, Nakamura K. In: UICC Fukuoka symposium on fundamental and clinical aspects of digestive tract tumors. Fukuoka, Japan: Tsukushi Kaikan, 1984: 23.
268. Rhodes JB, Holmes FF, Clark GM. JAMA 1977; 238: 1641.
269. Wood DA, Robbins GF, Zippin C, Lum D, Stearns M. Cancer 1979; 43: 961.
270. Falterman KW, Hill CB, Markey JC, Fox JW, Cohn I. Cancer 1974; 34: 951.
271. Drasar BS, Hill MJ. In: Human intestinal flora. London: Academic Press, 1974.
272. Drasar BS. In: Sircus W, Smith AN, eds. Scientific foundations of gastroenterology. London: Heinemann, 1980: 67.
273. Cruse JP, Lewin MR, Clark CG. Lancet 1979; i: 752.
274. Davidson M, Yoshizawa CN, Kolonel LN. Br Med J 1985; 290: 1868.
275. Burkitt DP. Cancer 1971; 28: 3.
276. Haenszel W, Berg JW, Segi M et al. J Nat Cancer Inst 1973; 51: 1765.
277. Cummings JH. In: Polak JM, Bloom SR, Wright NA, Butler AG, eds. Basic science in gastroenterology. Physiology of the gut. Glaxo Group Research, 1984: 371.
278. Thornton JR. Lancet 1981; i: 1081.
279. Jass JR. Med Hypoth 1985; 18: 113.
280. Newmark HL, Wargowich MJ, Bruce WR. J Nat Cancer Inst 1984; 72: 1323.
281. Nelson RL. Dis Col Rect 1984; 27: 459.
282. Veale AMO. In: Intestinal polyposis. London: Cambridge University Press, 1965.
283. Burt RW, Bishop T, Canon LA, Dowdle NA, Lee RG, Skolnick MH. New Engl J Med 1985; 315: 1540.
284. Lovett E. Br J Surg 1976; 63: 13.
285. Lynch HT, Lynch J, Guirgis HA. In: Lynch HT, ed. Cancer genetics. Springfield: Thomas, 1976: 326.
286. Pero RW, Miller DG, Lipkin M et al. J Nat Cancer Inst 1983; 70: 867.
287. Konishi F, Morson BC. J Clin Pathol 1982; 35: 830.
288. Muto T, Ishikawa K, Kino I et al. Dis Col Rect 1977; 20: 11.
289. Muto T, Bussey HJR, Morson BC. Cancer 1975; 36: 2251.
290. Eide TJ. Cancer 1983; 51: 1866.
291. Heald RJ, Bussey HJR. Dis Col Rect 1975; 18: 6.
292. Gilbertsen VA, Nelms JM. Cancer 1978; 41: 137.
293. Bussey HJR, Wallace MH, Morson BC. Proc Roy Soc Med 1967; 60: 208.
294. Bussey HJR. In: Cancer and aging. Thule International Symposia. Stockholm: Nordiska Bokhandelns Forlag, 1968: 1.
295. Shorter RG. Bull NY Acad Med 1984; 60: 980.
296. Ming-Chai C, Chi-Yuan C, P'ei-Yu C, Jen-Chun H. Cancer 1980; 46: 1661.
297. Cipolla R, Garcia RL. Am J Gastroenterol 1984; 79: 453.
298. van der Linden W, Katzenstein B, Nakayama F. Cancer 1983; 52: 1265.
299. Bundred NY, Whitfield BCS, Stanton E, Prescott RS, Davies GC, Kingsnorth AN. Br J Surg 1984; 71: 989.
300. Rubio CA, Nylander G, Wallin B, Sveander M, Alun M-L, Duvander A. Dis Col Rect 1984; 27: 468.
301. Filipe MI. J Clin Pathol 1972; 25: 123.
302. Jass JR, Morson BC. In: Glass GBJ, Sherlock P, eds.

Progress in gastroenterology, vol IV. New York: Grune & Stratton, 1983: 345.

303. Vobecky J, Leduc C, Devroede G. Cancer 1984; 54: 3065.
304. Welch JS, Dockerty JB. Dis Col Rect 1958; 101: 339.
305. Lui IOL, Kung ITM, Lee JMH, Boey JH. Pathol 1985; 17: 31.
306. Gibbs NM. Histopathol 1977; 1: 77.
307. Sanerkin NG. J Path Bact 1968; 95: 947.
308. Wattenberg LW. Am J Pathol 1959; 35: 113.
309. Czernobilsky B, Tsou K-C. Cancer 1968; 21: 165.
310. Vatn MH, Tjora S, Arva PH, Serck-Hanssen A, Stromme JH Gut 1982; 23: 194.
311. Reid PE, Culling CFA, Dunn WL, Ramey CW, Magil AB, Clay MG. J Histochem Cytochem 1980; 8: 117.
312. Boland CR, Montgomery CK, Kim YS. Proc Nat Acad Sci 1982; 79: 2051.
313. Magnani JL, Brachaus M, Smith DF et al. Science 1981; 212: 55.
314. Shi ZR, McIntyre LJ, Knowles BB, Solter D, Kim YS. Cancer Res 1984; 44: 1142.
315. Blaszczyk M, Ross AH, Ernst CS et al. Int J Cancer 1984; 33: 313.
316. Brown A, Ellis IO, Embleton MJ, Baldwin RW, Turner DR, Hardcastle JD. Int J Can.
317. McKinley M, Budman D, Caccese W et al. Am J Gastroenterol 1985; 80: 47.
318. Reddy EP, Reynolds RK, Santos E, Barbacid M. Nature 1982; 30: 149.
319. Alitalo K, Winqvist R, Lin CC, de la Chapelle A, Schwab M, Bishop JM. Proc Natl Acad Sci USA. 1984; 81: 4534.
320. Calabretta B, Kaczmarek L, Ming P-M, Au F, Ming SC. Cancer Res 1985; 45: 6000.
321. Kerr IB, Lee FD, Quintanilla M, Balmain A. Br J Cancer 1985; 52: 695.
322. Wolmark N, Fisher ER, Wieand HS, Fisher B. Cancer 1984; 53: 2707.
323. Jass JR, Atkin WS, Cuzick J et al. Histopathology 1986; 10: 437.
324. Symonds DA, Vickery AL. Cancer 1976; 37: 1891.
325. Jass JR. J Clin Pathol 1986; 39: 585.
326. Pretlow TP, Keith EF, Cryar AK et al. Cancer Res 1983; 43: 2997.
327. Grinnell RS. Ann Surg 1939; 109: 500.
328. Dukes CE. Proc Roy Soc Med 1937; 30: 371.
329. Dukes CE, Bussey HJR. Br J Cancer 1958; 12: 309.
330. Isaacson P. J Clin Pathol 1982; 34: 14.
331. Arends JW, Wiggers T, Thijs CT et al. Am J Clin Pathol 1984; 82: 267.
332. Hamada Y, Yamamura M, Hioki K, Yamamoto M, Nagura H, Watanabe K. Cancer 1985; 55: 136.
333. Dukes CE. J Path Bact 1940; 50: 527.
334. Astler VB, Coller FA. Ann Surg 1954; 139: 846.
335. Grinnell RS. Ann Surg 1966; 163: 272.
336. Patt DJ, Brynes RK, Vardiman JW et al. Cancer 1975; 35: 388.
337. Talbot IC, Ritchie S, Leighton M, Hughes AO, Bussey HJR, Morson BC. Histopathol 1981; 5: 141.
338. Ossowski L, Reich E. Cell 1983; 33: 616.
339. Sunter JP, Higgs MJ, Cowan WK. J Clin Pathol 1985; 38: 385.
340. Morson BC, Vaughan EG, Bussey HJR. Br Med J 1963; ii: 13.
341. Sanders GB, Hagen WH, Kinnaird DW. Ann Surg 1958; 147: 796.
342. Miln DC, McClaughlin IS. Br J Surg 1969; 56: 143.

343. Berardi RD. Dis Col Rect 1972; 15: 383.
344. Dawson IMP. Curr Topics Pathol 1976; 63: 221.
345. Jones RA, Dawson IMP. Histopathol 1977; 1: 137.
346. Bates HR. Dis Col Rect 1962; 10: 467.
347. Quan SHQ, Bader G, Berg JW. Dis Col Rect 1964; 7: 197.
348. O'Briain DS, Dayal Y, DeLellis RA, Tischler AS, Bendron R, Wolfe HJ. Am J Surg Pathol 1982; 6: 131.
349. Burke M, Shepherd NA, Mann C. Br J Surg (in press).
350. Shousha S. Histopathol 1982; 6: 341.
351. Gaston EA. Dis Col Rect 1967; 10: 435.
352. Zirkin RM, McCord DL. Dis Col Rect 1963; 6: 370.
353. Drennan JM, Falconer CWA. J Clin Pathol 1959; 12: 175.
354. Pemberton M, Lendrum J. Br J Surg 1969; 55: 273.
355. Rees BI, Okwonga W, Jenkins IL. Clin Oncol 1976; 2: 113.
356. Shoemaker CP, Hoyle CL, Levine SB, Farman J. Am J Surg 1970; 120: 99.
357. Fraser AM, Naunton Morgan M. Br J Surg 1969; 56: 317.
358. Olsen BS, Carlisle RW. Cancer 1970; 25: 219.

Non-epithelial tumours

359. Cornes JS, Wallace MH, Morson BC. J Path Bact 1961; 82: 371.
360. Louw JH. J Pediatr Surg 1968; 3: 195.
361. Atwell JD, Burge D, Wright D. J Pediatr Surg 1985; 20: 25.
362. Shaw EB, Hennigar GR. Am J Clin Pathol 1974; 61: 417.
363. Berg JW. Nat Cancer Inst Monogr 1969; 32.
364. Culp CE, Hill JR. Dis Col Rect 1962; 5: 426.
365. Dawson IMP, Cornes JS, Morson BC. Br J Surg 1961; 49: 80.
366. Renton P, Blackshaw AJ. Br J Surg 1976; 63: 542.
367. Pinkus GS, Wilson RE, Corson JM. Cancer 1974; 34: 2103.
368. Blackshaw AJ. In: Wright R, ed. Recent advances in gastrointestinal pathology. London: Saunders, 1980: 213.
369. Papadimitriou CS, Papacharalampous NX, Kittas C. Cancer 1985; 55: 870.
370. Asselah F, Crow J, Slavin G, Sowter G, Sheldon C, Asselah H. Histopathol 1982; 6: 631.
371. Isaacson PG, Maclennan KA, Subbuswamy SG. Histopathol 1984; 8: 641.
372. Association of Clinical Pathologists: Broadsheet 96, January 1981.
373. Walsh TH, Mann CV. Br J Surg 1984; 71: 597.
374. Ranchod M, Kempson RL. Cancer 1977; 39: 255.
375. Nemer FD, Stoeckinger JM, Evans OT. Dis Col Rect 1977; 20: 405.
376. Freni SC, Keeman JN. Cancer 1977; 39: 263.
377. Butler DB, Hanna E. Dis Col Rect 1959; 2: 291.
378. Grodsky L. Am J Surg 1958; 95: 474.
379. Raszkowski HJ, Hufner RF. Cancer 1971; 27: 134.
380. Staple TW, McAlister WH, Anderson MS. Am J Roent 1964; 91: 840.
381. Carney JA, Hayles AB. Mayo Clin Proc 1977; 52: 543.
382. Mendelsohn G, Diamond MP. Am J Surg Pathol 1984; 8: 515.
383. Wiedner N, Flanders DJ, Mitros FA. Am J Surg Pathol 1984; 8: 779.
384. Donnelly WH, Sieber WK, Yunis EJ. Arch Pathol 1969; 87: 537.

385. Castro EB, Stearns MW. Dis Col Rect 1972; 15: 441.
386. Yatto RP. Am J Gastroenterol 1982; 77: 436.
387. Ling CS, Leagus C, Stahlgren LH. Surg 1959; 46: 1054.
388. Swain VAJ, Young WF, Pringle EM. Gut 1969; 10: 587.
389. Elliott GB, Sandy JTM, Elliott KA, Sherkat A. Can J Surg 1968; 11: 179.
390. Gazet JC. Br J Surg 1964; 51: 371.
391. Cohen RS, Cramm RE. Dis Col Rect 1969; 12: 120.
392. Weitzner S, Lockard VG, Nascimento AG. Dis Col Rect 1976; 19: 675.
393. Russel IS, Hughes ESR. Aust NZ J Surg 1964; 34: 27.
394. Bacon HE, Herabat T, Koohdary A, Villanueva RP. Dis Col Rect 1974; 17: 365.
395. Marino AWM. Dis Col Rect 1959; 2: 438.

Miscellaneous conditions

396. Spjut HT, Perkins DE. Am J Roent 1969; 82: 1070.
397. Edwards DAW, Lennard-Jones JE. Proc Roy Soc Med 1960; 53: 877.
398. Schuffler MD, Beegle RG. Gastroenterol 1979; 77: 664.
399. Toffler AH, Hukill PB, Spiro HM. Ann Intern Med 1963; 58: 872.
400. Krisnamurty S, Schuffler MD, Rohrmann CA, Pope CE. Gastroenterol 1985; 88: 26.
401. Pearse AGE. In: Histochemistry, theoretical and applied. 3rd ed. Edinburgh: Churchill Livingstone, 1972: 1091.
402. Schrodt GR. Dis Col Rect 1963; 6: 277.
403. Ghadially FN, Parry EW. J Path Bact 1966; 92: 313.
404. Heizer WD, Washaw AL, Walkman TA. Ann Intern Med 1968; 68: 4.
405. Smith B. Gut 1968; 9: 139.
406. Smith B. Proc Roy Soc Med 1972; 65: 288.
407. Ecker JA, Williams RG, Clay KL. Am J Gastroenterol 1971; 56: 125.
408. Ramos AJ, Powers WE. Am J Roent 1957; 77: 678.
409. Rosenbaum HD. Am J Roent 1957; 78: 681.
410. Koss LG. Arch Pathol 1952; 53: 523.
411. Yale CE, Balish E, Wu JP. Arch Surg 1974; 109: 89.
412. Keyting WS, McCarver RR, Kovarik JL, Daywitt AL. Radiol 1961; 76: 733.
413. Haboubi NY, Honan RP, Hasleton PS et al. Histopathol 1984; 8: 145.
414. Coello-Remirez B, Gutierres-Topete G, Lifshitz F. Am J Dis Child 1970; 120: 3.
415. Radin DR, Chandrasoma P, Halls JM. Gastrointest Radiol 1984; 9: 359.
416. Di Silvo TV, Bartlett EF. Arch Pathol 1971; 92: 167.
417. Abdou NI, Napombejara C, Sagawa A et al. NEJM 1977; 297: 1413.
418. Ghosh S, Bilton JL. Dis Col Rect 1968; 11: 457.
419. Elliott GB, Freigang B. Ann Surg 1963; 155: 501.
420. Azzopardi JG, Evans DG. J Clin Pathol 1966; 19: 368.
421. Caravati CM, Litch M, Weisiger BB, Ragland S, Berliner H. Ann Intern Med 1963; 58: 166.

The anal canal and anus

ANATOMY

The anal canal is about 3.5 cm long and extends from the upper to the lower border of the internal sphincter (Fig. 9.1). About halfway down the mucosal surface of the anal canal is a series of small, crescentic folds, the anal valves. These are separated from one another by small papillae which represent the lower ends of the vertical mucosal folds or anal columns of the upper anal canal. The line of the anal valves is also known as the pectinate

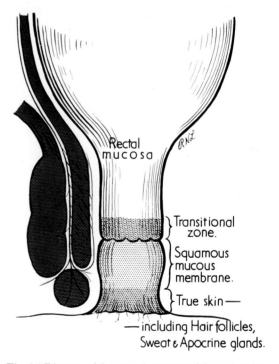

Fig. 9.1 Diagram of the normal anatomy of the anal region. The position of the pectinate line is indicated at the junction of the transitional zone with the squamous mucous membrane.

or dentate line and marks the site of the anal membrane in the fetus. It lies just below the middle of the internal sphincter.

Above the anal valves the mucosa is plum-coloured, due to the underlying internal haemorrhoidal plexus. The submucous tissues here are loose, but at the line of the valves the epithelium is firmly anchored down to the internal sphincter, creating a submucosal barrier which is important in the spread of cancer in this region. Below the valves, the external haemorrhoidal plexus of veins lies in the loose submucous connective tissue at the junction of the squamous membrane of the pecten and the skin of the anal margin.

The veins of the internal haemorrhoidal plexus drain into the portal system via the superior rectal vein. The external haemorrhoidal plexus, which has only very poor connections with the internal plexus, is drained into the systemic venous system by the inferior rectal vein. The lymphatic drainage of the anal canal above the dentate line goes to the superior haemorrhoidal group of lymph nodes, whereas the superficial inguinal glands drain the tissue below this line.

The lining of the anal canal below the pectinate line is of ectodermal origin, and so possesses a somatic type of nerve supply. This area is extremely sensitive to touch and pain, whereas the mucosa above the dentate line is insensitive, being supplied by autonomic nerves.

The anal canal above the pectinate line is lined by a continuation of the rectal mucosa, except for a narrow zone seldom more than a centimetre long immediately above the line and covering the lower part of the internal haemorrhoidal plexus. This is variously termed the 'junctional', 'transitional', or 'cloacogenic' zone of the upper anal canal because it represents the junction of the endoderm and ectoderm in the developing fetus. The type of epithelium lining the junctional zone varies with age and pathological conditions. Rectal mucosa, stratified columnar epithelium, transitional epithelium resembling that seen in the urinary tract and squamous mucosa are all seen in this area (Fig. 9.2).

Below the line of the anal valves is the pecten which is covered by squamous mucous membrane from which hair follicles and sebaceous and sweat glands are absent. At the lower border of the internal sphincter the squamous mucous membrane of the pecten merges into the true skin of the anal margin, which possesses hair follicles and sweat and apocrine glands.

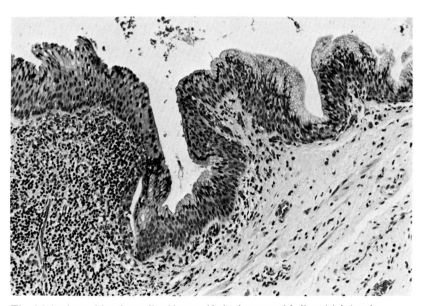

Fig. 9.2 Anal transitional zone lined by stratified columnar epithelium (right) and transitional epithelium (left). A collection of lymphocytes is present beneath the latter and represents a normal component of this region.

Haematoxylin-eosin   × 100

The orifices of the anal glands, about eight in number, lie behind the cusps of the anal valves. These glands are really branching ducts which pass into the submucosa and sometimes into and through the internal sphincter. They are lined by stratified columnar epithelium and act as a channel through which infection can reach the peri-anal tissues and ischiorectal fossae. The ducts are sometimes surrounded by lymphoid tissue.

The internal sphincter is composed of smooth muscle (involuntary) fibres and is really only an enlarged portion of the circular muscle of the rectum, with which it is continuous. The external anal sphincter is conveniently described in three parts: subcutaneous, superficial and deep. The superficial and deep parts are scarcely separable from one another. All three parts are composed of striated (voluntary) muscle.[1-3]

CONGENITAL ABNORMALITIES

Atresia and congenital stenosis of the rectum, anal canal and anus

Atresia (congenital absence of the lumen) or congenital stenosis (organic constriction of the patent lumen) of this region of the alimentary tract occurs in about one in 5000 live births. Atresia accounts for about 90% of these cases and anal stenosis for the rest.[4]

In 75% of cases of atresia there is wide separation between the blind lower end of the rectum and the exterior. The site of the anus may be apparent on the surface as a small dimple, the proctodaeal pit. In about 10% of atresias the anus is normally developed. The rectum, however, ends blindly well above the anus. In only 5% or fewer cases is there no more than a thin anal membrane separating the rectum from the exterior.

An alternative classification of these congenital obstructions divides them into 'high' and 'low' abnormalities.[5] In cases of 'high' abnormalities the end of the bowel ends above the pelvic floor and the levator ani muscles are absent. In 'low' abnormalities the end of the bowel is below the pelvic floor: the levatores ani are present, a potential sphincter being available and the functional prognosis after corrective surgery correspondingly better. The *'low' abnormalities* are classified in four groups: (1) covered anus, a condition in which a bar of skin covers the opening of the anal canal, which communicates with the exterior by a track running forward deep to the bar to open on the perineal raphe; (2) ectopic anus, which opens forward of its normal position—in the perineum in boys or within the vulva or vagina in girls; (3) stenotic anus, which may have an orifice so small as scarcely to admit the finest probe, and (4) anal membrane, the normally-sited anus being closed by a membrane so thin that it may bulge with the pressure of the meconium that is seen through it as a dark mass.

The *'high' abnormalities* form three groups: (1) anorectal agenesis, in which the anus, anal canal and lower part of the rectum are lacking—there is often a fistula connecting the developed part of the rectum to the urinary bladder in boys and to the posterior fornix of the vagina in girls; (2) rectal atresia, in which the bowel ends blindly above the pelvic floor and the normally-formed anal canal begins blindly at the level of the pelvic floor— fistula formation is not a feature of this anomaly, and (3) cloacal persistence—this form occurs only in girls, the rectum and the urinary and genital tracts opening into a common cloacal cavity.

INFLAMMATORY DISORDERS

Anal fissure

The typical anal fissure is found in the midline posteriorly and is very infrequent in other quadrants of the anal canal. It forms an elongated triangular ulcer in the squamous mucous membrane of the lower anal canal overlying the internal sphincter and the subcutaneous part of the external sphincter. The pathogenesis of anal fissure is not clear.[6] Predisposing factors include loss of the normal elasticity and mobility of the mucosa due to fibrosis accompanying chronic infection. Superficial fissures may heal spontaneously but the condition usually becomes chronic, probably because associated muscle spasm and constant exposure to infection interfere with healing. Microscopic appearances are those of non-specific inflammation. The edges of the chronic fissures are often thickened and somewhat undermined, and the tissues immediately adjacent are oedematous and heavily infiltrated by lymphocytes and plasma cells. The oedematous skin at the lower end of a fissure may form a little polypoid projection, the 'sentinel tag'.

Non-specific anal fissure is a common condition but must be distinguished from other causes of lower anal canal ulceration such as Crohn's disease, tuberculosis, primary syphilis and squamous cell carcinoma.

Anal fistula and anal abscess

Fistula in ano is recorded in the oldest medical literature and still remains a very common condition. Four main types are described, although the distinction between them is not exact. In most cases there is an internal opening at the level of the dentate line in the anal canal, although clinically this is often difficult to detect. This internal opening represents the orifice of an infected anal gland. The four main types are:

1. *Anal fistula.* In this common type, the fistulous track passes from the internal opening at the dentate line through the internal sphincter to the ischiorectal space and thence to the circumanal skin, where it opens.

2. *Subcutaneous fistula.* In this type the track passes downward from the dentate line to the external opening in the skin of the circumanal region and is wholly subcutaneous throughout its course.

3. *Submucosal fistula.* The track of this rare variety of fistula passes upward, deep to the rectal mucosa from the opening at the level of the dentate line; sometimes there is a second opening into the rectum at the upper end of the fistula.

4. *Anorectal fistula.* This is another rare type in which the track starts at an external opening in the circumanal skin below the level of the anal sphincters and passes through the levator ani muscle; in some cases it opens into the rectum above the anorectal ring.

An alternative and more scientific classification has been described which takes the normal anatomy of the pelvic floor into account.[7] This consists of two funnel-shaped structures, one situated within the other. The inner one consists of the rectum and anal canal with its smooth muscle layers including the internal sphincter. The outer one is composed of the striated muscle of the pelvic floor namely the levatores ani, puborectales and external sphincter. Between these muscular funnels lies the 'intersphincteric plane', composed of connective tissue. Most fistulous tracts spread in this plane; some extend into the fat surrounding the outer funnel of muscles, that is the ischiorectal fossa. They can be divided into low intersphincteric (low anal) fistula and high intersphincteric (submucous) fistula. A trans-sphincteric fistula spreads across the external sphincter mass into the ischiorectal fossa, whence it passes out on to the perianal skin. These can also be subdivided into low and high varieties. An extrasphincteric (perirectal) fistula passes from the perineal skin through the ischiorectal fossa and levator ani muscles into the rectum. It is rare and is usually due to some specific inflammatory condition like Crohn's disease or tuberculosis.

Pathogenesis

In the past, the most widely accepted theory of the cause of anal fistula was that the wall of the anal canal became infected through a fissure or wound and that faecal contamination kept the condition from healing. However, other evidence suggests that infection of the anal glands is probably the commonest cause.[8] Various authors have demonstrated infection in and around anal glands in cases of fistula and have suggested that the chronicity of the condition is due to persistence of the anal gland epithelium in the part of the track adjoining the internal opening. The presence of this persisting epithelium keeps the opening patent and healing can not take place.

Histology

During the exploration and surgical treatment of anal fistulae and abscesses, it is important that representative pieces of tissue from the tracts should be sent for histological examination, particularly to exclude carcinoma. Various patterns can be seen. In the great majority of cases sections will show an ordinary pyogenic type of inflammatory reaction. Giant cells of the foreign-body type are frequently encountered; presumably they are a reaction to the presence within the fistulous track of material derived from the faeces (Fig. 9.3). An

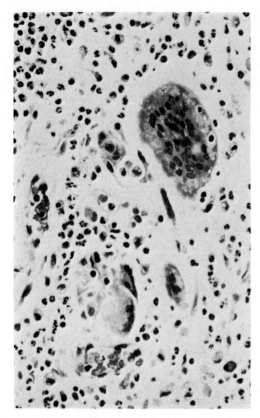

Fig. 9.3 Foreign-body granuloma within granulation tissue lining a fistulous tract. This must be distinguished from the granulomas of Crohn's disease (Fig. 9.5) and tuberculosis (Fig. 9.6).

Haematoxylin-eosin   × 250

oleogranulomatous reaction is occasionally present and is probably due to treatment of the condition with vaseline-impregnated gauze or to the escape of oily substances used for softening the faeces from the rectum into the fistulous track. A foreign-body reaction should be distinguished from tuberculosis or the granulomatous response of Crohn's disease. The most valuable distinguishing features are the absence of a compact epithelioid cell reaction in the foreign-body type of response and the appearance of the giant cells in Crohn's disease, which are usually of Langhans' type. The spread of infection in and around fistulous tracks can provoke tissue damage such as fat necrosis, secondary vasculitis and degenerative changes in striated muscle with the formation of giant hyperchromatic nuclei. The lymphoid tissue of the 'anal tonsils' may be hyperplastic (Fig. 9.4).

Crohn's disease

The diagnosis can be made by histological examination of pieces of tissue taken for biopsy or during surgical treatment of the anal lesion. However, it will only be helpful in those 60% of cases of Crohn's disease in which non-caseating tuberculoid granulomas are present. In patients without such a tissue response, the diagnosis rests on the clinical appearance of the anal lesion, together with any evidence of intestinal involvement. Because the clinical features are not always distinctive and a granulomatous histology is absent in some 40% of cases, it is probable that anal lesions due to Crohn's disease will continue to remain unrecognized until the abdominal disease becomes manifest. Apart from lack of the characteristic clinical and histological features the failure to biopsy all anal lesions at the time of surgical treatment must be a frequent cause of failure to recognize the pathology. It is probable that Crohn's disease often

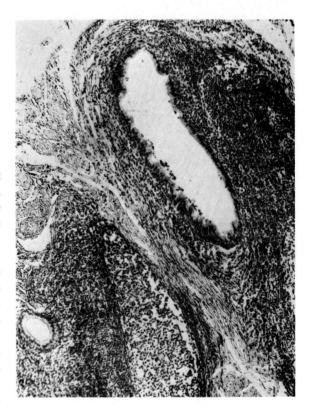

Fig. 9.4 Marked hyperplasia of lymphoid tissue surrounding anal glands which are lined by stratified columnar epithelium.

Haematoxylin-eosin   × 105

affects the anus because of the aggregations of lymphoid tissue ('anal tonsils') around the anal glands. The disorder likewise affects the terminal ileum because of the great amount of lymphoid tissue there.

A non-caseating tuberculoid reaction is a purely descriptive term applicable to any collection of epithelioid cells, sometimes giant cells, without central caseation (Fig. 9.5), although a little central necrosis with preservation of the reticulin pattern is permissible. In some cases of Crohn's disease of the anus the granulomas are few in number and very sparsely distributed. In other cases the tissues of the dermis, subcutaneous fat and fistulous track are riddled with lesions. The chances of finding granulomas are dependent on the amount of tissue available for examination.

A confident distinction between a sarcoid reac-tion due to Crohn's disease, sarcoidosis or tuber-culosis is impossible on histological evidence alone.[9] The presence of caseation is suggestive of tuber-culosis but examination by Ziehl-Neelsen staining is often negative, in which case culture or guinea-pig inoculation of fresh tissue is required.

Giant cells of the foreign-body type are com-monly seen in tissue removed from anal fistulae (see above).

Anorectal tuberculosis

Tuberculosis of the anorectal region is now a rare disease in Great Britain, having steadily declined over the past 50 years.[9] However, it is seen in those countries where pulmonary and intestinal tuber-culosis are still common.[10,11] There are two different clinical types. Firstly, there are the patients presenting with anal ulceration who have active pulmonary tuberculosis; tubercle bacilli can be readily demonstrated in smears from the surface of the ulcer or in biopsy material. Secondly, there are those who have anal fistulae or chronic anorectal abscesses.[12,13] The fistulae are often anatomically complex and may be associated with stricture of the lower rectum. There is a history of pulmonary tuberculosis in most cases, but this is often of a mild or chronic character. The histological diag-nosis can be difficult, especially the distinction from Crohn's disease (Fig. 9.6). The only certain way to establish it is by demonstrating the tubercle bacillus in biopsy material or by using guinea-pig inoculation or culture of fresh tissue from the anal lesion.

Ulcerative colitis

Although anal lesions do occur in patients with ulcerative colitis, they are less frequent than, and have a different character from, the anal lesions of Crohn's disease. Ordinary anal and retrovaginal fistulae are seen, but the inflammatory changes in the anal canal and anal margin are usually more superficial, presenting as acute anal fissure or excoriation of the skin around the anus. Acute peri-anal or ischiorectal abscesses are more fre-quent in ulcerative colitis. The histology shows no special features.

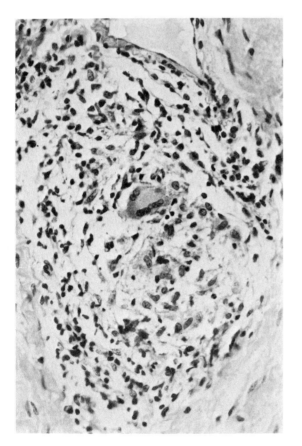

Fig. 9.5 Non-caseating granuloma of anal Crohn's disease, with Langhans' giant cell.

Haematoxylin-eosin   × 250

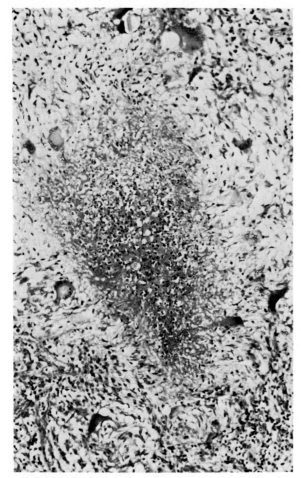

Fig. 9.6 Caseating granuloma from case of anal tuberculosis. Haematoxylin-eosin   × 100

Fungal infections

Anal and perianal lesions, including ulcers, inflammatory masses or sinuses, may accompany systemic mycoses including histoplasmosis, cryptococcosis, coccidioidomycosis, paracoccidioidomycosis and blastomycosis. The anal lesions may be the presenting feature. One case report describes involvement of the tongue and anal region by granulomatous lesions in a patient with disseminated histoplasmosis,[15] but anal lesions due to systemic infection by *Histoplasma capsulatum* often take the form of a pure histiocytosis. These infections may in future be encountered with a greater frequency in the United Kingdom and other low-incidence countries, not only because of

increased travel but as a result of their association with immune deficiency.

Syphilis

The primary lesion of anal syphilis can be easily confused with anal lesions due to other causes, in particular simple anal fissure.[16] The clinical distinction from carcinoma, the anal lesions of Crohn's disease and tuberculous ulcer, can also be difficult. The diagnosis should be confirmed by appropriate serological tests.

Manifestations of secondary syphilis can also be seen in the anal region. They include dermatitis of the peri-anal skin and, at a later stage, condyloma lata. The latter are moist, reddened hypertrophic warty lesions and are distinguishable clinically from condylomata acuminata (viral warts), although both types can be present together. Histologically, they show a hyperkeratotic epidermis covering a connective-tissue core that is heavily infiltrated by plasma cells.

Granuloma inguinale (granuloma venereum)

This condition is characterized by a slowly progressive ulceration of the tissues of the perianal and genital region. It is widespread in the tropics but very rare in Great Britain and Europe, USA, Japan and Australasia.

The early lesion is a papule which enlarges and then ulcerates to form a spreading lesion with a necrotic centre and a raised border. On microscopic examination a well-circumscribed mass of chronic inflammatory cells is seen, mainly polymorphs and plasma cells, a few lymphocytes, and occasional large, round macrophages in which the causative Donovan bodies can be demonstrated by Leishman's method or the stains of Giemsa or Wright.[17] The organism, *Calymmatobacterium granulomatis* (*Donovania granulomatis*), is frequently but by no means exclusively conveyed by sexual contact. When it is sparsely present it may be most readily demonstrated in sections by use of silver impregnation methods such as the Warthin-Starry procedure.

Lymphogranuloma venereum

The anal manifestations include confluent nodules with fissuring, multiple anal fistulae and peri-anal elephantiasis. Involvement of the rectum is described on page 329.

Hidradenitis suppurativa

This is a chronic inflammatory condition which affects the skin and subcutaneous tissues of those parts where apocrine sweat glands are found, namely the axilla, areola of the breast, umbilicus, genitalia and peri-anal area. Peri-anal hidradenitis is an uncommon condition which is more frequent in males than females. The affected area of skin has a red and white blotchy appearance; it is thickened and oedematous with watery pus draining from multiple openings of sinus tracks. The persistent chronic nature of the disease leads to ulceration and scarring. Lesions can be localized or involve large areas of peri-anal skin extending on to the buttocks. Microscopic examination of excised specimens shows an inflammatory exudate consisting of plasma cells, lymphocytes and occasional giant cells of the foreign-body type, with the formation of sinus tracks. The latter become lined by squamous epithelium by downgrowth from the surface skin. Ordinary sweat glands are present in normal numbers but apocrine glands are usually absent. This has led to the view that hidradenitis suppurativa is a primary infection of apocrine glands.

Other studies indicate that these glands are infected secondarily rather than primarily and that the hidradenitis can affect skin in sites other than apocrine gland-bearing areas.[18] The cause of the disease is not understood but, like acne, it seems to have some relationship to endocrine activity. Other aetiological factors may include excessive local moisture in apposing skin surfaces and the difficulty of maintaining cleanliness in the region involved. Peri-anal hidradenitis suppurativa has been complicated by squamous cell carcinoma.[19]

Pilonidal sinus

A typical pilonidal sinus consists of single or multiple pits in the skin crease of the natal cleft which extend into subcutaneous abscess tracks lined by granulation tissue containing a mass of loose hair. The tracks branch, most often in a cephalad direction and laterally into the buttocks, but occasionally towards the anus. Pilonidal sinus is most common in young adults, mostly men. Hirsutism, chronic irritation and intertrigo are precipitating factors. Pilonidal sinuses may be acquired by puncture of the skin of the natal cleft by ingrowing hair shafts.[20] An inflammatory reaction then results, leading to the formation of a pit lined by squamous epithelium into which more hair and skin debris penetrate. Further secondary infection causes the formation of subcutaneous abscess tracks. Alternatively, the condition could be due to a congenitally-misplaced pubic hair follicle, which would account for the age of presentation. Microscopic examination of surgically-excised pilonidal sinuses shows chronic inflammatory granulation tissue lining abscess tracks, which usually, though not invariably, contain numerous hair shafts, around which there is a florid foreign-body giant cell reaction. The development of squamous cell carcinoma has been reported.[21]

The anus in homosexual men

A constellation of inflammatory, infective, traumatic and neoplastic lesions may be observed in the anal canal and peri-anal region. Herpes lesions may be observed in the anal canal and peri-anal region. Herpes simplex virus infection may produce florid peri-anal ulceration in the acquired immune deficiency syndrome (AIDS). Viral warts, dysplasia and squamous cell carcinoma are being described with increasing frequency in homosexual men.

VASCULAR DISORDERS

Haemorrhoids

It has been suggested that haemorrhoids (piles) represent a downward displacement of specialized cushions of the submucosal tissue lining the anal canal, which consists of a plexus of veins receiving a rich arterial supply and supported by a scaffold of smooth muscle and elastic tissue.[22,23] The cushions are important in the maintenance of anal continence and haemorrhoids are the result of excessive straining at stool. This concept accounts for the characteristic sites of haemorrhoids, the arterial bleeding associated with surgery and the rarity of haemorrhoids as a complication of portal hypertension.

Microscopic examination of excised haemorrhoids shows a plexus of dilated vascular spaces some of which have rather more smooth muscle in their walls than would be expected for ordinary veins of the same size. Varying degrees of haemorrhage and thrombosis are seen and the overlying mucous membrane is thickened. There may be squamous metaplasia of the overlying transitional zone. The whole appearance can have a close resemblance to a cavernous haemangioma.

The most important complication of haemorrhoids is bleeding, which over a period of time may account for a serious degree of anaemia. Other complications are prolapse of the piles out of the anus, strangulation, thrombosis, necrosis and infection. The so-called fibrous polyp of the anal canal is the end-result of thrombosis and organization of an internal haemorrhoid.

Peri-anal haematoma

This presents as a tender lump beneath the skin of the anal verge, and is due to rupture and thrombosis of a peri-anal vein. It is a painful but harmless condition.

Oleogranuloma

This is a foreign-body reaction to unabsorbable oily substances within tissue. The usual cause of anorectal oleogranuloma is oil used as a vehicle in the injection treatment of haemorrhoids.[24] The degree of reaction depends upon the type of oil used. Vegetable oils produce the least severe reaction, followed by animal fat, with mineral oils causing the most extensive changes. Oleogranuloma can present as a rounded submucous tumour in the anal canal just above the dentate line, but annular and even ulcerating lesions have been described. Unless biopsy is performed in such cases the clinical diagnosis of carcinoma may be made leading to unnecessary radical excision of the rectum.[25] Oleogranulomatous inflammation can be found in any part of the rectum and even as high as the rectosigmoid junction.

The histology of oleogranuloma is characteristic. In the early stages there is an acute inflammatory response, including many eosinophils. This is followed by increasing fibrosis and a variable degree of inflammation which subsides with increasing age of the lesion. Rounded spaces lined by large mononuclear or multinucleate histiocytes are scattered throughout (Fig. 9.7). These spaces contained the oil which is removed from the tissues during the course of histological preparation but can be demonstrated in frozen sections of formalin-fixed material. The histological appearance can be confused with lymphangioma and with cystic pneumatosis, although the latter does not show any fibrous or inflammatory reaction.

TUMOURS OF THE ANAL REGION

BENIGN EPITHELIAL TUMOURS AND PRECANCEROUS LESIONS

Small, polypoid benign squamous cell and transitional cell tumours arising from the epithelium of the anal canal below or above the dentate line are only rarely seen.

Varying degrees of epithelial dysplasia, sometimes amounting to carcinoma-in-situ, are occasionally seen during histological examination of excised haemorrhoids or other clinically benign conditions.[26] Leukoplakia and carcinoma-in-situ are also seen in flat epithelium and near the margin of proven cancers.

Leukoplakia

There are two different conditions to which the term leukoplakia may be applied in the anal region. Firstly, white plaques of tissue may be present over the lower pole of prolapsing internal haemorrhoids as a result of squamous metaplasia with hyperkeratosis of the transitional zone of the anal canal. There is no evidence that this type of leukoplakia is precancerous. Secondly, the term can be applied to a white, thickened peri-anal skin which microscopically shows thickening of the epidermis, with hyperkeratosis, acanthosis and an underlying chronic inflammatory cell infiltration. Leukoplakia of the peri-anal area seems to be uncommon but may be associated with dysplasia and carcinoma-in-situ.

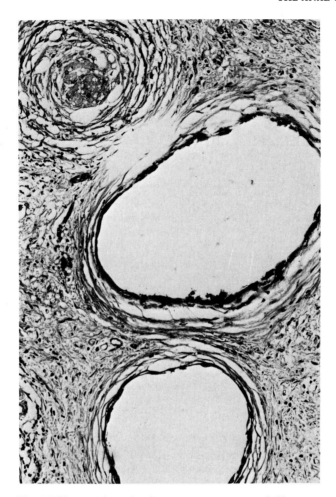

Fig. 9.7 Oleogranuloma showing empty spaces surrounded by multinucleate giant cells and fibroblasts. The spaces contained fat which was lost during tissue processing.

Haematoxylin-eosin   × 100

Dysplasia and carcinoma-in-situ

Dysplasia (intra-epithelial neoplasia) of the anal canal is found in the transitional epithelium above the dentate line, including the anal crypts, more frequently than in the squamous mucous membrane of the lower anal canal.[27,28] This observation corresponds with the relative incidence of invasive carcinomas above and below the dentate line. It seems certain that an intra-epithelial stage commonly exists for anal canal cancer.

The microscopic appearance of dysplasia in the anal canal is indistinguishable from the analogous lesion of the cervix. There is acanthosis, loss of the regular stratification of the nuclei and prominent palisading of basal cells. Varying degrees of nuclear pleomorphism and an increased number of mitotic figures are present. The changes extend right through to the surface in severe dysplasia or carcinoma-in-situ (Fig. 9.8). Such changes can be diffuse or patchy and are best treated by local excision.

Viral warts (condylomata acuminata)

These red, papilliferous and warty growths are found in the peri-anal region as well as other parts of the perineum, the vulva and penis. They are

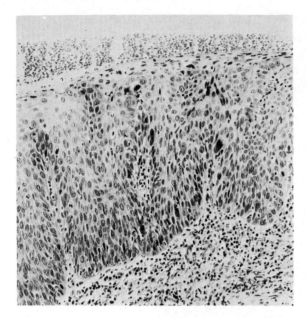

Fig. 9.8 Severe dysplasia within squamous epithelium of anal canal. The epithelium is acanthotic and almost the entire thickness is occupied by atypical basal cells showing nuclear enlargement, hyperchromatism and pleomorphism.

Haematoxylin-eosin   × 100

usually multiple and can cover a wide area of perianal skin. Exceptionally, they extend up the anal canal and can be found in the transitional zone but not in the rectal mucosa. Condylomata acuminata are due to the human papillomavirus which is apparently identical or closely related to the virus causing the common skin wart (verruca vulgaris).[30]

Microscopically, anal warts show marked acanthosis of the epidermis with hyperplasia of prickle cells, parakeratosis and an underlying chronic inflammatory cell infiltration. They are noted for the vacuolation of cells in the upper layers of the epidermis (Fig. 9.9). The occasional dyskeratotic cell may be observed. There is usually no sign of carcinoma-in-situ,[31] but it would appear that malignant change can occur. It is possible also that viral warts are part of a spectrum of squamous cell tumours which includes this common benign and easily curable lesion as well as the giant condyloma and verrucous carcinoma.

Giant condyloma

Giant condyloma of Buschke and Löwenstein is a

rare penile lesion which presents as a large warty growth and characteristically penetrates and burrows into the deeper tissues.[32] Similar, rare tumours have been described in the lower rectum and anal canal.[33] These lesions may show relentless invasion of the ischiorectal fossae, perirectal tissues and even the pelvic cavity. In spite of this aggressive behaviour the giant condyloma is cytologically bland and invasion of blood and lymphatic vessels is absent. The histology is essentially that of the usual condyloma acuminatum, but with accentuation of the acanthosis, papillomatosis and elongation of the rete ridges (Fig. 9.10). Vacuolation of epithelial cells has been described, suggesting a viral aetiology. The clinical picture or gross appearance may therefore provide the best guide to the nature of the lesion.

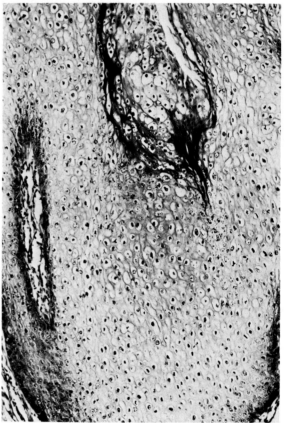

Fig. 9.9 Condyloma acuminatum or viral wart of anal region, showing characteristic cytoplasmic vacuolation.

Haematoxylin-eosin   × 100

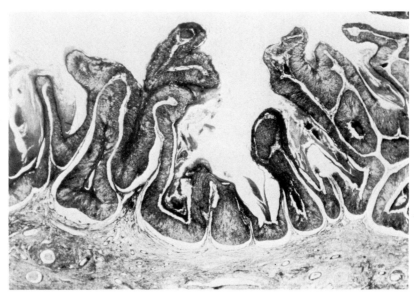

Fig. 9.10 Giant condyloma of anal canal, showing marked papillomatosis.
Haematoxylin-eosin   × 10

Verrucous carcinoma

This term has probably included two conditions. Some such designated lesions are comparable to tumours bearing the same name which occur in the mouth and respiratory tract and also to the family of tumours arising in the sole of the foot (carcinoma cuniculatum), penis (giant condyloma of Buschke and Löwenstein) and anal canal and vulva (giant condyloma; see above). These lesions show extensive local invasion but little propensity, if any, to metastasize.

Others represent low-grade squamous carcinomas, showing a verrucous appearance due to their predominantly exophytic growth (Fig. 9.11).[34] They are capable of metastasis, but do not exhibit relentless local invasion.

Some members of this second group may, as well-differentiated squamous carcinomas, show bland histology and therefore be indistinguishable from giant condyloma. However, unlike giant condyloma, they usually arise at the anal margin. An inverted verrucous carcinoma originating within a pilonidal sinus has been described.[35]

Keratoacanthoma

This is not premalignant, but an incision biopsy of this tumour may easily be misdiagnosed as a well-differentiated squamous carcinoma. The rare occurrence of this lesion in the peri-anal region should therefore be appreciated.[36]

Pilar tumours may also occur in the perianal skin and must be distinguished from both keratoacanthoma and squamous carcinoma. Pilar tumours, more commonly described in the scalp, present as slowly growing nodular masses that may ulcerate. They resemble pilar cysts histologically, but have been regarded by some as a form of low-grade squamous carinoma.

Sweat gland tumours

The least rare is the benign hidradenoma papilliferum, derived from apocrine sweat glands.[37] It usually occurs in white middle-aged women and presents as a circumscribed, firm nodule rarely greater than 1 cm in diameter. On section, it is often cystic. Microscopically, the tumour shows a glandular, papillary pattern. Two cell types are present (Fig. 9.12). One is columnar with apical blebs. This rests on a layer of cuboidal eosinophilic cells, which contain PAS-positive, diastase-resistant material.

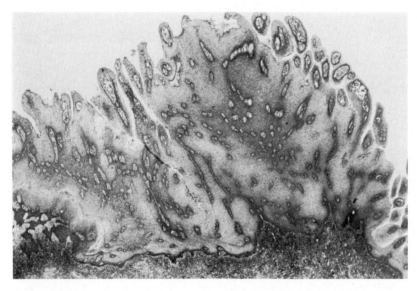

Fig. 9.11 Verrucous carcinoma of the anal margin. This large exophytic growth shows a bland histology and invades with a broad front. There is a marked lymphocytic infiltrate at the growing margin.

Haematoxylin-eosin   × 40

Bowen's disease

This occurs rarely in the peri-anal skin.[38] If numerous vacuolated cells are present, the appearances may simulate Paget's disease. The condition is clinically and histologically indistinguishable from counterparts arising in skin elsewhere.

Bowenoid papulosis

This presents as a papular eruption in the anogenital region. There is a relatively orderly maturation of squamous epithelium showing acanthosis and papillomatosis, but with a scattering of dyskeratotic cells and mitotic figures throughout, giving a 'salt and pepper' effect (Fig. 9.13).[39] It is generally stated that Bowenoid papulosis has no malignant potential, but it is possible that early removal pre-empts the development of this complication.

Extramammary Paget's disease

Paget's disease of the peri-anal skin is an extremely rare condition which presents clinically as a slightly raised, soft scaly and moist area with a red and grey colour.[40,41] The presence of induration usually indicates that an underlying invasive carcinoma is already present. The condition is most commonly found in elderly persons of either sex and is histopathologically identical with Paget's disease of the breast. The diagnosis is established by biopsy which reveals the characteristic Paget cells in the epidermis and sometimes in the lining epithelium of the ducts of underlying apocrine glands. These

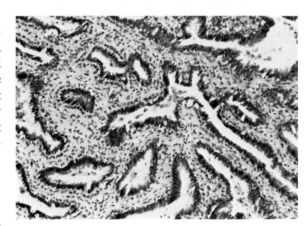

Fig. 9.12 Benign hidradenoma papilliferum of peri-anal region. The glands show papillary infolding and are lined by two cell layers.

Haematoxylin-eosin   × 100

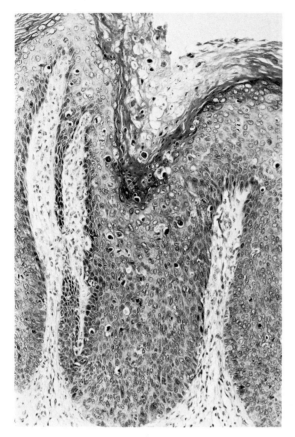

Fig. 9.13 Bowenoid papulosis of peri-anal region showing the 'salt and pepper' effect of scattered dyskeratotic cells and mitoses.

Haematoxylin-eosin × 100

are large cells with a foamy vacuolated cytoplasm and a vesicular nucleus which is often displaced to the periphery of the cell, giving a signet-ring appearance (Fig. 9.14). Paget cells contain a sialomucin which stains with PAS and alcian blue at pH 2.5. It is important that true Paget's disease of the peri-anal skin should not be confused with downward intra-epidermal spread of the signet-ring cell carcinoma of the rectum (Fig. 9.15) or with Bowen's disease of the peri-anal skin.

Electron microscopic and histochemical studies suggest that Paget cells originate from the epithelium of apocrine gland ducts and migrate into the epidermis.[42] If many sections are taken during the examination of surgical specimens, evidence of intraduct carcinoma will often be found. Paget's disease of the peri-anal skin has a long pre-invasive phase, but if the patient lives long enough an adenocarcinoma of apocrine gland type will develop.

Adenocarcinoma of the peri-anal apocrine glands without Paget's disease is referred to on p. 414.

MALIGNANT EPITHELIAL TUMOURS

Squamous carcinoma of the anal canal

Cancer of the anal region is uncommon in Europe and the USA. There are probably no more than 100 deaths per annum in England and Wales, but it is impossible to be precise because cancer of the anal margin is registered with other malignant neoplasms of the skin and many deaths from anal canal carcinoma are probably registered under rectal cancer. A better picture of the incidence is obtained from the study of surgical patients, in whom anal cancer as a whole comprises only 3% of carcinomas of the rectum.[43] However, carcinoma of the anal margin is much more common in parts of the world where conditions of extreme poverty are found. Under these circumstances there is a relatively high incidence of carcinoma of the penis, vulva and cervix as well as the anus, at least partly due to extremely poor personal hygiene. The practice of anal intercourse and the materials with which cleansing of the perineal area is carried out could also be significant in the aetiology. In low-risk countries there may be an increased incidence amongst homosexual males[44] and the role of a transmissible agent such as the human papillomavirus should be investigated.

The importance of distinguishing between squamous carcinoma of the anal canal and squamous carcinoma of the anal margin was emphasized many years ago.[45] They should be considered as two quite separate types of cancer, differing in their pathology, treatment and behaviour. Cancer of the anal canal is nearly three times more common than cancer of the anal margin in the population of England and Wales. The age incidence is the same (average 57 years), but anal canal cancer is more common in women than men (3:2) whereas anal margin cancer is more common in men (4:1).

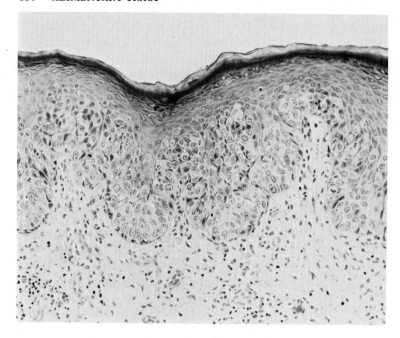

Fig. 9.14 Paget's disease of the peri-anal skin showing characteristic pale cells with large vesicular nuclei.

Haematoxylin-eosin   × 75

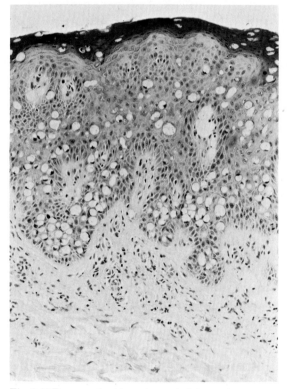

Fig. 9.15 Downward epidermal spread of signet-ring carcinoma of the rectum into the anal canal. The nuclei are small and hyperchromatic, in contrast to those of Paget's disease.

Haematoxylin-eosin   × 100

Site

The majority of squamous carcinomas of the anal canal arise above, or mainly above, the dentate line (Fig. 9.16). This represents the region of the transitional zone and is a site of predilection for dysplasia. Probably only about one quarter arise from the squamous mucous membrane of the lower canal.

Histology

Squamous carcinomas of the anal canal show a diversity of histological structure which reflects the variability and instability of the epithelium in this area. Ordinary squamous cell carcinoma, which closely resembles cancer of the cervix histologically, accounts for about one third of all cases. These do not show intercellular cytoplasmic bridges or prickle-cell formation and generally produce less keratin than is seen in typical skin cancers. However, prickle-cell carcinomas are occasionally seen in the anal canal, particularly when there has been a long history of benign anorectal disease, leukoplakia or granuloma inguinale. The commonest type of squamous carcinoma of the anal canal is the so-called basaloid[46] or cloacogenic carcinoma.[27,28] It accounts for about

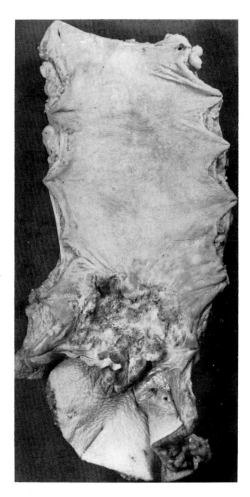 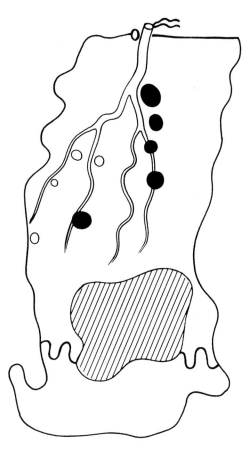

Fig. 9.16a, b (a) Ulcerating squamous carcinoma of the anal canal, which is arising above the dentate line. (b) Chart showing spread of carcinoma, illustrated in (a) to the superior rectal group of lymph nodes.

two-thirds of all cases. Mucoepidermoid carcinoma of the upper anal canal is rare. Detailed examination of the anal canal tumours will frequently reveal a mixed histological pattern containing elements of ordinary squamous, basaloid or transitional and even mucoepidermoid differentiation, but usually with a predominance of one histological type. It has been shown that these different features do not greatly influence prognosis independently of the grade of differentiation although some basaloid structure in an ordinary squamous cell carcinoma is a favourable factor in relation to prognosis.

Well-differentiated basaloid carcinomas are distinguished by the presence of palisading at the periphery of the clumps of tumour cells (Fig. 9.17).

Other features resembling basal cell carcinoma of the skin (rodent ulcer) are a pseudo-acinar pattern, which is really a manifestation of palisading, and the formation of small concentric whorls of squamoid cells undergoing incomplete keratinization. Sharply defined plugs of keratin scattered throughout the tumour are also reminiscent of the histology of rodent ulcer. One feature unlike basal cell carcinoma is the presence of masses of eosinophilic necrosis surrounded by a rim of tumour cells giving a 'Swiss cheese' appearance under the lower power of the microscope. In occasional cases there can be a striking resemblance to transitional carcinoma of the bladder.

In moderately-differentiated basaloid carcino-

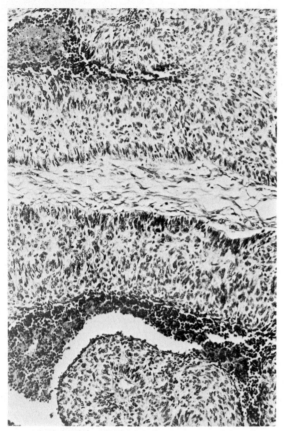

Fig. 9.17 Basaloid or cloacogenic carcinoma of anal canal showing characteristic palisading of cells at edge of tumour clumps and central necrosis.

Haematoxylin-eosin   × 100

mas the above features, especially the palisading, are less prominent and there is more cellular pleomorphism. Well-differentiated and moderately well-differentiated basaloid tumours have a 60–70% 5-year survival rate, even when regional lymph nodes are involved. However, the majority of basaloid carcinomas are poorly differentiated.

Poorly differentiated basaloid carcinomas have only a very superficial resemblance to rodent ulcers. Palisading is absent, there is loss of clumping of the tumour cells, eosinophilic necrosis may be prominent and the nuclei are hyperchromatic with much variation in size and shape and many mitotic figures. They are sometimes called 'basaloid small cell' carcinomas and have a very poor prognosis. Justification for the basal cell nature of basaloid carcinomas has come from electron microscopic

studies which confirm that these tumours arise from the basal cells in the epithelium of the transitional or junctional zone.[47] The propensity for basaloid carcinoma to invade regional lymph nodes marks an important distinction from basal cell carcinoma of the skin.

Spread and prognosis

Squamous cell carcinoma of the anal canal shows preferential direct spread upwards into the lower third of the rectum, which explains why many of these lesions present clinically as tumours of the lower rectum. This is probably because the line of least resistance is upwards in the submucous layer. Anal canal carcinoma also spreads to the superior haemorrhoidal lymph nodes and to nodes on the lateral walls of the pelvis as well as to the inguinal glands. Haemorrhoidal node involvement has been found in 43% of major operation cases of anal canal cancer seen at St Mark's Hospital, London, and clinical and pathological evidence of inguinal gland metastases occurs in 36% of cases. There is clinical evidence that in anal canal carcinoma the inguinal nodes are involved at a later stage than the haemorrhoidal nodes, the malignant cells possibly spreading backwards from within the pelvis.[43,45,48,49]

There is a relationship between differentiation of anal canal carcinoma and of the incidence of lymph node metastases as well as with survival after surgical treatment. Thus, in well-differentiated squamous cell carcinomas of all types, lymph node involvement is rare. However, it is present in about half of all the moderately- and poorly-differentiated grades. The 5-year survival rate is over 80%, for well-differentiated tumours, 50% for the moderately-differentiated group, and only about 30% for poorly-differentiated carcinomas. A detailed staging system has recently been proposed which takes heed of tumour size as well as depth of invasion, grade of differentiation and nodal status.[50]

Squamous carcinoma of the anal margin

Squamous cell carcinomas of the anal margin usually arise at the junction of the squamous mucous membrane of the lower end of the anal canal with the hair-bearing peri-anal skin. This junctional origin, the appearance of the tumours, and their histology and behaviour suggest a comparison with squamous carcinoma of the lip. At both sites one usually encounters a slowly-growing squamous cell carcinoma which metastasizes to regional lymph nodes at a late state in its natural history.

Squamous carcinoma of the anal margin is about one third as frequent as anal canal carcinoma.[48,51] It is more common in men than women but there is no significant difference in age incidence compared with adenocarcinoma of the rectum or squamous cell carcinoma of the anal canal. Macroscopically, it presents as an ulcerating, protuberant or verrucous carcinoma. Microscopically, it is usually a keratinizing, prickle-cell type of carcinoma which is well differentiated and of a relatively low grade of malignancy.[43] Poorly-differentiated tumours are very rare.

Inguinal lymph node metastases are found in about 40% of cases. The majority of anal margin cancers are treated by local excision of the primary tumour, but even in those cases which are so extensive as to require radical removal of the rectum, involvement of the haemorrhoidal group is rare.

The 5-year survival figures for anal margin cancer show that the prognosis is more favourable than for disease of the anal canal. Survival for anal margin cancer is about 50% and for anal canal cancer about 40%. Moreover, this better 5-year survival occurs despite the fact that most anal margin tumours are treated by local excision, whereas the majority of anal canal cancers have a combined excision operation which allows removal of the haemorrhoidal nodes.

Malignant melanoma of anal canal

Approximately one malignant melanoma of the anal canal will be seen for every eight squamous cell carcinomas of the anal region.[52] The age of incidence is about the same as for cancer of the rectum and the sex incidence shows a preponderance of men in some series,[53] though in others there has been no sex dominance.[52] Patients present clinically with a protuberant mass in the lower rectum, often very large, which can resemble thrombosed 'piles', particularly if the tumour is pigmented. The diagnosis is made by biopsy, but the distinction from undifferentiated adenocarcinoma of the rectum or undifferentiated squamous cell carcinoma of the anal canal can be very difficult unless obvious pigmentation is present.

Malignant melanoma invariably arises from the transitional zone above the dentate line and is therefore classified among the malignant melanomas of mucous membranes. Melanin-containing cells are present in small numbers in the normal anal canal.[54] Pigment is not always obviously present on macroscopic observation. As with squamous cell carcinomas of the anal canal, malignant melanomas show preferential upwards submucous spread, which is one reason why they present clinically as growths of the rectum.

The histological appearance of anorectal malignant melanomas is variable. They are often very invasive, with a marked degree of pleomorphism and large numbers of mitotic figures. They can be broadly divided into polygonal and spindle cell forms. The presence of tumour giant cells is valuable in the differential diagnosis from adenocarcinoma, malignant carcinoid and squamous cell carcinoma. Pigmentation can be found in H & E sections in about half of all cases, if searched for carefully, but it is not always readily discernible. Junctional change can be seen at the lower margin of the growth in many cases.

Malignant melanoma of the anal canal spreads rapidly in the anorectal tissues and may even ulcerate on to the peri-anal skin through the ischiorectal fossae. The superior haemorrhoidal group of lymph nodes is involved early in the course of the disease. Spread to the nodes on the lateral wall of the pelvis and to the para-aortic and the inguinal nodes then occurs. Death results from widespread blood-borne deposits, mostly in the liver and lungs. The survival rate after surgical excision of the rectum is measured in months rather than years[54] although there is one report of survival for over five years before the patient died from generalized metastases.[55]

Carcinoma of anal ducts

Adenocarcinoma of anal ducts or glands is extremely rare.[57] These tumours are flat, submucosal growths which spread widely within the tissues of the anal canal producing stenosis. Microscopically, they are adenocarcinomas in which the epithelium lining the glands bears a close resemblance to normal anal ducts. Certain diagnosis requires the demonstration of a transition from anal duct epithelium to carcinoma through an in situ stage. Otherwise the distinction from adenocarcinoma of the rectum, mucoepidermoid carcinoma of the anal canal and apocrine gland carcinoma of the peri-anal skin can be difficult if not impossible. Anal duct carcinomas should not be confused with colloid carcinomas arising in anorectal fistulae.[58] Histochemical methods may be useful in the differential diagnosis of anal gland carcinoma.[59] In contrast to normal rectal mucosa, the mucus of anal glands is characterized by strong PAS reactivity which is abolished after periodate borohydride saponification, indicating scarcity or absence of O-acylated sialic acids in the anal gland mucus.

Adenocarcinoma in anorectal fistulae

In this condition patients present with anorectal fistulae or recurrent abscesses around the anus. Mucus material can sometimes be clearly seen within abscesses or fistulous tracks but there is no visible mucosal lesion in the rectum or anal canal. Microscopic examination of biopsies obtained during surgical treatment of the fistulae show mucinous adenocarcinoma. It has been suggested that these mucinous carcinomas arise in duplications of the lower end of the hindgut.[60] Support for this view is provided by the fact that some of the fistulous tracks in such cases are lined by normal rectal mucosa including muscularis mucosae.[61] Indeed, it may be possible to demonstrate that rectal mucosa lines the upper part of the track only and gives way to squamous epithelium at the line of the anal valves. There are also cases of anal fistula in which it has been possible to demonstrate by biopsy that the track is lined by rectal mucosa without any evidence of carcinoma. This aberrant rectal mucosa can mimic invasive carcinoma, should it become misplaced into the wall of the fistulous track. Retained mucus secretions may then be forced into surrounding tissue spaces, and invasive mucinous carcinoma can be simulated.[61]

MISCELLANEOUS TUMOURS

The peri-anal skin is a rare site for *basal cell carcinoma*.[62] It is more commonly seen in men than in women, and the average age at diagnosis is between 60–65 years. The macroscopic appearances and histology are no different from the commonly-occurring lesions found elsewhere. There is one report of a basal cell carcinoma arising in an anal fistula.[63]

Rare examples of *adenocarcinomas of the peri-anal apocrine glands* without any evidence of extramammary Paget's disease may be found. They are ulcerating growths, the histology of which shows evidence of an apocrine gland origin as judged by the presence of PAS-positive cytoplasmic secretion at the free surface of the columnar cells.

Leiomyomas and *leiomyosarcomas* arising from the internal sphincter are very rare. The *granular cell tumour* (*myoblastoma*) may occasionally arise in the external anal sphincter, presenting as a painless lump. Overlying pseudo-epitheliomatous hyperplasia may simulate squamous carcinoma.[64] Peri-anal and anal *rhabdomyosarcoma* has been reported (Fig. 9.18).[65] *Benign lymphoid polyps* are not infrequently found in the upper anal canal just above the dentate line though they are more common in rectal mucosa. Malignant lymphoma involving the anus is very rare. Peri-anal abscess may be a presenting sign of leukaemia.[66] *Lipoma, liposarcoma* and *fibrosarcoma* are seen in the ischiorectal fossa. *Secondary carcinoma* can occasionally present in the anal canal as a manifestation of spread by implantation from an adenocarcinoma of the colon or rectum. *Endocrine tumours* have been classified as arising in the rectum, but could conceivably originate from the endocrine cell population normally present in the anal canal.[54]

Presacral tumours

A wide variety of conditions can present as a presacral tumour. Most of them fall into one of four categories: congenital anomalies, bone tumours, neurogenic tumours and a miscellaneous group of lesions including secondary carcinoma and connective-tissue tumours. Among the congenital anomalies dermoid cysts, teratomas, men-

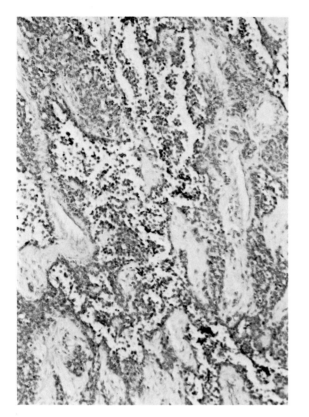

ingocele and pelvic kidney can be included. Among tumours found at this site are chordomas, osteochondroma, giant cell tumour and myeloma. Neurofibroma and ependymoma are also seen. So-called cystic hamartomas are composed of multiple cysts lined by columnar, transitional or ciliated epithelium and embedded in smooth muscle. These may be acquired as an inclusion of anal glands on an inflammatory basis. Some authors favour an underlying developmental defect.[67] A case of adenocarcinoma arising in a cystic hamartoma has been recorded.[67]

Fig. 9.18 Alveolar rhabdomyosarcoma arising in anal canal. This was an incidental finding within a resection for primary adenocarcinoma of the rectum. The patient was a man aged 108. He died three years later with secondary deposits of adenocarcinoma in the liver and of the alveolar rhabdomyosarcoma in the lungs. The sponge-like structure is illustrated with round tumour cells lining collagenous septa. These separate from one another as they lose their attachment to the stroma. Some of the tumour cells are multinucleate. Cross-striations were present.

Haematoxylin-eosin   × 150
Photograph provided by W. StC. Symmers.

REFERENCES

Anatomy

1. Walls EW. Br J Surg 1958; 45: 504.
2. Parks AG. Postgrad Med J 1958; 34: 360.
3. Fenger C. Acta Path Microbiol Scand Sect A 1979; 87: 379.

Congenital abnormalities

4. Ladd WE, Gross RE. Am J Surg 1934; 23: 167.
5. Partridge JP. Br J Surg 1961; 49: 37.

Inflammatory disorders

6. Gabriel WB. Principles and practice of rectal surgery. 5th ed. London: Lewis, 1963: 237.
7. Parks AG, Gordon PH, Hardcastle JD. Br J Surg 1976; 63: 1.
8. Parks AG. Br Med J 1961; 5: 510.
9. Jones-Williams W. Gut 1964; 1: 463.
10. Logan VStCD. Proc Roy Soc Med 1969; 12: 147.
11. Bremner CG. S Afr Med J 1964; 12: 147.

12. Terblanche J. S Afr Med J 1964; 38: 403.
13. Ahlberg J, Bergstrand O, Holmstrom B, Ullman J, Wallberg P. Acta Chir Scand 1980; 500 (suppl): 45.
14. Whalen TV, Kovalcik PJ, Old WL. Dis Col Rect 1980; 23: 54.
15. Earle JHO, Highman JH, Lockey E. Br Med J 1960; i: 607.
16. Samenius B. Dis Col Rect 1968; 11: 462.
17. Knight GH, Fowler W. Br Med J 1956; ii: 980.
18. Anderson MJ, Dockerty MB. Dis Col Rect 1958; 1: 23.
19. Humphrey LJ, Playforth H, Leavell UW. Arch Derm 1969; 100: 59.
20. Weale FE. Br J Surg 1964; 51: 513.
21. Gaston EA, Wilde WL. Dis Col Rect 1965; 8: 343.

Vascular disorders

22. Graham-Stewart CW. Dis Col Rect 1963; 6: 333.
23. Haas PA, Fox TA, Haas GP. Dis Col Rect 1984; 27: 442.
24. Graham-Stewart CW. Br Med J 1962; i: 213.
25. Hernandez V, Hernandez IA, Berthrong M. Dis Col Rect 1967; 10: 205.

Tumours of the anal region

26. Fenger C, Nielsen VT. Acta Path Microbiol Scand Sect A 1981; 89: 463.
27. Klotz RG, Pamukcoglu T, Souilliard H. Cancer 1967; 20: 1727.
28. Grodsky L. JAMA 1969; 207: 2057.
29. Morson BC, Jass JR. Precancerous lesions of the gastrointestinal tract. A histopathological classification. London: Baillière-Tindall, 1985.
30. Oriel JD, Almeida JD. Br J Vener Dis 1970; 46: 37.
31. Lee SH, McGregor DH, Kuziez MN. Dis Col Rect 1981; 24: 462.
32. Buschke A, Löwenstein L. Klin Wochenschr 1925; 4: 1726.
33. Knoblich R, Failing JF. Am J Clin Pathol 1967; 88: 46.
34. Gingrass PJ, Bubrick MP, Hitchcock CR et al. Dis Col Rect 1978; 21: 120.
35. Anscombe AM, Isaacson P. Histopathol 1983; 7: 123.
36. Elliott GB, Fisher BK. Arch Derm 1967; 95: 81.
37. Meeker JH, Neubecker RD, Helwig EB. Am J Clin Pathol 1962; 37: 182.
38. Bensaude A, Parturier-Albot M. Proc Roy Soc Med 1971; 64: 38.
39. Wade TR, Kopf AW, Ackerman AB. Cancer 1978; 42: 1890.
40. Helwig EB, Graham JH. Cancer 1963; 16: 387.
41. Linder JM, Myers RT. Am J Surg 1970; 36: 342.
42. Mazoujian G, Pinkus GS, Haagensen DC. Am J Surg Pathol 1984; 8: 43.
43. Morson BC, Pang LSC. Proc Roy Soc Med 1968; 61: 623.
44. Frederick PL, Osborn D, Cronin CM. Lancet 1982; ii: 391.
45. Gabriel WB. Proc Roy Soc Med 1941; 34: 139.
46. Pang LSC, Morson BC. J Clin Pathol 1967; 20: 28.
47. Fisher ER. Cancer 1969; 24: 312.
48. Morson BC. Proc Roy Soc Med 1960; 53: 416.
49. Hardcastle JD, Bussey HJR. Proc Roy Soc Med 1968; 61: 27.
50. Frost DB, Richards PC, Montague ED, Giacco CG, Martin RG. Cancer 1984; 53: 1285.
51. Kuehn PG, Beckett R, Eisenberg H, Reed JF. NEJM 1964; 270: 614.
52. Morson BC, Volkstadt H. J Clin Pathol 1963; 16: 126.
53. Mason JK, Helwig EB. Cancer 1966; 19: 39.
54. Fenger C, Lyon H. Histochem J 1982; 14: 631.
55. Pyper PC, Parks TG. Br J Surg 1984; 71: 671.
56. Berkley JL. Dis Col Rect 1960; 3: 159.
57. Wellman KF. Can J Surg 1962; 5: 311.
58. Winkelman J, Grosfeld J, Bigelow B. Am J Clin Pathol 1964; 42: 395.
59. Fenger C, Filipe MI. Acta Pathol Microbiol Scand Sect A 1977; 85: 273.
60. Dukes CE, Galvin C. Ann Roy Coll Surg 1956; 18: 246.
61. Jones EA, Morson BC. Histopathol 1984; 8: 279.
62. Nielson OV, Jensen SL. Br J Surg 1955; 90: 522.
63. Manheim SD, Alexander RM. Am J Surg 1981; 61, 856.
64. Johnston J, Helwig EB. Dig Dis Sci 1981; 26, 807.
65. Fagundes LA. Gastroenterol 1963; 44: 351.
66. Kott I, Urca I. Dis Col Rect 1969; 12: 338.
67. Marco V, Autonell J, Fare J, Fernandez-Layos M, Doncel F. Am J Surg Pathol 1982; 6: 707.

The peritoneum

ANATOMICAL CONSIDERATIONS

The peritoneum is a smooth, thin, elastic membrane that lines the abdominal cavity and covers the abdominal and pelvic viscera. Although the peritoneal cavity is a single, continuous space it is subdivided into four main potential compartments by serosal folds and by the attachments of the viscera. These compartments are: the *supracolic space*, or subphrenic (sub-diaphragmatic) region, which is bounded by the diaphragm above and by the transverse colon and transverse mesocolon below; the *right infracolic space*, which is bounded on the left by the small intestine and its mesentery and above by the corresponding part of the transverse colon and mesocolon; the *left infracolic space*, which is bounded on the right by the small intestine and its mesentery and above by the rest of the transverse colon and mesocolon; and the *pelvic cavity*.

The supracolic space is further subdivided into: the *right subphrenic space*, between the diaphragm and the right lobe of the liver; the *left subphrenic space*, between the diaphragm and the left lobe of the liver, the stomach and the spleen; the *right subhepatic space* (Rutherford Morison's pouch), between the undersurface of the right lobe of the liver and the gall-bladder above and the right adrenal and kidney, the duodenum and the hepatic flexure of the colon below; and the *left subhepatic space*, which is the omental bursa (lesser sac of the peritoneum).

When considering the spread of infection in the abdominal cavity it is important to realize that the barriers created by the peritoneal attachments of the viscera greatly influence the path followed by infected fluids from one region of the abdominal cavity to another and determine the 'drainage basins' in which they eventually collect.[1] In this context it is important to recognize that because of the obliquity of the small intestinal mesentery the right infracolic space is wide above, tapering downwards and to the right, while the left infracolic space is correspondingly narrow above and widens out below where it is continuous with the pelvic cavity. Adhesions between apposed peritoneal surfaces may obliterate the normal communications between the various compartments allowing localized accumulations of fluid.

In the male the abdominal cavity is entirely closed. In the female there is a communication between the abdominal cavity and the exterior of the body through the uterine tubes, uterus and vagina: infections of the female genital tract may extend to the peritoneum by this route.

The peritoneal serosa consists of a single sheet of flattened mesothelial cells covering a narrow layer of dense collagenous tissue that includes conspicuous elastic fibres. Deep to this is a rich network of lymphatics and thin-walled blood vessels and some large deposits of fat. The peritoneal 'membrane' is freely permeable to water and small molecules, which accounts for the accumulation of fluid in cases of generalized oedema or passive venous congestion, but which also allows the successful treatment of renal failure with peritoneal dialysis.

Particulate matter, such as bacteria or extravasated red cells, is absorbed from the peritoneal cavity mainly through the lymphatics of the diaphragm and thus is carried to the intrathoracic lymph nodes.[2] A secondary route of absorption is through lymphadenoid structures in the omentum, the 'taches laiteuses' ('milk spots'), whence they pass quickly to the regional lymphatics and the cisterna chyli.[3]

The peritoneal cavity normally contains a small amount of clear, straw-coloured fluid that serves to lubricate the apposed serosal surfaces. This fluid has the characteristics of a transudate—low specific gravity and a low content of protein. It contains some cells, most of which are either detached mesothelial cells or phagocytic macrophages, but a few lymphocytes and neutrophil leukocytes may also be present.

The presence of an excess of fluid in the peritoneal cavity is known as *ascites* (see p. 434). Estimation of its protein content and specific gravity will establish whether it has formed by transudation or exudation. Examination of the centrifuged deposit may reveal malignant cells or microorganisms. Peritoneoscopy (laparoscopy) may be useful in the diagnosis of diseases that involve the peritoneum, especially if combined with biopsy.

PERITONITIS

Inflammation of the peritoneum is a common condition which, despite the widespread availability of antibacterial agents, continues to cause much morbidity and mortality. Infection usually reaches the abdominal cavity either from the alimentary tract, by far the commonest source, or from the outside as a result of paracentesis, laparotomy or penetrating trauma. Less commonly it may derive from the vagina, uterus and uterine tubes. Blood-borne infection is rare.

ACUTE DIFFUSE PERITONITIS

The two commonest causes of acute diffuse peritonitis are appendicitis (see p. 293) and perforated peptic ulcer (see p. 178). In appendicitis bacteria gain entry to the peritoneal cavity through the diseased wall of the appendix and the severity of the inflammation depends upon the number and virulence of the organisms. If the appendix perforates the peritoneal cavity is suddenly flooded with organisms, usually accompanied by tissue debris and foreign matter, and the result is often a severe, diffuse inflammation, associated with pain and shock. Perforation of a peptic ulcer releases gastric or duodenal contents, including gastric juice, bile, pancreatic juice and partly digested food, into the peritoneal cavity. The digestive juices and bile produce an immediate 'chemical' peritonitis by their irritant effects and this is commonly followed by bacterial infection. Other common causes of peritonitis include perforation of gastrointestinal carcinomas, intestinal perforation due to inflammatory bowel disease, ischaemia, obstruction or diverticular disease, or rupture of the gall-bladder in acute cholecystitis. Rupture of a pyosalpinx or a tubo-ovarian abscess, perforating wounds involving abdominal viscera, abdominal surgery, and more recently peritoneal dialysis are other important causes. In newborn infants direct spread of umbilical infection may result in peritonitis.

Acute diffuse peritonitis as a complication of gastrointestinal surgery has become much less frequent since the introduction of effective antibiotics to sterilize the bowel pre-operatively. Nevertheless, soiling of the abdominal cavity by spilled faeces remains a serious complication of emergency surgery and peritonitis may also follow elective operations if meticulous attention is not paid to asepsis and surgical technique or if there is breakdown of an intestinal anastomosis, either due to infection or ischaemia.

Acute diffuse peritonitis may also be precipitated by the escape of blood into the peritoneal cavity (*haemoperitoneum*) although the inflammatory reaction is seldom pronounced unless there is also an infective element. On the other hand, release of bile[4] or pancreatic juice, the latter especially in acute pancreatitis, produces a severe acute chemical peritonitis with fat necrosis.

Acute diffuse peritonitis without any apparent pre-existing focus of infection, so-called '*primary peritonitis*' or '*spontaneous bacterial peritonitis*' is uncommon. It may occur in children, especially those with the nephrotic syndrome,[5] and the causative organism is usually a pneumococcus. It is generally considered that the infection reaches the peritoneum via the blood-stream, although in girls infection from the genital tract via the uterine tubes is a possibility. Occasionally an occult or overlooked infection of the upper respiratory tract can be found. Adults with primary peritonitis nearly always have cirrhosis.[6] The infection is usually due to a single organism, usually of intestinal origin. It is uncertain whether the route of infection is direct bacterial invasion of the bowel wall or haematogenous spread. The latter possibility is supported by the frequent occurrence of bacteraemia by enteric organisms in patients with chronic liver disease, the result of defective host defence mechanisms.

Bacteriology of acute diffuse peritonitis

Peritonitis secondary to gastrointestinal disease is usually associated with infection by a mixture of the organisms that form the normal flora of the alimentary tract, with anaerobic bacteria and coliforms predominating.[7] So-called primary peritonitis, on the other hand, is usually due to a single bacterial species (see above). A variety of organisms, aerobic and anaerobic, may be responsible for peritonitis secondary to infections of the gynaecological organs and gonococcal or chlamydial peritonitis may also arise by this route. Peritonitis complicating puerperal fever is usually caused by a beta-haemolytic streptococcus.

Macroscopical and microscopical appearances

The appearance of the peritoneum in diffuse peritonitis varies with the stage of development of the disease. Initially there is engorgement of the subserosal capillary blood vessels, accompanied by dulling of the peritoneal surface. This is succeeded by an exudative reaction, with the formation of a thin film of fibrin on the surface: this film is very sticky, and causes loops of bowel to adhere to one another and to the parietal peritoneum. The exudate may be serous, fibrinous, purulent or haemorrhagic, according to the type and severity of the pathogenic agent. Microscopical examination in the initial stage of the inflammation shows swelling and desquamation of the mesothelial cells. Their place is soon taken by a thin layer of fibrin enclosing many neutrophils and some cellular debris (Fig. 10.1). Granulation tissue begins to form underneath and pleomorphism and mitotic activity in mononuclear cells in this zone can sometimes mimic a malignant infiltrate, especially in a frozen section of a small biopsy (Fig. 10.1).

The development of peritonitis is accompanied by the accumulation of fluid with a high protein content in the peritoneal cavity. It contains neutrophil polymorphs and variable numbers of bacteria and red blood cells. Estimation of the neutrophil count is a useful rapid method for confirming the diagnosis in an emergency.[6] The fluid tends to collect in the dependent parts of the abdominal cavity, such as the rectovesical pouch, the paracolic gutters and the subphrenic region. The infection spreads rapidly in the subserosal lymphatics as well as over the surface of the peritoneum and this spread is promoted by respi-

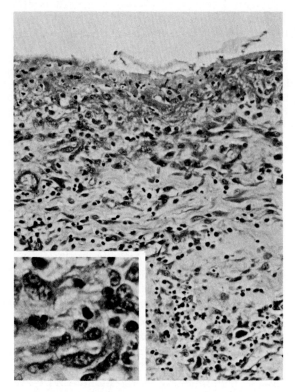

Fig. 10.1 Acute peritonitis. The mesothelium has been destroyed and replaced by a fibrinous exudate containing neutrophil leukocytes. Deep to this there is oedematous connective tissue containing mononuclear cells including fibroblasts, histiocytes and endothelial cells. Some of these are pleomorphic and even multinucleate (inset).

Haematoxylin-eosin   × 190; inset   × 500

ratory and bowel movements. In advanced cases of acute diffuse peritonitis septic thrombosis of veins in the mesenteries can occur; this may lead to portal pyaemia and the development of abscesses in the liver.

Complications

One of the most serious complications of diffuse peritonitis is *paralytic ileus* (adynamic ileus), a failure of peristaltic motility of the intestine that probably results from toxic damage to Auerbach's plexus. Later, possibly as a result of disturbances in electrolyte balance, the smooth muscle may lose its power of contraction. The paralysis usually develops three or four days after the onset of the peritonitis: it may affect much of the small intestine, but commonly it is confined to a short length of ileum or colon that has lain in a pool of purulent exudate in the pelvis.

The local paralysis produces a state of complete intestinal obstruction. The ensuing distension of the proximal loops with gas and secretions may in turn result in kinking, which adds to the obstruction. Even where the intestinal serosa itself is not inflamed, the dilated gut appears a dusky red as a result of venous stasis: the effects of partial anoxia may thus be added to those of intoxication. The accumulation of fluid in the distended intestinal loops leads both to the absorption of toxic products through the mucosa and to fluid and electrolyte imbalance. Death from acute diffuse peritonitis is more often brought about by paralytic ileus and intestinal obstruction than by septicaemia.

If the patient recovers from the acute effects of peritonitis, two serious complications may result—the formation of localized abscesses and the creation of peritoneal adhesions, with the danger of subsequent intestinal obstruction as a result of internal hernia or volvulus.

Localized abscess formation. The purulent exudate in acute diffuse peritonitis tends to accumulate in the subphrenic region, in the pelvis, and to a lesser extent in the paracolic gutters. The site of such localized abscesses depends largely on the original site of inflammation: following perforation of a peptic ulcer, for example, pus tends to accumulate in the subphrenic spaces or in the lesser sac of the peritoneum, whereas after appendicitis a pelvic collection of pus is more usual.

Subphrenic abscess (sub-diaphragmatic abscess) is much commoner on the right side than on the left. It develops insidiously, usually after a perforated peptic ulcer, cholecystitis, diverticulitis, pancreatitis or appendicitis. The pus collects in one of the anatomical compartments bounded by the diaphragm, the liver and the falciform ligament.[8] It becomes sealed off from the abdominal cavity by adhesions, and an abscess cavity lined by granulation tissue is formed. The abscess may then resolve, burst into the peritoneal cavity, or extend into adjacent structures.

A *pelvic abscess* may develop in the course of diffuse peritonitis or as a complication of local peritonitis elsewhere in the abdominal cavity. The pus accumulates in the rectovesical or recto-uterine pouch, where it becomes walled off by adhesions. The abscess may resolve spontaneously if it is not too large, or it may burst into the rectum, bladder or vagina.

Peritoneal adhesions

In most cases of acute diffuse peritonitis, resolution of the fibrinous or purulent exudate leaves a smooth serosal surface. The fibrinolytic properties of mesothelium, producing plasminogen activators,[9] are thought to play an important role in this resolution. If fibrin is not adequately removed there is fibroblastic invasion and organization of granulation tissue leading to collagen synthesis and the progressive formation of dense, fibrous adhesions.[10,11] Experimental mesothelial injury, and ischaemia in particular, is followed by a depression in fibrinolytic activity lasting for several days and during this time adhesion formation may be initiated, perhaps irreversibly.[12] Some patients seem to be particularly prone to develop peritoneal adhesions, even after a simple exploration of the abdominal cavity without any other inflammatory stimulus, while in others it is surprising how completely the peritoneum may return to normal after a severe diffuse infection. As well as the host response, the nature of the infective agent and the degree of chronicity of the peritonitis probably have considerable influence on the development of adhesions. In some instances there is evidence that adhesions are temporary and may gradually disappear.[13] Peritoneal adhesions may be localized or generalized. In either case they may cause obstruction later by constricting or strangling a segment of bowel, usually small intestine.

LOCAL PERITONITIS

Inflammation of the peritoneum may remain localized to the vicinity of the lesion that has given rise to it. For example, peritonitis resulting from perforation of a peptic ulcer may be localized by the formation of adhesions and, in particular, the enveloping action of the greater omentum.

The greater omentum plays an important part in limiting the spread of local infections, particularly in adults, in whom it is relatively larger than

in children. It is nearly always found to be adherent to a focus of peritonitis. There is little to support the old view that the omentum is directly attracted to sites of inflammation in the abdominal cavity, for it is incapable of independent movement. Nevertheless, it is constantly undergoing changes in its position as a result of intestinal movements and of alterations in posture, and when these passive movements bring it into contact with a focus of inflammation, fibrinous exudate forms on its serosal surface and anchors it to the site. The greater omentum is often found in the neighbourhood of an acutely inflamed appendix, surrounding it and hindering further spread of infection. Similarly, it becomes adherent to malignant tumours with peritoneal involvement, to the colon in diverticulitis with local peritonitis or the ileum in Crohn's disease, and to portions of infarcted bowel. It is commonly found, too, within hernial sacs, where it becomes attached to any inflamed bowel that is present.

The pathological appearances of local peritonitis are similar to those found in the diffuse form of the disease: the differences are essentially quantitative rather than qualitative. The reaction typically progresses from the serofibrinous stage of inflammation through the seropurulent to the frankly suppurative; in many instances, however, the condition is arrested before abscess formation has occurred.

SPECIAL FORMS OF PERITONITIS

Tuberculous peritonitis

With the striking decline in the general incidence of infection by *Mycobacterium tuberculosis* and *Mycobacterium bovis* in Western countries during the present century, peritonitis caused by these organisms has become rare. However, tuberculous peritonitis remains common in the Third World and occasional examples of both generalized and localized forms of the disease are found in Britain as a complication of infection of the intestines, the mesenteric lymph nodes, the female genital tract or the lungs.[14]

In generalized tuberculous peritonitis the peritoneum is sparsely or copiously studded with small glistening tubercles. In time, these may enlarge, coalesce to form plaques, and become caseous. There is a variable amount of exudate, which may be haemorrhagic or fibrinous, and in which lymphocytes are conspicuous. The greater omentum is often extensively affected, and may appear at necropsy as an elongated, retracted, fibrocaseous mass lying transversely across the abdomen. In wasted children this omental roll is often easily palpated during life. The diagnosis is best made by peritoneal biopsy,[15] in which typical caseating granulomatous inflammation is seen and in which mycobacteria may be recognizable on Ziehl-Neelsen staining. Culture of biopsy tissue should always be undertaken in order to confirm the diagnosis and establish the antibiotic sensitivity of the organisms. Should the disease become chronic, many adhesions form and the viscera become matted together (Fig. 10.2). Recurrent attacks of acute and subacute obstruction of the small intestine are then liable to occur.

Actinomycosis

Actinomycosis of the gastrointestinal tract, usually the appendix (see p. 298), or of the female genital tract, may lead to actinomycotic peritonitis. The inflammatory reaction is associated with much fibrosis and fistula formation such that the affected region of the peritoneal cavity is usually distorted in a localized inflammatory mass related to the appendix or an actinomycotic tubo-ovarian abscess.

Fungal peritonitis

Inflammation of the peritoneal surfaces by fungal organisms is uncommon and is often associated with immunosuppression or debilitation. *Candida albicans* peritonitis may follow intestinal perforation[16] or complicate peritoneal dialysis[17] and *cryptococcal peritonitis* has been described in immunosuppressed patients.[18] Coccidioidomycotic[19], blastomycotic and histoplasmic peritonitis may occur rarely in areas where these organisms are endemic.

Metazoal peritonitis

Chronic pelvic peritonitis can be caused in women by the pinworm (threadworm) *Enterobius vermi-*

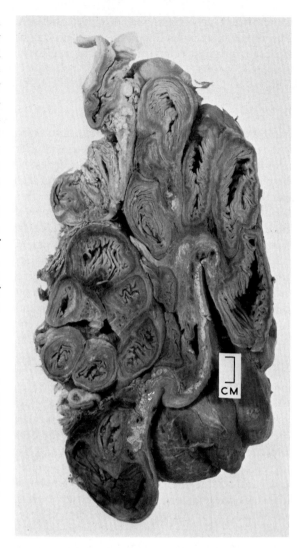

Fig. 10.2 Tuberculous peritonitis. The coils of small intestine are matted together by thick adhesions. Streaks and confluent rounded foci of caseation are seen as pale areas against the darker background of the fibrotic granulation tissue.

Specimen from the Gordon Museum, Guy's Hospital, London, reproduced by permission of the Curator, Mr J. D. Maynard. Photograph by Miss P. M. Turnbull, Charing Cross Hospital Medical School, London.

cularis which reaches the peritoneal cavity from the gastrointestinal tract by migrating from the rectum to the vagina and then ascending via the uterus and uterine tubes.[20] Having reached the peritoneum the worm (which is always a female) dies, sometimes releasing its ova. An eosinophil-rich granulomatous reaction is then formed, either to the dead adult or the ova (Fig. 10.3), which is later surrounded by a collagenous capsule. The lesions are usually found on the serosal aspect of the pelvic viscera, but they may occur anywhere within the peritoneal cavity. They are white or yellow in colour, generally rather less than a centimetre in diameter, and have a firm, fibrous capsule and a necrotic core. Clinical manifestations of this granulomatous peritonitis are extremely uncommon[21] and the lesions are usually discovered either during laparotomy for some unrelated condition, when they can be mistaken for tumour deposits, endometriosis or tuberculosis, or at autopsy.

Ascaris lumbricoides, in cases of heavy infestation of the small bowel, may cause intestinal obstruction (see p. 267). If this results in ulceration and perforation, large numbers of adult worms may escape into the peritoneal cavity: the accompanying septic peritonitis leads to laparotomy, disclosing

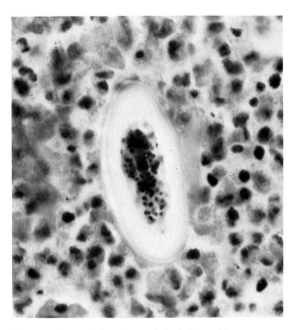

Fig. 10.3 Ovum of *Oxyuris vermicularis* (*Enterobius vermicularis*) in a localized granuloma in the recto-uterine pouch. The shape of the egg is characteristic, the curve at one end being of radius smaller than that at the other, and one side having a greater convexity. The ovum contains a larva. Most of the leukocytes forming the inflammatory exudate are eosinophils.

Haematoxylin-eosin   × 700

Photomicrograph provided by W. StC. Symmers.

the worms. It is important in such cases to make sure that all the worms are removed; any that are left will die, leading to persistent local peritonitis and eventual adhesion formation. The female worms may shed ova throughout the peritoneal cavity, and these can cause widespread adhesions, with a picture resembling tuberculous peritonitis. Recurrent episodes of intestinal obstruction may then develop. In the earlier stages the ascaris ova provoke the formation of discrete serosal granulomas, quite like single tubercles but readily recognized on microscopical examination because of the characteristic appearance of the ova (Fig 10.4). As the lesion ages, the ova gradually disintegrate and disappear and its origin may eventually become impossible to specify.[22]

In most cases of peritonitis due to ascaris ova there is no acute lesion. The serosal granulomatosis is then an incidental finding in the course of laparotomy for some other complaint, or is discovered when the exploration is undertaken because of obstructive symptoms caused by the adhesions. It is speculative how the ova reach the peritoneum in these cases. It has been said that an occasional ascaris may penetrate the bowel wall, the small perforation quickly healing after its passage without acute peritonitis resulting.

Peritonitis may also be produced when larvae of *Strongyloides stercoralis* or of the roundworm *Anisakis* escape into the peritoneal cavity.[23] An omental inflammatory mass in which eosinophil leukocytes are conspicuous may be formed.

Schistosomiasis may rarely produce a chronic granulomatous peritonitis with adhesions, but is better recognized as a cause of retroperitoneal fibrosis (see below), especially when there is infection with *Schistosoma haematobium*. Histological examination of scar tissue in such cases reveals the characteristic eosinophil-rich sclerosing granulomas around the ova (Fig. 10.5).

Hydatid cysts are occasionally found in the omentum or mesenteries. Linguatulid larvae may encyst in these tissues.

Traumatic peritonitis

Peritonitis due to surgical trauma is a common cause of localized adhesions. Incision of the peritoneum or bruising by ungentle handling of

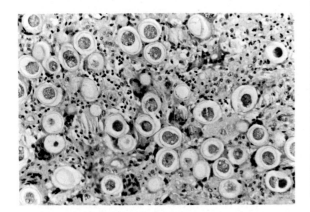
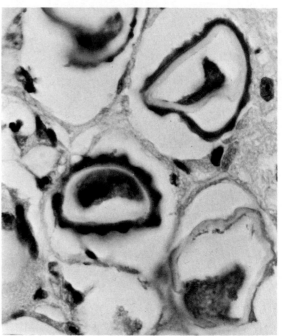

Fig. 10.4a, b The patient was a child who had spent a year in a tropical country where his parents were temporarily employed. While on holiday at home, in Europe, he developed acute intestinal obstruction from impaction of a large number of adult ascarids at the ileocaecal valve: the ileum had perforated and 14 ascarids were found free in the peritoneal cavity. Subsequently, he had a number of episodes of intestinal obstruction as a result of the adhesions that followed the acute ascaris peritonitis. It was during one of these episodes that the specimen illustrated was obtained: this shows that it was the presence of myriads of eggs throughout the peritoneal cavity that had led to the chronic fibrosing peritonitis. The patient eventually died during an episode of acute intestinal obstruction. (*a*) Chronic peritonitis due to the presence of ova of *Ascaris lumbricoides*, the common intestinal round worm. The ova, with the contained embryo and distinct hyaline wall, were initially mistaken for fungal cells. Compare with (**b**). (**b**) In this field, from the specimen illustrated in (**a**), some of the ova have the coarsely mamillate, dark outer shell that is characteristic of the ova of *Ascaris lumbricoides*.

Haematoxylin-eosin   (**a**) ×160; (**b**) ×630

Photomicrographs provided by W. St C. Symmers.

viscera damages the mesothelial surface and produces a local inflammatory response. Some experiments have suggested that blood at the site of damaged or dried serosal surfaces may promote the formation of postoperative adhesions,[12] although other investigations have shown that local ischaemia of the mesothelium (which markedly inhibits its fibrinolytic properties) along with the presence of foreign materials such as sutures, and not direct damage to the serosa, are mainly to blame.[24]

It is possible that mechanical violence to the abdominal wall may cause sufficient peritoneal irritation to provoke a sterile inflammatory reaction, but far more commonly traumatic perforation of an abdominal viscus is responsible for peritonitis following physical injury.

Peritonitis caused by foreign bodies

Foreign bodies, such as gauze left in the peritoneal cavity at operation, produce an inflammatory response: if these foreign bodies are infected, as is very commonly the case, particularly with surgical swabs, diffuse peritonitis generally results.

The contents of hollow viscera, particularly the stomach and appendix, may escape into the peritoneal cavity as a result of perforation. Granulomas are a frequent outcome of such an event, and they may contain a remarkable number of foreign bodies of vegetable or meat origin (Fig. 10.6).

Talcum powder, formerly used on surgeon's gloves, consists of magnesium silicate and calcium

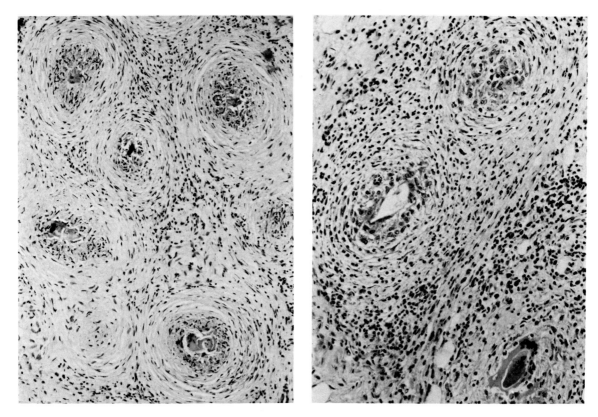

Fig. 10.5a, b (**a**) Sclerosing tuberculoid granuloma of the retroperitoneal tissues due to schistosomiasis. The histological picture in this case was at first taken to be that of sarcoidosis in its sclerosing stage; see (**b**). (**b**) Same specimen as illustrated in (**a**). Two of the tuberculoid foci in this field contain the remains of an ovum of *Schistosoma haematobium.*

Haematoxylin-eosin   (**a**) × 100; (**b**) × 160

Photomicrographs provided by W. St C. Symmers.

and magnesium carbonate. When introduced into the peritoneal cavity it causes a chronic fibrosing granulomatous reaction (*talc granuloma*).[25] Foreign-body giant cells are conspicuous in these granulomas, and the talc crystals that they contain can be demonstrated microscopically in polarized light (Fig. 10.7). Although talcum powder is very rarely used nowadays on surgeon's gloves, talc granulomas resembling miliary tubercles or tumour deposits macroscopically may still be found in patients who have had any form of intra-abdominal surgery in the past. While the clinical effects of this are usually trivial, some patients have developed extensive peritoneal adhesions with disastrous consequences.

Similar granulomatous nodules may be produced by the spores of the club-moss *Lycopodium,*

which was also once used as a dusting powder for gloves.[26] In this case the spores are acid-fast and can be stained by the Ziehl-Neelsen method.

In recent years epichlorhydrin-treated Indian corn or rice *starch* has been used on surgeon's gloves. It was originally hoped that absorption of the starch from the peritoneal cavity would abolish glove-powder peritonitis but this hope has not been fulfilled: starch is now known to be a rare but important cause of postoperative complications.[27] Starch peritonitis usually develops at any time from days to many weeks after an otherwise uneventful abdominal operation. Small amounts of starch powder can produce this effect, and it has even been recognized following vaginal examination without surgical exposure of the peritoneum: presumably in such cases powder from the surface

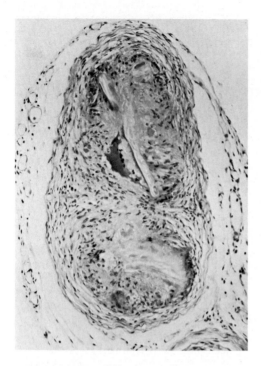
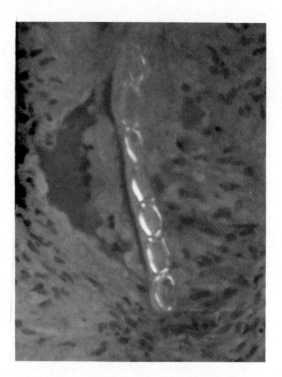

Fig. 10.6a, b (**a**) Tuberculoid foreign-body granuloma in the subserosa of the mesoappendix. The outline of foreign material can just be made out—for instance, lying obliquely below the multinucleate giant cell near the middle of the field; see (**b**). (**b**) Higher magnification of the giant cell and foreign body referred to in the caption of (**a**), photographed in polarized light. The foreign body is birefringent, and has the structure of vegetable matter. The specimen was obtained at appendicectomy, carried out after recovery from an appendix mass that had been treated by drainage. The foreign material must have escaped from the lumen of the appendix during the acute stage of the disease.

Haematoxylin-eosin   (**a**) × 120; (**b**) photographed in polarized light   × 325

Photomicrographs provided by W. StC. Symmers.

of the gynaecologist's gloves is carried by retrograde flow through the uterine cavity and along the lumen of the uterine tubes to set up typical starch granulomatosis of the pelvic peritoneum. In the severer cases abdominal pain, fever and signs of peritoneal irritation lead to laparotomy: this usually discloses some degree of ascites and a varying number of minute granulomas scattered over the serosal lining, and an inflammatory mass of omentum may sometimes be found. The granulomas consist of macrophages, often in a palisade arrangement, and multinucleate giant cells enclosing foci of necrosis (Fig. 10.8).[28] They predispose to the formation of adhesions. Starch granules are demonstrable as 'Maltese cross' figures of birefringence when examined under polarized light (Fig. 10.8): they are present both in the giant cells and in the necrotic matter. Delayed hypersensitivity to starch is regarded as the mechanism underlying starch granulomatosis in susceptible individuals[29] and treatment with corticosteroids may be helpful. The future development of starch-free surgical gloves coated by polymers may eventually abolish this important complication of surgery.

Not all starch granulomatosis of the peritoneum can be related to surgical-glove powder and a similar reaction to food-derived starch may occur following bowel perforation.[30] The histological appearances of the granulomatous reactions are identical but food-starch particles within the lesions can be recognized because they tend to be

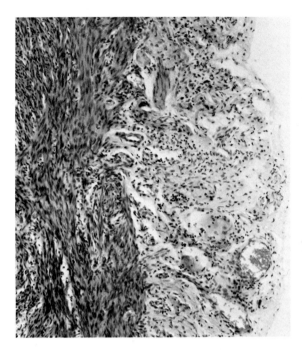 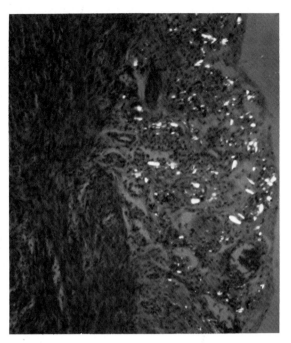

Fig. 10.7a, b (**a**) Serosal aspect of a uterus, showing localized thickening of the subserosa by fibrosis. A few inconspicuous multinucleate giant cells can just be seen, but no foreign bodies are visible; see (**b**). (**b**) The same field as in (**a**), photographed in polarized light. The bright particles are crystals of talcum powder. These findings show that the fibrotic focus is a talc granuloma. It dated from an earlier laparotomy.

Haematoxylin-eosin   (**a**) × 100; (**b**) photographed in polarized light × 100

Photomicrographs provided by W. StC. Symmers.

larger and more variable in size than those of glove powder. Furthermore, they are often oval rather than round in shape, and may be extremely resistant to salivary diastase digestion.

Escape of barium sulphate into the peritoneal cavity, usually due to colonic perforation during barium enema, may also be associated with peritonitis. There is nearly always an initial bacterial peritonitis due to the release of faecal organisms and laparotomy is often necessary at this stage to repair the perforation. A foreign-body granulomatous reaction to the barium sulphate particles may develop later, although this produces little fibrosis and is virtually never clinically significant, despite giving rise to extraordinary radiographic appearances.[31] The barium sulphate particles may have a variety of appearances when examined by polarized light.[32]

Insoluble antibiotic preparations, various oily substances such as liquid paraffin (which some surgeons formerly instilled into the abdominal cavity in the hope of preventing adhesions), and cellulose fibres from disposable surgical gowns and drapes[33] are among the rarer of potent causes of postoperative granulomatous peritonitis with extensive adhesions.

Meconium peritonitis

Meconium peritonitis is the result of intra-uterine or neonatal intestinal perforation causing spillage of meconium into the peritoneal cavity and inciting an inflammatory reaction.[34] It is associated with congenital abnormalities of the intestine including atresia, stenosis, intussusception, volvulus, and hernia, and also with cystic fibrosis (fibrocystic disease of the pancreas) in which there may be intestinal obstruction by abnormally viscid meconium. The spilled meconium contains swallowed amniotic fluid, mucus, bile and pancreatic and

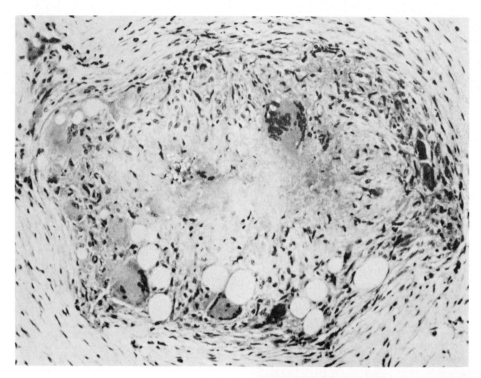

Fig. 10.8a, b (**a**) Starch granuloma of the peritoneum. Multiple peritoneal nodules, adhesions and ascites had developed in the interval of 11 weeks between consecutive laparotomy operations on a man in his 60s. The picture of one of the nodules shows a central area of necrosis surrounded by epithelioid macrophages, multinucleate giant cells and fibrosis. The field was photographed during illumination through partially crossed polarizing filters, enabling the general histological detail to be seen while the granules of starch show as bright structures, some free in the necrotic area and others in the cytoplasm of giant cells. The group of free-lying granules just above and slightly to the right of the centre of the picture is shown at higher magnification in (**b**). (**b**) Starch granuloma. Same preparation as that illustrated in (**a**). A group of starch granules is shown in fully polarized light, which gives the so-called Maltese cross appearance that is characteristic of their structure when viewed under these conditions.

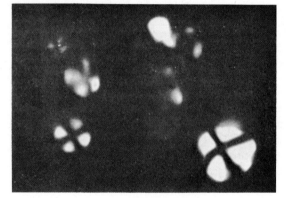

Haematoxylin-eosin (**a**) ×200; (**b**) ×1550

Photomicrographs provided by Dr J. D. Davies, University of Bristol.

intestinal secretions which are particularly irritant to the peritoneum, causing an intense peritonitis with fat necrosis. If the baby survives, a florid fibrosing granulomatous reaction often develops and extensive firm adhesions result. Occasionally the peritonitis is localized and a thick-walled inflammatory cyst may be formed by the fixed intestinal loops. Histological examination in the acute phase shows a florid peritonitis with fat necrosis and foreign-body giant cells. Later there is fibrosis which is often loose and myxoid and which contains areas of amorphous or granular calcification, haemosiderin deposition, histiocytes and foreign-body giant cells.[34] Healing of meconium peritonitis can result in a fibrous calcified mesenteric nodule. In boys it may extend into the tunica vaginalis and result in a scrotal nodule that can mimic a tumour, especially if there is no history of an acute episode of peritonitis in the neonatal period, as is sometimes the case.[35]

Peritonitis in the collagen diseases

Patients with collagen diseases, especially polyarteritis nodosa, rheumatoid arthritis and systemic lupus erythematosus, may develop peritonitis secondary to major intestinal complications such as ulceration or infarction. However, a low-grade primary peritoneal serositis may rarely occur in systemic lupus erythematosus and give rise to painless ascites: this may even be the first manifestation of the disease.[36]

Familial Mediterranean fever

Familial Mediterranean fever (familial paroxysmal polyserositis) is an inherited disorder of unknown aetiology that affects predominantly patients of Jewish (non-Ashkenazic), Armenian and Arabic ancestry. It is characterized by recurrent episodes of fever, peritonitis and pleurisy,[37] but there may also be arthritis, skin lesions and amyloidosis affecting blood vessels, the renal glomeruli and the spleen. The clinical manifestations of peritonitis frequently result in laparotomy being undertaken, revealing a diffuse fibrinous serositis. The pathological changes are non-specific; biopsy rarely reveals amyloid deposition in mesenteric blood vessels, the only potential clue to the correct diagnosis.

Sclerosing peritonitis

Practolol, a beta-adrenergic blocking agent that was introduced in Britain in 1970, was found to cause dense, progressive fibrosis of the peritoneum in some patients, with consequent obliteration of the peritoneal cavity by thick, vascular adhesions.[38] The condition, often called *sclerosing peritonitis*, affected the peritoneum of the small bowel predominantly, without involvement of the retroperitoneum. In some cases the peritoneal fibrosis did not become clinically evident until very many months after the patient stopped taking the drug. The pathogenesis of the condition is unknown. Histo-

logically, there is a deposition of laminated fibrous tissue immediately deep to the mesothelium (Fig. 10.9), with a focal mononuclear inflammatory cell infiltrate in the underlying tissue. Deposits of fibrin may be present focally on the surface of the mesothelium. Practolol was withdrawn from sale in the United Kingdom in 1976.

More recently there has been a case report of a similar sclerosing peritonitis in a patient receiving metoprolol,[39] another beta-receptor blocker, but the significance of this single case is dubious in view of the widespread use of the drug as an antihypertensive agent. There have also been a number of reports of retroperitoneal fibrosis (see p. 431) in patients receiving a variety of beta-

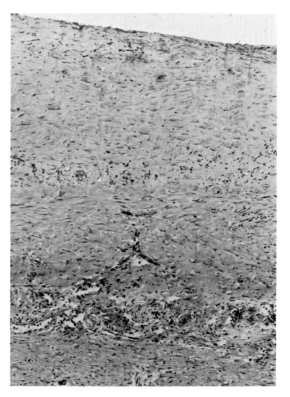

Fig. 10.9 Practolol peritonitis. This patient developed a sclerosing peritonitis while taking the beta-adrenergic receptor blocking agent practolol. Dense laminated fibrosis is seen immediately below the mesothelium while there is a focal chronic inflammatory cell infiltrate in the underlying connective tissue.

Haematoxylin-eosin × 55

Histological preparation provided by Dr J. A. Waycott, Medical Department, Imperial Chemical Industries. Photomicrograph by Mr Peter Langham, University of Wales College of Medicine, Cardiff.

blockers[40] but once again a causal relationship would seem unlikely.

A sclerosing obstructive peritonitis encasing the small intestine, very similar to that produced by practolol and different from ordinary postoperative adhesions, has recently been described in patients undergoing long-term continuous ambulatory peritoneal dialysis.[41] Recurrent attacks of bacterial peritonitis are common in such patients but it is uncertain whether the peritoneal thickening can be attributed to this, or to a reaction to some component of the dialysis solutions. Apparently identical lesions have been recorded in cirrhotic patients with ascites treated with LeVeen peritoneovenous shunts,[42] perhaps with a similar pathogenesis.

Polyserositis

Polyserositis (Concato's disease)[43] is a condition characterized by pearly-white thickening of the subserosa of the peritoneum, pericardium and pleurae. In the peritoneum the thickening may occur as discrete plaques, or it may form an almost continuous sheet over the serosal surface of the liver and spleen and of the underpart of the diaphragm. It is accompanied by an ascitic transudate.

The aetiology and pathogenesis of polyserositis are obscure. The condition has sometimes been regarded as tuberculous, but usually there is no evidence to support this view. It is even doubtful if the disease is inflammatory, but no convincing alternative explanation of its pathogenesis has been suggested.

Similar lesions are occasionally found accompanying asbestosis.

INFLAMMATORY CONDITIONS OF THE MESENTERIES AND RETROPERITONEUM

Mesenteric panniculitis and retractile mesenteritis

A rare inflammatory condition of the mesentery affecting individuals of all ages and manifesting a spectrum from acute inflammatory necrosis to exuberant and dense fibrosis has been given a variety of names. *Mesenteric panniculitis* is perhaps the most popular label for the inflammatory variant of the disease;[44] others include *mesenteric lipodystrophy*,[45] *isolated lipodystrophy*, and *mesenteric lipogranuloma*. The fibrotic, end-stage of the disease has been called *retractile mesenteritis*[46] or *multifocal subperitoneal sclerosis.*[47]

The macroscopical appearance in the inflammatory phase is one of oedematous or rubbery thickening of the mesentery or omentum, sometimes forming a discrete mass but on other occasions affecting a localized segment of the mesentery in a more diffuse fashion. The root of the mesentery is often particularly affected and multiple lesions may be found.[45] Later, in the fibrotic phase, there is a more sclerotic thickening of the mesentery with retraction, adhesion formation and distortion of the bowel. The aetiology and pathogenesis of the condition are unknown and progression from the inflammatory to the sclerotic form is not inevitable—in some cases the early lesion appears to resolve almost completely. Males are more commonly affected and there may be some association with obesity. Sometimes there is vascular thrombosis related to the lesion and ischaemic changes in nearby bowel, but whether ischaemia is the primary cause of the disease, or merely a secondary effect, is speculative. Occasional examples are associated with a more widespread panniculitis such as the Pfeifer-Weber-Christian syndrome (relapsing non-suppurative nodular panniculitis),[48] while in a few cases the condition has appeared to merge with idiopathic retroperitoneal fibrosis (see below).[49] The overall prognosis is very good.[44] A possible association with malignant lymphoma has been described in one report,[45] but this is not mentioned in other published series.

The histological appearances in the early stages of the disease are those of fat necrosis with neutrophil polymorphs, clusters of lipophages, foreign-body type giant cells and cholesterol clefts (Fig. 10.10). There is usually a serositis of the overlying peritoneum. Later there is dense mesenteric fibrosis and non-specific focal chronic inflammation.

Mesenteric fibrosis resembling retractile mesenteritis may sometimes be caused by neoplastic infiltration of the mesentery. While any malignancy may potentially produce this effect the mimicry is

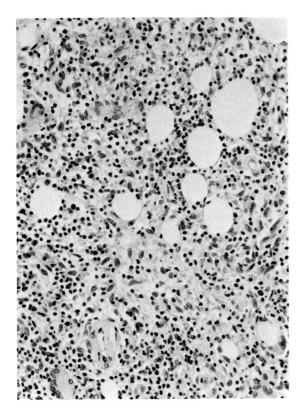

Fig. 10.10 Mesenteric panniculitis. There has been fat necrosis and the few surviving fat cells are separated by a mixed inflammatory infiltrate of lymphocytes, plasma cells, macrophages and occasional neutrophils and eosinophils. Some of the macrophages are multinucleate. There is also early fibrosis.

Haematoxylin-eosin   × 170

Photomicrograph provided by W. StC. Symmers.

greatest in cases of argentaffin carcinoid (endocrine cell) tumour of the ileum which frequently causes dense sclerosis, retraction and kinking when it invades the mesentery, along with a distinctive elastic sclerosis of the mesenteric blood vessels.[50]

Idiopathic retroperitoneal fibrosis

Idiopathic retroperitoneal fibrosis, also known as retroperitoneal sclerosis or sclerosing retroperitonitis, is an uncommon condition that affects middle-aged individuals, men more than women. It is a disease of slowly progressive fibrosis beginning around the lower abdominal aorta and extending laterally towards the ureters, anteriorly towards the root of the mesentery, upwards towards the diaphragm, and occasionally downwards into the pelvis (Fig. 10.11).[51,52] The result is an ill-defined fibrous mass, sometimes diffuse, sometimes nodular, which usually becomes clinically manifest when it reaches the ureters, obstructing them, drawing them medially, and eventually causing renal failure. More localized forms of the disease have also been described, in which the process is limited around one ureter, one renal pelvis, or one kidney.[53]

The histological features are variable and suggest that the disease is essentially an inflammatory condition that progresses to fibrosis. Thus at the periphery or at the advancing margin of the lesion there is a mixed infiltrate of lymphocytes, macrophages, and plasma cells, sometimes with conspicuous eosinophil and neutrophil leukocytes and occasionally with foci of fat necrosis with giant cells (Fig. 10.12). More centrally there is fibroblastic proliferation, which on rare instances may be sufficiently cellular to suggest a sarcoma (Fig. 10.13). The most mature areas show dense collagen deposition and relative hypocellularity.

One of the most characteristic histological features of idiopathic retroperitoneal fibrosis is a sclerosing phlebitis of small and medium-sized veins.[54] It is a useful diagnostic feature whose extent is often not appreciated in biopsy material unless elastic stains are performed (Fig. 10.14). In advanced cases the walls of major veins or the vena cava may be affected with clinical features of venous obstruction. It is important that the diagnostic histopathologist should appreciate that vascular invasion by lymphoid cells does not indicate malignancy in this context, especially when the differential diagnosis may include true malignant lymphoma. Other criteria, especially the cytology of the lymphoid cells and the polymorphous or monomorphous nature of the infiltrate, must be used to make the important distinction.

Idiopathic retroperitoneal fibrosis is sometimes associated with an inflammatory fibrosis of other organs and this also may be accompanied by similar phlebitis. These include idiopathic mediastinal fibrosis, Riedel's thyroiditis, sclerosing cholangitis, and inflammatory pseudotumour of the orbit: the five conditions have collectively been given the name *multifocal fibrosclerosis*.[55] A familial incidence of this syndrome has been reported. More recently fibrosis in the pituitary and testes has also been

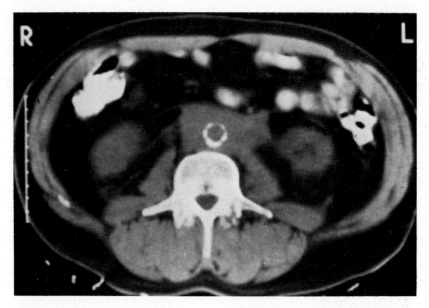

Fig. 10.11 Transverse computerized tomography radiograph, taken at the level of the lower poles of the kidneys, from a patient with obstructive renal failure due to idiopathic retroperitoneal fibrosis. The heavily calcified atherosclerotic abdominal aorta is surrounded by an abnormal cuff of soft tissue density. This extends laterally towards both kidneys, but is especially obvious on the left.

Radiograph provided by Dr Colin Evans, Department of Radiology, Cardiff Royal Infirmary. Photograph by the Department of Medical Illustration, University of Wales College of Medicine, Cardiff.

recognized with the retroperitoneal lesion.[56] An association with scleroderma and lupus erythematosus[52] has given support to the suggestion that idiopathic retroperitoneal fibrosis is an immunological disorder akin to other collagen diseases, with vascular damage as its basis. The frequent clinical improvement with corticosteroids would support this idea. Moreover, some patients may have polyarteritis nodosa-like lesions,[57] especially involving the coronary arteries.[58]

It is interesting that patients with atheromatous aneurysms of the aorta sometimes develop a pronounced adventitial chronic inflammatory reaction with fibrosis which can even extend in the retroperitoneum in a manner identical to idiopathic retroperitoneal fibrosis, with ureteric obstruction.[59] This, together with the occasional finding of either an aortitis or extrusions of atheromatous debris into the inflamed aortic adventitia in cases of idiopathic retroperitoneal fibrosis, has prompted Mitchinson to suggest that an immune reaction to atheromatous material may be the basis for the

disease.[57,58] However, while idiopathic mediastinal fibrosis could possibly be explained by a similar mechanism it is difficult to understand how the other associated lesions—Riedel's thyroiditis, sclerosing cholangitis and orbital inflammatory pseudotumour—could be caused by such a mechanism.

In view of the evidence that vascular changes are important in the aetiology of idiopathic retroperitoneal fibrosis, it is interesting to note that a number of vasoactive drugs have been linked with a similar condition. Thus there are isolated case reports of retroperitoneal fibrosis in patients receiving ergot derivatives, alpha-methyldopa, beta-adrenergic receptor blockers[40] and lysergic acid.[58] While these associations may very well be coincidental there can be no doubt that *methysergide maleate*, another vasoactive drug (an inhibitor of 5-hydroxytryptamine) used clinically for migraine prophylaxis, has produced retroperitoneal fibrosis, and also mediastinal, pulmonary, pleural and endocardial fibrosis, in a small but significant

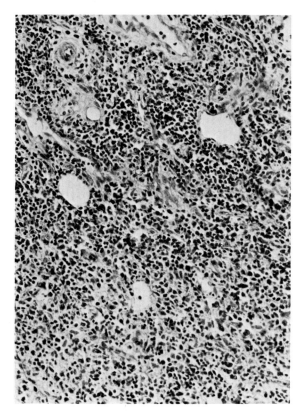

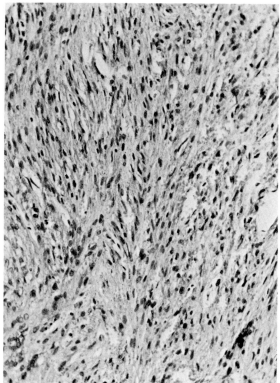

Fig. 10.12 Idiopathic retroperitoneal fibrosis. In the active, cellular phase of the disease there is a dense infiltrate of mature chronic inflammatory cells, along with smaller numbers of neutrophil and eosinophil leucocytes. Few fat cells remain.

Haematoxylin-eosin × 180

Fig. 10.13 Idiopathic retroperitoneal fibrosis. In this field the inflammation has faded away and has been replaced by an unusual degree of fibroblastic proliferation, mimicking a sarcoma. Other areas showed more typical features of idiopathic retroperitoneal fibrosis.

Haematoxylin-eosin × 140

Photomicrograph provided by W. StC. Symmers.

number of cases.[60] It has been estimated that, during a period when over half a million people were treated with this drug, about 100 were reported as having this complication. The risk to users of the drug would thus seem to be slight and perhaps concerns only those who take the drug regularly over long periods. Moreover, the fibrosis would appear to be reversible on methysergide withdrawal.

In addition to the above idiopathic and drug-induced varieties, retroperitoneal fibrosis can occur in a number of other conditions. Post-inflammatory fibrosis following infections rarely produces clinical effects although this may occur in tuberculosis and is well recognized in schistosomiasis due to *Schistosoma haematobium* (see above). Other granulomatous diseases, including *sarcoidosis*[61] and

malakoplakia,[62] and also post-radiotherapy scarring, may produce an identical picture.

Retroperitoneal infections

Infection in the retroperitoneal tissues may result from posterior perforations of the appendix or of the small or large intestine; spread of infections of the pancreas, biliary tree, kidneys or spine; or from secondary infection from a suppurative retroperitoneal lymphadenitis consequent upon infections of the lower limbs. The clinical features are often vague and progression to a retroperitoneal abscess may occur insidiously.[63] The bacteria responsible clearly depend upon the primary cause—mixed infections by enteric bacteria, frequently anaerobes, from intestinal perforations or pancreatitis;

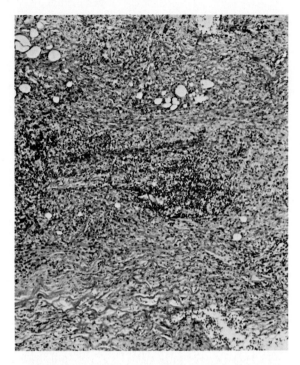 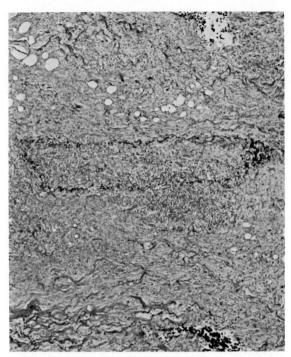

Fig. 10.14a, b (**a**) Idiopathic retroperitoneal fibrosis. In this routinely stained section there is fibrosis and patchy chronic inflammation. No hint of any vascular structure is seen. Compare with (**b**). (**b**) The same field as in (**a**), in a consecutive section stained for elastic fibres. The presence of a vein, obliterated by inflammatory fibrosis, is now obvious.

(**a**) Haematoxylin-eosin   × 80; (**b**) Miller's elastic-van Giesson   × 80

Escherichia coli or *Klebsiella* or *Proteus* species from renal infections; and streptococci from soft tissue infections of the lower limbs, especially in children. Salmonella infection of the wall of an abdominal aortic aneurysm has been reported to progress to a lumbar abscess.[64] Actinomycosis may also occur in the retroperitoneum while tuberculosis, usually secondary to vertebral infection, classically causes a 'cold' abscess which may extend within the psoas sheath to 'point' in the groin. Tuberculosis presenting in this way is now rare in the developed world, however, and nowadays psoas abscess is usually caused by a retroperitoneal intestinal perforation in Crohn's disease, appendicitis, diverticular disease or colonic cancer.[65]

ASCITES

Ascites is the accumulation of fluid within the peritoneal cavity. The character of the fluid varies in different conditions: a *transudate* is a fluid with a protein content of up to 25 g/l and a specific gravity of up to 1.016; an *exudate* has a protein content of more than 25 g/l and its specific gravity is greater than 1.016. An exudate is usually the result of peritoneal inflammation whereas a transudate is formed in consequence of a fall in the plasma colloid osmotic pressure or of portal hypertension, or a combination of both.

The conditions associated with *ascitic transudates* include cardiac failure and those forms of hepatic disease (cirrhosis, Budd-Chiari disease and veno-occlusive disease) that diminish the vascular bed of the liver. In these conditions, an excess of fluid collects in the abdominal cavity in consequence of a rise in the portal capillary pressure to a level that is higher than the osmotic pressure of the plasma proteins. In chronic liver disease two factors thus account for the development of ascites: (1) a diminished synthesis of albumin, and hence a fall in the plasma colloid osmotic pressure, and

(2) intrahepatic vascular obstruction leading to portal hypertension.[66] In cases of generalized oedema due to malnutrition, nephrotic syndrome or other causes of plasma protein deficiency, excess fluid accumulates in the peritoneal cavity because of the low colloid osmotic pressure of the plasma. Often there is also a fall in plasma volume or renal perfusion, in which case ascites may be further aggravated by retention of sodium and water.

The *exudative type of ascites*, typical of acute and other infective forms of peritonitis, is frequently seen when malignant tumours have involved the peritoneum. Wherever the secondary deposits develop in the serosa they excite an inflammatory reaction, and it is probably at these sites that the fluid escapes into the peritoneal cavity. In time some small blood vessels become involved by the tumour, and red blood cells may then escape and pass into the ascitic fluid. Tumour cells may be present in the fluid and can often be found in the deposit obtained by centrifuging it.

Chylous ascites refers to a turbid, milky peritoneal fluid due to the presence of lymph. It results from obstruction of the cisterna chyli or of the main lymphatic ducts, usually by neoplasms but sometimes in the course of infections, notably tuberculosis and filariasis: lymph containing absorbed fat then escapes into the peritoneal cavity, the result of rupture of distended lacteals (Fig. 10.15). Traumatic damage to the main lymphatics may, rarely, be responsible. Recurrent chylous ascites, and chylous pleural effusions, occur in *lymphangioleiomyomatosis*, a rare condition of young women related to tuberose sclerosis, in which proliferation of smooth muscle in the walls of lymphatics causes obstruction and rupture of these vessels. Similar, and often more florid, changes occur in the lung in this condition.[67]

MISCELLANEOUS CONDITIONS

Intraperitoneal loose bodies

Most of the loose bodies that are found in the peritoneal cavity are formed by torsion or infarction and detachment of appendices epiploicae (see p. 389); others originate as small, subserosal fibroids of the uterus that lose their attachment to the latter. Nearly always the loose bodies are symptom-

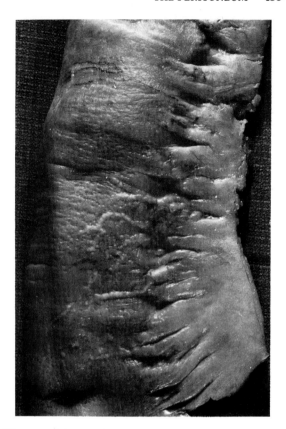

Fig. 10.15 Subserosal lymphatics permeated by tumour are clearly visible on the surface of the small intestine of an elderly man dying of carcinoma of the stomach. Rupture of obstructed peritoneal lymphatics in this case resulted in 3.5 litres of chylous ascites.

× 1

less, which perhaps accounts for their description as 'peritoneal mice'. Microscopically, they consist of a thick capsule of hyalinized fibrous tissue and a central core that may clearly show the pattern of adipose or myomatous tissue, although no cells survive, except in 'ghost' form.

Thin-walled translucent cysts containing clear fluid and measuring up to 6 cm in diameter are occasionally found lying loose within the peritoneal cavity, nearly always in women.[68] They are lined by mesothelium, sometimes of more than one cell thick.

Segmental infarction of the greater omentum

This is an uncommon condition in which a segment of the greater omentum, nearly always wedge-shaped and involving the inferior border on the right side, undergoes infarction for no apparent reason.[69] A local peritonitis develops and the infarcted tissue usually becomes adherent to the caecum, ascending colon and the anterior parietal peritoneum, with development of a serosanguinous exudate. Patients of all ages may be affected. In some cases there is a history of recent trauma while in others torsion or strangulation of the omentum in a hernial sac may be responsible for the infarction.

Retroperitoneal haemorrhage

Massive retroperitoneal haemorrhage is usually due to rupture of an aortic aneurysm or to trauma. So-called 'spontaneous' haemorrhage also occurs[70] and among the commoner causes for this are anticoagulant therapy, abnormalities of the renal vasculature, tumours (benign and malignant) of the kidneys, adrenal glands or of the retroperitoneum, and adrenal haemorrhage in relation to severe stress or systemic illness.

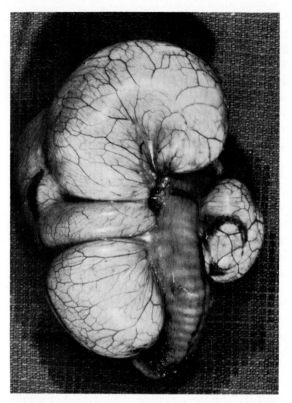

Fig. 10.16 A multicystic lymphangioma of the proximal ileal mesentery resected from a 3-week-old infant. A milky chylous fluid filled the cystic spaces. The lesion was an incidental finding during laparotomy for volvulus of the more distal ileum consequent upon congenital malrotation of the bowel.
× 1.5

TUMOURS

PRIMARY TUMOURS AND TUMOUR-LIKE CONDITIONS

Omental, mesenteric and retroperitoneal cysts

Most cysts of the omentum and mesenteries are chylous cysts which are considered to be developmental abnormalities derived from lymphatic tissue.[71] They are usually incidental findings at laparotomy or autopsy although clinical effects may be produced, especially in children. Chylous cysts are unilocular and have a smooth lining of flattened or cuboidal endothelial cells, and contain milky chylous fluid. Larger examples may be multilocular and contain smooth muscle bundles, in which case they are sometimes called cystic lymphangiomas or hygromas (Fig. 10.16). Foci of mature lymphoid tissue may be recognizable in the wall. They may rarely be found in the retroperitoneum.

Cystic mesotheliomas (see below) may have a similar appearance but they usually contain clear fluid and the mesothelial nature of the constituent cells is usually demonstrable by mucin histochemistry or electron microscopy. Their recognition is important because of their tendency to recur.[72] Other cysts of the omentum, mesentery and retroperitoneum include developmental cysts of enteric or urogenital origin, infestations (such as hydatid disease), inflammatory 'pseudocysts' (especially following pancreatitis), cystic change in metaplastic lesions of the serosa or subserosa (especially of Müllerian type—see below), or true cystic neoplasms.[71]

Infantile hamartoma

Multifocal nodular lesions consisting of plump mesenchymal cells in a vascular myxoid stroma may occur in the omentum or mesentery of infants.[73] The mesenchymal cells may be spindly or stellate, binucleate or even multinucleate, and the cytoplasm may be vacuolated. The mitotic rate is low. There may be a striking resemblance to a sarcoma, especially myxoid liposarcoma, but the clinical behaviour in the few reported cases has so far been benign and the lesion has been regarded as an infantile myxoid hamartoma.

Mesenteric and retroperitoneal fibromatosis

Firm, irregular and ill-defined masses measuring up to 15 cm in diameter and having the histological appearances of fibromatosis may occur in the small intestinal mesentery and retroperitoneum of patients with familial adenomatous polyposis coli, and especially in Gardner's syndrome (see p. 361).[74] They usually follow abdominal surgery and are aggravated by it, a feature they hold in common with fibromatoses in other parts of the body. Nevertheless, cases of spontaneous mesenteric fibromatosis, unrelated to surgery, have been described.[75] Although essentially a benign, non-metastasizing lesion, mesenteric fibromatosis may behave as an aggressive, locally-recurring proliferation causing intestinal obstruction or fistula formation. In the original Gardner kindred, two, and probably three, of five cases with mesenteric fibromatosis of greater than six years' duration died of complications directly attributable to it. However, a more indolent behaviour is recorded in other families.[74] Wide local excision would appear to be the treatment of choice. Isolated cases of mesenteric fibromatosis, apparently unrelated to colorectal polyposis, occur very rarely.

Inflammatory pseudotumour

Inflammatory pseudotumours may occur in the mesentery or retroperitoneum.[76] They are usually solitary, firm, well-circumscribed masses that are white or tan-coloured and measure up to many centimetres in diameter. Histologically, they consist of varying proportions of vascular fibrous tissue, fibroblasts, histiocytes, mature lymphocytes, plasma cells and sometimes eosinophils. Mitoses are sparse. A frequent abundance of plasma cells is responsible for the term *plasma cell granu-*

loma by which the lesions are also known. Apparently identical lesions are better recognized in the lungs, and also in other sites. The aetiology is unknown: some cases seem to be related to trauma or surgery while others may be related to mesenteric panniculitis (see above). In some patients abdominal pseudotumour has been associated with fever, weight loss and a hypochromic, microcytic anaemia and these features have usually resolved after removal of the mass.[77] Whilst the behaviour of these pseudotumours is usually benign, a small proportion may recur, with a return of the systemic symptoms, and may even prove lethal eventually.[77]

Splenosis

Rupture of the spleen may be followed by auto-transplantation of fragments of splenic tissue on to the serosa of the peritoneal cavity, so-called *splenosis.*[78] Adhesions may be associated with this.

Tumours and tumour-like lesions of female genital type

It is now widely believed that in females the connective tissue immediately deep to the peritoneal surface, the so-called subcoelomic mesenchyme,[79] is potentially responsive to hormonal influences and, either alone or in combination with proliferations of the overlying serosa, may give rise to tissues of Müllerian type in a manner similar to that which occurs during normal fetal development in the formation of the upper female genital tract. Decidual, endometrial, endosalpingeal and even endocervical differentiation may thus occur. Furthermore, neoplasia may arise within these tissues. It is felt that the pelvic peritoneum is especially prone to these changes, but similar effects may occur anywhere in the abdomen.

Deciduosis, endometriosis and endosalpingiosis

The appearance of a typical decidual stroma beneath the peritoneal mesothelium, so-called *deciduosis*, is usually, but not invariably, related to pregnancy (Fig. 10.17).[80] It is most commonly found on the serosal surface of appendicectomy specimens. It is highly unlikely that deciduosis

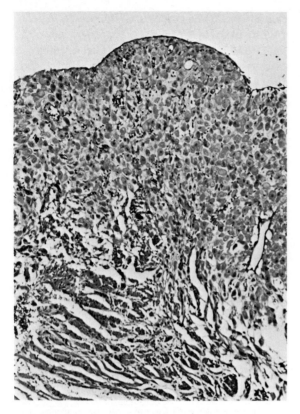

Fig. 10.17 Deciduosis of the mesoappendix in an appendicectomy specimen from a young woman who was 22 weeks pregnant. Typical decidual tissue occupies a zone immediately beneath the mesothelium.

Haematoxylin-eosin   × 80

causes clinical symptoms or is involved in the pathogenesis of appendicitis in such cases.

On the other hand, *endometriosis*, the appearance of endometrial tissue in the pelvic serosa, may produce symptoms. Haemorrhage may occur in relation to cyclical hormonal changes and this may be followed by a local peritonitis and the formation of adhesions. The lesions usually consist of both endometrial glands and stroma, and rarely endometriotic cysts may be found in the mesentery or retroperitoneum.

From time to time a uterine tubal type of epithelium is found lining some of the glandular components of endometriosis, so-called tubal metaplasia. However, on other occasions the peritoneum, mesentery or retroperitoneum are found to contain glandular inclusions of uterine tubal type without any associated stroma, a condition distinct

from endometriosis and called *endosalpingiosis*.[81] Endosalpingiotic inclusions usually have a round outline and the lining consists of a single layer of ciliated, secretory and peg cells with regular basal nuclei. Occasionally they may be pseudostratified and in some instances there may be more complex papillary structures with calcification in the form of psammoma bodies. Although a Müllerian metaplastic origin from coelomic mesothelium is usually given for this condition, a strong association with inflammation or trauma to the uterine tubes has suggested to some that it might arise by autotransplantation following inflammatory sloughing of the tubal epithelium.[81] Endosalpingiosis is probably asymptomatic but it is important to the surgical pathologist because it can mimic metastatic carcinoma. Indeed it may even co-exist with carcinoma of the ovary. A lack of nuclear pleomorphism and the absence of a desmoplastic reaction around the inclusions are the most useful distinguishing features.

Leiomyomatosis peritonealis disseminata

In this rare condition nodules of proliferating smooth muscle are scattered over the surface of the peritoneal cavity in a manner that resembles disseminated cancerous deposits macroscopically.[82] It occurs in women of childbearing age, nearly always in association with pregnancy or the use of an oral contraceptive. Histologically, the nodules are subserosal whorls of smooth muscle cells, nearly always bland in appearance with few mitotic figures, sometimes admixed with decidual cells. The nodules are considered to represent hormonally-induced proliferations of metaplastic Müllerian subserosal mesenchyme: smooth muscle cells and myofibroblasts are normally derived from this tissue in embryogenesis.[83] There are case reports of endometriosis occurring in leiomyomatosis peritonealis disseminata.[84]

Malignant tumours of female genital type

Primary extragenital malignant tumours of the peritoneum, mesentery or retroperitoneum, of a type commonly found in the female genital tract, occur rarely in women. Some arise in endometriosis, including endometrial adenocarcinomas, stromal sarcomas and malignant 'mixed' Müllerian tumours.[79,85] Others apparently arise *de novo*, or possibly in relation to endosalpingiosis, and are identical to primary tumours of the ovary arising from the ovarian surface. Papillary serous carcinomas, often containing conspicuous psammoma bodies, are commonest,[86,87] but mucinous adenocarcinomas are also described.[88]

Perhaps it is not altogether surprising that similar tumours should arise from the ovarian surface and the peritoneal mesothelium, since they have a common embryological origin. Moreover, non-invasive papillary carcinoma of the peritoneum may co-exist with 'borderline' serous papillary tumours of the ovary, raising the possibility of multifocal neoplasia in coelomic lining cells.[89] In this respect it is very interesting that disseminated intra-abdominal carcinoma, indistinguishable from ovarian carcinoma, has developed in female members of families with a high incidence of ovarian carcinoma despite prophylactic oophorectomy.[90] Nevertheless, not all papillary malignant tumours of the peritoneal serosa in women are ovarian type carcinomas: some are true mesothelial tumours (see below) while in others it is impossible to make the distinction with any certainty.[87]

Mesothelial hyperplasia

Benign, reactive hyperplasia of mesothelial cells is usually a localized phenomenon associated with chronic irritation of the peritoneum.[91] It may therefore be found in relation to an intra-abdominal abscess or tumour but it may also occur in ascites, in viral infections, in collagen diseases, or even in acute peritonitis associated with appendicitis or intestinal perforation. Nodular mesothelial hyperplasia has been described in hernia sacs, especially in children.[91] Hyperplastic mesothelium may have a papillary, tubular or solid configuration (Figs 10.18 and 10.19), the mesothelial cells being acidophilic with a variable degree of nuclear pleomorphism and occasional mitotic figures.[87,91] Psammoma bodies may be found in papillary areas and rarely multinucleated giant cells and eosinophilic 'strap' cells reminiscent of rhabdomyosarcoma may occur.[91]

The histological appearances of mesothelial hyperplasia may mimic metastatic carcinoma or

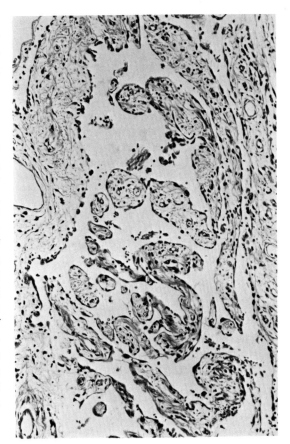

Fig. 10.18 Mesothelial hyperplasia showing a papillary pattern. Oedematous vascular stromal cores are covered by flattened or cuboidal mesothelial cells showing mild nuclear pleomorphism. The patient suffered from rheumatoid arthritis and was receiving corticosteroids. The mesothelial hyperplasia accompanied an acute peritonitis due to perforation of a duodenal ulcer which had probably occurred a few days before this biopsy was taken, the symptoms of peritonitis having been suppressed by the steroid therapy. Note the similarity with localized papillary mesothelioma (Fig. 10.20).

Haematoxylin-eosin   × 130

mesothelioma closely and sometimes it can be impossible to exclude either of these confidently (Fig. 10.19). The finding of neutral mucin production and the immunocytochemical demonstration of carcinoembryonic antigen in the cells is good evidence against a mesothelial origin, but negative results do not exclude carcinoma. Mesothelial cells classically produce hyaluronidase-sensitive acid mucopolysaccharides but experience shows that this is not completely reliable for their distinction from carcinoma cells. Moreover, many examples of mesothelial hyperplasia show no mucin production of any sort.[91]

The differentiation between mesothelial hyperplasia and mesothelioma can also be difficult (see below): the presence of inflammation and the absence of nuclear features of malignancy would tend to support a reactive lesion. However, there are reported cases of apparent mesothelial hyperplasia progressing to malignant mesothelioma, suggesting that a spectrum of appearances may exist.[92]

Mesothelioma

Mesotheliomas are uncommon neoplasms of the peritoneal serosa with a very wide spectrum of histological appearances. Most occur in the second half of life, although examples in childhood are described.[93] Like pleural mesotheliomas, many are related to asbestos exposure, almost invariably the amphiboles, and occur more commonly in men than women.[87,94,95] Sometimes mesotheliomas arise in a background of reactive mesothelial hyperplasia[92] and the boundary between these two conditions may become very blurred (see above).

Peritoneal mesotheliomas can be divided into a number of morphological types and grossly they may be localized or diffuse. Generally speaking the localized mesotheliomas are unrelated to asbestos exposure and have a benign, indolent behaviour while the diffuse, asbestos-linked tumours are aggressive, lethal malignancies.

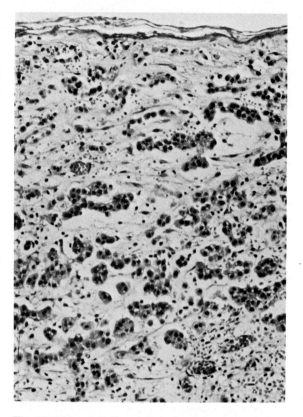

Fig. 10.19 Mesothelial hyperplasia showing a partly tubular, partly solid pattern. Collections of regular, acidophilic mesothelial cells forming solid nests or tubular structures are embedded in a fibrinous exudate. This appearance can mimic metastatic carcinoma closely. This particular example was related to an appendix abscess in a 55-year-old man. The patient is alive and well four years after the operation.

Haematoxylin-eosin   × 130

Papillary mesothelioma

Papillary mesotheliomas are usually solitary, localized, pedunculated lesions of the peritoneal surface that do not appear to be related to asbestos exposure. Although occasional examples have produced symptoms by torsion most are incidental findings at laparotomy or autopsy.[96] Histologically, they are made up of a delicate stroma covered by a single layer of regular cuboidal mesothelial cells with acidophilic cytoplasm and vesicular nuclei containing inconspicuous nucleoli (Fig. 10.20). The cells may have a brush border and a vacuolated cytoplasm and lie on a conspicuous basement membrane. Papillary mesotheliomas may be indistinguishable from papillary mesothelial hyperpla-

sia (see above and Fig. 10.18) and indeed they may be the same lesion. They always behave in a benign fashion.

Very rarely multiple papillary mesotheliomas are scattered over the peritoneal surface, sometimes in association with ascites. These cases also have a good prognosis.[87]

Fibrous mesothelioma

Fibrous mesotheliomas are localized, solitary, pedunculated or sessile tumours arising from serosal surfaces, usually the pleura, but occasionally from the peritoneum.[97] No relationship with asbestos exposure is known. They consist of bland, spindle-shaped fibroblasts and collagenous tissue

Cystic mesothelioma

Cystic mesotheliomas are rare, localized, solitary tumours of the peritoneum occurring mainly in women under the age of 50 years.[100] There is no association with asbestos exposure. The tumours are usually asymptomatic and grossly appear as gelatinous, multicystic masses measuring up to 20 cm in diameter. The cysts usually contain clear fluid and are lined by a single layer of flattened or cuboidal mesothelial cells with small uniform nuclei, sometimes with focal intracystic papillary proliferations. The lesions may mimic cystic lymphangiomas but can be distinguished from them by the production of hyaluronic acid-containing mucopolysaccharides and by their ultrastructural appearances.[72]

Cystic mesotheliomas, unlike most other localized mesotheliomas, are not completely benign lesions and in about 20% of reported cases there have been local recurrences within the peritoneal cavity.[100]

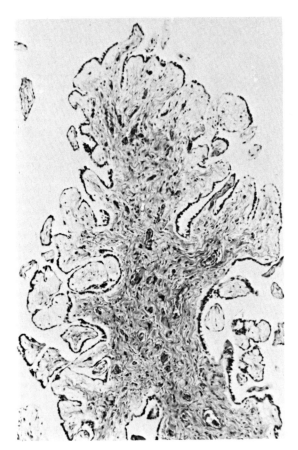

Fig. 10.20 A small, solitary, localized papillary mesothelioma on the serosal surface of the ileum which was an incidental finding during a staging laparotomy for Hodgkin's disease. Note the striking similarity with papillary mesothelial hyperplasia (Fig. 10.18).
Haematoxylin-eosin × 80

in varying proportions, sometimes covered by a layer of typical mesothelial cells (Fig. 10.21). There is debate over the origin of these benign lesions: a true mesothelial derivation is proposed by some, while others regard them as proliferations of subserosal mesenchyme.

Adenomatoid mesothelioma

Adenomatoid tumours, best recognized as tumours of the surface of the epididymis, uterus or uterine tubes, are now considered to be lesions of mesothelial origin.[98] Rare examples have been described in the mesentery of the small intestine, and may be regarded as adenomatoid mesotheliomas.[99] They are benign.

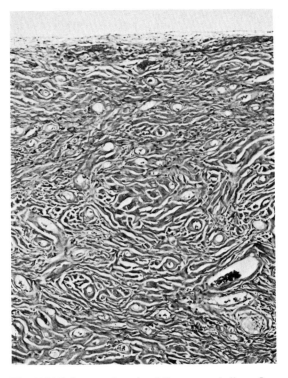

Fig. 10.21 Solitary, pedunculated fibrous mesothelioma. In this example the cellular component of regular, spindle-shaped fibroblasts is inconspicuous and the stroma is densely sclerotic.
Haematoxylin-eosin × 70

Diffuse malignant mesothelioma

Although diffuse malignant mesothelioma is probably the commonest of all peritoneal mesothelial tumours, it is nevertheless a very unusual disease in clinical practice. Men are affected far more commonly than women, and most are over 50 years old. A history of asbestos exposure is common, and some patients have pulmonary changes of asbestosis. The clinical presentation is usually insidious, consisting of abdominal discomfort, pain, weight loss, and ascites. The prognosis following diagnosis is poor, with only about half the patients surviving six months.

Macroscopically, diffuse malignant mesothelioma affects most or all of the peritoneum, both visceral and parietal, producing nodules, sheets and plaques of tumour, thickening of the omentum and mesenteries, and encasement of the liver and spleen. The appearance may be identical to diffuse carcinomatosis of the peritoneal cavity, a far commoner condition (Fig. 10.22). In the earlier stages of the disease there is an exudative ascites but as the tumour progresses adhesions form, leading eventually to obliteration of the peritoneal cavity. Invasion of the underlying viscera, notably the intestine, occurs in about one third of cases while metastatic spread to lymph nodes, the liver, the lungs and pleurae is found at autopsy in about one half.[94]

The histological appearances of malignant mesothelioma are variable. A number of patterns are recognized, however, including the epithelial type, the sarcomatoid type, and the mixed type (Fig. 10.23). Most peritoneal mesotheliomas are of epithelial type, about a quarter are of mixed type, while pure sarcomatoid mesotheliomas are very uncommon.[94]

Epithelial patterns of malignant mesothelioma can be further divided into papillary, tubular and solid forms, (Fig 10.23a, b and c) and mixtures of these within the same tumour are also common. The neoplastic mesothelial cells in these lesions are usually cuboidal but in neoplastic papillae they may be dome-shaped. They have an abundant glycogen-containing eosinophilic cytoplasm which is frequently vacuolated, sometimes to produce signet-ring-like cells and sometimes to give the tumour a lacy pattern. Hyaluronic acid in acidic

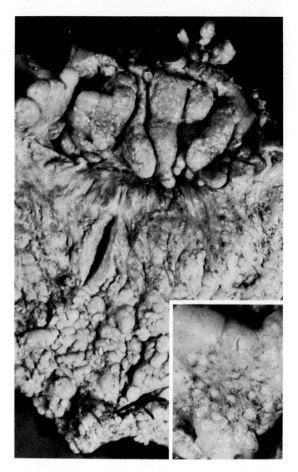

Fig. 10.22 Diffuse thickening of the greater omentum by secondary carcinoma of the ovary, so-called carcinomatosis peritonei. The tumour deposits vary in size from tiny excrescences (inset) to large nodules and plaques. An identical appearance may be produced by diffuse malignant mesothelioma.

×0.4; inset ×1.2

mucopolysaccharides is frequently demonstrable in such vacuoles by the abolition of a positive alcian blue or colloidal iron reaction by pretreatment with the enzyme hyaluronidase. The nuclei of 'epithelial' mesothelioma cells are often vesicular and pleomorphic, with conspicuous nucleoli; mitotic figures may be surprisingly few.

'Epithelial' malignant mesotheliomas produce diagnostic problems for the pathologist because they can mimic metastatic carcinoma (Fig. 10.23): sometimes a distinction cannot be made. Papillary lesions can be confused with metastatic ovarian cancer, tubular mesotheliomas having intracellular vacuoles can mimic metastatic tumours from the gastrointestinal tract, and the solid type of mesothelioma with its sheet-like pattern of poorly-differentiated mesothelial cells can resemble an undifferentiated carcinoma from any source. Mucin histochemistry can be useful—the demonstration of significant amounts of neutral mucin supports a diagnosis of carcinoma while the presence of hyaluronic acid suggests mesothelioma. Immunocytochemistry is only of limited value—demonstration of carcinoembryonic antigen probably negates a diagnosis of mesothelioma but most other epithelial markers so far tested are less useful.[101] Electron microscopy may help to make a diagnosis in difficult cases.[101] Papillary malignant mesotheliomas sometimes have psammoma bodies, but rarely in large numbers. In female patients, therefore, a papillary tumour containing numerous psammoma bodies is more likely to be a metastatic ovarian cancer than a mesothelioma. Malignant mesotheliomas can also resemble some forms of benign mesothelial hyperplasia (see above), especially the papillary lesions. The nuclear morphology of the mesothelial cells is the best discriminant in such difficult cases.

The *sarcomatoid* pattern of malignant mesothelioma (Fig. 10.23d) is rare in the peritoneum and takes the form of spindle or fusiform cells with elongated or oval nuclei, often in a parallel orientation. There may also be anaplastic cells with giant bizarre nuclei and pleomorphic giant cells.[94] Confusion with true sarcomas can occur, but the gross anatomical distribution of the tumour tissue usually allows the correct diagnosis to be made.

Malignant mesotheliomas of *mixed epithelial and sarcomatoid type* are generally diagnosed easily because the combination of patterns is typical of this tumour (Fig. 10.23e). Sometimes a transition between the two patterns can be seen while on other occasions different zones of the same tumour have strikingly different appearances.

Soft tissue tumours

Soft tissue tumours of the mesentery and retroperitoneum are relatively uncommon. While many types can occur, only a few are found with sufficient frequency to merit consideration here.

Smooth muscle tumours

Benign and malignant smooth muscle tumours may arise primarily in the mesentery or retroperitoneum while others may spread from the gastrointestinal or female genital tracts. Malignant tumours, leiomyosarcomas, form a very high proportion of smooth muscle tumours in the retroperitoneum[102] while similar tumours in the mesentery are very rare.[103]

Smooth muscle tumours are usually solitary, large, nodular, pale or tan-coloured masses. They may reach huge proportions, sometimes weighing several kilograms. They often show areas of cystic degeneration. Histologically, most have a typical spindle-celled pattern but areas of 'epithelioid' pattern, classically described in gastric smooth muscle tumours (see p. 214), or areas with a prominent vascular pattern may occur.[102] The histological assessment of malignancy in smooth muscle tumours in any site is difficult, and this is particularly true for retroperitoneal tumours. While a high mitotic rate (more than five per 10 high-power fields) is the best indicator, tumours of the retroperitoneum containing as few as one mitosis per 10 high-power fields have resulted in death of the patient. Multiple samples should be examined because of focal variations in the mitotic rate and it would seem prudent to consider any large (more than 7.5 cm) retroperitoneal smooth muscle tumour showing mitotic activity with suspicion. The overall prognosis of leiomyosarcomas at this site is not good, with only 50% surviving two years.[102]

Fibrohistiocytic tumours

Fibrohistiocytic tumours of the retroperitoneum present as large grey or yellow masses, usually in late adult life. Virtually all are malignant, and some may behave in a highly aggressive fashion.

Retroperitoneal xanthogranuloma, a tumour consisting predominantly of xanthoma and inflammatory cells, was once considered a benign lesion but it is now recognized as an inflammatory variant of *malignant fibrous histiocytoma*.[104,105] While many of the xanthomatous histiocytes in this lesion have a bland appearance, careful scrutiny will usually reveal nuclear atypia and mitotic figures in some,

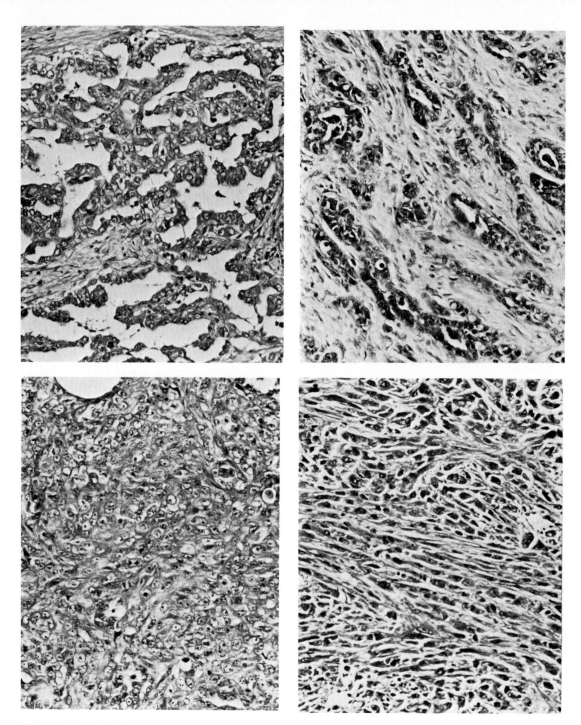

Fig. 10.23a–d (a) Malignant mesothelioma of papillary 'epithelial' pattern. The neoplastic papillae consist of acidophilic cells with large, mildly pleomorphic vesicular nuclei. There is a close resemblance to papillary carcinoma. **(b)** malignant mesothelioma of tubular 'epithelial' pattern. Irregular tubules are formed by neoplastic mesothelial cells, some of which contain cytoplasmic vacuoles. There is a close resemblance to tubular adenocarcinoma. Same case as **(a)**.**(c)** Malignant mesothelioma of solid 'epithelial' pattern. Closely-packed polygonal neoplastic mesothelial cells form solid sheets, mimicking undifferentiated carcinoma. They have large, vesicular pleomorphic nuclei with very conspicuous nucleoli. **(d)** Malignant mesothelioma of 'sarcomatoid' pattern. The tumour is made up of fascicles of parallel spindle-shaped malignant mesothelial cells, clearly imitating a soft tissue sarcoma.

Haematoxylin-eosin   × 180

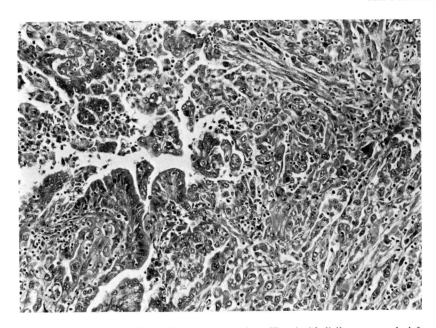

10.23e Malignant mesothelioma of mixed pattern. A papillary 'epithelial' pattern on the left merges with a 'sarcomatoid' pattern on the right, the latter containing occasional deeply eosinophilic giant cells. This combination is reminiscent of synovial sarcoma, but in the context of an abdominal mass is virtually diagnostic of malignant mesothelioma.

Haematoxylin-eosin   × 180

Histological preparations provided by: (**a, b**) *Dr A. R. Gibbs, University of Wales College of Medicine, Cardiff;* (**d**) *Dr J. C. Wagner, Llandough Hospital, Penarth.*

signalling their true malignant nature. While it seems that this 'inflammatory' variant of malignant fibrous histiocytoma has a better prognosis than other types which occur more commonly in other sites, it nevertheless recurs frequently and may eventually cause death.[104]

Other malignant fibrous histiocytomas of the retroperitoneum have a more typical storiform, pleomorphic or myxoid histological pattern and often behave aggressively.[105]

Lipomas and liposarcomas

While benign lipomas of the mesentery and retroperitoneum do occur, they are uncommon. Care must be taken to distinguish them from well-differentiated liposarcomas which occur more frequently in the retroperitoneum and which may be multicentric.[106] These tumours are large, fatty, partly gelatinous masses measuring 20 cm or more in diameter. Histologically, they contain mature adipose tissue, fibrous tissue and sometimes myxoid areas. Sclerosis may be conspicuous.[106,107] While many of the constituent cells are bland, a variable proportion have atypical hyperchromatic nuclei or mitoses and occasional lipoblasts are present. Well-differentiated liposarcomas of this type virtually never metastasize, but troublesome local recurrence is common.

Large liposarcomas of the more usual myxoid, round cell and pleomorphic types also occur in the retroperitoneum. They are often aggressive, having a very high rate of local recurrence. Metastasis is not infrequent and a 5-year survival rate of 39% has been quoted.[107]

Haemangiopericytoma

The retroperitoneum is recognized as one of the major anatomical locations for haemangiopericytoma. The tumour has usually reached a large size before the diagnosis is made, and hypoglycaemia due to the production of an insulin-like substance may be the presenting feature (Fig. 10.24). The characteristic histological pattern is one of tightly-packed cells with oval nuclei surrounding thin-walled endothelium-lined vascular channels, but looser degenerative areas are common. Most haemangiopericytomas behave in a benign fashion, but local recurrence or metastasis may occur, especially in tumours with a high mitotic rate and areas of necrosis.[108]

Other primary tumours

Primary germ cell tumours of the retroperitoneum are uncommon but well recognized. The commonest is the *mature cystic teratoma*, usually a tumour

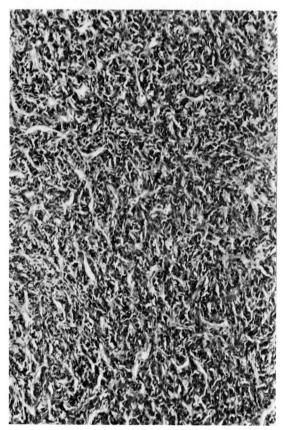

Fig. 10.24 A typical haemangiopericytoma of the retroperitoneum that presented with hypoglycaemic attacks. A fine network of capillary channels is separated by regular neoplastic spindle-shaped cells.

Haematoxylin-eosin × 160

of young children with a benign behaviour that frequently involves the sacrococcygeal tissues.[109] Rupture of the cyst may produce an intense foreign-body granulomatous reaction with fibrosis. Rare examples of omental teratoma are also described.[110] *Malignant teratomas* of any histological pattern may also arise primarily in the retroperitoneum, but care must be taken to exclude a metastasis from an occult primary tumour of the testis or ovary before making the diagnosis.[111] Similarly, primary retroperitoneal *seminomas* may be diagnosed after careful exclusion of a testicular primary tumour.[111] A retroperitoneal *endocrine cell tumour* has also been described.[112] Whether or not this represented single tissue differentiation in a teratoma was unclear to the authors.

Paragangliomas of the retroperitoneum with cytoplasmic argyrophilia may arise outside the adrenal gland, either from the sympathetic chain or from the organ of Zuckerkandl.[113] Local recurrence and metastasis is commoner in these tumours than in paragangliomas occurring at other sites. An association between multiple extra-adrenal paragangliomas, gastric smooth muscle tumours and pulmonary chondromas has been described.[114]

Malignant lymphomas occurring in the retroperitoneum represent extension from locally involved lymph nodes. All varieties of Hodgkin's and non-Hodgkin's lymphoma may occur. The differentiation from the cellular phase of idiopathic retroperitoneal fibrosis (see above) can be difficult, particularly in malignant lymphomas of follicle centre cell origin which are themselves frequently sclerotic when they infiltrate the retroperitoneum.[115] Attention to the cytological detail of the cellular components is essential to making the distinction.

Sinus histiocytosis with massive lymphadenopathy[116] and *giant lymph node hyperplasia* (Castleman's disease)[117] have been recorded as causes of retroperitoneal and mesenteric masses respectively.

SECONDARY TUMOURS

The peritoneum may be involved by carcinoma or sarcoma in three ways: by direct extension, for example of a tumour of the stomach or large intestine; by transcoelomic dissemination; and by permeation of subperitoneal lymphatics. Malignant tumours arising in the gastrointestinal tract need to spread only a short distance before they involve the visceral peritoneum. This malignant invasion of the peritoneal covering is preceded by the local deposition of fibrinous exudate on the serosal surface, and this may lead to the organ becoming adherent to some other intra-abdominal structure, such as the greater omentum or loops of small intestine. This opens the way for neoplastic infiltration of the adherent structures and the formation of gastrocolic, vesicocolic or other intra-abdominal fistulae.

Such a sequence is characteristic only of the more slowly growing tumours. Those that grow rapidly, such as most gastric and ovarian carcinomas, usually give rise to extensive transcoelomic dissemination once they penetrate through the serosa, and this results in the development of ascites. Carcinomatous deposits become implanted throughout the abdominal cavity and appear first as minute firm, white nodules in the serosa. Later, these nodules coalesce to form plaques of growth (Fig. 10.22). Invasion of the viscera underlying secondary deposits is unusual; in contrast there may be extensive invasion of tissue spaces and lymphatics in the greater omentum. Sometimes the peritoneal lymphatics are permeated by tumour and appear as a network of fine white lines (see Fig. 10.15).

Secondary tumours in the retroperitoneum may arise either by direct local spread or by extension from lymph node deposits. Primary tumours of the pancreas, kidneys, adrenal glands or the spine may involve the retroperitoneum by direct spread while carcinomas of the testis, prostate, cervix, endometrium or breast may reach there via the lymph nodes.

Pseudomyxoma peritonei

Pseudomyxoma peritonei is defined as the presence of masses of mucinous material within the peritoneal cavity, caused by the rupture of a mucus-containing viscus. It is a description of an appearance, and not a diagnosis. The natural history of the condition is governed by the nature of the underlying disease. If it is a benign lesion, such as a mucinous cystadenoma of the appendix, gall-

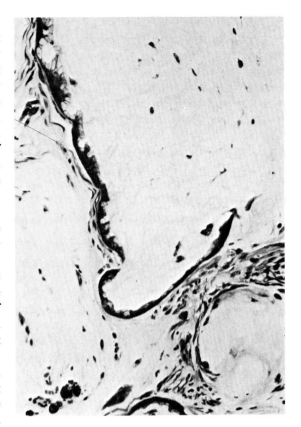

Fig. 10.25 Pseudomyxoma peritonei due to a ruptured cystadenocarcinoma of the appendix. Islands of neoplastic mucus-secreting epithelial cells are seen floating in lakes of extracellular mucus in this peritoneal biopsy.

Haematoxylin-eosin   × 180

bladder or ovary then a localized pseudomyxoma peritonei, confined to the relevant part of the peritoneal cavity, is formed; this resolves after surgical excision of the primary condition, albeit sometimes with adhesion formation. If, on the other hand, the cause is a ruptured mucus-producing malignant tumour, such as a cystadeno-carcinoma of the ovary or appendix, a progressive pseudomyxoma peritonei affecting the whole peritoneal lining will develop, often with a fatal outcome from intestinal obstruction.[118,119] This is due to seeding of mucinous adenocarcinoma over the peritoneum, which often extends into the underlying mesentery or omentum to form a thickened, gelatinous mass. Histological examination in such cases will demonstrate pools of mucus within which islands of neoplastic epithelial cells may be floating (Fig. 10.25). These may have the cytological features of malignancy, but sometimes they are deceptively bland. The demonstration of such cells in mucus from cases of pseudomyxoma peritonei is of dubious prognostic value because exfoliated cells from a recently ruptured appendiceal cystadenoma may show the atypical features of dysplasia and yet the pseudomyxoma will almost certainly resolve. Histological examination of the underlying lesion to establish the presence or absence of invasive malignancy is far more reliable for determining prognosis.

Gliomatosis peritonei

Gliomatosis peritonei is the name given to miliary implantation on the peritoneal surface of mature glial tissue. It is a rare complication of solid ovarian teratomas that contain glial elements and, provided it is not accompanied by implants of other less mature teratomatous elements, it almost invariably behaves in a benign manner.[120] On rare occasions other mature tissues, such as cartilage or bone, may also be present but this does not affect the

excellent prognosis. It is clearly essential to scrutinize biopsy material from gliomatosis peritonei very carefully for other immature elements because their presence will influence the prognosis and management significantly.[120]

'Parasitic fibroids'

The rare implantation of a benign uterine leiomyoma (fibroid) on to the surface of the peritoneum has been termed a 'parasitic fibroid'. It is generally considered that it arises as a result of ischaemia of a pedunculated subserosal fibroid, probably by torsion. This leads to an inflammatory reaction in the overlying serosa, causing the tumour to become adherent to the peritoneum elsewhere—for example, to one of the broad ligaments, the colon or the greater omentum. A fresh blood supply may then be derived from this new attachment, and the so-formed 'parasitic' fibroid may then lose its connection with the uterus. If no attachment is formed the fibroid will continue to degenerate and will form a peritoneal loose body.

REFERENCES

1. Mitchell GAG. Br J Surg 1940–41; 28: 291.
2. Yoffey JM, Courtice FC. Lymphatics, lymph and the lymphadenoid complex. London: Academic Press, 1970: 295.
3. Bangham AD, Magee PN, Osborn SB. Br J Exp Path 1953; 34: 1.
4. Ellis H, Adair HM. Postgrad Med J 1974; 50: 713.
5. Harken AH, Shochat SJ. Am J Surg 1973; 125: 769.
6. Crossley IR, Williams R. Gut 1985; 26: 325.
7. Parker MT. In: Wilson GS, Miles AA, Parker MT, eds. Topley & Wilson's principles of bacteriology, virology and immunity, vol 3. 7th ed. London: Arnold, 1984: 183.
8. Barnard HL. Br Med J 1908; 1: 429.
9. Whitaker D, Papadimitriou JM, Walters MN-I. J Pathol 1982; 136: 291.
10. Williams DC. Br J Surg 1954–55; 42: 401.
11. Buckman RF, Woods M, Sargent L, Gervin AS. J Surg Res 1976; 20: 1.
12. Ryan GB, Grobety J, Majno G. Am J Pathol 1971; 65: 117.
13. Boys F. Surg 1942; 11: 118.
14. Bhansali SK. Am J Gastro 1977; 67: 324.
15. Singh MM, Bhargava AN, Jain KP. N Engl J Med 1969; 281: 1091.
16. Solomkin JS, Flohr AB, Quie PG, Simmons RL. Surg 1980; 88: 524.
17. Boyer AS, Blumenkrantz JS, Montgomerie JS, Gralpin JE, Cobur JW, Guze LB. Am J Med 1976; 61: 832.
18. Watson N, Johnson A. South Med J 1973; 66: 387.
19. Chen KTK. Am J Clin Path 1983; 80: 514.
20. Symmers WStC. Arch Path (Chicago) 1950; 50: 475.
21. Pearson RD, Irons RP, Irons RP. JAMA 1981; 245: 1340.
22. Cooray GH, Panabokke RG. Trans Roy Soc Trop Med Hyg 1960; 54: 358.
23. Rushovich AM, Randall EL, Caprini JA, Westenfelder GO. Am J Clin Pathol 1983; 80: 517.
24. Ellis H. Surg Gynec Obstet 1971; 133: 497.
25. Postlethwait RW, Howard HL, Schanker PW. Surg 1949; 25: 22.
26. Antopol W. Arch Path (Chicago) 1933; 16: 326.
27. Neely J, Davies JD. Br Med J 1971; 3: 625.
28. Davies JD, Neely J. J Pathol 1972; 107: 265.
29. Grant JBF, Davies JD, Espiner HJ, Eltringham WK. Br J Surg 1982; 69: 197.
30. Davies JD, Ansell ID. J Clin Pathol 1983; 36: 435.
31. Kay S. Arch Pathol 1954; 57: 279.
32. Levison DA, Crocker PR, Smith A, Blackshaw AJ, Bartram CI. J Clin Pathol 1984; 37: 481.
33. Tinker MA, Burdman D, Deysine M, Teicher I, Platt N, Aufses AH. Ann Surg 1974; 180: 831.
34. Forouhar F. Am J Clin Pathol 1982; 78: 208.

35. Berdon WE, Baker DH, Becker J, De Sanctis P. N Engl J Med 1967; 277: 585.
36. Jones PE, Rawcliffe P, White N, Segal AW. Br Med J 1977; 1: 1513.
37. Sohar E, Gafni J, Prass M, Heller H. Am J Med 1967; 43: 227.
38. Marshall AJ, Baddeley H, Barritt DW et al. Quart J Med 1977; NS 46: 135.
39. Clark CV, Terris R. Lancet 1983; 1: 937.
40. Pryor JP, Castle WM, Dukes DC, Smith JC, Watson ME, Williams JL. Br Med J 1983; 287: 639.
41. Bradley JA, McWhinnie DL, Hamilton DNH et al. Lancet 1983; 2: 114.
42. Greenlee HB, Stanley MM, Reinhart GF. Gastroenterol 1979; 76: 1282.
43. Concato L. G Int Sci Med 1881; NS 3: 1037.
44. Durst AL, Freund H, Rosenmann E, Birnbaum D. Surg 1977; 81: 203.
45. Kipfer RE, Moertel CG, Dahlin DC. Ann Intern Med 1974; 80: 582.
46. Tedeschi CG, Botta GC. N Engl J Med 1962; 266: 1035.
47. Black W, Nelson D, Walker W. Surg 1968; 63: 706.
48. Milner RDG, Mitchinson MJ. J Clin Pathol 1965; 18: 150.
49. Binder SC, Deterling RA, Mahoney SA, Patterson JF, Wolfe HJ. Am J Surg 1972; 124: 422.
50. Anthony PP, Drury RAB. J Clin Pathol 1970; 23: 110.
51. Mitchinson MJ. J Clin Pathol 1970; 23: 681.
52. Anonymous (Editorial). Br Med 1981; 282: 1343.
53. Harbrecht PJ. Ann Surg 1967; 165: 388.
54. Meyer S, Hausman R. Am J Clin Pathol 1976; 65: 274.
55. Comings DE, Skubi KB, van Eyes J, Motulsky AG. Ann Intern Med 1967; 66: 885.
56. Grossman A, Gibson J, Stansfeld AG, Besser GM. Clin Endocrinol 1980; 12: 371.
57. Mitchinson MJ. In: Anthony PP, MacSween RNM, eds. Recent advances in histopathology, no 12. Edinburgh: Churchill Livingstone, 1984; 223.
58. Mitchinson MJ. J Clin Pathol 1972; 25: 287.
59. Serra RM, Engle JE, Jones RE, Schoolwerth AC. Am J Med 1980; 68: 149.
60. Graham JR, Suby HI, LeCompte PR, Sadowsky NL. N Engl J Med 1966; 274: 359.
61. Godin M, Fillastre J-P, Ducastelle T, Hemet J, Morere P, Nouvet G. Arch Int Med 1980; 140: 1240.
62. Hamdan JA, Ahmad MS, Sa'adi AR. Pediatrics 1982; 70: 298.
63. Harris LF, Sparks JE. Dig Dis Sci 1980; 25: 392.
64. Kanwar YS, Malhotra V, Anderson BR, Pilz CG. Arch Int Med 1974; 134: 1095.
65. Hardcastle JD. Br J Surg 1970; 57: 103.
66. Sherlock S. Diseases of the liver and biliary system. 6th ed. Oxford: Blackwell Scientific, 1981: 116.
67. Carrington CB, Cugell DW, Gaensler EA et al. Am Rev Resp Dis 1977; 116: 977.
68. Lascano EF, Villamayor RD, Llauro JL. Ann Surg 1960; 152; 836.
69. Crofoot DD. Am J Surg 1980; 139: 262.
70. Swift DL, Lingeman JE, Baum WC. J Urol 1980; 123: 577.
71. Vanek VW, Phillips AK. Arch Surg 1984; 119: 838.
72. Mennemeyer R, Smith M. Cancer 1979; 44: 692.
73. Gonzalez-Crussi, deMello DE, Sotelo-Avila C. Am J Surg Path 1983; 7: 567.
74. Simpson RD, Harrison EG, Mayo CW. Cancer 1964; 17: 526.
75. Richards RC, Rogers SW, Gardner EJ. Cancer 1981; 47: 597.
76. Wu JP, Yunis EJ, Fetterman G, Jaeschke WF, Gilbert EF. J Clin Path 1973; 26: 943.
77. Case records of the Massachusetts General Hospital, Case 13–1984. N Engl J Med 1984; 310: 839.
78. Garamella JJ, Hay LJ. Ann Surg 1954; 140: 107.
79. Ober WB, Black MB. Arch Path 1955; 59: 698.
80. Bassis ML. Am J Obstet Gynecol 1956; 72: 1029.
81. Zinsser KR, Wheeler JE. Am J Surg Path 1982; 6: 109.
82. Valente PT. Arch Pathol Lab Med 1984; 108: 669.
83. Scully RE. Arch Pathol Lab Med 1981; 105: 505.
84. Kuo T, London SN, Dinh TV. Am J Surg Path 1980; 4: 197.
85. Brooks JJ, Wheeler JE. Cancer 1977; 40: 3065.
86. Kannerstein M, Churg J, McCaughey WTE, Hill DP. Am J Obstet Gynecol 1977; 127: 306.
87. Foyle A, Al-Jabi M, McCaughey WTE. Am J Surg Path 1981; 5: 241.
88. Roth LM, Ehrlich CE. Obstet Gynecol 1977; 49: 486.
89. McCaughey WTE, Kirk ME, Lester W, Dardick I. Histopathol 1984; 8: 195.
90. Tobacman JK, Greene MH, Tucker MA, Costa J, Kase R, Fraumeni JF. Lancet 1982; 2: 795.
91. Rosai J, Dehner LP. Cancer 1975; 35: 165.
92. Riddell RH, Goodman MJ, Moossa AR. Cancer 1981; 48: 134.
93. Talerman A, Chilcote RR, Montero JR, Okagaki T. Am J Surg Path 1985; 9: 73.
94. Kannerstein M, Churg J. Hum Path 1977; 8: 83.
95. Craighead JE, Mossman BT. N Engl J Med 1982; 306: 1146.
96. Goepel JR. Histopathol 1981; 5: 21.
97. Chan PSF, Balfour TW, Bourke JB, Smith PG. Br J Surg 1975; 62: 576.
98. Said JW, Nash G, Lee M. Hum Path 1982; 13: 1106.
99. Craig JR, Hart WR. Cancer 1979; 43: 1678.
100. Katsube Y, Mukai K, Silverberg SG. Cancer 1982; 50: 1615.
101. Whitaker D, Shilkin KB. J Pathol 1984; 143: 147.
102. Shmookler BM, Lauer DH. Am J Surg Path 1983; 7: 269.
103. Dixon AY, Reed JS, Dow N, Lee SH. Hum Path 1984; 15: 233.
104. Kahn LB. Cancer 1973; 31: 411.
105. Enzinger FM, Weiss SW. Soft tissue tumors. St Louis: Mosby, 1983: 166.
106. Evans HL, Soule EH, Winkelmann RK. Cancer 1979; 43: 574.
107. Enzinger FM, Weiss SW. Soft tissue tumors. St Louis: Mosby, 1983: 242.
108. Enzinger FM, Smith BH. Hum Path 1976; 7: 61.
109. Arnheim EE. Pediatrics 1951; 8: 309.
110. Ordonez NG, Manning JT, Ayala AG. Cancer 1983; 51: 955.
111. Montague DK. J Urol 1975; 113: 505.
112. Yajima A, Toki T, Morinaga S, Sasano H, Sasano N. Cancer 1984; 54: 2040.
113. Lack EE, Cubilla AL, Woodruff JM, Lieberman PH. Am J Surg Path 1980; 4: 109.
114. Carney JA, Sheps SG, Go VLW et al. N Engl J Med 1977; 296: 1517.

115. Waldron JA, Newcomer LN, Katz ME, Cadman E. Cancer 1983; 52: 712.
116. Wright DH, Richards DB. Histopathol 1981; 5: 697.
117. Neerhout RC, Larson W, Mansur P. N Engl J Med 1969; 280: 922.
118. Qizilbash AH. Arch Path 1975; 99: 548.
119. Cariker M, Dockerty M. Cancer 1954; 7: 302.
120. Truong LD, Jurco S, McGavran MH. Am J Surg Path 1982; 6: 443.

Index